Intensive Care Nursing

Intensive care is one of the most rapidly developing areas of healthcare. This introductory textbook is written specifically for qualified nurses who are working in intensive care units and also for those undertaking post-registration courses in the speciality. *Intensive Care Nursing* is structured in four parts. 'Fundamental Aspects' explores patient-focused issues of bedside nursing; 'Monitoring' describes the technical knowledge necessary to care safely for ICU patients; 'Pathophysiology and Treatments' illustrates the more common and specialised disease processes and treatments encountered; 'Developing Practice' looks at how nurses can use their knowledge and skills to develop their own and others' practice. This accessible text is:

- Comprehensive: it covers all the key aspects of intensive care nursing.
- User-friendly: it includes fundamental knowledge sections, introductions, chapter summaries, a glossary of key terms, extensive and up-to-date references and a comprehensive index.
- Clearly written: by an experienced university lecturer with a strong clinical background of working in intensive care nursing. He has also published widely in the nursing press.
- Practically-based: end-of-chapter clinical scenarios provide stimulating discussion and revision topics.

Intensive Care Nursing will be welcomed by ICU nurses throughout the world.

Philip Woodrow, MA, RGN, Dip.N., Grad. Cert. Ed., is a Senior Lecturer at Middlesex University, where he is responsible for ENB 100 courses in intensive care nursing.

Jane Roe is a Lecturer-Practitioner at St George's Hospital Medical School and Kingston University, St George's Hospital Intensive Therapy Unit.

What the reviewers said:

'An informed, well written and clinically focused text that has ably drawn together the central themes of intensive care course curricula and will therefore be around for many years. ... Revision activities and clinical scenarios should encourage students to learn as they engage in analysing and reflecting on their everyday practice experiences. More experienced nurses will also find it a valuable reference source as a means of refreshing their ideas or in developing practice.'

John Albarran, *Faculty of Health and Social Care, University of the West of England*

'An excellent book which will be useful to nurses working in ICUs in many countries. The writers have managed to integrate theory with practice to produce an easy-to-read practical text which will be useful to both beginning and experienced ICU nurses.'

Kathy Daffurn, *Associate Professor and Co-Director Division of Critical Care, Liverpool Health Service, Liverpool, Australia*

'Incredibly comprehensive ... this text should meet Woodrow's goal of contributing to the "further growth of intensive care nursing". It should find a place on the shelves of intensive care units, as well as in Higher Education institutions providing critical care courses. It will also be a welcome source of reference for nurses caring for critically ill patients outside of the intensive care unit.

Woodrow provides a balance between pathophysiology oriented aspects of nursing practice and the relationship between patient/family and nurses that is the very essence of intensive care nursing. The text is helpfully punctuated with activities for the reader, whilst the extensive references also enable the reader to pursue specific aspects in greater depth.'

Ruth Endacott, *Adviser and Researcher in Critical Care*

'A book geared for practical use, it will be helpful to many intensive care nurses, especially those new to the discipline.'

Pat Ashworth, Editor, *Intensive and Critical Care Nursing*

Intensive care nursing

A framework for practice

ROUTLEDGE

To the States or any one of them, or any city of the States,
Resist much, obey little,
Once unquestioning obedience, once fully enslaved,
Once fully enslaved, no nation, state, city, of this earth, ever afterwards resumes its liberty.

Walt Whitman

Fashion, even in medicine.

Voltaire

First published 2000
by Routledge
11 New Fetter Lane, London EC4P 4EE

Simultaneously published in the USA and Canada
by Routledge
29 West 35th Street, New York, NY 10001

Reprinted 2001 (twice)

Routledge is an imprint of the Taylor & Francis Group

Typeset in Sabon and Futura by Taylor & Francis Books Ltd
Printed and bound in Great Britain

British Library Cataloguing in Publication Data
A catalogue record for this book is available from the British Library

Library of Congress Cataloging in Publication Data
Woodrow, Philip, 1957–
Intensive care nursing: a framework for practice / Philip Woodrow; clinical scenarios by Jane Roe.
Includes bibliographical references and index.
1. Intensive care nursing. I. Roe, Jane. II. Title.
[DNLM: 1. Critical Illness – Nursing. 2. Intensive Care – methods.
WY 154 W893i 2000]
RT120.I5W66 2000
610.73'61–dc21
DNLM/DLC 99–33382

ISBN 0–415–18456–8

Contents

Illustrations

Figures

Tables

Preface

This book is for intensive care nurses. Intensive care nursing is a diverse speciality, and a text covering its every possible aspect would neither be affordable nor manageable to most clinical staff. This text, therefore, is necessarily selective, and will probably be most useful about 6 to 12 months into intensive care nursing careers. It assumes that readers are already qualified nurses, with experience of caring for ventilated patients, who wish to develop their knowledge and practice further. Discussion of clinical issues is therefore followed by implications for practice.

Knowledge develops and changes; controversy can, and should, surround most issues. Some controversies are identified, others are not. But every aspect of knowledge and practice should be actively questioned and constantly reassessed. If this book encourages further debate among practising nurses it will have achieved its main purpose.

Since a novice (Benner 1984) has little knowledge or experience, 'basic' nursing texts tend to explain almost everything. This book is for competent and advanced practitioners, however, whose knowledge and experience will vary. To help readers, 'fundamental knowledge' is listed at the start of many chapters, so that readers can pursue anything they are unsure about. Much 'fundamental knowledge' is related anatomy and physiology, and it would be a disservice to readers to displace other material for superficial summaries when there are many excellent anatomy and physiology texts available.

Any book is necessarily a pragmatic balance between the author's priorities and interests; this book represents mine. Part I concentrates on values and some of the 'basic' aspects of care that can be lost in the dehumanised technological ICU environment. Part II reviews various means of monitoring, including application to relevant problems (e.g. intracranial hypertension). The more common pathologies seen in ICUs are included in Part III as nurses need an understanding of pathophysiologies and treatments. Many more topics could be covered (some were removed during writing), but this is not fundamentally a book about pathophysiology and the cost of comprehensiveness would be the book remaining largely unused and unread. Finally, Part IV explores aspects of career development.

Any stage of professional development is a beginning rather than an end;

to help readers develop further, each chapter concludes with 'further reading', which is generally restricted to recent and easily accessible books and articles. Full publication details are given in the References, pp. 539–67. A few classic key texts are also included in the further reading sections and, where the original year of publication provides a historical context for material, I have included this with the year of the edition consulted (for example, Nightingale 1980 [1859]). The large numbers of specialist, general nursing and other medical journals means that new material is frequently appearing and readers should pursue current material through their libraries.

The clinical scenarios by Jane Roe provide an opportunity for nurses to apply the knowledge acquired in each chapter to a clinical situation.

I have tried to adopt Eliot's 'the word precise, but not pedantic'. The glossary explains technical terms that are likely to cause problems and the first occurrence of these have been highlighted in the text. Few laws of physics or medical formulae are included unless frequently used in clinical nursing practice. Many chapters identify issues surrounding families; this implicitly includes friends and all other significant visitors. A few chapters include references to statute and civil law; these are usually English and Welsh law, and so readers in Scotland, Northern Ireland and outside the United Kingdom should check applicability to local legal systems. I have tried to minimise errors, but some are almost inevitable in a text of this size; like any other source, this text should be read critically.

Although intensive care nursing is younger than most healthcare specialities, it already possesses a wealth of nursing knowledge and experience. I hope this book contributes to further growth of intensive care nursing, and enables readers to develop their own specialist practice.

Acknowledgements

I am grateful to everyone who has helped in the development of this text, especially Jane Roe (who has contributed so much as both author of the clinical scenarios and who has been a particularly conscientious reviewer of every chapter) and Fidelma Murphy (whose experience of both paediatric and general intensive care is combined in the chapter about nursing children in general ICUs). I would also like to thank all the reviewers who read and assisted with comments on the developing typescript: John Albarran, University of the West of England; Kate Brown and Maureen Fallon, Nightingale Institute, King's College University; Kay Currie, Glasgow Caledonian University; Lynne Harrison and Mandy Odell, University of Central Lancashire. Thanks also to Jane Fellows, who illustrated the book.

All reasonable efforts have been made to contact the copyright holders of material reproduced in this book. Any omissions brought to the attention of the publishers will be remedied in future editions.

I am grateful to everyone at Middlesex University for the support given towards this book, and for the sabbatical leave which enabled me to complete it. I would especially like to thank Sheila Quinn (Senior Lecturer, Middlesex University), who has helped me at so many stages of my career, and who first suggested I should write a textbook. I am grateful to Sue MacDonald (RM) for her comments toward the obstetrics chapter.

I would also like to thank everyone who has helped develop my ideas, especially past and present staff of the Whittington Hospital and all my past students and colleagues and clinical staff at Chase Farm and North Middlesex Hospital.

And of course this book would not have been possible without the encouragement and support of Routledge, in particular Alison Poyner and Moira Taylor.

Philip Woodrow, March 1999

Abbreviations

ACE	angiotensin converting enzyme
ACT	activated clotting time
ACTH	adrenocorticotrophic hormone
ADH	antidiuretic hormone
AF	atrial fibrillation
AIDS	acquired immune deficiency syndrome
AMV	assisted mandatory ventilation
ANF	atrial natriuretic factor (also called atrial natriuretic peptide = ANP)
ANP	atrial natriuretic peptide (also called atrial natriuretic factor = ANF)
APRV	airway pressure release ventilation
APSAC	anisolylated plasminogen streptokinase activator complex
ARDS	acute respiratory distress syndrome
AST	asparate transaminase
ATP	adenosine triphosphate
BE	base excess
BiPAP	biphasic/bilevel positive airway pressure
BMI	body mass index
BMR	basal metabolic rate
BNF	British National Formulary
BSA	body surface area
BUN	blood urea nitrogen
c/cal	calorie
CABG	coronary artery bypass graft
cAMP	cyclic adenosine monophosphate
CAPD	chronic ambulatory peritoneal dialysis
CAT	computerised axial tomography (see also CT)
CAVH	continuous arteriovenous haemofiltration (= ultrafiltration); rarely now used in ICU
CAVHD	continuous arteriovenous haemodialysis
CAVHDF	continuous arteriovenous haemodiafiltration

CCUs	coronary care units (US: critical care units)
CD4, CD8	CD = cluster designation, the numbers refer to different types
CFAM	Cerebral Function Analysing Monitor
CFM	Cerebral Function Monitors
CK	creatine kinase (formerly, creatine phosphokinase: CPK)
CMV	(1) cytomegalovirus; (2) controlled minute volume (depending on context)
COP	colloid osmotic pressure
COPD	chronic obstructive pulmonary disease
COSHH	Containment of Substances Hazardous to Health
CPAP	continuous positive airway pressure
CPB	cardiopulmonary bypass
CPK	creatine phosphokinase
CPP	cerebral perfusion pressure
CRRT	continuous renal replacement therapy
CSF	cerebrospinal fluid
CT	computerised tomography (see also CAT)
CVA	cerebrovascular accident (stroke)
CVP	central venous pressure
CVVH	continuous venovenous haemofiltration
CVVHD	continuous venovenous haemodialysis
CVVHDF	continuous venovenous haemodiafiltration
Da	dalton (kilodalton: kDa)
DHHNK	diabetic hyperosmolar hyperglycaemic nonketotic coma
DIC	disseminated intravascular coagulation
E coli	*Escherichia coli*, a lactose-fermenting species of bacteria
$ECCO_2R$	extracorporeal carbon dioxide removal
ECMO	extracorporeal membrane oxygenators
EDRF	endothelium derived relaxing factor
EEG	electroencephalogram
EMD	electromechanical dissociation
EMRSA	epidemic strains of MRSA (see below)
EPIC	European Prevalence of Infection in Intensive Care
ERCP	endoscopic retrograde cholangiopancreatography
ESR	erythrocyte sedimentation rate
ESRF	endstage renal failure
ETT	endotracheal tubes
FDPs	fibrin degradation products
FEV	forced expiratory volume (so FEV1 = forced expiratory volume at one second)
FFP	fresh frozen plasma
FiO_2	fraction of inspired oxygen (see Glossary)
FVC	functional ventilatory capacity
GABA	gamma aminobutyric acid
GBS	Guillain Barré syndrome

GCS	Glasgow Coma Scale
GI	gastrointestinal
GTN	glyceryl trinitrate
GvHD	graft-versus-host disease
HAI	hospital acquired infection (nosocomial)
HAS	human albumin solution (ie albumin for infusion)
HAV	hepatitis A virus
HbA	adult haemoglobin
HbF	fetal haemoglobin
HbS	sickle cell haemoglobin
HBV	hepatitis B virus
HCV	hepatitis C virus
HDU	high dependency unit
HDV	hepatitis D virus
HELLP	haemolysis elevated liver enzymes and low platelets
HES	hydroxyethyl starch
HEV	hepatitis E virus
HFJV	high frequency jet ventilation
HFOV	high frequency oscillatory ventilation
HFV	high frequency ventilation
HITTS	heparin-induced thrombocytopaenia and thrombosis syndrome
HIV	human immunosuppressive virus
HLA	human leucocyte antigen
HME	heat moisture exchanger
HUS	haemolytic uraemic syndrome
IABP	intra-aortic balloon pumps
ICP	intracranial pressure
Ig	Immunoglobulin (eg IgA = immunoglobulin A)
IL	interleukin
IMA	internal mammary artery
IMV	intermittent mechanical volume
iNO	inhaled nitric oxide
INR	international normalised ratio (of prothrombin time)
IPPB	intermittent positive pressure breathing
IPPV	intermittent positive pressure ventilation
IPR	individual performance review
IRDS	infant respiratory distress syndrome (see also RDS)
IRV	inverse ratio ventilation
IVOX	intravenous oxygenators
kPa	kilopascal
LDH	lactate dehydrogenase
LIMA	left internal mammary artery
LMAs	laryngeal mask airways
LVAD	left ventricular assist device
m/s	metres per second

MAP	mean arterial pressure
MCL	modified chest lead
MDMA	3–4 methylenedioxymethamphetamine (Ecstasy)
MI	myocardial infarction
mmol	millimole (unit for measuring chemicals)
MMV	mandatory minute ventilation
MODS	multiorgan dysfunction syndrome
MOF	multiorgan failure
MRSA	multiresistant (or methicillin resistant) *Staphylococcus aureus*
MSSA	methicillin sensitive *Staphylococcus aureus*
mv	millivolt
NAPQI	N-acetyl-p-bezoquinone imime
NIRS	near infrared spectroscopy
NPPV	noninvasive positive pressure ventilation
NSAID	nonsteroidal anti-inflammatory drug
PAC	pulmonary artery (Swan Ganz) catheters
PACP	pulmonary artery capillary pressure
PAFC	pulmonary artery flotation catheters
PaO_2	partial pressure of arterial oxygen
PAWP	pulmonary artery wedge pressure
PBC	primary biliary cirrhosis
PCA	patient controlled analgesia
PCOP	pulmonary capillary occlusion pressure
PCP	*Pneumocystis carinii* pneumonia
PCWP	pulmonary capillary wedge pressure
PDIs	phosphodiesterase inhibitors
PEEP	positive end expiratory pressure
PEG	percutaneous endoscopic gastrostomy
PFC	perfluorocarbon
PGE_2	prostaglandin E_2
PGI_2	prostaglandin I_2, also known as prostacyclin
pHi	intramucosal pH
ppm	parts per million
PS	pressure support
PSV	pressure support ventilation
PTCA	percutaneous coronary angioplasty
PTT	prothrombin time
PUFAs	polyunsaturated fatty acids
PVR	pulmonary vascular resistance
QALYs	Quality Adjusted Life Years
RAP	right atrial pressure
RDS	respiratory distress syndrome
REM	rapid eye movement
RNA	ribonucleic acid
RQ	respiratory quotient

RR	respiratory rate
RVEDP	right ventricular end diastolic pressure
SA	sinoatrial (node)
SBC	standardised bicarbonate
SBE	standardised base excess
SCUF	slow continuous ultrafiltration removal of ultrafiltrate, usually using a small-pore filter, so minimising solute removal; used only for removing/reducing fluid overload
SD plasma	solvent detergent plasma
SDD	selective digestive decontamination
SGOT	serum glutamic oxaloacetic transaminase
SIADH	syndrome of inappropriate antidiuretic hormone
SIMV	synchronised intermittent minute volume
SIRS	systemic inflammatory response syndrome; (formerly called septic inflammatory response syndrome)
SNP	sodium nitroprusside
SV	stroke volume
SVR	systemic vascular resistance
SWOT	strengths, weaknesses, opportunities, threats
TCNS	transcutaneous nerve stimulation (see TENS)
TENS	transcutaneous electrical nerve stimulation (see TCNS)
TIPS	transjugular intrahepatic portosystemic shunt
TMP	transmembrane pressure
TMR	total metabolic rate
TNF	tumour necrosis factor
t-PA, TPA	tissue plasminogen activator
TPN	total parenteral nutrition
TTP	thrombotic thrombocytopenia purpura
TV	tidal volume (also written at Vt)
UKTSSA	United Kingdom Transplant Support Service Authority
VAD	ventricular assist devices
VAP	ventilator associated pneumonia
V/Q	ventilation to perfusion ratio
VRE	vancomycin resistant enterococci
vWF	von Willebrand's Factor

Part I

Fundamental aspects of ICU nursing

Part I explores issues that are fundamental to ICU nursing and can be read sequentially or used as a resource for later chapters.

It develops issues that may have been introduced during pre-registration courses, but which can too easily be lost in the technical demands of intensive care. The first chapter therefore explores the values underlying intensive care nursing; the second chapter develops these through outlining two influential moments in psychology. The third chapter examines issues about the environment in which intensive care patients are nursed. Intensive care units (ICUs) developed primarily from respiratory units, and so Chapters 4 and 5 discuss respiratory management while Chapter 6 reviews sedation. The human needs and problems of nursing rituals are explored in the chapters on pain management, pyrexia, nutrition, mouthcare, eyecare and skincare. The next two chapters then explore the extremes of age: paediatrics and older adults. Most ICU patients are immuno-compromised, and infection control is discussed in Chapter 15. The final chapter of this section applies ethical principles and theories to ICU nursing practice.

Chapter 1

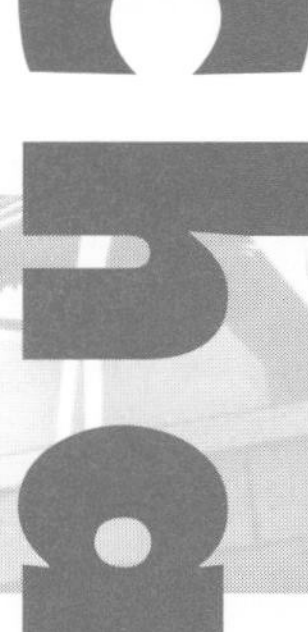

Nursing perspectives

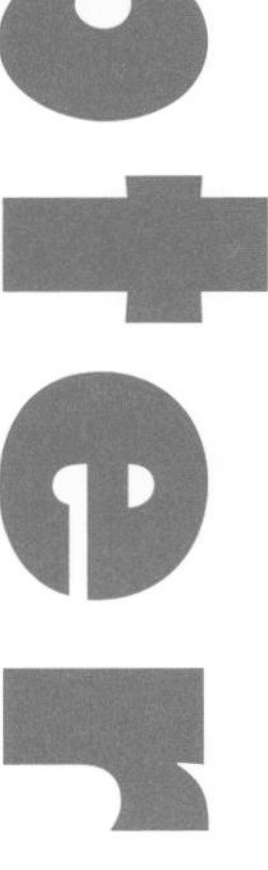

Contents

Introduction

This book explores issues for intensive care nursing practice, and this first section establishes its core fundamental aspects. Nurses' salaries have always formed a major part of healthcare budgets: Endacott (1996) estimates that nursing accounts for three-quarters of ICU costs. Thus it is important for ICU nurses to clarify their roles in, and value to, healthcare in order to be able to 'articulate the importance of their role in caring for patients and their relatives' (Wilkinson 1992: 196). To help readers to do this, this first chapter explores what nursing means in the context of intensive care and the following chapter outlines two schools of psychology (behaviourism and humanism) that have influenced healthcare and society.

The Department of Health publication *A Strategy for Nursing* (DoH 1989) identified four possible roles for nurses:

1 as surrogate parent
2 as technician
3 as contracted clinician
4 as advocate

Previously, Ashworth (1985) had identified similar role conflicts within ICUs:

1 the technician
2 the doctors' assistant
3 the carer for patients while others deal with technical treatment and maintenance
4 the 'prickly' professional

Both these documents raise issues of values and beliefs. Acknowledging and continuously re-evaluating our individual values and beliefs is part of human growth, so that examining nursing's values and beliefs within the context of our own area of practice is part of our professional growth. This is something that each nurse can usefully explore and there are a number of published exercises available in this respect (e.g. Manley 1994), but essentially it means working out a nursing philosophy for oneself. What is meant by this is not some esoteric message hung neatly on a wall and seldom read or practised – such as 'man is a bio-psycho-social being' – but, rather, simple values which may be more meaningful – such as 'remember our patients are human'.

This question of values is well illustrated by the semantic dilemma of whether to call the speciality 'Intensive Therapy' (ITU) or 'Intensive Care' (ICU) – in practice, the terms are often interchangeable, and many ICU staff value cure rather than care (Steel & Hawkey 1994). Care can (and should) be therapeutic, but therapy (cure) without care is almost a contradiction in terms. Thus, in order to emphasise the caring human role of critical care nurses (and other staff), this book refers to 'intensive care (ICUs)'.

Technology

Intensive care is a young speciality. Respiratory units for mechanical ventilation developed from the polio epidemic of 1952–3 (Edwards 1994), and the first purpose-built intensive care units (ICUs) in the UK opened in 1964 (Ashworth, personal communication). These units offered potentially life-saving intervention during acute physiological crises, with the emphasis on medical need and availability of technology. As the technology and medical skills of the speciality developed, so technicians were needed to maintain and operate machines.

Although many ICUs employ technicians, technology-related tasks are still delegated to nurses – such as managing bedside machines, recording observations from them and changing regimes as prescriptions change. However, the fact that technology provides a valuable means of monitoring and treatment should not allow it to become a substitute for care. For nursing to retain a patient-centred focus, it is the patients themselves and not the machines that must remain central to the nurse's role. Therefore, technology should not justify the role or presence of nurses. Healthcare assistants (and, potentially, robots) can be trained to perform technological tasks – and are cheaper to employ. While acknowledging the need for technical roles, then, ICU nurses need to be more than just technicians.

Doctor–nurse relationships

Ford and Walsh (1994) observed that nurses working in high dependency areas often have good relationships with medical staff. Most ICU nurses would agree with, and value, this. But Ford and Walsh suggest this good relationship is on the terms of the medical staff. Some Canadian studies (Grundstein-Amado 1995; Cook *et al.* 1995) suggest that values differ between doctors and nurses (influenced by profession rather than gender), and this can lead to potential communication breakdown. For example, nursing's focus on the emotional costs to intensive care patients may limit the wider recognition of nursing as a profession (Phillips 1996).

Nurses should collaborate with doctors (and other members of the healthcare team) (UKCC 1992a), but how that collaboration is achieved will vary between units and individuals. However, while recognising and respecting the valuable and unique role of doctors, this collaboration by nurses should not mean subservience (i.e. 'doctor's handmaiden'). The roles of technician and doctors' or contracted assistant should be only part of ICU nursing. ICU nurses need to define their unique role and contribution actively and positively within the specialty, and this can be achieved through exploring nursing values.

Psychology

The increasing emphasis by the nursing profession on psychology and the psychological needs of patients, whether conscious or unconscious, makes psychological care an essential part of holistic care – a focus noticeably absent in the medical and technological perspectives above.

Cochran and Ganong (1989) suggest that ICU nurses are more concerned with the psychosocial stressors, while patients are more concerned with their physical care. Patients' needs and nursing care vary between units and individuals, but, if Cochran and Ganong are right, there is cognitive dissonance between ICU nurses and their patients.

Since patients are admitted to ICU with acute physiological crises, intervention must necessarily focus care on their physical needs – for instance, considerations about needle phobias are obviously inappropriate during a cardiac arrest. However, psychology and physiology are not two separate and distinct pigeon-holes that some nursing (and other) course timetables might suggest, and the subject of homeostatic imbalances from psychological distress is explored in Chapter 3. Rather than ritualistically following lists of pre-ordained cues (e.g. assessment forms), nurses should actively evaluate the holistic needs of their patients; by acknowledging these individual psychological needs, ICU nurses can complement the valuable physiological care offered by the other professions. In recognising both the physical and psychological needs of patients, nurses can add a humane, holistic perspective into their care, preparing their patients for recovery and discharge. The importance of assessing and planning nursing care is a recurring theme in many of the later chapters of this book.

Care or torture?

Following Ashworth's seminal study of 1980, psychological stresses specific to, or accentuated by, intensive care have been widely discussed in nursing literature. Dyer (1995) arguably makes the most poignant exploration, comparing ICU practices to torture. ICU patients, often deprived of the ability to speak, make decisions or alter their own environment, are confronted not only with a barrage of unusual sensory inputs, but also suffer a deficit of normal inputs when some of the most basic human physiological functions – such as breathing and movement – are replaced. Admittedly, ICU environments present the ingredients for successful psychological (and physical) torture, but whereas the normal purpose of torture is to enforce the victim to serve the torturer (such as through confession), the aim of ICU treatment is to overcome the patient's physiological disease and restore health. To this end, it is often necessary, unfortunately, to add knowingly to the patient's suffering, but this is one of the costs of critical illness (Carnevale 1991). However, much suffering can be prevented or minimised through good nursing care.

Since suffering is inevitable in ICUs, the admission of any patient unlikely to survive becomes inappropriate (cruelty), since that patient will in effect be tortured to death. The rationing of ICU care is often financially determined, but there can also be valid humanitarian reasons for refusing inappropriate admissions.

Holistic care

The intrinsic needs of patients derive from their own physiological deficits, including many 'activities of living' (e.g. communication, comfort, freedom from pain); meeting these needs is fundamental to nursing, and this provides the focus of the first part of this book.

People are influenced by, and interact with, their environment; their extrinsic needs, which define each person as a unique individual, rather than just a biologically functioning organism, include:

- dignity
- privacy
- psychological support
- spiritual support

It is within the nurse's scope to promote, proactively and creatively, a therapeutic environment, and accounts of patients' own experiences in ICUs, such as those provided by Watt (1996) and Sawyer (1997), make salutary reading. Waldmann and Gaine (1996) describe one patient, unable to drink, feeling tortured by hearing a can opened – opening cans of enteral feed away from a patient's hearing may reduce such unintentional, but unnecessary, suffering. Again, probably few ICU nurses would wish to sleep naked (with only a single sheet) in a mixed ward, yet many ICU nurses subject their patients to this potentially degrading experience. Thus, nurses need to question every nursing action proactively, no matter how small and apparently insignificant it may seem to be. Patients are dehumanised by admission to ICUs (Calne 1994); nurses can restore that humanity (Ball 1990; Mann 1992).

Psychological approaches to nursing should be individually planned and implemented according to each patient's needs. These needs can be assessed through the patients themselves and augmented by information from families and friends. Different nurses will feel comfortable with different approaches, but all should recognise the individual human being within each patient.

Unlike the other medical and paramedical professions, nurses do not treat a problem or a set of problems. Unique among healthcare workers, ICU nurses remain with patients throughout their hospital stay. A fundamental role of a nurse, therefore, is to be with and for the patient; this is compatible with the advocacy role promoted by *A Strategy for Nursing* (DoH 1989). This role is facilitated by making patients the focus in the organisation of care (such as through primary/named nursing). As the one member of the multidisciplinary team continuously present in the patient's environment, an ICU nurse is ideally placed to put the patient (as a person) first.

The recommended one-to-one nurse–patient ratio (DOH 1996a) in the UK reflects the higher dependence of ICU patients here than elsewhere (Silvester 1994); it also highlights the unique role of ICU nurses in the UK. Although an ideal (at times most ICU nurses care for more than one ventilated patient at the same time), the overall nurse–patient ratio in the UK is 0.85 (Ryan 1997a). Depasse *et al.* (1998), profiling six European countries, found that the UK had the highest number of nurses per bed (4.2), and on average the sickest patients. This constant presence of a specific nurse at the patient's bedside should allow more holistic, patient-centred care.

Relatives

Relatives, together with friends and significant others, form an important part of each person's life, and they too are similarly distressed by the patient's illness. The psychological crises experienced by relatives necessitate skilful psychological care, such as the provision of information to allay anxiety and make decisions, and facilities to meet their physical needs (Curry 1995). Relatives should be offered the opportunity to be actively involved in the patient's care (Hammond 1995) without being made to feel guilty or becoming physically exhausted, rather than left sitting silently at the bedside, afraid to touch their loved ones in case they interfere with some machine. Whether units should permit 'open' visiting, and how open 'open' this should be, is a matter for debate; ICUs might become more humane if visiting were individualised to meet, first, the individual needs of each patient and, second, the needs of families and friends (Simpson 1991). Despite some recent interest in the care of relatives (e.g. Jones and Griffiths 1995; Plowright 1995), ICU nursing still has much to learn from other specialities (in particular, paediatrics).

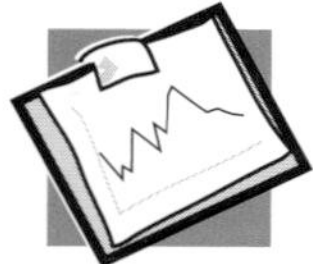

Implications for practice

- a nurse needs technical knowledge and skills, but nursing is more than being a technician
- ICU nurses have a unique role in the holistic, patient-centred perspectives that humanise a technology-orientated environment
- nursing values underpin each nurse's actions; the clarification of values and beliefs helps each nurse and each team to increase their self-awareness
- since patients' experiences are central to ICU nursing, nurses need to consider what their patients are experiencing

Summary

Intensive care is labour intensive; nursing costs consume considerable portions of hospital budgets. Therefore, ICU nursing needs to assert its value by:

- recognising nursing knowledge
- valuing nursing skills
- offering holistic patient/person-centred care

Person-centred care involves nurses being there for each patient, rather than the institution. Having recognised the primacy of the patient, nurses can then develop their valuable technological skills, together with other resources, in order to fulfil their unique role in the multidisciplinary team for the benefit of patients. ICU nurses should value ICU nursing on its own terms – namely, to humanise the environment for their patients. The beliefs, attitudes and philosophical values of nurses will ultimately determine nursing's economic value. Much of this book necessarily focuses on the technological and pathological aspects of the knowledge needed for ICU nursing. This chapter is placed first in order to establish fundamental nursing values, prior to considering individual pathologies and treatments; nursing values can (and should) then be applied to all aspects of holistic patient care.

Further reading

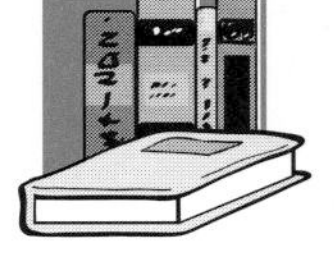

Much has been written on what nursing is or should be. Henderson, famous for her earlier definition of the unique role of the nurse, wrote a classic article about nursing in a technological age (Henderson 1980). More recent perspectives from ICU nurses include Ball (1990), Calne (1994), Carnevale (1991), Mann (1992) and Wilkinson (1992). Manley (1994) offers a useful framework for clarifying values and beliefs.

Over the years, many accounts of patients' experiences have been written; Watt (1996) and Sawyer (1997) are recent, easily accessible and vivid articles, while Dyer (1995) offers further challenging perspectives.

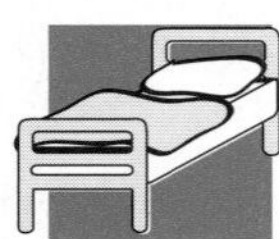

Clinical scenario

Q.1 Identify environmental, cultural, behavioural and physiological factors that may (potentially) contribute to the suffering and dehumanisation of patients in ICUs.

Q.2 Outline specific nursing strategies which can minimise the range of factors identified in Q.1. Examine the potential conflicts between these strategies and the more technical, physiologically necessary interventions.

Q.3 Reflect on the role of specialist nurses within ICU. What is their role (or range of roles) and how did this develop? What do they contribute to actual patient care, and how is their effectiveness evaluated?

Chapter 2

Humanism

Contents

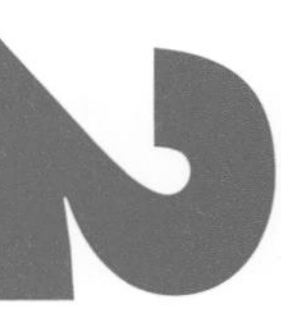

chapter 2

Introduction

Philosophical beliefs affect our values, and so influence our approaches to care. Chapter 1 identified the need to explore values and beliefs about ICU nursing. This chapter describes and contrasts two influential philosophies to supply a context for developing individual beliefs and values. As this is not a book about philosophy, descriptions of these movements are brief and simplified, and readers are encouraged to pursue their ideas through further reading.

The label 'humanism' has been variously used throughout human history, probably because its connotations of human welfare and dignity sound attractive. The Renaissance 'humanistic' movement included such influential philosophers as Erasmus and Sir Thomas More. In this text, however, 'humanism' is a specifically twentieth-century movement in philosophy led primarily by Abraham Maslow and Carl Rogers.

The humanist movement, sometimes called the 'third force' (the first being psychoanalysis, the second behaviourism), was a reaction to behaviourism. Our beliefs, even if we are unaware of their source, influence our practice. Playle (1995) suggests that the art-versus-science debate within nursing is an extension of the humanistic-versus-mechanistic (i.e. behaviourism) debate of philosophy. The art of ICU nursing – the process of bringing humanity into intensive care – can be optimized by

- being there
- sharing
- supporting
- involving
- interpreting
- advocating (Andrew 1998)

This chapter begins therefore by describing behaviourism.

Behaviourism

The behaviourist theory was largely developed by John Broadus Watson (1878–1958) who, drawing on Pavlov's famous animal experiments, stated that if each stimulus eliciting a specific response could be replaced by another (associated) stimulus, the desired response (behaviour) could still be achieved ('conditioning') (1998 [1924]).

The behaviourist theory enabled social control and so became influential when society valued a single socially desirable behaviour. Thus behaviourism focuses on outward, observable behaviours and for behaviourists, learning *is* a change in behaviour (Reilly 1980).

Holloway and Penson (1987) have suggested that nurse education contains a 'hidden curriculum' controlling the behaviour of students and their socialisation into nursing culture. Through Gagne's (1975, 1985) influence, many nurses have accepted and been acclimatised into a behaviouristic culture without always being made aware of its philosophical framework. Hendricks-Thomas and Patterson (1995) suggest that this behaviouristic philosophy has often been covert, masked under the guise of humanism. Thus using aspects from humanism, such as Maslow's hierarchy of needs in Roper *et al.*'s model of nursing (1996), does not necessarily reflect the adoption of a humanistic philosophy. For instance, the debate surrounding nursing uniforms and their replacement in ICU with theatre-style 'pyjama suits' can reflect values about outward appearance.

Whether from cause ('types' of nurses attracted to work in ICU) or effect (values learned from others), similar covert socialisation among ICU nurses encourages adoption of such defensive mechanisms as limiting communication to under one minute (even with conscious patients), and providing nurse-led information, questions and commands (Leathart 1994).

Behaviourist theory draws largely on animal experiments; but humans do not always function like animals, especially where cognitive skills are concerned. Focus on outward behaviour does not necessarily change inner values. People can adopt various behaviours in response to external motivators (e.g. senior nursing/medical staff), but once stimuli are removed, behaviour may revert; when no external motivator exists, people are usually guided by internal motivators, such as their own values. Thus if internal values remain unaltered, desired behaviour exists only as long as external motivators remain (see Chapter 48).

Behaviourism in practice

Time out 1

A patient in ICU attempts to remove his endotracheal tube. There have been no plans to extubate as yet.
Options:

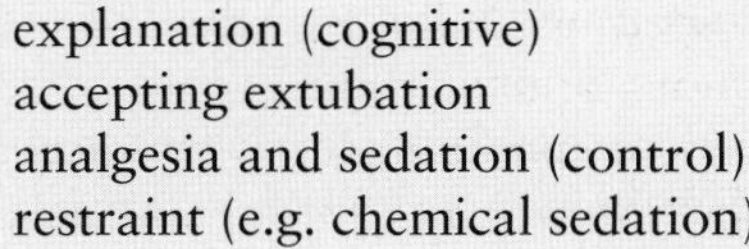
explanation (cognitive)
accepting extubation
analgesia and sedation (control)
restraint (e.g. chemical sedation)

Comment:
Here, 'pure' behaviourism has already been tempered with humanitarianism: to try and comfort. Nevertheless, description remains deliberately behaviouristic, seeing the problem as behaviour (extubation). While extubation causes justifiable concern, behaviour is a symptom of more complex psychology. The patient attempts extubation

because the tube causes distress. Until underlying problems are resolved, they remain problems; restraint only delays resolution.

No philosophy is ideal for all circumstances, and few are without some merit. In this scenario, behaviourism may justifiably 'buy time' until underlying pathophysiology is resolved or reduced, when extubation will no longer be a problem, and may be medically desirable. Behaviourial approaches can be useful, but they can also be harmful by dehumanising others to a list of task-orientated responses. Smith (1991) found that preregistration courses still emphasised task-orientated, rather than holistic, nursing. Nurses should analyse their values and beliefs, understanding the implications they have for practice, and selecting appropriate approaches to each context; this is, after all, an extension of individualising care.

Humanism

The humanist movement was concerned that behaviourism overemphasised animal instincts (and relied too heavily on animal experiments) in an attempt to control outward behaviour. Hence humanism emphasises inner values that distinguish people from animals and is a 'person-centred' philosophy; rather than emphasising society's needs, humanism emphasises the needs of the individual self. Maslow's *Motivation and Personality* (1987 [1954]) popularised the concept of 'holism' (the whole person). Humanists believe that people have a psychological need to (attempt to) achieve and to realise their maximum potential. Maslow (1987[1954]) described a hierarchy of needs, self-actualization being the highest of these; Roper *et al.*'s (1996) adoption of this in their model of nursing illustrates the influence of humanistic philosophy in nursing. However, adopting primacy of the individual, inherent in humanism, conflicts with the objective decontextualisation of traditional scientific methodologies (Playle 1995), raising difficulties when undertaking humanist research, as exemplified by debate surrounding qualitative and quantitive nursing research.

Emphasis on inner values led humanist educationalists to concentrate on developing and/or attempting to change inner values: values that are internalised will continue to influence actions after external motivators are removed. Thus, changes in nursing practice made in order to conform with the desires of another may not continue after that person has left, or even when absent (e.g. days off), but changes made because staff concur with them will continue as long as that consensus remains.

Concern for inner values and holistic approaches to care makes humanism compatible with many aspects of healthcare and nursing, although overfamiliarity with terms can reduce them to clichés. Humanism has much to offer nurses in the process of analysing their philosophies of care and practice, but ideas should not be accepted uncritically.

Lifelong learning

Where the aim of behaviourist education was to achieve conformity, humanist education sought to promote individuality, and these differences are reflected in the training-versus-education debate. Training seeks to equip learners with a repertoire of responses to specific stimuli, and is, by implication, time-limited. In animals, stimulus–response reactions are often simple (as with Pavlov's dogs); in humans, more complex responses may be learned. Such subconscious (conditioned) responses can be valuable: a cardiac arrest requires rapid action and follows protocols shared by other team members. However, for many nursing interventions, 'training' fails to provide the higher skills to work constructively through actual and potential problems. Training equips the learner to be reactive to problems (stimuli) rather than proactive (to prevent potential problems occurring).

For humanist education, facts and ideas are quickly outdated (Rogers 1983) and so are less valued by humanists than the development of skills to enable personal growth (Maslow 1971) and learning (Rogers 1983). Humanism seeks to develop higher cognitive and affective skills in order to analyse issues according to individual needs – most valuable human interactions occur above the stimulus–response levels. For healthcare, humanism promotes a person-centred philosophy that enables learning to continue beyond designated courses; each clinical area becomes a place for learning, and nurses should be extending and developing their skills through practice.

The current trend away from the teaching of factual information to the emphasis on individualised learning (e.g. learning contracts), reflection and lifelong learning will be familiar to nurses. This pragmatic hybrid not only values factual knowledge (e.g. research), but also recognises the individuality of the learning process, which is determined less by behaviourist outcomes than by what is meaningful for each individual. The UKCC's PREP requirements (UKCC 1997) emphasise that attendance at a study day does not ensure learning has taken place.

The more radical aspects of humanistic education (e.g. Neill 1992), which in recent years have been largely discredited, have not been applied to nursing. Many nursing actions can have (literally) vital effects and professional safety has to be ensured (Rogers 1951); humanistic elements, as with any other valuable philosophy, have been adapted to meet professional needs, and most countries have professional bodies, such as the UKCC, to regulate nursing education and registration.

Problems

Humanism has a weak research base, and so acceptance or rejection of its philosophy remains largely subjective. Arguably, research-based approaches conflict with humanism's fundamental beliefs in individualism; Rogers' early work did attempt to adapt traditional scientific research processes to humanism, but his later work adopts more discursive, subjective approaches.

A great deal of learning occurs through making mistakes, and individualistic learning necessarily means making mistakes. Accepting the possibility of errors involves taking risks, and human fallibility does need to be recognised; the expection that mistakes will not occur, thus treating them as unacceptable, is unrealistic. However, errors with critically ill patients can cause significant and potentially fatal harm. Staff in ICU, particularly at managerial level, need to achieve the difficult balance between facilitating a positive learning environment and the maintenance of safety for patients and others.

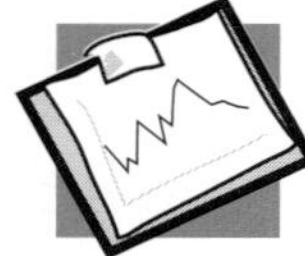

Implications for practice

- philosophy (our beliefs and values) influence our practice; in order to understand our practice, we need to understand our underlying beliefs and values
- changing inner values, rather than just outward behaviour, ensures continuity when external stimuli are removed
- healthcare, nursing and ICU retain behaviouristic legacies that can undermine individualistic, patient-centred care
- humanism emphasises inner values and individualism, and humanistic nursing helps to humanise ICU for patients

Summary

Philosophy is not an abstract theoretical discipline, but something underlying and influencing all aspects of practice. Hence it is relevant to each chapter in this book. This chapter has outlined two influential and opposing philosophies: behaviourism and humanism; applying these beliefs to nursing values (see Chapter 1) helps to clarify our own and others' motivation.

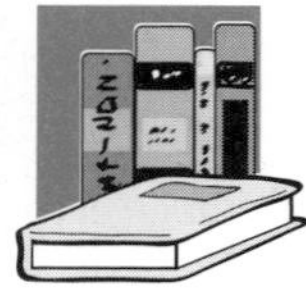

Further reading

Much has been written on behaviourism, including within the context of nursing. Skinner (1971) gives interesting late perspectives on behaviourism, while Gagne (1975, 1985) significantly influenced nurse education.

Maslow (1987 [1954]) is a classic text on humanistic philosophy. Rogers is equally valuable, and possible more approachable; his 1967 text synthesises his ideas, while his 1983 book gives a useful discussion of educational theory.

Many texts identified in Chapter 1 (for example, Ball 1990) reflect (often unacknowledged) humanistic philosophy. Andrew (1998) offers valuable applications of humanistic principles to intensive care nursing.

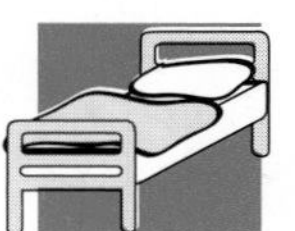

Clinical scenario

Mr Oliver is orally intubated, awake and being weaned from positive pressure ventilation. He moves his hand towards the endotracheal tube (ETT). This movement causes the nurse to respond.

Q.1 Describe a behaviourist response by the nurse to Mr Oliver reaching for his ETT.

Q.2 Explain how a humanistic response would differ from a behaviourist response in this interaction. Consider the values that underpin each response, e.g. safety, duty of care, motivation of Mr Oliver, needs of Mr Oliver.

Q.3 Reflect on your own practice, evaluate typical responses to the above patient gesture, your own and others motivating values.

Chapter 3

Sensory imbalance

Contents

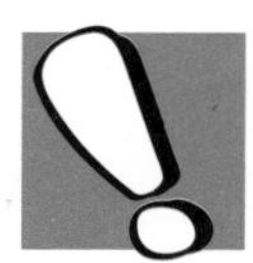

Fundamental knowledge

Sensory receptors and nervous system
Motor nervous system
Autonomic nervous system

Introduction

Sensory balance and psychological health are threatened by exogenous (e.g. environmental) and endogenous (e.g. body rhythms) factors. Sensory imbalance includes overload and deprivation, although literature may use other names (ICU syndrome, ICU psychosis/delirium, sleep disturbance/deprivation). Confusion may have many causes:

- sensory imbalance
- acute cerebral hypoxia/ischaemia/damage
- chronic cerebral damage

Physiological as well as psychological causes of confusion should therefore be assessed.

Sensory imbalance, like so many aspects of intensive care, initiates a stress response, which causes many physiological and psychological problems. The stress response is described in this chapter, but is referred to in many later chapters.

Sedatives can provide comfort and **anxiolysis** (see Chapter 6), but are also a means of (chemical) restraint, and so should not become substitutes for nursing care. Despite sedation, most patients remember being in intensive care (Green 1996), even if memories are incomplete and compressed. ICU environments are abnormal, exposing patients both to excessive and deficient sensory stimulation, and causing psychological and physiological problems.

Intubation severely limits interactive communication with ICU patients; even if conscious, most ICU patients experience difficulty writing, due to psychomotor weakness, impaired vision, or both, and asking closed questions limits quality of information. Patients' gestures, facial expression and physiological signs (e.g. tachycardia) can indicate comfort, pain or anxiety. Isolation can be physical (e.g. side rooms) or social; social isolation may be overt (e.g. gowns and masks, emphasising subhuman 'untouchable' status, restricting visiting) or covert (e.g. deprivation of quality touch and meaningful conversation). Solitary confinement is an established and effective measure for torture (Dyer 1995), often unwittingly imitated on many ICUs.

The five senses (sight, hearing, touch, taste, smell) supply raw materials for interpreting environments. Misinterpretation or imbalance of sensory inputs may cause confusion/delirium ('rubbish in – rubbish out'). To approach this topic experientially, first work through these exercises:

Time out 1

Take 2–3 minutes to list your own impressions of your environment at this moment; complete this before reading any further.
Review your list, noting down beside each item whether impressions were perceived through sight, hearing, touch, taste or smell. Some items may be perceived by more than one sense. How often was each sense used?
Most items are probably listed under sight, followed by a significant number under hearing. Touch is probably a poor third, with few (if any) under taste or smell. This reflects usual human use of senses: most input is usually through sight and hearing, with very limited inputs perceived from other senses.

Time out 2

Imagine yourself as a patient in your own ICU. Jot down under each of the five senses any inputs you are likely to receive.
When finished, review your lists analysing how many of these inputs are 'normal' for you. Remember that people usually rely most on visual and auditory inputs.

Sensory input

Even if their eyes are/can open, ICU patients often have distorted *vision* from

- drugs causing blurred vision
- absence of glasses (if normally worn).

Absence of vision may be caused by

- periorbital oedema (preventing eye opening)
- coverings to prevent corneal drying (see Chapter 11: Eyecare)

Those able to see may be nursed supine: ceilings are usually visually unstimulating; overhead equipment may be frightening. Attempts to rationalise such sensory inputs, especially if unprepared for this environment before admission, are likely to cause bizarre interpretation. Watching overhead monitors detracts from eye contact (non-verbal communication), and becomes dehumanising. Nurses should actively develop non-verbal skills (e.g. open body language, quality touch). Windows (with beds placed to give patients a view) help maintain orientation to normality.

Patient recall of ICU suggests that *hearing* remains unaltered by critical illness, so staff and visitors should assume patients can hear normally, although hearing may be impaired by

- absence of hearing aids
- **ototoxic** drugs (e.g. gentamicin, frusemide); many accentuate high pitches (e.g. alarms), blurring lower pitches (e.g. voices), so causing pain and further isolation

Normal conversation or other human interaction relies heavily on response ('cueing') (Eastabrooks & Morse 1992), which few ICU patients can give. Auditory input is too often confined to either instructions or others' conversation (e.g. medical/nursing/team discussions, sometimes spoken across patients). Both are detrimental; instructions, although valid in themselves, should be supplemented by quality conversation. Patients learning about their own condition and progress (or misinterpreting conversation as being about them) may become understandably anxious; half-heard discussions and misunderstood terms are likely to compound anxieties.

Touch is a major means of non-verbal communication, especially with disordered vision; touch deprivation is the most remembered deprivation in ICU (MacKellaig 1990), while overload of abnormal tactile sensations may be caused by:

- heavily starched (and sometimes patched) sheets (few nurses living in nurses' accommodation tolerate them, yet expect patients to be comfortable)
- pulling from tubes/drains/leads
- oral endotracheal tubes
- endotracheal suction
- pressure area care

Most touch in ICU remains task-orientated (Verity 1996a). Task-orientated touch is necessary, but reduces individuals to commodities, reinforcing their dehumanisation. Patients appreciate having their pillows turned and their head stroked in a comforting manner (affective touch).

Affective touch is individual, and may become threatening (e.g. invading personal space; overload); as with any aspect of care it should be assessed. Factors such as culture and gender affect how touch is interpreted (Eastabrooks & Morse 1992); touching some body parts can suggest inappropriate intimacy (Lane 1989) or power (Davidhizer *et al.* 1995). Touching hands, forearms and shoulders is usually acceptable (Schoenhofer 1989). Massage offers valuable opportunities for developing qualitative touch (see Chapter 47), but spontaneous affective touch can rehumanise care.

Few ICU patients receive oral diets, thus *taste* is limited to drugs (e.g.

intravenous cephalosporins cause a metallic taste) and anything remaining in the mouth:

- blood
- vomit
- mucus
- mouthwash (reminiscent of dentists)
- toothpaste (difficult to rinse out with supine patients)
- thrush

Air turbulence over four nasal conchae (or tubinates) exposes *smells* to olfactory chemoreceptors. Intubation largely bypasses this mechanism, but it remains intact and presumably functional, and so total absence should not be presumed. ICU smells are often abnormal:

- 'hospital' smells (disinfectant, diarrhoea, body fluids)
- human smells (perfume, body odours, cigarette smoke)
- putrefying wounds
- nasogastric feeds

Reaching across patients (e.g. for thermometers or suction equipment) places the axilla near the patient's nose.

'Normal' smells (e.g. food/drinks, entering through windows, ventilation systems or from bedsides) may reinforce perceptions of deprivation, while vitamin deficiencies can alter taste.

Patient experiences

Abnormal sensory inputs (both overload and deprivation) results in abnormal interpretation of environments; hallucinations, 'ICU psychosis', frequently occur (Mackellaig 1990). Psychological imbalance is twice as likely on ICUs as on general wards (Green 1996), and may remain undetected (Hopkinson & Freeman 1988).

Hallucinations and psychosis are a form of psychological pain (stress), a response to a stimulus, and in humanistic nursing should receive similar attention to physiological pain. Responses depend on both *reception* (sensory stimuli) and *perception* (sensory transmission to, and interpretation by, higher centres). Hallucinations vary, often being vivid, and usually terrifying. Since Ashworth (1980), many authors have described patients' experiences. Jones *et al.* (1994) record a range of hallucinations, many bizarre and horrific, from being in hell, trapped in fireplaces and buried alive, to being on a cross-channel ferry. Healthy adults suffering eight hours sensory deprivation can experience acute psychotic reactions, delusions and severe depression for several days, and anxiety for several weeks (Hudak *et al.* 1998) – the duration of one 'traditional' nursing shift.

Understanding patients' perceptions and interpretations is not always possible, but it can make sense of hallucinations and bizarre actions – for instance, lying on alternating mattresses may resemble cross channel ferries. Reported experiences often suggest profound fear; nurses (and other health-care professionals) can appear as devils/tormentors, so that nurses attempting to explore fears or reassure patients may meet resistance.

Stress response

Stress, however initiated, causes physiological responses to enable 'fight or flight'. Catecholamine release and sympathetic stimulation make circulation hyperdynamic:

- tachycardia
- vasoconstriction
- hypertension

and so increase oxygen consumption. Neuroendocrine release includes

- catecholamines (primarily adrenaline; also noradrenaline): as above
- cortisol (immunosuppression, impaired tissue healing)
- antidiuretic hormone: fluid retention, oedema (including pulmonary)
- growth hormone: anabolism (tissue repair)
- glucagon: hyperglycaemia (also peripheral insulin resistance from catecholamines)
- insulin.

Sodium and water retention, with plasma extravasation, cause oedema formation (including pulmonary). Stress also activates intrinsic clotting pathways.

Barrie-Shevlin (1987) describes classic studies in which healthy volunteers, exposed to sensory deprivation, experienced hallucinations, impaired intelligence and psychomotor skills, and body water and electrolyte imbalance. For critically ill (hypoxic) patients, these demands may exceed homeostatic reserves, provoking myocardial infarction or other crises; even moderate hyperglycaemia aggravates immunocompromise (Torpy & Chrousos 1997).

Reticular activating system

This dense cluster of neurons between the medulla and posterior part of the midbrain selects which stimuli reach the cerebral cortex, preventing overload and so maintaining internal balance (biorhythm). Repetitive, familiar or weak signals are filtered out, and so loud, but unimportant, sounds may remain unnoticed (e.g. constant heavy traffic). Quieter, meaningful noises may be noticed (parents sleeping through heavy traffic may waken with small noises from their children). As the reticular activating system filters out progressively more, or receives progressively fewer/abnormal sensory stimuli, the cortex attempts to rationalise remaining stimuli, resulting in hallucinations and progressively disorganised behaviour.

Reticular activating system function can be altered by:

- reduced sensory input
- relevance deprivation
- repetitive stimulation
- unconsciousness (O'Shea 1997)

All may occur in ICU.

The reasons behind nursing actions may appear mysterious to many patients (relevance deprivation), and explanations can reduce anxiety and psychological (and so physical) pain (Hayward 1975). (Meaningless stimuli and the enforcement of meaningless petty rules are often used in torture procedures (Dyer 1995).) Reality orientation can be useful, but may provoke aggression (most people react negatively to being contradicted).

Repetitive stimulation can make actions appear meaningless and irritating. Patients often quickly forget so that nurses should not assume patients will remember rationales given previously. Environmental stimuli can also become annoyingly repetitive (e.g. flickering lights). Ashworth (1980) describes one patient interpreting a monitor as fluorescent light displays in Piccadilly Circus. Alarms are deliberately irritating (to nurses) to ensure prompt response; patients' responses vary (from fearing something is wrong to using alarms to control attention), but the purposes of alarms should be explained to patients and families, and the parameters selected should balance safety against stress.

Reticular activating system dysfunction may cause failure to filter out stimuli, bombarding the cortex with excessive, often meaningless, inputs. Sensory filters can be removed by drugs (e.g. lysergic acid (LSD), Ecstasy; see Chapter 41), causing sensory overload ('psychedelic' effects); sensory overload in ICU may result from dysfunction through critical illness.

Sleep

The purpose of sleep remains unclear; Canavan (1984) observes that some people sleep little without consequent impairment, alluding obscurely to one (unidentified) author's suggestion that sleep is merely an instinct. Most literature suggests sleep is restorative (physically and psychologically), although precise benefits from each stage remain disputed, and (cerebral) hypoperfusion may limit applicability of information from sleep research on healthy volunteers to ICU patients (Turnock 1990).

Sleep patterns vary widely, most people sleeping 6–9 hours each night (Atkinson *et al.* 1996), although the amount of sleep required usually decreases with age (Canavan 1984). Each patient's normal sleep pattern should therefore be individually assessed. Sleep cycles are controlled by the suprachiasmatic nucleus ('biological clock') in the hypothalamus, which regulates the preoptic nucleus (sleep-inducing centre). Precise mechanisms of sleep remain debated; theories of passive control by the reticular activating system have been largely discounted in favour of active inhibitory hormone control (Guyton & Hall 1997), especially by **serotonin**. Other hormonal changes with sleep include:

- melatonin increases twentyfold overnight (production is suppressed by light)
- most growth hormone is produced during stages 3 and 4, or orthodox sleep (Lee & Stotts 1990); this stimulates protein anabolism, contributing to tissue repair
- most ACTH is produced overnight
- ADH increases overnight (until 4 a.m.), concentrating urine (hence the value of early morning urine samples

Hormone changes regulate **circadian rhythm** (below, p.27).

Full sleep usually consists of 4–5 cycles, each lasting about 90 minutes (Hodgson 1991). Each cycle consists of a number of stages. Terminology varies, but most authors identify two main parts:

- orthodox or non-REM sleep
- paradoxical or REM sleep

Orthodox (non-REM) sleep

Names, length and function of sleep stages vary; McGonigal's (1986) influential description is followed here. Timings of stages vary between individuals and over subsequent sleep cycles. McGonigal (1986) describes orthodox (non-rapid eye movement, slow-wave) sleep as having four stages (see Table 3.1).

Orthodox sleep reduces metabolism, respiration, heart rate (Atkinson *et al.* 1996), and so oxygen demand. Whether orthodox sleep achieves emotional healing (Evans & French 1995), protein synthesis, physical restoration and leucocyte production (Krachman *et al.* 1995) is disputed, but deprivation causes a stress response (Krachman *et al.* 1995), reduced pain tolerance and central nervous system exhaustion (Lee & Stotts 1990). Dreams during

***Table 3.1* Stages of sleep**

Stage	*Duration*	*Description*
1	few minutes	aware of surroundings; muscle jerking
2	15–20 minutes	sleep becoming deeper; oblivious of surroundings, but remains easily aroused
3	15–20 minutes	progressively deeper
4	10–20 minutes	deep sleep

***Source*: After McGonigal 1986**

orthodox sleep are usually realistic, resembling thought processes (Turnock 1990), and often forgotten on waking (Guyton & Hall 1997). The duration of stage 4 reduces steadily from birth, and often disappears altogether by about 60 years of age, contributing to poor sleep and muscle atrophy in older people.

Paradoxical (REM) sleep

As cerebral metabolism (and oxygen consumption) increases, EEG patterns reflect consciousness (McGonigal 1986), hence 'paradoxical'. Paradoxical sleep has two stages: initial rapid eye movement (REM) and muscle twitching gives way to profound muscle relaxation (McGonigal 1986).

Dreams during REM sleep are often dramatic, emotional and illogical (Turnock 1990; Atkinson *et al.* 1996), being remembered only if interrupted (Atkinson *et al.* 1996). Arousal level varies (Krachman *et al.* 1995), but disturbing someone after one hour's sleep probably interrupts REM dreams, causing mental frustration; frequent recall of illogical dreams may contribute to emotional instability and personality disorders (Marieb 1995).

If woken during paradoxical sleep, the person returns to stages 1 and 2 orthodox sleep, thus being deprived of the later stages. Sleep deprivation may impair tissue repair (Krachman *et al.* 1995), although Landis and Witney's (1997) animal study found skin healing unimpaired after 72 hours sleep deprivation.

Paradoxical sleep occupies about one-half of an infant's sleep cycles, but by adulthood forms only about one-fifth of total sleep (Atkinson *et al.* 1996). Overnight paradoxical sleep progressively replaces stage 4 orthodox sleep (Guyton & Hall 1997), providing mental restoration. Topf and Davies (1993) found significant deprivation of REM sleep occurred in patients in intensive care.

Sleep disturbance

Orthodox stages 3 and 4, and REM sleep are seriously disturbed or absent following major surgery (Aurrell & Elmqvist 1985) and presumably any critical illness. Exogenous factors can also disturb sleep, including pain (ibid.) and noise. Whenever possible, clustering nursing actions to minimise physical disturbance can help to ensure undisturbed stretches of 2 hours (one sleep cycle). Barrie-Shevlin (1987) cites classic studies showing that two-fifths of ICU nurses failed to distinguish non-essential from essential tasks between 10 p.m. and 6 a.m., and that some critically ill patients slept for only 2.6 hours in a day. Awareness of the need for sleep has increased, and lights are now usually dimmed overnight to maintain circadian rhythm, but commencing nursing activities early each morning (e.g. 6 a.m.) may deprive patients of their final sleep cycle (Davis *et al.* 1997; Cureton-Lane & Fontaine 1997). One of the most valuable nursing interventions at night is usually to allow patients to sleep.

Family and close friends may also suffer sleep deprivation from prolonged overnight vigils (Hodgson 1991); nurses should encourage visitors to get adequate sleep.

Daytime sleep

Sleep patterns alter during the day, although generally the quality of daytime sleep is poorer than night sleep (Wood 1993). Morning sleep contains more orthodox stage 4 and REM than afternoon sleep (Turnock 1990), making morning sleep more useful for patients with head injuries, while increased stages 3 and 4 during afternoon/evening sleep assists wound healing (e.g. after surgery or myocardial infarction (MI)). Since the length of stage 2 sleep increases during daytime, less daytime sleep provides less tissue recovery than night-time sleep (Turnock 1990).

Although not usually identified in literature, nightwork may alter hormone and sleep patterns; individual assessment of patients' normal patterns will help nurses to plan appropriate individualised care (e.g. maintaining daytime sleep patterns for permanent night workers).

Circadian rhythm

Circadian rhythm (change in body function over a day) is individual to each person, with slight variations normal between each day; however critical illness and abnormal environments (ICU) can severely disrupt the circadian rhythm. Times and figures given here are 'averages', and should be treated as guides rather than absolutes.

The circadian cycle usually peaks at about 6 p.m. and ebbs between 3 a.m. and 6 a.m. (Clancy & McVicar 1995). Since most nurses working night duties experience the ebb stage, high-risk actions (such as extubation) should be avoided during this period when they and their colleagues are likely to be least efficient.

The release of catecholamine peaks around 6 a.m. (Todd 1997) causing sympathetic stimulation (including increased heart rate and vasoconstriction) in preparation for increased physical activity. The risk of myocardial infarctions and strokes is therefore increased between 6 a.m. and 10 a.m. (Todd 1997). Early morning stimulation (e.g. washes, physiotherapy) are best avoided with vulnerable patients.

Reduced peripheral circulation may cause ischaemia ('night cramps'); assessment should identify whether patients normally suffer from night cramps, and what they do for relief.

Circadian rhythm adapts to environments; dimming lights can mimic day/night cycles, but 'dimmed' lighting often exceeds levels most nurses would choose for their own bedrooms at night. Night-time environments should generally be as dark as is safely possible. Daylight, rather than artificial light, helps psychological wellbeing, so fluorescent lighting is a poor substitute for lack of windows.

Drug benefits may be increased by coinciding with circadian rhythm (**chronotherapy**); leucocyte count peaks and bacterial reproduction ebb make once daily antibiotics most effective in the early morning.

Other 'natural' body rhythms may also exist. For example, seasonal affective disorder (SAD) (Ford 1992) affects emotions, causing more depression and suicides during winter.

Noise

Noise (undesired sound) is subjective: what is useful or enjoyable for one person can annoy others (e.g. overloud 'personal' cassettes). Noise impairs both quality and quantity of sleep (Topf *et al.* 1996). ICUs are noisy; much noise is unavoidable, inevitably continuing overnight. However, 'unnecessary noise is the most cruel absence of care which can be inflicted on either sick or well' (Nightingale [1859] 1980: 5); nurses should actively seek to reduce unnecessary noise.

Physical pain results at levels from 130 decibels (dB); while equipment and interventions in ICU rarely reach this level, they constantly exceed the International Noise Council's recommended upper limit of 45 dB for ICU during daytime and 20 dB overnight (Granberg *et al.* 1996), and often exceed the UK upper legal limit of 85 dB for noise at work. Reading *et al.* (1977) measured 71 dB from cardiac alarms ten feet away, 70 dB from endotracheal suction and 68 dB from physicians talking fifteen feet away (further than distances between most ICU beds).

Studies consistently show staff conversation (potentially reaching 90 dB) as a major cause of ICU noise (Kam *et al.* 1994). Even whispers usually cause 30 dB, enough to disturb sleep (Wood 1993), and exceeding the International Noise Council's night-time limit of 20 dB. Conversation cannot be avoided, and appropriate conversation can benefit patients, but volume, tone and pitch of speech vary between individuals, and nurses coordinating care should ensure that both content and timing of conversation is appropriate.

Suction catheters (with vacuum running) under pillows places noise near patients' ears; suction units are also usually near patients' heads. Suction should therefore normally be switched off when not in use.

Environmental noise combines all these (and other) activities. Citing 1977 material, Krachman *et al.* (1995) suggest that total ICU noise levels range from 53 dB (day average) to 42.5 dB (night average). Recent measurements are higher: 61.3–100.9 dB (McLaughlin *et al.* 1996), 84.8 dB (day) and 79.9 dB (night) (Meyer *et al.* 1994), and 55 dB on a paediatric ICU (Lane and Fontaine 1992). An average quiet bedroom at home might measure 20–30 dB overnight (Krachman *et al.* 1995). Sound and interruption levels on ICU are severely disruptive, preventing patients from maintaining normal circadian and sleep cycles (Meyer *et al.* 1994).

Children have fewer coping mechanisms than adults (Bood 1996) and so may be more susceptible to disturbed sleep. Scothern *et al.* (1992) found that nearly one-quarter of mothers reported anxiety and phobias among children for three months after discharge from (general) ICUs.

Childrens' normal circadian rhythm and psychological health may be helped by play, an essential need during prolonged admissions (Palmer 1996), but adult nurses are often less able than paediatric nurses to meet children's play and other needs, and may have less access to play therapists.

Music

Sensory inputs can be pathways for pleasure. Music therapy can be positively developed in ICU, reducing heart rate and pain (O'Sullivan 1991; Zimmerman *et al.* 1996), although haemodynamic effects may be minimal (Coughlan 1994).

Music should:

- reflect the patients' choices (rather than staff's)
- use comfortable volume levels (this varies between individuals, choosing the right level for someone unable to speak can be problematic)
- include prompt side changes (especially if single pieces last more than one side of the tape)
- be varied rather than repeated
- allow rest periods (especially if using headphones, which can quickly become uncomfortable)

Memories of ICU

Dyer (1995) compares many ICU nursing actions with Amnesty International's categories of torture (see Chapter 1). ICU is only one episode in a patient's healthcare needs, but can cause significant residual complications; follow-up clinics and studies can identify/resolve problems for individual patients, while gathering valuable information to develop practice. (For instance, abdominal girth measurements may be misinterpreted as coffin measurements (Waldmann & Gaine 1996)). Transfer from ICU can increase psychological stress, and so introducing liaison nurses can facilitate discharge planning (Hall-Smith *et al.* 1997), although significant numbers of 'mild to moderate' problems may remain unresolved, some necessitating referral to mental health teams (Daffurn *et al.* 1994).

Post-discharge support may include:

- follow-up clinics
- discharge liaison nurses
- inviting patients to return or telephone the unit

While potentially easing psychological trauma, nurses should be confident that they have the knowledge and skills needed to provide adequate support, including providing psychologically 'safe' environments (confidentiality, privacy) and meeting local ethical requirements; unit managers should be able to guide staff on such issues.

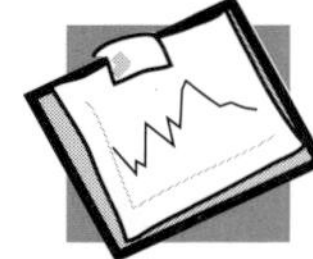

Implications for practice

- sensory imbalance is a symptom of psychological pain, provoking a stress response; alleviating pain provides both humanitarian and physiological benefits, so should be fundamental to nursing assessment and care
- monitors should be sited unobtrusively
- facilitating sleep is usually the nurse's most important role overnight
- sleep is individual, so each patient's normal sleep pattern should be assessed
- whenever possible, planned care should include 4 sleep cycles, each lasting at least 90 minutes (patients remaining undisturbed during this time)
- circadian rhythm can be facilitated through daylight, interesting views and, overnight, by dimming lights as much as is safely possible
- relatives should be encouraged to participate in care, and encouraged to share news and use touch. They should not be made to feel guilty or exhausted. Open visiting, facilities and information can give relatives much-needed support
- patients should be offered psychological support following ICU discharge
- information gained from post-discharge surveys can valuably develop practice
- continuing education raises staff awareness of sensory imbalance

Summary

Sensory imbalance includes both sensory overload and sensory deprivation. Maintaining sensory balance helps to maintain psychological health and reduces complications from stress responses.

Many factors contribute to sensory imbalance, including sleep deprivation (quality or quantity) and noise. Nurses should assess each individual patient's needs; while safety and physiological needs of critically ill patients necessarily compromise psychological care, nurses can humanise even the most technological environments.

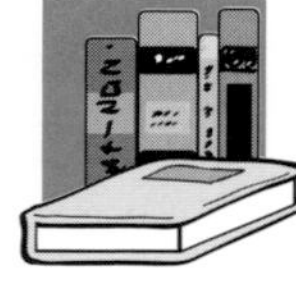

Further reading

Much has been written on sensory imbalance: West (1996) and Granberg *et al.* (1996) offer reliable and recent overviews; Barrie-Shevlin's (1987) classic paper remains useful. Detrimental physiological effects of stress are described by Torpy and Chrousos (1997). Dyer (1995) is valuably provocative. Jones *et al.* (1994), Waldmann and Gaine (1996) and Green (1996) offer insights from post-discharge interviews/clinics.

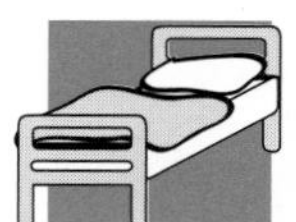

Clinical scenario

Edward Creighton is a 20-year-old university student admitted with bacterial meningitis. He has a fever of 39.2°C, a variable level of consciousness with deteriorating respiratory function, which has necessitated intubation and ventilation. He is sedated, paralysed and given intravenous antibiotics (Cefotaxime 2 g, 8 hourly). This is Edward's first ever hospital admission.

Q.1 Examine the structure of current sensory/psychological assessment used in your clinical practice area. Does this structure allow for documentation or give a scale rating of patient's psychological risk factors; previous history, time on ICU, prescribed drugs that may adversely effect cognition, memory, sleep, etc.

Q.2 Identify Edward's risk factors and potential for developing ICU psychosis. How can these risks be minimised?

Edward recovers, but *may* be left with some long-term neurological complications (e.g. deafness, visual and behavioural disorders) from bacterial meningitis and psychological imbalances from his ICU experience.

Q.3 Evaluate strategies which ICU nurses can implement to help Edward understand and transcend his residual sensory imbalances (e.g. referral to specialists, follow up ICU visits and use of discharge clinics, etc.).

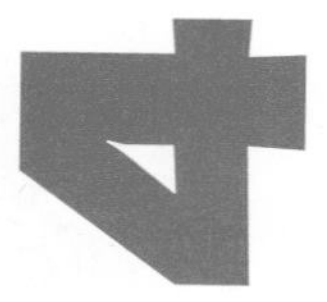
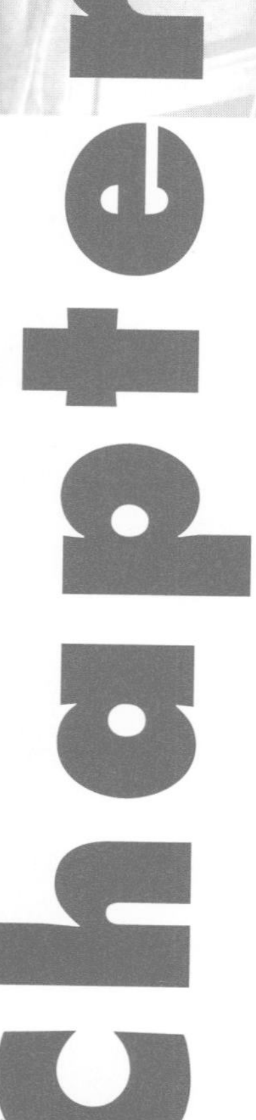

Chapter 4

Artificial ventilation

Contents

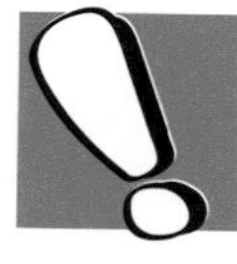

Fundamental knowledge

Respiratory physiology
Normal (negative pressure) breathing
Dead space
Normal lung volumes
Experience of nursing ventilated patients

Introduction

Intensive care units developed from respiratory units: the provision of mechanical ventilation, and thus the care of ventilated patients, is fundamental to intensive care nursing. In this chapter a brief revision of nursing care is given.

Nurses should have a safe working knowledge of whichever ventilators they use – manufacturers' literature and company representatives are usually the best source for this. This chapter discusses the main components of ventilation (tidal volume, **I:E ratio**) and the more commonly used modes. Additional ventilatory options are discussed in Chapter 29. Since negative pressure ventilation is rarely used in ICUs, it is not discussed in this book. The chapter ends by identifying the complication of positive pressure ventilation on other body systems.

The UK terminology of 'ventilator' is used throughout the chapter, although outside the UK other terms, such as 'respirator', may be used; 'respiration' is used wherever possible for self-ventilating breaths and 'ventilation' for mechanically initiated breaths.

Artificial ventilation should meet physiological deficits (metabolic oxygen demand and carbon dioxide elimination). Early positive pressure ventilators were simple and basic – driven by gas or electrical bellows, delivering gas at a set rate (time), volume or pressure – and so ventilators were classified as:

- time cycled
- volume cycled
- pressure cycled

Although these terms are still used, modern ICU ventilators (e.g. Servo® 300, Puritan-Bennett® 7200ae) are arguably too sophisticated for such crude categories: when controlled minute volume (CMV; volume-cycling) modes are used, upper pressure limits are normally set (pressure-cycling). These terms are therefore not used here, but readers should be aware of their existence and meanings.

Oxygenation relies on functional alveolar surface area, so is determined by

mean airway pressure
inspiration time
PEEP
FiO_2
pulmonary blood flow.

Carbon dioxide removal requires active tidal ventilation and so is affected by

inspiratory pressure
tidal volumes
expiratory time.

Manipulating these factors can optimise ventilation while minimising complications.

Normal adult alveolar ventilation is about four litres each minute; normal cardiac output is about five litres each minute. This creates a ventilation:perfusion (**V/Q**) ratio of 4:5, or 0.8 (Pierce 1995). Perfusion without ventilation is called a **shunt**. Shunting can also occur at tissue level (reduced oxygen extraction ratio, see Chapter 20).

Care of ventilated patient

The care of ventilated patients should be holistic – the sum of many chapters in this book, especially in Part I. This chapter identifies only those aspects specifically related to ventilation.

Artificial ventilation causes potential problems with:

- safety
- replacing normal functions
- system complications

Ventilated patients have respiratory failure, so ventilator failure or disconnection may be fatal. Modern ventilators include alarms and default settings, but each nurse should check, and where appropriate reset, alarm limits for each patient; Pierce (1995) recommends a 'rule of thumb' margin of 10 per cent for alarm settings.

Alarms do not replace the need for nursing observation. Alarms may fail and so nurses should observe ventilated patients both aurally and visually. This necessitates appropriate layout of bed areas to minimise the need for nurses to turn their backs on their patients.

Back-up facilities in case of ventilator, power or gas failure should include:

- manual rebreathing bag, with suitable connections
- oxygen cylinders
- equipment for reintubation

Additional safety equipment may also be needed (e.g. tracheal dilators). Nurses should check all safety equipment at the start of each shift.

Positive pressure ventilation is unphysiological; increased intrathoracic pressure compromises many other body systems (especially cardiovascular), causing problems identified later in this and many other chapters.

Fighting ventilation (dysynchrony between ventilator and patient-initiated breaths) should not occur, almost all modern ventilators incorporate trigger modes. However patient discomfort from ventilation (coughing, gagging – often from oral tracheal tubes, including biting on tubes) may cause problems. Nurses should monitor effects of ventilation, providing comfort where possible (e.g. endotracheal suction to remove secretions), and reporting problems they cannot resolve.

Physical restraint is used in some countries to prevent self-extubation and ensure safety, but is generally unacceptable in the UK and unnecessary with ICU staffing levels. Nurses using unnecessary restraint are liable to civil prosecution for assault. When physical restraint cannot be avoided, it is best limited to manual restraint, using the minimum force necessary, which should be released as soon as possible. The use of chemical restraint (sedation) is discussed in Chapter 6.

Tidal volume

Tidal volume affects gas exchange, but can also cause shearing damage to lungs; settings should therefore balance immediate needs of oxygenation and carbon dioxide removal against potential lung damage/healing. Many texts still recommend 8–10 ml/kg (i.e. 700 ml for the 'average' 70 kg patients). While not too dissimilar to peak flow volumes, normal respiration preferentially distributes air to dependent lung bases (especially when standing) (Ryan 1998), matching maximal ventilation with optimum perfusion; lying down reduces the functional residual capacity by about one-third, thus artificial ventilation distributes gas unevenly, overdistending upper lung zones (Ryan 1998).

High intra-alveolar pressure (from PEEP or high peak airway pressure) diverts further blood away from apices, causing shunting, but lung volume, rather than airway pressure, appears to cause most ventilator-associated lung injury (Manning 1994), alveolar distension (**volotrauma**) damaging alveoli (Keogh 1996). Reducing peak pressure (e.g. pressure limited ventilation, pressure controlled ventilation, small tidal volumes such as 6 ml/kg) limits gaseous exchange so that $PaCO_2$ is likely to rise (**permissive hypercapnia** – see Chapter 27). Patients at greatest risk from alveolar trauma usually have poor compliance, low functional lung volumes and hypoxia, creating dilemmas between adequate oxygenation and risks of lung damage. However, gas exchange can be improved through manipulating other aspects (e.g. inspiratory flow, mean airway pressure).

Triggering

Trigger (sensitivity, assisted mandatory ventilation – AMV) is the mechanical equivalent of sensing patient-initiated breaths with manual rebreathing bags before delivering manual inflation. When patient-initiated negative pressure exceeds the set trigger level, patients can 'breath through' the ventilator. With most ventilatory modes, triggered breaths are in addition to preset volumes, but included in measured expired minute volume. Incorporating triggering/sensitivity into ventilators aids weaning and facilitates patient comfort by overcoming the problems of 'fighting'.

Intermittent positive pressure breathing (IPPB – e.g. the 'Bird') is effectively a ventilator cycled solely by triggering. IPPB encourages deep breathing and alveolar expansion, and remains a useful physiotherapy aid.

At rest, self-ventilation negative pressure is approximately −3 mmHg (Adam & Osborne 1997); trigger levels below this can cause discomfort (fighting). Settings close to zero are usually used (e.g. 0.5–2.0); settings of zero can cause autocycling, the ventilator triggering itself at the end of each expiratory phase. Trigger/sensitivity settings normally allow for PEEP (but manufacturer's information should be checked), and so setting a trigger of −0.5 cmH_2O with PEEP of 5 allows triggering at +4.5 cmH_2O.

Inspiratory volume modes (IMV/SIMV)

Intermittent minute volume (IMV) was an early weaning mode, enabling reduction of frequency of ventilator breaths without changing tidal volume. As $PaCO_2$ rises, the respiratory centre is stimulated and the patient breathes more; as respiratory muscles grow stronger, triggered tidal volumes increase and the ventilatory support can be further weaned.

Dysynchrony between ventilator and triggered breaths with IMV allowed possible delivery of ventilator tidal volumes before triggered breaths were exhaled, causing breath stacking, hyperinflation and pneumothoraxes. Thus IMV was synchronised (SIMV) to inhibit ventilator breaths before triggered breaths were exhaled. SIMV, once the main mode of ICU ventilation, remains widely used, although pressure support ventilation is increasingly replacing it.

Positive end expiratory pressure (PEEP)

As respiratory muscles relax passively with expiration, airways close, leaving residual gas (and residual pressure) within airways (usually 2.0–2.5 cmH_2O). This is variously called 'auto-PEEP', 'intrinsic PEEP', 'natural PEEP', 'air trapping' and 'breath stacking'. Intubation prevents upper (but not lower) airway closure, and so measured airway pressure returns to *zero-PEEP* at the end of expiration. PEEP prevents alveolar collapse and increases mean airway pressure, improving alveolar gas exchange. Low levels of PEEP (e.g. 2.5 cmH_2O) may replace physiological auto-PEEP. However PEEP can also

- increase the work of breathing (Ruggles 1995)
- reduce venous return (so increasing cardiac workload)
- cause gas trapping and hypercapnia
- overdistend alveoli (Naik *et al.* 1996).

Positive End Expiratory Pressure (PEEP) creates resistance to expiratory flow. Early methods of immersing expiratory port tubing into water (hence measurement in cmH_2O) have been replaced by resistance valves (usually incorporated into ventilators). The mechanics of PEEP can be seen on CPAP valves (see Figure 4.1). Valves close when airway pressure falls below preset levels.

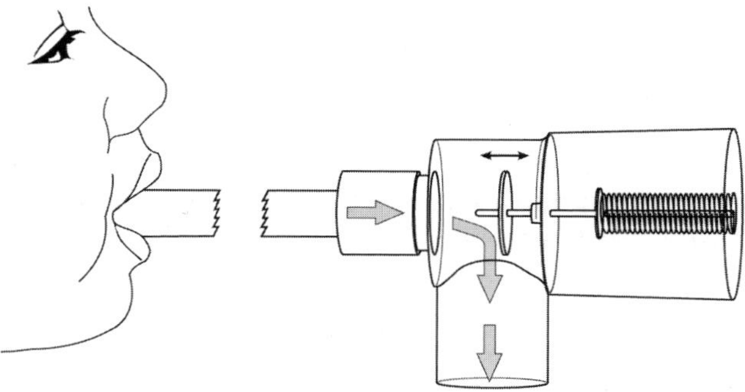

Figure 4.1 Continuous positive airway pressure (CPAP) valve

Mandatory minute volume (MMV)

If triggered breaths are sufficiently large, SIMV minute volumes can be excessive; MMV limits minute volume. However, frequent small tidal volumes may achieve minute volume limits without clearing airway dead space. MMV is rarely used now, and there appears to be little indication for future use.

BiPAP

BiPAP (Biphasic/BiLevel positive airway pressure) combines two levels of pressure and so resembles CPAP with periodic deflation (Pierce 1995). To overcome the problems of PEEP (see above), periodic release of higher expiratory pressure enables trapped gas to escape (Calzia & Radermacher 1997), so reducing barotrauma (Ryan 1998). BiPAP is sometimes called airway pressure release ventilation (APRV); some authors used the terms interchangeably, others apply 'BiPAP' for modes supporting conscious patients with respiratory drive (using face masks or nasal cannulae) and APRV for technologies used when respiratory drive is limited or absent.

Pressure limited/support ventilation

PRESSURE LIMITED VENTILATION This is a form of volume cycling which rapidly achieves, and then maintains, preset upper airway pressure (Rappaport *et al.* 1994); this increases mean airway pressure, so optimising gas exchange while limiting baro/volo-trauma.

PRESSURE SUPPORT VENTILATION (PSV) This is flow-cycled, relying on spontaneous effort ('triggering') (Beale 1994) – although most modern ventilators have default settings to initiate volume-controlled ventilation during apnoea. Once a breath is triggered, pressure support delivers gas until the preset peak airway pressure is reached. Thus pressure support encourages patients to initiate breaths, but replaces shortfall in volume from weak respiratory muscles.

Inspiratory time and tidal/minute volumes vary as other factors (e.g. external pressure on chest) affect peak airway pressure. However tidal volumes are sufficiently consistent; alveolar ventilation is optimised (Bohm & Lachmann 1996) with minimal barotrauma. Spontaneous negative pressure also reduces cardiac compromise.

Low levels of PSV are usually used; ACCP (1993) suggest 5–10 cmH_2O; higher levels are normally weaned with recovery.

Pressure support (PS) can also be combined with modes such as SIMV to increase spontaneous tidal volume.

Flow-by

Triggering (and pressure support) require sufficient negative pressure to open a closed valve, causing a delay in ventilation, increasing work of breathing and causing possible distress to patients. Flow-by provides a continuous flow of gas (5–20 litres per minute) through ventilator circuits (Kalia & Webster 1997) to prevent these problems occurring.

Inspiratory:expiratory ratio

A breath has three potential parts:

- inspiration
- pause/plateau
- expiration

Oxygen transfer occurs primarily during inspiration and plateau; incomplete expiration (e.g. short expiratory phase; gas trapping) increases alveolar carbon dioxide concentrations, so reducing diffusion from blood. Changing inspiration to expiration (I:E) ratio therefore manipulates alveolar gas exchange.

Poor lung compliance (e.g. chronic airflow limitation) reduces airflow speed into lungs, necessitating relatively longer inspiratory time. Prolonging pause/plateau time has similar effects to PEEP – increasing gas exchange, but also increasing intrathoracic pressure. Bronchospasm (e.g. asthma) reduces expiratory flow, needing longer expiratory time.

Some ventilators determine breath pattern by adjusting two of the parts as percentages of the whole breath; other ventilators set an I:E (inspiratory to expiratory) ratio, with separate control for pause/plateau time. Whichever is used, these are different ways to express the same equation. This text uses I:E ratios.

Normal I:E ratios are about 1:2.

Inverse ratio ventilation

Inverse ratio ventilation (IRV) uses ratios below 1:1 (ACCP 1993), so inspiratory exceeds expiratory time. The advantages of IRV are:

- alveolar recruitment from prolonged inspiration time
- reduced alveolar collapse from shorter expiratory time (like PEEP)
- increased mean airway pressure (increased ventilation) without raising peak pressure (barotrauma)

However Mercat *et al.* (1997) found IRV with ARDS reduced carbon dioxide levels without benefit to oxygenation.

The adverse effects of IRV include:

- air-trapping (increased intrathoracic pressure) (ACCP 1993)
- hypercarbia (reduced carbon dioxide clearance)
- breath stacking
- discomfort (Fawcett 1997), possibly requiring more sedation, and possibly paralysis (ACCP 1993)
- further reduction in cardiac return (Mercat *et al.* 1997)

Haemodynamic effects of IRV can be monitored by pulmonary artery catheters (ACCP 1993).

Sigh

Normal respiration includes a physiological **sigh** every 5 to 10 minutes (Hough 1996). Ratios between intra-alveolar pressure and volume differ between inspiration and expiration (**hysteresis**); lung expansion during inspiration increases alveolar surface area, facilitating adsorption of new surfactant adsorbed onto alveolar surfaces; this reduces surface tension during deflation by up to one-fifth (Drummond 1996). Occasional hyperinflation (sigh) prevents atelectasis during shallow respirations (Hough 1996), increases compliance, and so prevents infection.

Since physiological sighs are lost with unconsciousness (Hough 1996), mechanical sighs were incorporated into ventilator technology, often delivering double tidal volumes. However, the mechanical sigh has no proven benefit – hysteresis depends on surfactant production, which is often impaired in ICU patients (e.g. ARDS). The sigh may cause barotrauma and volotrauma and so is not normally used in the UK, but it may be switched on accidentally (occasional but regular peak pressure alarm).

Bersten and Oh (1997) suggest that with use of smaller tidal volumes, sigh use requires reassessment.

Independent lung ventilation

With single-lung pathology, patients may benefit from different modes of ventilation being used to each lung. Independent lung ventilation requires double lumen endotracheal tubes, one lumen entering each bronchus. Independent ventilators, each using any available mode, may then be used for each lung.

Independent lung ventilation may be impractical due to:

- insufficient ventilators available
- increased costs and workload (e.g. ventilator observations are doubled)
- detrimental to safety (access to patient, consuming more nursing time)

Noninvasive ventilation

Noninvasive (e.g. nasal) ventilation avoids endotracheal intubation, using close-fitting masks (similar to CPAP) and relying on normal airway resistance; it therefore reduces the complications of artificial ventilation. However, as air leaks are invariably present and the airway is unprotected, with no access for suction (Elliott *et al.* 1990) unless a minitracheostomy is performed, patients must be able to clear their own secretions (Pierce 1995).

Noninvasive ventilation is not intended for prolonged use, although it may facilitate weaning (Wedzicha 1992). The availability of non-invasive ventilation extends ethical dilemmas about decisions not to ventilate. Such decisions should be taken by the multidisciplinary team, nurses being potentially valuable patient advocates.

Physiological complications

All body systems are affected by artificial ventilation. Although this description is reductionist, and further complications are identified in Chapter 5 and elsewhere, it should be remembered that there are cumulative effects on the whole person.

CARDIOVASCULAR Normal respiration aids cardiac return through negative intrathoracic pressure, entraining blood from the lower inferior vena cava. Conversely, positive pressure ventilation

- impedes venous return
- increases right ventricular workload
- causes cardiac tamponade

resulting in reduced arterial pressure and extravasation of plasma into interstitial spaces (oedema, including pulmonary). Cardiac compromise reduces perfusion to all systems.

RESPIRATORY In addition to infection risks and abnormal gas distribution (see above) from intubation and ventilation, peak airway pressures of 35 cmH_2O may cause **barotrauma** (damage from excessive airway pressures) (ACCP 1993), volotrauma (damage from excessive lung volume), and tension pneumothorax.

Although maintaining patency of airways, rigid endotracheal tubes (and other ventilator circuitry) create resistance, usually of 5–10 cmH_2O (Bersten & Oh 1997). Airway resistance increases work of breathing with patient-initiated breath, unless compensated (e.g. PEEP, pressure support).

The work of breathing at rest consumes 1–3 per cent of total oxygen consumed; with respiratory failure, the work of breathing may consume one-quarter of total body oxygen (Hinds & Watson 1996), depriving other vital organs of oxygen. Modes incorporating some patient-initiated breaths increase work of breathing so that patients showing signs of exhaustion, or who are tachypnoeic but with low tidal volumes, should be given more artificial support.

RENAL PERFUSION This is reduced with systemic hypotension, potentially causing prerenal failure. Renin-angiotensin-aldosterone and inappropriate ADH release increase tubular reabsorption of sodium and water, predisposing to systemic and pulmonary oedema. Impaired toxin/metabolite removal prolongs the effects of drugs and toxins (e.g. uraemia can cause confusion).

HEPATIC DAMAGE AND DYSFUNCTION This results from:

- physical (diaphragmatic) compression from raised intrathoracic pressure
- portal congestion and hypertension from impaired venous return
- ischaemia from arterial hypotension

The liver has many functions, but three especially complicating critical illness are:

- drugs/metabolite clearance (prolonged effects, confusion)
- clotting factor production (coagulopathies)
- complement production (infection)

NEUROLOGICAL COMPLICATIONS Impaired venous return increases intracranial oedema and intracranial pressure causing various psychological and neurological complications, including SIADH (see Chapter 22).

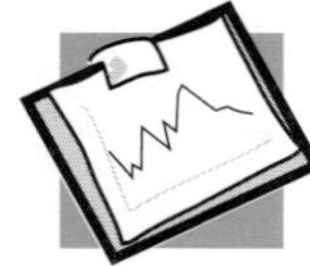

Implications for practice

- any machine can be inaccurate or fail; nurses should check all alarms and safety equipment at the start of each shift; ventilator function should be checked through recorded observations (at least hourly) and continuously by visual observation and setting appropriate alarm parameters (often within 10 per cent); remember alarms may also fail
- check monitor circuits for leaks by assessing air entry
- most modern ventilators include default settings – know your machine and check these
- familiarise yourself with all ventilators used on your unit
- positive pressure ventilation affects all body systems; function of other systems should be continuously and holistically assessed
- ventilation often increases the need for fundamental aspects of care (e.g. mouthcare: oral intubation encourages mouth drying; eyecare: increased intraocular pressure may prevent eye closure)
- all intubation/mask equipment can cause damage – ties/tapes can occlude venous flow or cause direct trauma (e.g. tapes across open corneas); CPAP or other close-fitting masks and endotracheal cuffs can cause pressure sores

Summary

Sophisticated ventilator technology continues to develop rapidly in response to increasingly complex pathologies. This chapter has discussed the main principles of ventilation design; material on specific models should be available on units where they are used. Despite technological development, artificial ventilation continues to cause many problems for patients, which are identified in this and many later chapters.

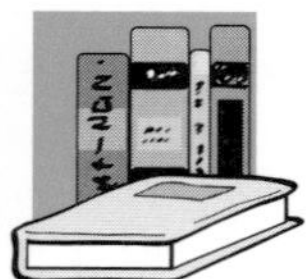

Further reading

Manuals/information on machines used on your unit should be read. Most specialist texts include sections on ventilators and ventilation. Pierce (1995) and ACCP (1993) give comprehensive overviews. Moxham and Goldstone's (1994) book is also useful. Robb (1997) and Ashurst (1997) review nursing care of ventilated patients.

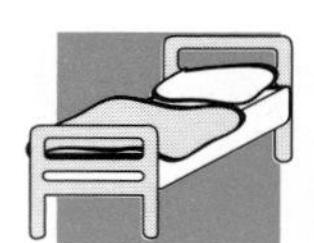

Clinical scenario

Anthony Webb is a 58-year-old taxi driver with emphysema (COPD). He has recently quit a smoking habit of over 30 cigarettes per day. Mr Webb was admitted to ICU for artificial ventilation following acute exacerbation of COPD, hypercarbia and deteriorating respiratory function from chest infection. He is orally intubated and receiving positive pressure ventilation.

The ventilator settings include:		*Arterial Blood Gas results following 12 hours invasive ventilation*		*Other results*	
Mode SIMV		*pH*	*7.51*	*Sputum culture: Streptococcus pneumonia*	
V_T	600ml	PaO_2	7.07 kPa		
Pressure Support	20 cmH_2O	$PaCO_2$	4.5 kPa	WCC	13.5 g/dl
PEEP	+ 8 cmH_2O	HCO_3^-	26.2 mmol/l	Hb	16.2 g/dl
I:E ratio	2:1	BE	3.6 mmol/l	K	3.2 mmol/l
Inspired O_2	40%	SaO_2	89%	Na	148 mmol/l
				PO_4^{2-}	1.8

Q.1 Interpret these results and identify any abnormal values in relation to those expected for patients with COPD.

Q.2 From the above data, analyse and rate potential complications of invasive ventilation for Mr Webb. What nursing strategies can minimise potential complications (suggest changes to ventilator settings)?

His family brings in an Advanced Directive signed by Mr Webb stating that he does not wish to be invasively ventilated. Mr Webb confirms this non-verbally and indicates he would like to be extubated.

Q.3 Justify the nurse's role (and any conflicts) and responsibilities in withdrawing invasive ventilation. Select alternative therapies to support Mr Webb's respiratory function.

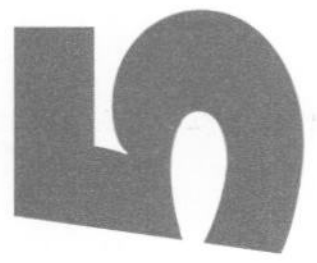
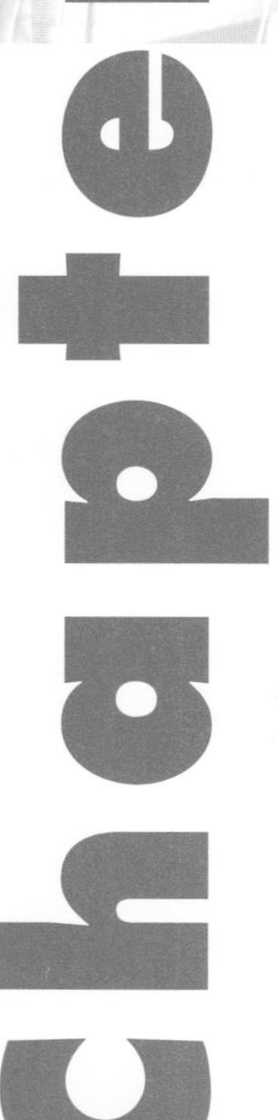

Chapter 5

Airway management

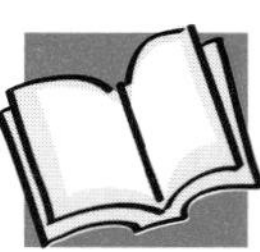

Contents

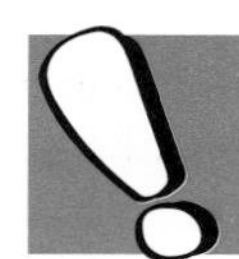

Fundamental knowledge

Tracheal anatomy, function of cilia and mucus
Cricoid anatomy
Carina plus positions of right and left main bronchi
Differences between paediatric and adult trachea
Alveolar physiology

Introduction

Most patients admitted to ICUs receive ventilatory support, normally necessitating endotracheal tubes (ETTs) or tracheostomies. ICU nurses are therefore responsible for ensuring patency of, and minimising complications from, endotracheal tubes. This chapter describes the types of tubes usually used in ICUs, the main complications of intubation and the controversies surrounding endotracheal suction.

Despite the frequency of endotracheal suction, substantive evidence for many aspects is usually lacking or not translated into practice. The lack of substantive evidence makes many recommendations for practice in this chapter necessarily tentative.

Intubation

Traditionally intubation could be:

- oral
- nasal
- tracheostomy

Unless specific surgery or pathophysiology necessitated a specific route, oral tubes were usually used for short-term, nasal tubes for medium-term and tracheostomies for prolonged intubation, practice often being guided by protocols that specified time limits for each method.

Oral tubes cause gagging, but are easier to insert. ETTs are rigid, limiting lumen size and increasing airway resistance (especially nasal tubes). The sharply angled nasal cavity (see Figure 5.1) makes trauma and bleeding almost unavoidable during intubation (especially if patients have coagulopathies), and suction difficult.

Tracheostomy avoids many complications of oral and nasal intubation, and reduces dead space by up to half (Pritchard 1994), but necessitates surgery, leaving a residual wound. Heffner (1993) suggests tracheostomies should ideally be performed after 21 days, but most intensivists now determine changes by the individual needs of patients rather than by protocols.

Mini-tracheostomies, initially developed to facilitate the removal of secretions, can also be used for high frequency ventilation. Non-invasive positive pressure ventilation and laryngeal masks (see below) may avoid the necessity for intubation.

Nurses may be requested to assist with intubation by applying cricoid pressure. The cricoid cartilage (just below the 'Adam's apple') forms a complete ring, so cricoid pressure (pressing the cricoid cartilage down with three fingers towards the patient's head) compresses the pharynx against cervical vertebra, preventing gastric reflux and aspiration. Pressure is maintained until the endotracheal tube cuff is inflated.

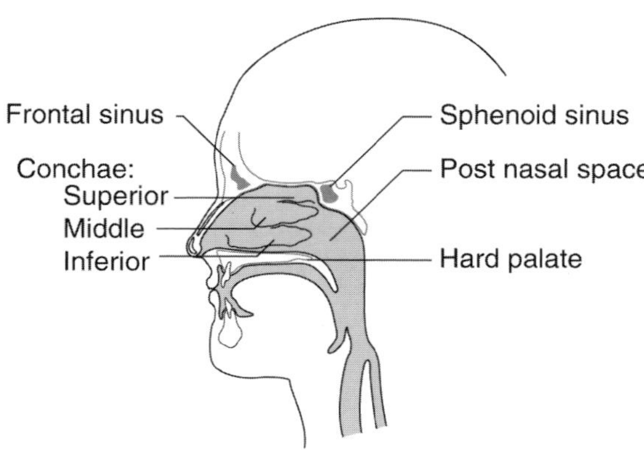

Figure 5.1 Main anatomy of the nasal cavity

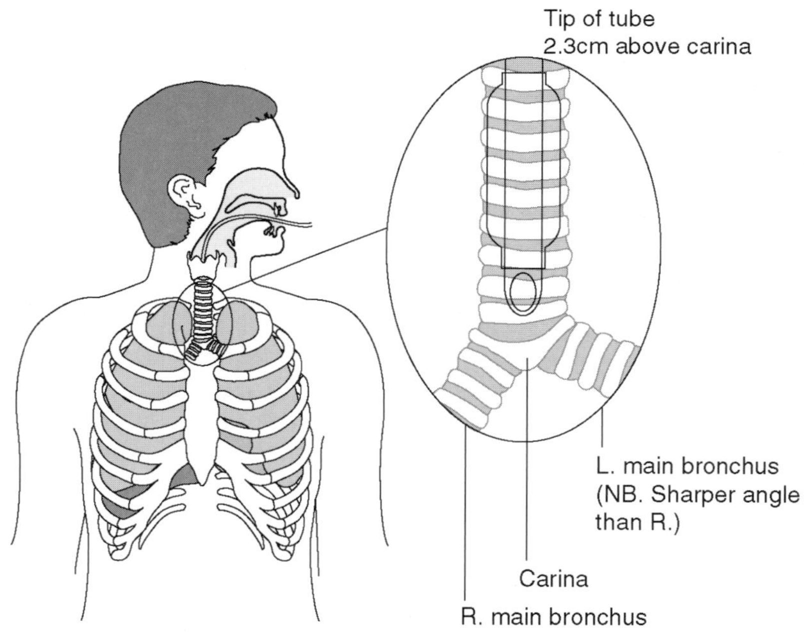

Figure 5.2 Placement of an endotracheal tube (ETT) showing end of tube just above the carina

To ventilate both lungs, ETTs should end above the carina (see Figure 5.2); this should be checked by

- X-rays
- auscultating for air entry
- ensuring chest movement is bilateral.

Accidental single bronchus intubation usually occurs in the right main bronchus, due to its gentler angle from the carina. Mulvey *et al.* (1993) cite right tracheal intubation rates of 9 per cent. Malplaced tubes should be repositioned by anaesthetists and reassessed.

Endotracheal tubes are manufactured in a single (long) length and so almost invariably require cutting to minimise ventilatory dead space, usually to 21 cm (female) and 23 cm (male).

Potentially prolonged intubation on ICU necessitates

- hypoirritant material
- low pressure ('profile') cuffs

Hypoirritant materials (e.g. silastic, polyvinylchloride (PVC)) prevent granuloma formation.

Childrens' airways differ from those of adults (see Chapter 13) and so, in order to prevent excessive pressure on tracheal tissue, uncuffed endotracheal tubes should be used with children under 8 years old (James 1991); nasal intubation with Tunstall connector fixation can prevent damage from tube movement.

Laryngeal mask airways (LMAs), which remain above the vocal cords, are easy to insert, thus making them useful for operating theatre and emergency use (Janssens & Lamy 1989); they do not isolate the trachea from the oesophagus so that aspiration may still occur, making laryngeal masks essentially modified face masks (Raphael & Langton 1995) rather than replacements for ETTs (Janssens & Lamy 1989). They may be used for short-term ICU ventilation, weaning and in combination with mini-tracheostomy (Brimacombe *et al.* 1997), but are more often seen with patients admitted unexpectedly from other departments.

Problems

Intubation is often a necessary medical solution which creates various nursing problems.

Airway sensory nerve stimulation causes a *cough reflex*, involving vagal afferent pathways, the cough centre and motor nerves of the diaphragm, abdomen, intercostal muscles and larynx. Coughing is a protective mechanism, removing foreign bodies (including respiratory pathogens) from the airway at up to 100 mph. This reflex can be initiated by oral endotracheal tubes and suction catheters, causing discomfort (antitussive drugs, such as codeine phosphate, can suppress gag reflexes). Many critically ill patients have impaired gag reflexes, causing possible aspiration (including past low-pressure endotracheal cuffs).

Impaired cough and swallowing reflexes may cause *aspiration* of saliva and gastric secretions. ETT cuffs should provide a reasonable seal between lower and upper trachea to prevent aspiration, without causing tracheal tissue damage. Seals are usually incomplete; cuffs often develop slow leaks, usually from external valves, but sometimes from cuff permeability to gases or chemicals. ETT cuffs should state recommended air volumes so that 'topping up' should only be performed when checking residual cuff volume (before deflating cuffs, remove tracheal secretions to prevent aspiration). If excessive cuff volumes or pressures are needed, the tube probably needs replacing.

While cuff pressure should be sufficient to minimise risks from aspiration, excessive pressure on tracheal epithelium may occlude capillary perfusion causing *tracheal ulcers*; unlike pressure sores on skin, these are not directly visible. The average capillary occlusion pressure is about 30 mmHg, but can be as low as 25 mmHg (see Chapter 12); as most ICU patients are hypotensive, recommending cuff pressure ranges of 14–30 mmHg (Crimlisk *et al.* 1996) seems cavalier.

Wound healing (e.g. from pressure sores) leaves inelastic scar tissue; ring-shaped tracheal scars from ETT cuffs cause tracheal stenosis (potential respiratory distress). Mulvey *et al.* (1993) cite post-extubation stenosis rates of 19 per cent, using 1981 texts; while availability of profile cuffs and greater awareness of the problem should have reduced these rates, their recommendation of 25 mmHg maximum cuff pressures remains reliable. Jones *et al.* (1997) suggest that tracheal stenosis may be associated with reintubation, although the incidence in reintubated patients who had remained on ICUs for over five days was only 3 per cent, and they do not indicate cuff pressures. 'High volume low pressure' 'profile' cuffs (see Figure 5.3) achieve a (reasonable, but incomplete) seal by exerting low pressure over an extended area, but may still cause ulcers. Assessing cuff pressures by squeezing the external balloon is unreliable, but commercially available manometers are available and reliable, and so nurses should, as part of their individual accountability, check cuff pressures at least once each shift, and whenever cuff volume is changed.

Oral ETTs cause *hypersalivation* and impairment of swallowing reflexes (see Chapter 10), with drying of mucosa near the lips and saliva accumulation (and potential aspiration) at the back of the throat. 'Bubbling' sounds during inspiratory phases of ventilation indicate the need to remove secretions and to check cuff pressure. Nasal intubation and tracheostomy prevent hypersalivation, but tracheal secretions may still accumulate.

Tubes can cause mechanical *tissue damage*. Like cuff pressure sores (above), pressure from tubes can damage any surrounding tissue (lips, gums, nostril). Tubes also damage cilia and mucus-producing goblet cells (non-specific immunity). Laryngeal oedema often causes hoarseness following extubation.

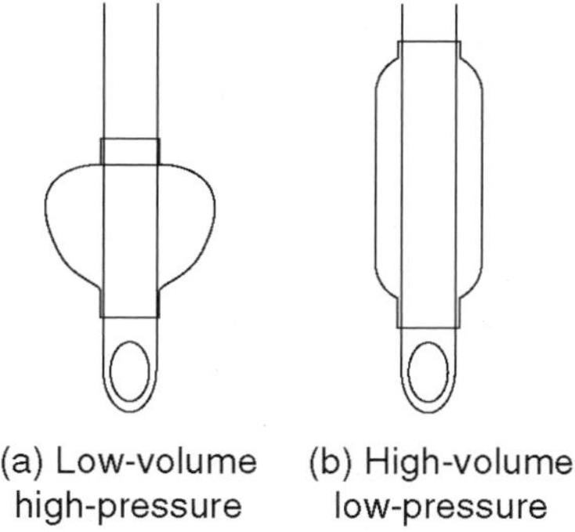

Figure 5.3 High and low pressure cuffs on endotracheal tubes

Bypassing and damage to non-specific immune defences (e.g. cilia) causes *immunocompromise* which, together with impaired cough reflex, predisposes patients to infection.

Sympathetic nervous stimulation from intubation and suction initiates *stress responses* (see Chapter 3); suction-induced stress responses can cause intracranial hypertension (Brucia & Rudy 1996). Direct vagal nerve stimulation (anatomically close to the trachea) can cause bradycardic dysrhythmias and blocks, especially during intubation.

Oral ETTs cause discomfort and *anxiety* (Cochran & Ganong 1989); nasal tubes and tracheostomies are usually better tolerated and so tend to be used more with conscious patients. Patients' inability to speak due to intubation through their vocal cords should be explained.

Humidification

Nasal epithelium has a rich venous supply covering the nasal conchae; air turbulence maximises exposure for heat and moisture exchange, inspired air normally reaching body temperature just below the carina (Jackson 1996); thus the human airway (a) warms, (b) moistens, and (c) filters inspired air.

Endotracheal intubation bypasses these normal physiological mechanisms, necessitating artificial replacement. Since oxygen is a dry gas, inadequate humidification dehydrates exposed membranes (below the endotracheal tube), potentially causing necrotising tracheobronchitis (ACCP 1993). Hot air transports more water vapour than cold air and so fully saturated room air/gas (100 per cent relative humidity) will not be fully saturated once warmed to body temperature. Gas not fully saturated absorbs moisture from airway surfaces, causing dehydration, making mucus more viscid. Viscid mucus increases:

- risk of chest infection
- risk of airway encrustation/obstruction
- airway resistance and work of breathing
- surfactant dysfunction

Gas should therefore be heated and fully saturated exogenously; tracheal gas temperature should be 32–36°C.

Humidifiers use either exogenous water or hydrophobic membranes. Heated *water baths* provide an ideal medium for bacterial incubation, particularly pseudomonas. Closed circuit systems reduce, but do not remove, this risk. Water bath humidifiers may cause overhumidification, mucosal burns, hyperthermia and water intoxification (Jackson 1996). Where exogenous heat is used, temperature of inspired air should be continuously monitored.

Heat moisture exchangers (HMEs) use hydrophobic membranes to repel airway moisture; they are efficient bacterial filters, but less satisfactory at achieving adequate humidification (Martin *et al.* 1990). Current dilemmas between humidification and infection control lack an ideal solution. Saline lavage to remove encrusted secretions can cause various problems (discussed below). Ackerman *et al.* (1996) argue that encrustations resulting from systemic dehydration should be prevented by increasing hydration. However pulmonary oedema from increased capillary permeability may limit hydration of critically ill patients.

Suction

Intubation bypasses non-specific mucus and cilial defences, while impaired cough reflexes from critical illness, antitussives and sedation, enable accumulation of lower respiratory tract secretions, reducing/obstructing airway patency (increasing work of breathing) and providing media for bacterial growth. Endotracheal suction can remove accumulated secretions, but can also cause:

- infection
- trauma
- hypoxia
- atelectasis

Post-discharge surveys consistently identify patient anxiety and discomfort from suction (e.g. Puntillo 1990), and so it should never be a ‘routine’ procedure (Ashurst 1997); nurses should evaluate benefits against dangers. The changes made in endotracheal suction practice in the 1980s necessitate caution when reading older literature. Indications for suction include:

- rattling/bubbling on auscultation
- sudden increases in airway pressure
- audible ‘bubbling’ from the back of the throat
- sudden hypoxia (e.g. sudden fall in SpO_2)

To help later staff make informed decisions, time and efficacy of suctioning should be recorded, together with any problems or other relevant information.

Disconnecting ventilation (inevitable unless closed-circuit suction systems are used) causes arterial desaturation, especially when patients are dependent on high levels of oxygen; preoxygenating all patients (3–5 minutes of 100 per cent oxygen) minimises risks.

Although intended to remove bacteria, suction catheters can introduce/displace bacteria into lower airways. During suction, equipment (e.g. HMEs, catheter mounts) should be stored in a clean area to minimise contamination.

Respiratory pathogens sprayed into the environment through patients' coughing or from suction catheters can infect others (e.g. staff) up to one metre away (Cobley *et al.* 1991). Gowns, gloves, masks and goggles may protect staff, but efficacy of each needs evaluation, and their use delays suction procedures.

Negative (suction) pressure damages delicate tracheal epithelium, causing possible

- haemorrhage
- oedema
- stenosis
- metaplasia.

Negative pressure should be sufficient to clear secretions, but low enough to minimise trauma. Bronchial stenosis occurs in 1.2 per cent of infants (Knox 1993); adult epithelium is less friable, but trauma remains unseen until bleeding occurs. Suction pressures, usually measured in kilopascals (kPa) but sometimes in millimetres of mercury (mmHg), should be displayed on equipment. Odell *et al.* (1993) recommend maximum pressures of 27 kPa (200 mmHg); Ashurst's (1997) 16 kPa (120 mmHg) recommendation reflects current evidence-based practice. Intermittent release of negative pressure during suctioning has no advantage (Czarnik *et al.* 1991).

Disconnection from ventilation and negative pressure from suction can cause hypoxia through

- removal of oxygen supply
- removal of oxygen-rich air from airways
- alveolar collapse.

Suction passes should therefore be as brief as possible (maximum 15 seconds), with rapid reconnection of ventilation. Nurses are recommended to hold their own breath during each pass: when they need oxygen, so will their patient.

Hypoxia from bronchoconstriction (sympathetic stress response) usually follows endotracheal suction. Although Wood's review (1998) found no proven benefit to routine preoxygenation, evidence is sparse, and failure to preoxygenate is probably more dangerous than routine preoxygenation. Many ventilators include time-limited control for delivery of 100 per cent oxygen; using these prevents inadvertent delivery of toxic levels continuing after stabilisation. If FiO_2 is increased manually, it should be returned to baseline levels once PaO_2 is restored.

Catheters

Removing oral secretions is easiest and safest with Yankauer catheters; angling the head to enable drainage of secretions into the cheek avoids trauma to the delicate soft palate.

Endotracheal (soft) catheters should remove the maximum amount of secretions in the quickest possible time with minimal trauma. Many texts (usually anecdotally) recommend catheters should not exceed one-half to two-thirds ETT diameter; for ETTs above 6 Ch size, Odell *et al.* (1993) recommend:

$$\text{catheter size} = (\text{endotracheal tube size} - 2) \times 2$$

Removing tenacious secretions with small catheters (below FG 12) can be difficult.

'Atraumatic' catheters with a lip preventing direct contact between the suction port of catheters and epithelium have been marketed, but Fiorentini (1992) found them of no benefit; few units now use them.

The practice of reusing disposable catheters for more than one pass seems to be based on anecdotal evidence that infection risks are not increased. Without substantive evidence, nurses reusing catheters should consider their professional accountability, and the legal liabilities of reusing equipment labelled by manufacturers as single-use (de Jong 1996).

Gloves: sterile or clean?

Using clean (rather than sterile) gloves for suction similarly appears based on anecdotal claims that infection rates are not significantly increased. Gloves of any sort protect (universal precautions) nurses, and clean gloves are both quicker to put on and cheaper; with gloved hands not touching catheter tips, infection risks appear small, but any substantive evidence to support this is lacking (Odell *et al.* 1993), and so again nurses should consider their professional and legal liabilities.

Closed circuit suction

Closed circuit suction systems are commercially available. These enable ventilation and PEEP to continue until negative pressure is applied, thus improving mixed venous oxygenation saturation following suction (Clark *et al.* 1990) – although this probably has only a significant benefit for a few patients. Ventilation continues during catheter insertion and so catheters should be advanced more carefully to reduce trauma (passes should not be slowed so much that patient discomfort is increased). Closed systems also prevent environmental contamination (Cobley *et al.* 1991; Graziano *et al.* 1987), reducing infection risk to staff and patients (especially eye infections). Concerns that they create reservoirs for microbial colonisation appear to be unfounded (Adams *et al.* 1997), although users' hands may be contaminated (Blackwood 1998); perhaps 'closed' is a relative term.

Nurses' concerns that closed circuit catheters may be more difficult to manipulate (Graziano *et al.* 1987; Blackwood 1998) are not supported by either radiological analysis (Graziano *et al.* 1987) or anecdotal reports from staff familiar with using these systems.

Closed circuit systems can be cost effective if they replace sufficient numbers of disposable items. Most manufacturers recommend replacement after 24 hours; Quirke (1998) found 48-hour changes safe and suggests that further research may support weekly changes; however, staff should remember their legal liability if flouting manufacturer's recommendations.

Saline

Encrustations from dried secretions appear to have increased since HMEs largely replaced water humidifiers. Widespread practice of saline instillation to loosen secretions has little support beyond anecdotal literature. Mucus is not water soluble and so will not easily mix with saline; encrustations on dentures can be difficult to remove after soaking overnight, and a few seconds contact with saline seems unlikely to significantly loosen airway encrustations. The cough reflex elicited by instillation may clear mucus and debris (Gray *et al.* 1990), but coughs can be stimulated without saline.

Benefits from instilling saline are dubious. Hanley *et al.* (1978) found that bolus saline did not reach distal bronchioles after thirty minutes, and they only recovered up to one-fifth of fluid instilled. Hagler and Travers (1994) found saline dislodged up to 310,000 viable bacteria from ETTs, compared to 60,000 from catheter insertion, exposing patients to significant reinfection risks. Ackerman (1993) found saline instillation reduced PaO_2, possibly from bronchospasm or creating a fluid barrier to gas perfusion. However Ackerman's methodology alternated use and non-use of saline in the same patients, ignoring possible late complications of consolidation through inadequate removal of mucus. Temperature differentials between cold fluids and airways may trigger bronchospasm so that warming fluids (from hand heat) may reduce complications (Gunderson & Stoeckle 1995).

Bolus volumes range between 0.5–5.0 ml, with little beyond anecdotal literature for evidence. The frequency between installations also varies greatly. Increasingly, Ackerman's prolonged campaign to abandon saline installation (e.g. Ackerman *et al.* 1996) is echoed by other writers, such as

Haggler and Travers (1994) and Knox (1993). There may be individual cases where saline is indicated, but what those indications currently are remains unclear. Substantial research evidence is needed before saline instillation can be recommended.

Nebulisation produces smaller droplets which should reach distal bronchioles, but Asmundsson *et al.* (1973) found very little reached the lungs.

Hyperinflation

Hyperinflation ('bagging', to loosen secretions) can be achieved with manual ('rebreathe') bags or through most modern ventilators (e.g. manual sigh). Muscle recoil following hyperinflation mimics the cough reflex and so loosens secretions. It also potentially

- removal raises intrathoracic pressure
- removal reduces cardiac return
- causes (mechanical) vagal stimulation (resulting in bradycardia)
- causes barotrauma.

Manual rebreathe bags are available in various sizes; adult systems should include

- pressure escape valves
- oxygen reservoirs if patients normally receive high concentration oxygen
- 2-litre bags (ideal hyperinflation volume is 1.5 preset tidal volume).

Grap *et al.* (1994) found manual hyperinflation did not significantly affect heart rate, mean arterial pressure or SaO_2, but vital signs should be closely monitored. Glass *et al.* (1993) found that manual hyperinflation usually failed to deliver the ideal 1.5 times ventilator tidal volume, although Clapham *et al.* (1995) recorded significantly better results, provided preset tidal volume was below 700 ml. Despite underinflation, Clapham *et al.* (1995) found manual hyperinflation caused surprisingly high peak pressures compared with mechanical sigh. Relative merits of manual and mechanical hyperinflation remain debated (Robson 1998), but ventilator-controlled hyperinflation leaves nurses' hands free while ensuring hyperinflation volume is both controlled and measured (limiting barotrauma).

Extubation stridor

Mulvey *et al.* (1993) suggest that 5 per cent of patients experience extubation stridor, but draw their evidence from 1981 texts (when there was less awareness of problems with high cuff pressures). Marley (1998) cites more recent post-operative evidence showing a 0.1 incidence of post-extubation oedema, although ICU incidence is presumably higher due to prolonged intubation. Children's tracheas are smaller and so where 1 mm of oedema might cause slight hoarseness in adults, it would obstruct three-quarters of a child's airway (Marley 1998). Should croup/stridor occur, Mulvey *et al.* (1993) recommend 1 mg of nebulised adrenaline in 5 ml of saline, or helium–oxygen inhalation.

Implications for practice

- ETT cuff pressures should be checked by each nurse caring for an intubated patient, and whenever any change in pressure is suspected; pressures should not exceed 25 mmHg (3.3 kPa)
- suction should never be 'routine', but performed when indicated
- negative pressure should not exceed 16 kPa (120 mmHg)
- practices lacking substantive evidence (reuse of catheters, clean rather than sterile gloves and bolus saline instillation) cannot be supported
- closed circuit suction should be considered if
    - hypoxia from suction causes significant problems
    - spread of respiratory pathogens exposes others to significant risks
    - where frequent suction is needed
- hyperinflation is more safely performed through ventilators

Summary

While the intubation route remains a medical decision, bedside nurses monitor and manage artificial airways. Despite the frequency and long history of mechanical ventilation, many dilemmas of nursing management remain unresolved, influenced more by tradition or small-scale (often in-house) studies than substantial research and meta-analysis. No aspect of airway management should be considered routine; as with all other aspects of care, frequent assessment enables the individualisation of care in order to meet the patient's needs.

Further reading

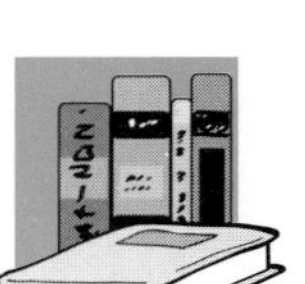

Much is written about aspects of respiratory management. Overviews are usually best obtained from books, but many articles usefully pursue aspects in detail. Fiorentini (1992), Odell *et al.* (1993) and Grap *et al.* (1994) describe hazards of suctioning. Wood (1998) provides an extensive literature review on dilemmas of endotracheal suction.

Ackerman *et al.* (1996) highlight problems from saline instillation. Reviewing literature for developing departmental guidelines, McKelvie (1998) gives a reliable overview. James (1991) and Knox (1993) offer useful paediatric perspectives.

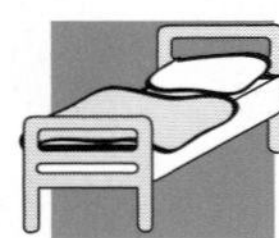

Clinical scenario

Q.1 List the main adverse effects of ETT suctioning to the ICU patient. Identify those effects that you have observed in your own clinical practice and those from the literature.

Q.2 From the literature and experiences of colleagues (including respiratory physiotherapists), critically analyse the use of saline installation to promote tracheal clearance. Examine the evidence base to justify (or support) this practice.

Q.3 Reflect on your professional responsibilities when instructed/asked to use saline instillation whilst suctioning a patient with normal tracheal secretions. Consider: Duty of Care; Advocacy; Scope of Professional Practice (UKCC 1992b), paragraph 9, and any other relevant material.

Chapter 6

Sedation

chapter 6

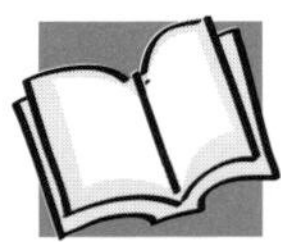

Contents

Introduction

In the 1980s ICU practice changed from 'heavy' (deeply unconscious) to 'light' sedation, reflecting changes in both philosophy and ventilator technology. Lighter sedation

- enables patients to remain semiconscious, thus reducing psychoses while promoting autonomy
- reduces hypotensive and cardioinhibitory effects caused by most sedatives

Light sedation is a narrow margin between over- and under-sedation. Increasingly, ICUs have used assessment tools to optimise sedation.

Evidence-based practice has encouraged the questioning of traditional rituals. This chapter explores benefits and problems from sedation assessment tools, and discusses issues surrounding the nursing of conscious patients in ICUs in order to enable nurses to develop evidence-based practice. The focus is therefore a nursing one rather than pharmacological, although some widely used sedatives are described. Neuromuscular blockade, once a common adjunct of sedation therapy, is also mentioned.

Shelly (1998) stresses that comfort (in its widest sense) can be achieved through sedation. Bion and Ledingham's (1987) post-discharge survey found over half of ICU patients remembered pain, anxiety and lack of rest, and so there are sound humanitarian arguments for sedation; however, physiological effects of stress (see Chapter 3) also delay recovery. Sedation is now usually only necessary for ventilation if patients have:

- *tachypnoea*, which will cause exhaustion
- *discomfort* from artificial ventilation (usually from oral endotracheal tubes; also for brief procedures such as cardioversion and bronchoscopy).

There are some specific pathologies, such as intracranial hypertension, where sedation is therapeutic. Where relevant, these are identified in Part III of this book.

Some authors suggest that potential line displacement justifies sedation (Shelly 1994). Restraint (including chemical, i.e. sedation) is ethically questionable.

Problems of sedation

Adverse effects vary between sedatives, but problems include:

- hypotension
- prevention of REM sleep (Shelly 1993)
- amnesia (patients waking from induced sedation experience only a void of time, without the usual recall of normal sleep); 'missing time' can cause anxiety. Amnesia prevents recall of often horrific procedures, but

inability to recall experiences, however horrific, may cause greater psychological trauma (Perrins *et al.* 1998); the deliberate (non-consensual) deprivation of life experiences of others is arguably paternalistic.

GABA receptors

Gamma-aminobutyric acid (GABA), the main cerebral cortex inhibitory neurotransmitter, prevents excessive exposure to stimuli (Park & Navapurkar 1994). GABA stimulation (by benzodiazepines) therefore induces sedation, anxiolysis and hypnosis (Eddleston *et al.* 1997). Prolonged benzodiazepine use causes receptor growth and down-regulation (tolerance), necessitating higher doses (Eddleston *et al.* 1997). Endorphins (endogenous opiates) contribute to sedative effects of critical illness.

Some GABA receptors are also found in the heart, kidney, mast cells, platelets and adrenal glands (Park & Navapurkar 1994). Cardiovascular receptors may cause hypotension with benzodiazepines.

Benzodiazepines (diazepam, lorazepam, midazolam)

Midazolam, which has largely superseded other benzodiazepines in ICU, has the shortest **half-life** (two hours with short-term use (Viney 1996)). Midazolam is largely hepatically metabolised and renally excreted, so failure of these organs may cause accumulation of active metabolites (especially with older people, who usually have reduced renal clearance); causing unpredictable increases in half-life with critical illness (Bion & Oh 1997).

GABA receptor growth can cause dependence, leading to convulsions if benzodiazepines are suddenly withdrawn (Eddleston et al. 1997); if benzodiazepine use exceeds two weeks, Hudak et al. (1998) recommend weaning by 20–25 per cent each day.

Being relatively cheap, midazolam is still used by many units for prolonged sedation. Anxiolytics (e.g. lorazepam, haloperidol) may also be given enterally (Hall-Smith et al. 1997).

The antagonist for benzodiazepines is flumazenil. Flumazenil's effect is far shorter than benzodiazepines (half-life under one hour (Armstrong *et al.* 1992)) and so although it is useful to assess underlying consciousness, resumption of sedation necessitates caution if changing any treatments (e.g. extubation).

Opiates

Most opiates have sedative effects; as analgesia is usually necessary, this 'side effect' can be beneficial, provided it is remembered when assessing sedation. Opiates may become the most important part of sedative regimes (Bion & Oh 1997). Morphine remains one of the most powerful opiates, but newer drugs, such as fentanyl, achieve rapid sedation with strong respiratory depression (which facilitates ventilation).

Propofol

Propofol's lipid emulsion facilitates transfer across the blood–brain barrier, achieving rapid sedation. Inactivity of metabolites (Sherry 1997) and rapid redistribution into fatty tissue (Eddleston *et al.* 1997) limits half-life to between 34 and 64 minutes, although like midazolam, hepatic failure may prolong half-life (Sherry 1997). Widely used for short-term sedation, Propofol is relatively expensive and so some units restrict use to circumstances where sedation is planned to last less than one day.

Propofol depresses cerebral metabolism, thus reducing both cerebral oxygen consumption and intracranial pressure (Viney 1996). It may also have bronchodilatory properties (Viney 1996), which are potentially beneficial to many ICU patients.

A number of disadvantages have been reported with propofol:

- **bradycardia** from resetting of carotid receptors (Sherry 1997)
- **hypotension** from resetting of baroreceptors, sympathetic inhibition and increased venous capacitance (Robinson *et al.* 1994); stroke volume is reduced by 10–15 per cent (Sear 1996)
- **hypertriglyceridaemia** (causing delay in return of cerebral function) has been reported when used for more than 72 hours (Eddleston *et al.* 1997)
- *convulsions* have been reported in patients with no previous history of epilepsy (e.g. Valente *et al.* (1994)), although Smith (1994) claims it is the ideal sedative agent for intracranial pathologies
- *unpleasant psychiatric side-effects*, including nightmare-like hallucinations (Hall-Smith *et al.* 1997)
- '*creaming*' – accumulation of emulsifying fat in lungs and serum (Spencer & Willats 1997); although visible with blood samples, it can affect analyses (e.g. blood gases) and damage analysers
- *impaired immunity* from inhibition of phagocytosis (Krumholz *et al.* 1995)
- *infection*: propofol contains no preservative, and so asepsis is especially important

Prolonged use can cause greenish urine (Sherry 1997); although probably clinically insignificant, relatives and staff should be aware of this effect. Some anecdotal reports suggest propofol may perish giving sets.

Currently propofol is licensed for adult use only for a period of up to 72 hours. Use of any drug or equipment beyond a manufacturer's licence places the onus of legal liability on the users (see Chapter 45).

Since propofol does not have any analgesic effect, concurrent analgesia should be given.

Bolus sedation

The introduction of shorter-acting sedatives together with the improvement of infusion pump technology has largely replaced the use of bolus sedation with continuous infusions. Like analgesia, bolus sedation can cause fluctuations between under- and over-sedation (Shelly 1998). Where sedative effects are prolonged, constant infusion can result in over-sedation (Shelly 1998).

Assessing sedation

Over- and under-sedation are relative concepts. The lighter levels of sedation now preferred create relatively narrow margins between over-sedation and under-sedation. Over-sedation is arguably inhumane, depriving patients of life awareness, but it also causes respiratory and cardiovascular depression (compromising tissue perfusion) and so it potentially prolongs recovery. Drugs also increase the costs of patient care, placing further burdens on (usually) stretched unit budgets. Thus unnecessary drugs are psychologically, physiologically and financially undesirable.

Under-sedation exposes patients to noxious stimuli (e.g. pain) and so may be considered inhumane. Increased protein (muscle) breakdown from stress-induced hypermetabolism (see Chapter 3) prolongs ventilatory weaning and (eventual) ambulation, thus increasing the risk of later complications such as pneumonia and thromboses.

Assessing sedation, therefore, and so titrating prescribed drugs is an important ICU nursing role. However, sedation is difficult to measure, both because the needs of patients vary (Shelly 1998) and because of the discrepancies between different assessors (Westcott 1995). Haemodynamic changes are an unreliable sign as most ICU patients are already haemodynamically labile (Shelly 1998). Electroencephalogram (EEG) measurements (Crippen 1992) and oesophageal contractility (Sinclair & Suter 1988) have not been widely adopted (O'Sullivan & Park 1990). Gently brushing the tips of eyelashes can usefully identify if someone is sedated deeply enough to tolerate traumatic interventions (e.g. intubation) since corneal reflexes remain until deep coma (Myburgh & Oh 1997). However, a more precise measurement is desirable for evidence-based nursing assessment and the search for precision has created various sedation scales, most developed in this country, many initially for drugs research.

Some scales, such as Bion and Ledingham, are too complex and time-consuming for routine use, and few have been tested for reliability (Olleveant *et al.* 1998). However most lists are relatively simple, if potentially subjective; Shelly (1998) suggests that the choice between tools is less important than using one to ensure regular assessment. Reliable assessment necessitates familiarity and confidence with whatever is used, and so limiting the number of tools used on one unit promotes reliable assessment. However, many scales necessitate inflicting pain and so, for regular assessment, observation-orientated tools may be more appropriate. Many scales are known both by their developer's names and the place where they were developed.

Paralysis, whether from paralysing agents or pathology, prevents patients expressing awareness so that infusions of any paralysing agents should be stopped long enough before sedation assessment to ensure they will not influence the result. Achieving optimum sedation is a humanitarian necessity; professional autonomy and accountability make each nurse responsible for ensuring their patients are appropriately (i.e. not over- or under-) sedated. The only reasonable way to ensure patients are adequately sedated is by objective assessment.

The Ramsay scale

Originally designed for drugs research rather than clinical use, this scale (see Table 6.1) has influenced designs of many scoring systems and remains widely used in practice. Like many systems, it is simple, offering a choice between five categories. However these categories remain open to subjective interpretation.

Table 6.1 **The Ramsay sedation scale**

Awake levels:	
1	patient anxious and agitated or restless or both
2	patient cooperative, orientated and tranquil
3	patient responds to command only
Asleep levels:	
4	brisk response
5	sluggish response
6	no response

***Source*: Ramsay *et al.* (1974)**

The Bion and Ledingham scale

This score uses three linear analogue scales (depth of sedation, degree of distress, level of comprehension) which are then plotted in a prism (Olleveant *et al.* 1998) three times a day in association with APACHE II scores (O'Sullivan & Park 1990). Bion suggests that patients should be observed for 10–15 minutes before assessment (Olleveant *et al.* 1998). While triangulation increases reliability, this cumbersome assessment tool has not been widely adopted into ICU nursing practice. Use of APACHE II (see Chapter 50) introduces a further variable.

The Cohen and Kelly scale

Like the Ramsay scale, this scale (see Table 6.2) was devised for drugs research, and uses a similar numerical scale. Although this makes it relatively easy to use, like Bion and Ledingham's scoring system, it is not widely used in ICU.

Table 6.2 The Cohen and Kelly sedation scale

0	asleep, no response to tracheal suction
1	rousable, coughs with tracheal suction
2	awake, spontaneously coughs or triggers ventilator
3	actively breathes against ventilator
4	unmanageable

***Source*: Cohen & Kelly (1987)**

The Newcastle scale

Adapted from the Glasgow Coma Scale (Viney 1996), this scale (Table 6.3) was developed to evaluate propofol (Olleveant *et al.* 1998), although descriptors are applicable for any sedated patient. Being based on a tried and trusted neurological assessment tool, it has proved reliable. The scoring system is more complex than Ramsay and Ramsay-like scales, which can make it time-consuming, but makes it more comprehensive.

Table 6.3 The Newcastle sedation scale

eyes open	spontaneously	4
	to speech	3
	to pain	2
	none	1
responds to nursing procedure	obeys commands	4
	purposeful movement	3
	non-purposeful movement	2
	none	1
cough	spontaneously strong	4
	spontaneously weak	3
	on suction only	2
	none	1
respirations	extubated	5
	spontaneous intubated	4
	SIMV triggering respiration	3
	respiration against ventilator	2
	no respiratory effort	1
loading for spontaneous communication		+ 2
Interpretation of score:		
	awake	17–19
	asleep	15–17
	light sedation	12–14
	moderate sedation	8–11
	deep sedation	5–7
	anaesthetise	4

***Source*: Cook & Palma (1989)**

The Addenbrookes/Cambridge scale

Unlike most of the above scales, this was developed for clinical practice and from substantial clinical experience, although it is derived from the Ramsay scale. The last two categories (paralysed, asleep) were added to the initial four-point scale following comments by nursing staff; the fourth category (roused by tracheal suction) was also added (see Table 6.4).

Table 6.4 The Addenbrookes sedation scale

agitated
awake
roused by voice
roused by tracheal suction
paralysed
asleep

***Source*: O'Sullivan & Park (1990)**

O'Sullivan and Park (1990) recommend scoring sedation every hour; their scale facilities scoring as part of nursing care, although potential trauma from hourly suction cannot be supported just to assess sedation.

The New Sheffield scale

This scale (Table 6.5), which was developed for ICU nursing practice, also adapts the Ramsay scale (Viney 1996). However, the subjectivity of Ramsay is replaced by descriptions of each level, enabling greater objectivity (descriptions are omitted from Table 6.5). Olleveant *et al.*'s (1998) evaluation resulted in minor modifications, the Modified New Sheffield. They claim this modification is more reliable, although potential researcher bias necessitates further objective measurement to support their claim.

Table 6.5 The New Sheffield sedation scale

1	awake
2	agitation
3	optimal level (i)
4	optimal level (ii)
5	sluggish level
6	flat level

***Source*: Laing (1992)**

Note: The scale includes a description of each level.

The Bloomsbury scale

This Ramsay-derived scale (Table 6.6) has not been widely discussed or studied; nor does it appear to have been widely adopted, although Saggs' (1998) small-scale comparison found this more useful than the Addenbrooks scale.

Table 6.6 The Bloomsbury sedation scale

3	agitated and restless
2	awake and uncomfortable
1	awake but calm
0	roused by voice, remains calm
−1	roused by movement or suction
−2	roused by painful stimuli
−3	unrousable
A	natural sleep

***Source*: Armstrong *et al.* (1992)**

Awake patients

Patients in intensive care are usually sedated, but lighter sedation has raised questions about whether patients should be sedated at all. Monger (1995) compares the practice between a UK unit and a Dutch unit. The Dutch unit does not normally use sedation, arguing that very sick patients are naturally sedated, and that chemical sedation overpowers useful compensatory mechanisms. Sedatives cause problems such as hypotension. Many of the patients Monger describes are clearly not as sick as most patients in ICUs in the UK, and this lower dependency, typical of non-UK ICUs, inevitably reduces the need for sedation.

Monger's (1995) article makes passing mention of the use of physical restraints to maintain safety. The choice between chemical (sedation) and physical restraint is an ethical dilemma with no absolute answer. Physical restraint is generally avoided by UK nursing, and so Monger's 'awake patients' seems unlikely here.

Hudak *et al.* (1998) describe 'conscious sedation' combining analgesia with amnesia so that patients remain conscious but relaxed. As with Monger's awake patients, this allows response to both verbal and physical stimuli (Hudak *et al.* 1998). Ensuring amnesia while allowing consciousness implies that this is merely an extension of lighter sedation. While amnesia is arguably beneficial from humanitarian perspectives, nurses should ensure that patients are not exposed to unnecessary pain (physical or psychological), however soon that pain may be forgotten.

Paediatric sedation

As with analgesia, usually children have traditionally received little sedation, presumably for similar (unfounded) reasons (see Chapter 7). Propofol is not licensed for use with children below 5 years, but other sedatives are available; chloralhydrate, a serotoninergic receptor agonist, is one of the most widely used paediatric sedatives in ICU, although morphine and other opiates can also have useful sedative effects. Unless drugs are specifically contraindicated for children, approaches to sedation should be similar: humanitarian arguments for sedating adults should apply equally to children. However, the higher metabolic rate of children may cause more rapid clearance, necessitating larger doses; Sherry (1997) suggests that children may need up to 50 per cent more sedation (relative to weight) than adults.

Neuromuscular blockade

Blocking release of acetylcholine (a neurotransmitter) at the neuromuscular junction causes skeletal (but not smooth) muscle relaxation. Paralysing agents cannot cross the blood–brain barrier, so have no sedative or analgesic effects. Once the standard conjunct therapy with sedation, the use of paralysing agents (also called muscle relaxants) showed a similar reversal between the three studies cited at the start of this chapter. The routine use of paralysing agents fell from nearly all units in Merriman's 1981 study to only 16 per cent regularly using it by 1987 (Bion & Ledingham 1987), with little change (15 per cent) by Reeve and Wallace's 1991 study. The reasons for reduced use of paralysis reflect those for reduced use of chemical sedatives.

If adequately sedated, neuromuscular blockade does not further reduce oxygen consumption or energy expenditure (Sheridan *et al.* 1997). Paralysing agents should only be given where there are specific therapeutic indications, such as hyperpyrexia (see Chapter 8) and intracranial hypertension (see Chapter 22). Where patients are receiving paralysing agents, these will need to be stopped to assess sedation. With paralysing agents normally being given for therapeutic benefits (to prevent aggravating intracranial hypertension), the removal of paralysis for sedation assessment may cause undesirable physiological effects. When paralysing agents are being used, frequency of assessment should therefore be a multidisciplinary team decision, with paralysing agents being stopped for no longer than is pharmacologically necessary.

Similarly, the use of paralysing agents should be assessed to ensure full therapeutic benefit (other than when sedation is being assessed). Paralysis is usually tested by absence of reflexes, such as electrical nerve stimulation. A relatively low (unpainful) voltage is usually sufficient to stimulate nerve reflexes; users can benefit by trying out such tests on themselves so that they know what they are inflicting on their patients.

Implications for practice

- the sedation needs of each patient should be individually assessed by the multidisciplinary team to meet each patient's need, evaluating
  - humanitarian needs
  - therapeutic benefits
  - side effects (e.g. hypotension)
- nurses have a particularly valuable contribution for their continuing observation of each patient
- assessment scoring systems reduce subjectivity of nursing assessment, although there is no universally accepted system for ICU
- adoption of a single or limited number of assessment tools on each unit enables staff to become competent and consistent
- professional accountability necessitates assessment of sedation at least once per shift
- daily total dose of sedation exceeding recommended upper limits indicates tolerance has developed and sedation regimes need review
- for brief procedures (e.g. intubation), absence of blink reflexes confirms patients are adequately sedated
- any paralysing agents should be stopped for sufficient time prior to assessment sedation to enable reliable assessment
- removing paralysis may affect therapy, so should be agreed by the multidisciplinary team
- paralysing agents are given for therapeutic benefits, so nurses should similarly ensure patients are sufficiently paralysed
- paralysis assessment being potentially painful/uncomfortable, nurses can assess what they are subjecting their patients to by trying out tests on themselves (where it is safe to do so)

Summary

Appropriate use of sedation can remove much psychological trauma caused by ICU admission, potentially providing physiological as well as humanitarian benefits (e.g. limiting intracranial hypertension). However, side effects can cause problems such as cardiovascular depression, while deep coma inhibits orientation and compliance with requests, as well as removing patient autonomy. Critical illness often produces natural sedation. How far, if at all, this should be compounded by chemical sedation is a question of balancing benefits and burdens. These issues cut across professional boundaries and plans for sedation should be agreed by nurses and doctors, using the advice of pharmacists and other appropriate disciplines.

Although chemical sedatives are prescribed by doctors, they are (normally) given by nurses, and so the professional accountability of each nurse ensures that patients receive adequate (but not excessive) sedation. This requires assessment. Commonly used assessment tools have been discussed.

The use of paralysing agents has declined; where they are used, there are usually specific therapeutic indications. Nurses should therefore similarly assess paralysis.

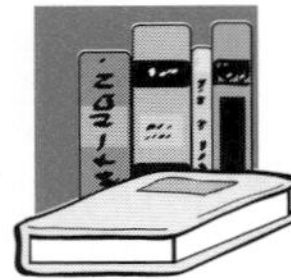

Further reading

Sedation has been widely studied and written about in both nursing and medical journals. Shelly has written many reliable articles, his 1998 being among the more recent. Westcott (1995) offers useful nursing perspectives on sedation. Monger (1995) provides a thought-provoking article well worth reading, but it should be read critically. Readers are also advised to follow up source articles and any subsequent studies on the scoring system used on their unit identified above.

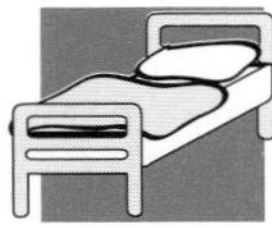

Clinical scenario

Joanna Tomlinson is 38 years old and was on holiday with her family when their hired car became involved in a tragic road traffic accident. Her husband and two children were mortally injured and Joanna was admitted to ICU with multiple fractures and crush injuries. She was sedated with a continuous intravenous infusion of midazolam (1 mg/ml) in order to facilitate ventilation and other treatments.

Q.1 Explain the sedative actions (pharmodynamics) of midazolam and how it differs from analgesic and paralysing agents.

Q.2 Select an appropriate Sedation Scoring Tool or Scale for assessing the effectiveness of Joanna's sedation:

(a) justify choice of Sedation Score
(b) note its main limitations and
(c) consider other factors (e.g. environmental, events, pathophysiology) which may influence Joanna's level of sedation and accuracy of score.

The midazolam infusion was administered at titrated rate of between 2 and 4 ml/h for 10 days. During this period Joanna developed rhabdomyolysis and acute renal failure.

Q.3 Appraise the amount of midazolam given in relation to the recommended dosage, drug metabolism and elimination (pharmokinetics). Evaluate any potentially longer-term effects and outline some nursing strategies which can minimise these.

Chapter 7

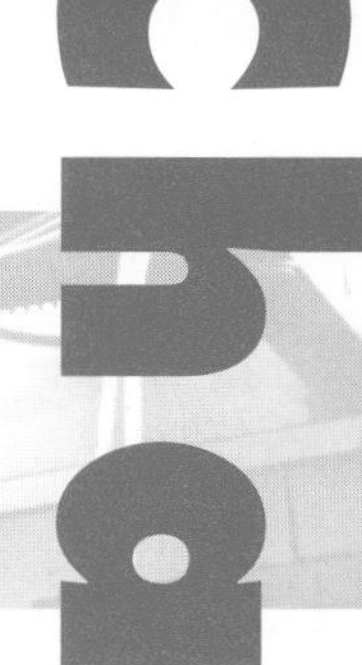

Pain management

Contents

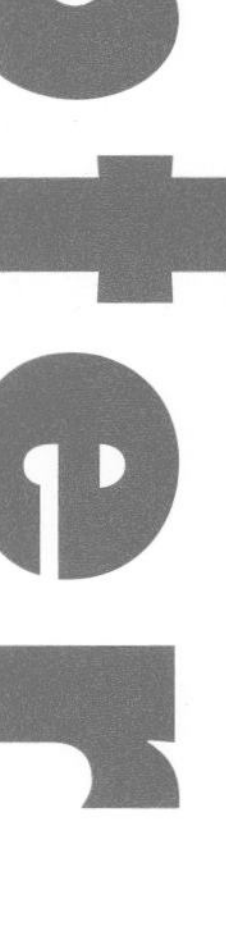

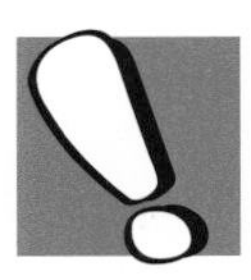

Fundamental knowledge

Nerve pathways – sympathetic, parasympathetic, motor, sensory
Spinal nerves
Stress response (see Chapter 3)

Introduction

Much literature on pain management focuses on pharmacology. While pharmacological interventions are necessary to ICU pain management, most opiates have broadly similar effects, and so this chapter concentrates on mechanisms of pain, psychological effects, nursing attitudes to and assessment of pain. Specific information on individual drugs (indications, contraindications, usual doses, preparation, benefits and adverse effects) can be found in the manufacturer's data sheets and pharmacopaedias (e.g. British National Formulary), both of which should be available in all clinical areas.

Causes of acute pain may be obvious (e.g. surgery), but patients may also suffer pre-existing chronic pain (e.g. arthritis). Pain can also be caused by nursing/medical interventions; Puntillo's (1990) post-discharge survey found most ICU patients remembered suffering moderate to severe pain from:

- surgery
- intubation
- suction
- chest drain removal
- potassium infusions

Waldmann and Gaine's (1996) patients similarly reported pain from oximeter probes. Individual nursing assessments may identify ways to minimise discomfort – information which should be shared with colleagues (verbally, nursing records).

Pain should be controlled for humanitarian reasons, but pain also initiates all the detrimental physiological effects of stress response (see Chapter 3), while reluctance to breathe deeply (if self-ventilating) contributes to atelectasis (Puntillo & Weiss 1994).

Many ICU patients are unable to perform even the fundamental activities of living and so managing pain should include promoting comfort:

- smoothing creases in sheets
- relieving prolonged pressure
- turning pillows over
- limb placement (e.g. with arthritis)

Complementary therapies, which may relieve pain, are discussed in Chapter 47.

What is pain?

Pain is a response to stimuli which can be physical or psychogenic. How the stimuli are perceived by the cerebral cortex determines whether pain exists and, if so, its type and intensity ('quality'). If signals are blocked, pain cannot be sensed. Pain is therefore necessarily individual to each sufferer, a complex interaction between physiology and psychology. The individuality of pain experiences underlies McCaffery's widely quoted definition: 'pain is whatever the experiencing person says it is, existing whenever the experiencing person says it does' (McCaffery & Beebe 1994:15). Pain relief can therefore block either reception or perception of pain signals.

However some patients may deny pain, even if experiencing it (possibly due to social expectations – 'stiff upper lip'). McCaffery and Beebe (1994) add that nurses should not accept denial of pain, but explore reasons for that denial. Assessing pain, perceptions and needs can be difficult with most ICU patients due to intubation, sedation and/or impaired psychomotor skills, but pain relief and the provision of comfort are fundamental to nursing.

Sternbach (1968) described pain in terms of 'hurt' and 'tissue damage', but 'hurt' merely replaces one word by another without clarifying concepts. Pain as a signal of tissue damage (defence mechanism) also ignores psychological stressors, individual interpretations, or powerlessness to prevent tissue degeneration causing chronic pain (e.g. arthritis).

Nerve fibres

Pain is sensed by nociceptors which exist throughout almost all body tissue, especially the skin. Two main types of nerves (A and C fibres) transmit pain signals.

A fibres are large; their thick myelin sheaths enable rapid conduction – up to 20 m/s (Grubb 1998). Four subgroups have been identified: alpha, beta, gamma and delta. A-delta fibres are found mainly in skin, skeletal muscle and joints, producing *sharp* and well-localised impulses and defensive motor reflex withdrawal (Melzack & Wall 1988).

C fibres are small and unmylinated, conducting impulses at less than 2.5 m/s (Grubb 1998). C fibres transmit *dull*, poorly localised, deep and prolonged pain signals, resulting in guarded movements and immobility. Sharp impulses from the fast A-delta fibres are superseded by slower, dull and prolonged impulses from C fibres.

Pain may be described in these or other terms, and descriptions may indicate the sources of pain (e.g. *cramps* suggests ischaemia). Pain may be *referred* (e.g. phantom limb pain, cardiac pain in left arm – see Figure 7.1) where embryonic nerve pathways were shared or where residual nerve pathways remain intact.

Gate control theory

Ancient associations of pain with the heart bequeathed linguistic concepts and images (e.g. 'broken heart'). Descartes' description of direct pain pathways to the brain, although now recognised as grossly oversimplistic, influenced many subsequent theories. While pain mechanisms remain unproven, Melzack and Wall's 'gate control' theory is widely accepted.

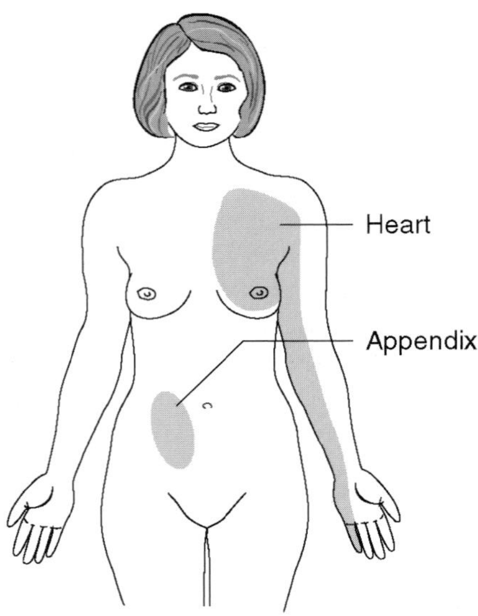

Figure 7.1 Examples of referred pain

Melzack and Wall (1988) describe a 'gate' (in the *substantia gelatinosa* capping grey matter of the spinal cord dorsal horn) which may be

open
closed
blocked.

When open, impulses pass to higher centres (where they are perceived). A closed gate prevents impulses passing and so no pain is perceived. Endogenous chemicals control this gate (e.g. serotonin increases pain tolerance), and so manipulating, supplementing or replacing these chemicals can control pain. Hopes that neuropeptide *endorphins* (*end*ogenous m*orphin*es) would achieve better pain control than exogenous narcotics have been disappointed (McCaffery & Beebe 1994). The gate can also be blocked by other signals. A-delta and C fibres share pathways, and so A-delta stimulation (e.g. skin pressure) can block the slower, dull, prolonged C-fibre pain; this explains how scratching an itch, pressure bracelets and transcutaneous electrical nerve stimulations can relieve pain.

Psychology

The perception of signals received is influenced by various psychological factors, including

culture
anticipation (past experience, fear, misinterpretation)
distraction.

The word 'pain' derives from the Latin *poena* (punishment) (Schofield 1994), and the perception of pain as retribution may be partly a psychological coping mechanism, but it also encourages stoic attitudes of endurance that can be physiologically harmful. Cultures can also influence whether, when and how it is acceptable to admit to pain.

Anticipation is influenced by previous exposure to similar stimuli (e.g. endotracheal suction) and expectations, and fear can create self-fulfilling prophecies – something hurts because we expect it to hurt; in addition uncertainty increases fear and so clear, honest explanations before actions help to prepare patients for pain and warn them how long they can expect to endure it; thus preparation reduces pain, analgesia needs, and recovery time (Hayward 1975).

Distraction may help people cope with pain (Puntillo 1988) by blocking the gate with other impulses and stimulating serotonin release. Distraction and guided imagery can be useful nursing strategies, although impaired consciousness and verbal responses can limit their value in ICU; non-pharmacological interventions are reviewed by Carroll (1997).

Stereotypes

While recognising cultural influences (especially when pain is denied), stereotyping people is unhelpful and dehumanising; the examples below illustrate some of the dangers.

Men are expected to tolerate more pain than women (McCaffery & Beebe 1994), and so are less likely to report it (Puntillo & Weiss 1994), but in fact pain tolerance is similar between the genders (Phillips 1997).

Older people may require less analgesia due to slower metabolism of analgesics and reduced pain sensation (Puntillo & Weiss 1994), but older UK adults grew up before the NHS existed and when stoicism was more widely expected.

Children used to receive little analgesia, even though pain pathways are intact by 30 weeks gestation (Tatman & Ralston 1997); misconceptions may still prevent children receiving adequate analgesia (see Table 7.1).

Table 7.1 Some misconceptions about pain in children

infants cannot feel pain
children cannot feel as much pain as adults
an active or sleeping child cannot be in pain
children always tell the truth about pain

***Source:* Twycross (1998)**

Stereotypes have also created myths about how painful certain conditions or operations for adults can be, and the type and amount of analgesia they deserve. Even if pain impulses were comparable, pain experiences are unique to each individual necessitating individual assessment, which should be a nursing priority (Doverty 1994).

Assessing pain

Pain assessment, together with nursing knowledge and attitudes, is fraught with problems. Compared with patients' own assessments, nurses consistently underestimate pain (Seers 1987; Ferguson *et al.* 1997) and overestimate fears of addiction (McCaffery & Beebe 1994). Since it is impossible to judge what others are experiencing, it is better to give too much analgesia rather than too little (McCaffery & Beebe 1994).

Pain control is improved through using assessment tools (Scott 1994). Most patients stay in ICUs for only a few days and yet pain experiences and analgesia needs are often volatile, so that assessment tools should be flexible and relevant. Currently, there is no ideal ICU pain assessment tool.

Complex and time-consuming questionnaires may be postponed or completed superficially, so that the McGill pain questionnaire is impractical for ICU (even in its short form). *Verbal* assessment may be influenced by a nurse's choice of words and so 'hurt', 'discomfort', 'ache' and 'soreness' may identify discomforts that would be denied as 'painful' (McCaffery & Beebe 1994). *Pain rulers* and thermometers rely on consciousness, vision and psychomotor skills which are often impaired in ICU patients. The Bourbonnais (1981) pain assessment tool (see Figure 7.2) relies more on visual assessment and so is potentially useful for ICUs, although the latter parts of it may need adaption/omission – for example, by replacing Section 4 (Questions a nurse should ask herself) by the following and omitting Section 5:

- How tired is the patient?
- Is the patient in a sensory deprived environment?
- Is the patient anxious?
- Does the patient have an altered level of consciousness?

Other *visual* signs (e.g. sudden hypertension, facial expression, position and other body language) should be assessed, although they may be absent through conditions/treatments (e.g. paralysis) and, since interpretation is subjective, on their own such signs are unreliable (Briggs 1995).

Pharmacological interventions

Although the actions of drugs are often complex, including significant psychological/placebo components, analgesics can be divided between those with peripheral actions (e.g. aspirin, paracetamol, nonsteroidal anti-

1. Observe for skeletal muscle response
   - (a) body movement
     immobility
     purposeless or inaccurate body movements
     protective movements include withdrawal reflex
     rhythmic movements
   - (b) facial expression:
     clenched teeth
     wrinkled forehead
     biting of lower lip
     widely opened or tightly shut eyes
2. Autonomic nervous system response
   - (a) sympathetic nervous system activation:
     increased pulse
     increased respiration
     increased diastolic and systolic blood pressure
     cold perspiration
     pallor
     dilated pupils
     nausea
     muscle tension
   - (b) parasympathetic activation in some visceral pain
     low blood pressure
     slow pulse
3. Verbal report of pain
   Questions to elicit from the patient
     location of pain
     intensity of pain (scale 1–10)
     onset and duration
     precipatating and aggravating factors
     nature of pain (i.e. sharp, dull)
4. Questions nurses should ask themselves
   - (a) How long has it been since the fresh postoperative patient was medicated for pain?
   - (b) How fatigued is the patient?
   - (c) Is the patient in an environment of sensory restriction?
   - (d) Are you reaching the true cause of the patient's pain?
   - (e) Are you aware of your biases?
   - (f) Is the patient anxious?
   - (g) What is the patient's past experience of pain?
   - (h) Does the patient have an altered level of consciousness?

Figure 7.2 **The Bourbonnais pain assessment tool**
***Source*: Bourbonnais (1981)**

inflammatory drugs – NSAIDs) and those acting on the central nervous system (e.g. opiates).

ICU nurses should monitor both the delivery and effects (benefits, complications) of all drugs given.

Peripheral analgesics

The peripheral transmission of pain can be blocked by inhibiting the neurotransmitter prostaglandin E_2 (PGE_2). Most peripheral analgesics are anti-inflammatory, making them effective against musculoskeletal pain. Since prostaglandin inhibition impairs platelet aggregation, coagulopathies may be aggravated. NSAIDS may also cause bronchoconstriction. Although their place in ICU is limited, they may provide relief for some conditions, and may usefully supplement opiates. NSAIDs (e.g. ibuprofen) are mainly used for chronic musculoskeletal pain; they can cause renal failure.

Opiates

Opiates bind to receptors in the central nervous system; three types of receptors have been identified: mu, kappa and sigma. Most opiates bind to mu (μ) receptors (causing constipation (Sear 1996)). Since fats and fat soluble molecules readily cross the blood–brain barrier, lipid soluble (lipophilic) analgesics act quickly. Differences between opiates are relatively small and so choice largely depends on the personal preference of prescribers/users (Bergman & Yate 1997).

Opiates are usually given in ICUs through continuous intravenous infusions, although other routes may also be used (especially epidural). Continuous infusions can cause accumulation if drugs have prolonged action or if renal or hepatic metabolism is impaired (renal failure, hepatic failure). Duration depends on metabolic rate, which declines with age.

MORPHINE As the primary active ingredient of opium, it remains the opiate against which derivatives and synthetic alternatives are judged. It suppresses impulses from C fibres, but not A-delta fibres, and so relieves dull, prolonged pain. Its poor lipid solubility prolongs its effect and makes it unsuitable for epidural analgesia (McCaffery & Beebe 1994). Adverse effects include:

- respiratory depression
- histamine release (causing hypotension) (Viney 1996)
- nausea (concurrent antiemetics may be needed)
- euphoria

Most other opiates also cause these effects. Morphine can be used with children; by the age of six, clearance and half-life have reached adult levels (Knight 1997).

DIAMORPHINE (HEROIN) This is chemically engineered morphine, and being highly lipophilic it is more powerful than morphine (Pinger *et al.* 1995).

FENTANYL This lasts 2–5 hours, but long-term accumulation can cause problems (Viney 1996). It has few cardiovascular effects, but analgesia remains unpredictable (Viney 1996). Its high lipid solubility makes it useful for epidural infusions (McCaffery & Beebe 1994). Transcutaneous patches are also available, but impaired peripheral perfusion may limit absorption in the critically ill. Fentanyl derivatives include: alfentanil, sufentanil and remifentanil.

ALFENTANIL This has a shorter duration of action (1–2 hours (Viney 1996)) which makes continuous infusion safer; its metabolites are inactive, making it useful for patients in renal failure (Viney 1996).

PETHIDINE This is similarly short acting (2–3 hours (McCaffery & Beebe 1994)), and being highly lipophilic, epidural infusion is effective (McCaffery & Beebe 1994).The metabolite nor-pethidine is a highly toxic central nervous system stimulant, causing twitches, tremors, muscle jerks and fits (McCaffery & Beebe 1994). The half-life of nor-pethidine exceeds fifteen hours (McCaffery & Beebe 1994); the antagonist for pethidine is naloxone hydrochloride. However, although naloxone eliminates pethidine, it does not eliminate nor-pethidine (McCaffery & Beebe 1994).

CODEINE This is not widely used; it can only be given intramuscularly or orally, and can cause constipation.

Patient controlled analgesia (PCA)

Patient controlled analgesia empowers patients to control their own pain management. The underlying pain stimuli remain unaltered, but conscious patients prefer PCA (Snell *et al.* 1997). Patient control devices can be used for intravenous or epidural analgesia, but most ICU patients cannot use control devices due to:

- inability to move (sedation/paralysis)
- impaired psychomotor function
- muscle weakness
- visual deficits
- confusion/forgetting how to control machine

Novel routes

The search for safer and more effective ways to relieve pain has encouraged trials with novel routes of administration; Alexander-Williams and Rowbottom (1998) found intranasal, inhalational and transdermal opiates to be as effective as intravenous fentanyl for relief of postoperative pain. Intubation (preventing nasal absorption) and poor peripheral perfusion (limiting transdermal distribution) may limit applicability to ICU nursing, but such routes are simpler and reduce infection risk.

Transcutaneous nerve stimulation (TCNS/TENS)

The benefits from the use of TCNS may result from

- endorphin stimulation (McCaffery & Beebe 1994)
- blocking the spinal 'gate' (McCaffery & Beebe 1994)
- placebo effects (Johnson 1998).

Success is difficult to predict (Seymour 1995a), and excessive electrical stimulation may cause pain. TCNS relies on patient control and so has the same limitations as PCA.

Placebos

As pain perception is influenced by psychology, chemically inactive substances may relieve pain if patients believe they will work. However, if caregivers appear sceptical, patients will probably lose trust in a placebo's effectiveness, and because the drug is a placebo, this necessitates lying to patients (directly or by implication), which is ethically questionable. Consequentialists might justify such lies by the benefits obtained from pain relief, but deontologists are less likely to consider any lie acceptable. Placebos are discussed further in Chapter 47.

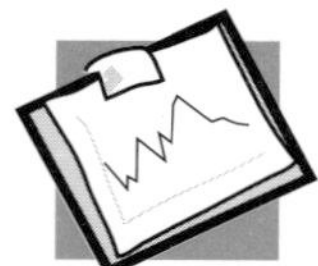

Implications for practice

- promoting comfort and removing/minimising pain are fundamental to nursing
- pain is individual to each person and so requires individual nursing assessment
- currently there is no ideal pain assessment tool for ICU, but Bourbonnais' scale can be effective; additional observations (mainly visual) can provide additional information
- nociceptor signals (reception) are interpreted as pain in the cerebral cortex (perception); pain can be managed by removing either component
- opiate analgesics remain the mainstay of pain management in ICU, but supplementary ways to relieve pain and provide comfort should also be used
- psychological comfort usually reduces the pain experienced, and so holistic nursing care is a valuable part of multidisciplinary team pain management

Summary

Suffering is an almost inevitable part of critical illness. Nurses can do much to alleviate the pain experienced by almost every patient. Nurses have various roles in pain management, ranging from provision of simple comforts to administering and observing controlled drugs. In all aspects of care, holistic and humanistic approaches can reduce patient suffering.

Further reading

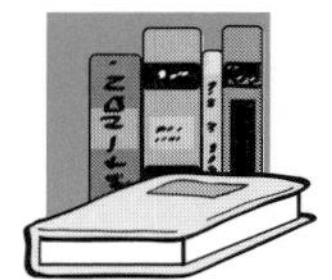

Classic books on pain management include Melzack and Wall (1988) or McCaffery and Beebe (1994); Hayward's (1975) classic study on postoperative pain remains valuable. Wall and Melzack (1994) is a comprehensive reference text.

Since Puntillo (1990), many articles have appeared in ICU journals, often relating to subgroups of patients (Thompson has written some valuable articles about cardiac pain); a useful nursing overview is provided by Viney's (1996) chapter. Baillie (1993) gives a comprehensive review of pain assessment tools.

Although Melzack's own work on the gate control theory is authoritative, Davis (1993) gives a clear summary.

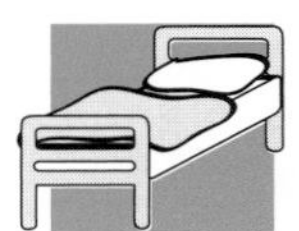

Clinical scenario

William Hunt is a 62-year-old retired civil servant who was admitted to ICU following coronary artery bypass grafts via midline sternotomy incision. In addition to acute postoperative pain, Mr Hunt is known to suffer with chronic back pain from kyphotic scoliosis in his thoracic vertebrae. Mr Hunt is initially ventilated and sedated. Analgesia is administered via continuous intravenous infusion of morphine.

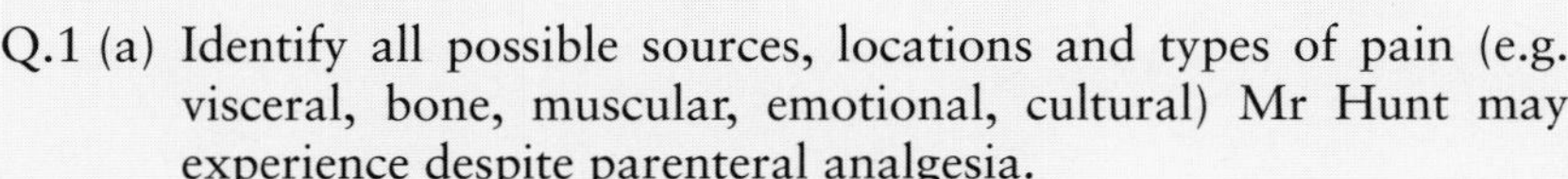

Q.1 (a) Identify all possible sources, locations and types of pain (e.g. visceral, bone, muscular, emotional, cultural) Mr Hunt may experience despite parenteral analgesia.

(b) Until he becomes fully conscious what signs and symptoms (physiological, behaviourial etc.) are used to assess Mr Hunt's level of pain?

Q.2 Analyse the range of pharmacological and non-pharmacological nursing interventions needed to manage Mr Hunt's pain effectively. Consider the appropriate NSAID/opiate and administration route, and the use of comfort therapies, e.g. supporting chest on coughing, positioning, guided imagery, etc.).

Q.3 Review the variety of approaches that can be used to administer analgesia to Mr Hunt. These should include patient-controlled infusions, epidural and interpleural techniques. Using the literature, your own, colleagues' and patients' experiences debate the most effective approach to manage Mr Hunt's pain.

Chapter 8

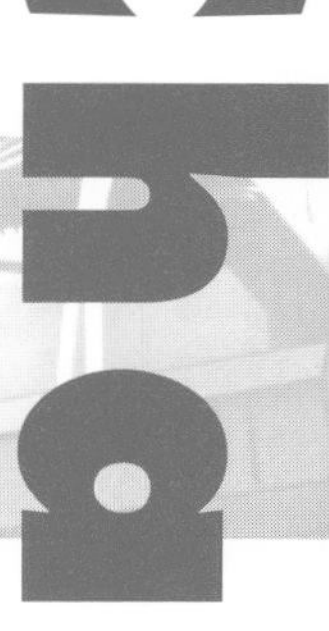

Pyrexia and temperature control

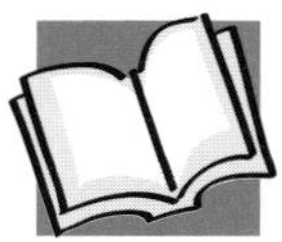

Contents

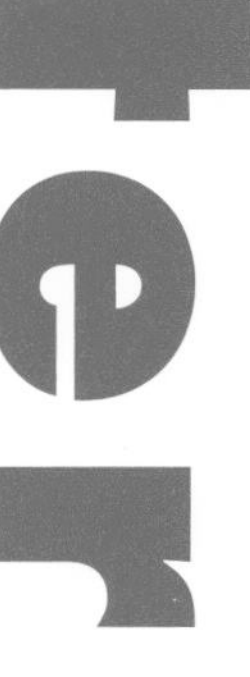

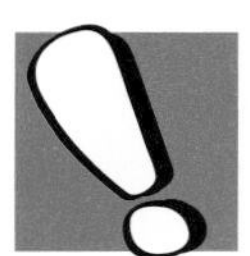

Fundamental knowledge

Sweat production and function

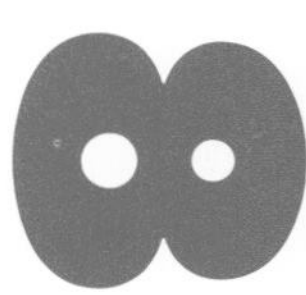

Introduction

Howie (1989) suggests that nurses treat pyrexia immediately, regardless of causes or severity. Pyrexia (fever) is a homeostatic elevation of body temperature which may be problematic. This chapter describes benefits and problems, together with ways to monitor and treat pyrexia.

Heat is produced through metabolism (especially hepatic). Human bodies can only function healthily within a narrow temperature range. The thermoregulatory centre (anterior hypothalamus) responds to central and peripheral thermoreceptors to conserve heat (vasoconstriction) and increase heat production (shivering) when cold and heat loss when hot (sweating, vasodilation). The thermoregulatory setpoint varies between individuals, but in health maintains body temperature, usually at 36–37°C).

Pyrogens (e.g. TNFα, **interleukin**-1) increase the thermoregulatory setpoint (usually peaking at 40.5°C), initiating heat production to achieve the higher level (= fever). Hypermetabolism to produce heat increases oxygen consumption. Despite being pyrexial, the person feels cold, so attempts to keep warm (e.g. by extra bedding/clothing).

Heat damages living tissue; as most bacteria and viruses are more susceptible to heat than human cells, pyrexia can be a defence mechanism so that temperatures up to 40°C may be best untreated. The management of pyrexia should be guided by individual assessment rather than rigid protocols. Hyperpyrexia (heatstroke; above 40°C) damages human cells and so should be treated before reaching the limits of life (at about 43–44°C).

Circadian rhythm causes metabolism and temperature to peak at around 6 p.m. (making this the most suitable time to detect pyrexia (Samples *et al.* 1985)), although normal fluctuations rarely exceed 1°C over the course of a day (Marieb 1995).

Infants are especially prone to rapid pyrexial fluctuations due to hypothalamic immaturity, higher metabolic rates and more brown fat (insulation). Since thermoregulatory impairment may cause febrile convulsions, pyrexial children should be monitored frequently.

Older people may have impaired thermoregulation due to reduced metabolism; thus when feeling cold, they may appreciate additional bedding.

Pyrexia

Body temperature fluctuates during each day (circadian rhythm) and in different parts of the body so that monitoring temperature trends is more important than absolute figures; the sites chosen affect measurement (e.g. removing pulmonary artery catheters may cause recorded temperatures to fall simply because different sites are used for measurement). Analysing blood gases by different body temperatures will give different results, even though the only change may be the removal of a pulmonary artery catheter.

Holtzclaw (1992) describes three stages to the febrile response:

- chill phase: discrepancy between existing body temperature and the new hypothalamic set point; the person feels cold, shivering to increase hypermetabolism
- plateau: temperature overshoots the new set point, triggering heat loss mechanisms; endogenous pyrogen levels also start to fall
- diaphoresis and flushing: heat loss through evaporation, with massive reduction in endogenous pyrogen levels, which causes uneven resolution of pyrexia

Fever is a symptom, not a disease; attempts to cool patients, whether by reducing bedding or through active interventions such as tepid sponging, may stimulate further hypothalamus-mediated heat production (Bartlett 1996) and so become self-defeating. Shivering increases metabolism three- to five-fold, consuming oxygen and nutrients needed for tissue repair, while increasing carbon dioxide production. Since many ICU patients are already hypoxic, compounding hypoxia by peripheral cooling may prolong recovery.

Some disease processes (e.g. immunocompromise) and treatments (e.g. chemotherapy) inhibit fever, while artificial cooling may mask clues for diagnosis. Thus the patient, rather than the thermometer, should be treated (Kramer 1991).

Fever can be protective as it:

- *inhibits bacterial and viral growth* by restricting supply of iron and zinc (needed for cell growth) (Ganong 1995); most micro-organisms cannot replicate in temperatures above 37°C (Murray *et al.* 1994)
- promotes *tissue repair* through hypermetabolism
- promotes *immunity* (T-lymphocyte replication, interferon production) and phagocytosis (but not with hyperpyrexia) (Styrt & Sugarman 1990; Rowsey 1997b)

Pyrexia is a defence mechanism against infection. Mortality from sepsis increases when fever is absent (Styrt & Sugarman 1990). Mild to moderate fevers are therefore beneficial and should remain untreated (Rowsey 1997b). However, fever and hypermetabolism create physiological stress because:

- each 1°C *increases oxygen consumption* by 13 per cent (Nowak & Handford 1994); more carbon dioxide is also produced;
- *increased intracranial pressure* from hypermetabolism (Morgan 1990) may compound problems for patients with neurological pathologies and head injuries;
- permanent *brain damage* may be caused by protein denaturation (the mechanism inhibiting bacterial growth) (Closs 1992), although there is no evidence of neural damage from brief pyrexias of up to 42°C (Styrt & Sugarman 1990).

Hyperpyrexia

Hyperpyrexia (also called 'heatstroke' and 'severe hyperthermia') is a temperature of 40.5°C or more for one hour. Incidence of hyperpyrexia is increasing, largely due to use of the recreational 'ecstasy' (see Chapter 41). Problems with pyrexia that are accentuated by hyperpyrexia are:

- *disseminated intravascular coagulation* (DIC) (Hinds & Watson 1996)
- impaired myocardial contractility (Hinds & Watson 1996)
- convulsions (especially above 41°C) (Marieb 1995).

At 42°C autoregulation fails, enzymes become dysfunctional and membrane permeability increases (causing electrolyte imbalance and further cell dysfunction – see Chapter 23).

Measurement

Hypothalamic temperature (site of the thermoregulatory centre) is the ideal core measurement. However, being impractical, other choices are a necessary compromise.

Pulmonary artery temperature, the closest measurable site to hypothalamic temperature (Bartlett 1996), remains the 'gold standard' (Fulbrook 1993), although catheter calibration is rarely checked on insertion, and impractical afterwards. Since pulmonary artery catheters are highly invasive, temperature measurement alone does not justify their use. Studies assessing accuracy of other sites frequently identify drifts of about 1°C from the pulmonary artery temperature, leaving the choice largely to personal preference. Debate about the accuracy of alternative sites and equipment continues.

Mercury-in-glass thermometers were banned by Sweden in 1992 (Woollons 1996). Mercury is listed in COSHH (Health & Safety Executive 1989), its vapour being neurotoxic; broken glass is also a hazard.

Electronic thermometers provide quick, less subjective (digital) measurement. Smith's (1998) paediatric study found significant differences between mercury-in-glass and electronic/tympanic thermometers, but since neither were compared with pulmonary artery temperature, Smith's conclusions about the unsuitability of electronic thermometry are unfounded. Erickson and Kirklin (1993) found good correlation between tympanic and pulmonary artery measurement.

Any non-disposable equipment can cause cross-infection if inadequately cleaned. Disposable *chemical thermometers* are cheap and prevent cross-infection. Some anecdotal reports suggest inaccuracies, although Board's (1995) small study found them to be accurate; Erickson *et al.* (1995) found axillary measurements to be 0.4°C higher than electronic measurements, but oral temperatures 0.4°C lower. The chemical thermometer range is limited to 35.5–40.4°C (O'Toole 1997), making these thermometers unsuitable for measuring hypothermia. Being disposable, chemical thermometers may prove expensive if frequent measurement (common practice in ICU) is needed (O'Toole 1997). Like mercury-in-glass thermometers, chemical thermometers rely on visual interpretation and so can be subjective.

Schmitz *et al.* (1994) found *rectal* temperature measurement closest to core temperature, but hypotension and gut ischaemia reduce rectal blood supply, and faeces will delay conduction of blood heat, so that rectal temperatures are unreliable with critical illnesses (Holtzclaw 1992). Konopad *et al.* (1994) found tympanic measurement correlated well with rectal temperature, and so rectal measurement should rarely be necessary.

Rectal temperature measurement causes emotional trauma for children (Rogers 1992) and should therefore be avoided, while with adults it is undignified and so should only be used if benefits can be justified.

The proximity of the *axillary* artery to the skin surface should make axillary temperature similar to central temperature provided the thermometer tips maintain skin contact (hollow axillary pockets, more frequent in older people, make contact difficult).

Fulbrook (1993) found axillary measurement compared favourably with pulmonary artery temperature provided thermometers were left in place for 12 minutes (Rogers (1992) cites only 5 minutes), but Fulbrook subsequently (1997) identified discrepancies of between 1.2°C above to 1.6°C below pulmonary artery temperature, claiming that axillary measurement was clinically unreliable for ICUs. The latter study used chemical dot thermometers.

Leaving thermometers in place is not as problematic in ICUs as elsewhere, but forgetting to remove thermometers can become irritating for patients (Bauby 1997), and displacement may prevent sufficient skin contact time.

Since the *tympanic* membrane shares carotid artery blood supply with the hypothalamus (Klein *et al.* 1993), it should reflect core temperature. Tympanic thermometers use infrared light to detect thermal radiation, and many devices include facilities to allow readings to be adjusted to equivalent core temperatures.

The accuracy of tympanic measurement remains controversial with some authors (e.g. Klein *et al.* 1993) finding them reliable substitutes for pulmonary artery measurements, while others (e.g. Fulbrook 1997) find them clinically unreliable for ICUs; as both studies identify drifts of about 1°C, their opposing conclusions raise pragmatic dilemmas about how accurate measurement should be.

Fulbrook (1997) questions whether cerumen (earwax) affects readings, citing Doezema *et al.*'s (1995) finding that cerumen lowered readings by 0.3°C; such differences would be difficult to differentiate on many glass and mercury thermometers, and seldom significantly affect management.

Bladder temperature can be measured by probes attached to urinary catheters; Earp and Finlayson (1992) and Bartlett (1996) found good correlation with pulmonary artery temperature. Since nearly all ICU patients have urinary catheters, this method avoids additional invasive equipment. Oliguria presumably makes measurement unreliable.

Noninvasive skin probes, usually on patients' feet, can measure *peripheral* temperature; when compared with central temperature, the difference indicates perfusion/warming. If well perfused, skin to core differences should be under 2°C. Following vascular surgery to the leg (e.g. saphenous vein harvest), the differences between two right and left pedal probes indicate the effects of surgery on limb perfusion.

Treatment

The appropriateness of treating pyrexia necessitates individual assessment and evidence-based practice. With pyrexias of infective origin, microorganisms can often be destroyed more safely by antibiotics than by endogenous pyrexia.

Cooling may be

- central (altering hypothalamic setpoint)
- peripheral (increasing heat loss)

Practices for cooling owe more to ritual than research; what little research does exist is mainly from children and/or community practice and so it would be problematic if applied to ICU nursing (Shackell 1996). As pyrexia is controlled by the hypothalamus, peripheral cooling increases stimuli for centrally regulated heat production/conservation. Vasoconstriction increases differences between core and peripheral temperatures, pooling heat centrally, and so exposing the main organs to further protein denaturation and damage.

Pyrexia is a symptom. Masking symptoms does not resolve problems, although reducing metabolic rate decreases oxygen consumption. Peripheral cooling (e.g. tepid sponging, fans) is fundamentally illogical, and animal studies show that a hypothalamic-induced hypermetabolic response (Styrt & Sugarman 1990) restores pyrexia.

Sweating is effectively tepid sponging, although clean water may provide more psychological comfort than human sweat. If employed, tepid sponging should use tepid (not cold) water as cold water produces both discomfort and vasoconstriction.

Skin surface heat conduction can be increased by the use of cooling blankets and mats, although some of these are hard and uncomfortable, thus predisposing to pressure sore formation with prolonged use (and vasoconstriction) (Shackell 1996); if used, nurses should observe any detrimental effects. Shackell (1996) recommends using cooling blankets for hyperpyrexia. Ice packs are best avoided since they may cause cold burns (Shackell 1996) and cannot be (easily) regulated.

Antipyretic drugs (e.g. aspirin, paracetamol, nonsteroidal anti-inflammatory drugs – NSAIDs) inhibit hypothalamic prostaglandin synthesis, so can reverse pyrexia caused by infection, but not pyrexia from hypothalamic damage (e.g. head injuries). Most studies with antipyretics are paediatric (Shackell 1996); anecdotal reports suggest less consistent benefits with adults.

Sweat evaporation, vasodilation and increased capillary permeability cause hypotension, necessitating fluid replacement. Electrolyte imbalances, acid–base imbalance and hyperglycaemia should be monitored and treated where appropriate.

Malignant hyperpyrexia

Malignant hyperpyrexia may be caused by drugs (e.g. anaesthetic agents such as suxamethonium, ecstasy) and stress (e.g. massive skeletal injury, strenuous exercise). Untreated malignant hyperpyrexia is fatal.

Precipitating causes should be removed. Dantrolene sodium is the only available drug treatment (Miranda *et al.* 1997); this relaxes skeletal muscle, thus preventing contraction. Dinsmore and Hall (1997) suggest that while dantrolene decreases cooling time, it does not affect outcome. Neuromuscular blockade (paralysis) may be used to prevent shivering (heat production).

Body systems should be closely monitored to enable appropriate system support.

Implications for practice

- pyrexia is a symptom, not a disease; managing pyrexia should be evidence-based, using individual holistic nursing assessment rather than ritualised practice
- pyrexia may be a useful defence mechanism, but it will increase oxygen consumption
- peripheral cooling is usually illogical and counterproductive
- central cooling (antipyretic drugs) can restore normal hypothalamic thermoregulation
- mercury-in-glass thermometers are potentially hazardous
- thermometers should be left in place for sufficient time to obtain reliable readings; discomfort/dangers to patients from their use should be remembered

Summary

Legacies from rituals and folklore have left a range of inappropriate reflexes to pyrexia. This chapter has explored the benefits and burdens of fever, mentioned some of the more commonly used means and sites of measurement, together with ways of managing fever to enable nurses to develop evidence-based practice. Malignant hyperpyrexia has been described. The importance of holistic, individualised nursing care has been emphasised.

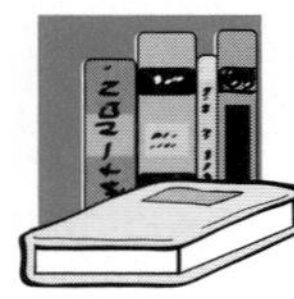

Further reading

Much material is written from general nursing or paediatric experience, sometimes relying more on tradition than research. Styrt and Sugarman (1990) remains a thorough review of the issues to consider before responding to fever. Holtzclaw's (1992) classic article remains useful. Those building on Holtzclaw's work include Bartlett (1996) and Shackell (1996). Fulbrook's (1993, 1997) research on pyrexia in ICU is especially valuable. O'Toole (1997) offers a comprehensive overview of ways to measure temperature.

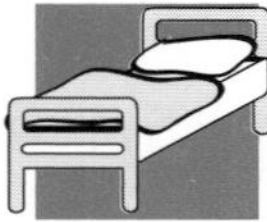

Clinical scenario

Frank Cockburn, a 55-year-old taxicab driver was admitted to ICU for postoperative monitoring following aortofemoral bypass graft surgery. On the first postoperative day (24 hours) Frank's core (central) body temperature is 38.4°C and his shell (skin) temperature is 31°C. He has started to shiver.

Q.1 (a) List potential causes of his increased core temperature.
(b) Identify the blood cells and mediators responsible.
(c) Explain his shivering response and its effects on his metabolism.

Q.2 Compare various approaches to temperature assessment in your own clinical practice area; include common sites used in temperature assessment as well as the equipment available. Which would be the most appropriate method to monitor Frank's core temperature (consider accuracy, time resources, safety, comfort, minimal adverse effects)?

Q.3 Review effective nursing strategies for managing Frank's temperature, select the most suitable pharmacological interventions, laboratory investigations, physical cooling methods (their value, limitations, necessity) and comfort therapies.

Chapter 9

Nutrition

Contents

Introduction

Nutrition is fundamental to health, yet Nightingale's (1980 [1859]) claim that thousands starve in hospitals in the midst of plenty still has some validity. Despite improvements since the 1992 Kings Fund Report, nutrition often receives low priority in ICUs, with feeds often being delayed and incomplete (Adam 1994; Briggs 1996a); incomplete administration of antibiotics would be considered unacceptable.

Prescription practices for nutrition vary widely between different hospitals and feeds; multidisciplinary teams can bring together a wealth of knowledge, but a lack of identified leadership can also cause inaction. ICU nurses therefore need to understand nutrition and the effects of critical illness in order to coordinate optimal care for their patients (Say 1997), provide health education for others together with care of their own health.

Mortality rates reflect malnutrition (Kennedy 1997). One single day's severe catabolism can take one week's nutrition to reverse (Horwood 1990).

Nitrogen, the major source of amino acids, is essential for the production of body proteins. One gram of nitrogen provides 6.25 grams of protein, creating 30 grams of lean body mass (Hudak *et al.* 1998), so hypercatabolism (or starvation) causes significant muscle weakness, delaying weaning. Most serum nitrogen is carried as ammonia (NH_3), converted hepatically to urea (hence 'blood urea nitrogen' – BUN). Nitrogen waste is excreted in urine, mainly as urea. Thus:

neutral nitrogen balance = dietary nitrogen matches urinary nitrogen
negative nitrogen balance = excess urinary nitrogen from breakdown of body protein for energy (catabolism)
positive nitrogen balance = protein building (anabolism)

Nitrogen balance is normally measured by 24-hour urine collections; however abnormal nitrogen metabolism and nitrogen loss (e.g. through wounds) makes urinary nitrogen unreliable during critical illness (Walters & Brooks 1996). Faecal loss of nitrogen, normally about 4 gm/day, increases with diarrhoea, and decreases with parenteral nutrition (Adam 1994), so that the value of routine 24-hour urine collections in ICUs is questionable.

Metabolism

Metabolic rate is the energy produced by all chemical reactions and mechanical work in the body. It may be measured in **calories** (cal), **kilocalories/kiloCalories** (kcal/kCal) or **joules/kilojoules** (J/kJ). One kilocalorie (kcal) is approximately equal to 4.2 joules (J) (Nightingale & Campbell 1998).

Basal metabolic rate (BMR), usually 60–90 per cent of total metabolic rate (Nightingale & Campbell 1998), is energy consumed at rest to maintain only essential activities of living. It is measured by number of calories consumed each hour per square metre of body surface area or per kilogram of body weight (see Schofield equation: Table 9.1). Adult basal metabolic rates usually consume about 1,400 calories each day (Marieb 1995), although this increases with

- body surface area
- muscle mass
- fever (1°C increases BMR 6–7 per cent (Campbell 1997))

and decreases with

- body fat

Women usually have lower basal metabolic rates than men because they have proportionally more body fat (Nightingale & Campbell 1998). At rest, most body heat is generated by vital organs (liver, heart, brain, endocrine).

***Table 9.1* The Schofield Equation (kcal/day)**

Age (years)	*male*	*female*
15–18	17.6 × kg + 656	13.3 × kg + 690
18–30	15.0 × kg + 690	14.8 × kg + 485
30–60	11.4 × kg + 870	8.1 × kg + 842
60+	11.7 × kg + 585	9.0 × kg + 656

***Source:* Bettany and Powell-Tuck (1997)**

Notes: Bettany and Powell-Tuck cite additional factors; the only significant ones for ICU are ventilation: +15%
bedbound and awake: +10 per cent
each 1°C above 37°C: +10 per cent

Total metabolic rate (TMR) is basal metabolic rate together with body heat produced by additional activities. Thus

energy expenditure = physical activity
+ growth (including healing)
+ basal metabolic rate

As metabolism produces heat, high metabolic rates can cause pyrexia.

Direct measurement of metabolism (direct calorimetry) is currently clinically impractical. However, nearly all energy used is derived from reactions involving oxygen (4.825 calories per litre of oxygen ± 3 per cent (Guyton & Hall 1997)), and so some ventilators incorporate indirect calorimetry (metabolic monitors). Otherwise formulae such as the Harris Benedict equation (Nightingale & Campbell 1998) can measure energy expenditure:

male BMR = 66.5 + (13.8 × kg weight) + (5 × cm height) − (6.8 × age in years)

female BMR = 655 + (9.6 × kg weight) + (1.8 × cm height) − (4.7 × age in years)

Obesity

Obesity is endemic in most Western societies – UK rates have doubled since 1980 (O'Meara & Glenny 1997). Fatty acids and cholesterol are essential for cell membranes, hormones and immunity. The liver metabolises fat; elsewhere, the body uses glucose rather than fat for energy production. Since dietary fat, and hence cholesterol production, usually exceeds demand, most fat is stored. Obesity can be measured by body mass index (BMI) (DoH 1994a):

BMI = weight (kg)/height^2 (metres)

The Department of Health (DoH 1994a) defines BMI below 20 as underweight, 20–25 as normal, 25–30 as overweight, and above 30 as obese. However, these figures ignore the effects of dehydration and fluid retention (Wallace 1993) that often complicate critical illness.

Being under- or overweight significantly increases health risks (Gibbs 1996) as extra fat increases vasculature, systemic vascular resistance and the risk of pathologies such as hypertension, arteriosclerosis, cardiomyopathy and diabetes mellitus.

Fats can be classified by saturation – the number of atoms joined by single bonds – and so **saturated fatty acids** (usually animal fat) have univalent bonds joining all atoms; valency determines the hydrogen binding capacity of molecules, and so saturated fatty acids contribute to hypercholestrolamia and cardiovascular (especially coronary) disease. *Monounsaturated fatty acid* (e.g. olive oil) molecules have one bi/tri-valent bond. *Polyunsaturated fatty acids* (PUFAs, e.g. soya) have multiple covalent bonds, and can be positively healthy (e.g. omega 3, found in fish oils, inhibits platelet aggregation and promotes cell-mediated immunity (Schears & Deutschman 1997)).

The Krebs' cycle ('Citric Acid Cycle')

Fat metabolism, which is the combination of pyruvate and coenzyme A (CoA), produces adenosine triphosphate (for energy) together with various waste products – ketone and other metabolic acids, carbon dioxide, water.

Each stage of this complex chain reaction releases energy (ATP) and two carbon atoms which combine with coenzyme A to form acetyl-CoA; this then re-enters the cycle.

The **Krebs' cycle** contributes to metabolic acidosis and hypercapnia.

Hypoperfusion (shock) deprives tissues of sufficient glucose, necessitating (anaerobic) fat metabolism.

The ratio between carbon dioxide produced and oxygen consumed during the Krebs' cycle is the *respiratory quotient* (RQ), which indicates the source of energy: carbohydrate metabolism gives an RQ of 1.0; fat gives an RQ below 1.0. Thus feeds formulated with fewer carbohydrate calories may reduce respiratory acidosis in critically ill patients.

Enteral nutrition

Immunoglobulins in the gut wall (IgA, IgM) protect against translocation of gut bacteria, but gut villi necrose within minutes of splanchnic hypoperfusion (shock), structure and function markedly deteriorating within one week of starvation (Buckley & McFie 1997). The gut is thus a major mediator of sepsis. Although most evidence for this is from animal studies (rodent cells migrate from villi crypts to tips in 1–2 days; in humans, this takes 6–7 days (McFie 1996)), enteral feeding assists wound healing (Heyland 1998), immunity and reduces infection. Moore *et al.*'s (1992) meta-analysis found sepsis rates of 17 per cent with enteral feeding compared to 44 per cent with parenteral nutrition (not from line infection).

Wide-bore tubes (e.g. Ryles®) are easier to insert than fine bore tubes, but cause more upper airway/gastrointestinal inflammation, erosions and haemorrhage (Bettany & Powell-Tuck 1997). As fine-bore tubes cannot be aspirated, residual volumes cannot be measured to test absorption and require X-ray confirmation of placement before use (Briggs 1996b). Marking nasogastric tubes enables any external tube migration to be detected (Methany 1993).

The absence of bowel sounds does not necessarily indicate absence of function (Methany 1993); most bowels sounds are from swallowed air (Raper & Maynard 1992), which is reduced by intubation.

Paralytic ileus seldom affects ileal motility (Adam & Osborne 1997), and so postpyloric tubes (percutaneous endoscopic gastrostomy (PEG)), although more difficult to insert, facilitate absorption while decreasing the risks of pulmonary aspiration (Zainal 1994).

Physiological gut secretions often exceed 9 litres/day, and so absorption may be present despite aspirate volumes of up to 200 ml. If larger volumes are aspirated, drugs can increase gut motility (e.g. cisapride, metaclopramide). Discarding aspirated volumes may cause electrolyte imbalance, although research evidence is currently inconclusive (Methany 1993).

The stomach is normally sterile, but gastric pH above 4.0 enables colonisation with anaerobic gram negative organisms (Clarke 1997). Unlike normal oral diets, continuous enteral feeding maintains reduced gastric acidity. Gastric colonies migrating up nasogastric tubes readily cause pneumonia: uninterrupted enteral feeding increases ventilator-associated pneumonia by over 54 per cent (Lee *et al.* 1990). Rest periods from enteral feeds enable gastric emptying and return to below pH 3 (Rennie 1993a). Even with reduced absorption, gastric emptying should occur within one hour; Zainal (1994) and Lee *et al.* (1990) recommend 8-hour rests, but practice varies with four hours being common; some units rest for more than one period per day, opting for relatively short periods (e.g. 4 one-hour periods). Substantive research is needed to clarify the ideal length of rest periods.

Diarrhoea

Many ICU patients develop diarrhoea. Diarrhoea is an imbalance between fluid entering the colon and reabsorption, and may be caused by:

- excessive fluid (colonic absorption is limited to about 4.5 litres/day)
- hypoalbuminaemia (common in ICU) and low colloid osmotic pressure reducing absorption (Payne-James & Silk 1992)
- sorbitol (used in drugs, e.g. sucralfate suspension): this exerts higher osmotic gradients than plasma, drawing fluid into the bowel
- antibiotics (destroy gut flora): 41 per cent of patients on antibiotics develop diarrhoea with enteral feeds; the incidence falls to 3 per cent without antibiotics (Guenter *et al.* 1991)
- diluting feeds (Rennie 1993a)
- hyperosmolar feeds (> 2 kcal/ml)

Diarrhoea can be a homeostatic way to remove pathological bowel bacteria, and so reducing motility (e.g. with metaclopramide) may facilitate pathogen translocation. Bulking agents fail to prevent diarrhoea (Payne-James & Silk 1992).

Enteral feeds should not cause diarrhoea unless hyperosmolar, or volumes exceed 275 ml/hour (Adam & Osborne 1997). Feeding should not usually be stopped if diarrhoea occurs.

Parenteral nutrition

While enteral nutrition is preferable, some patients are unable to absorb sufficient enteral nutrition, and so supplementary or (total) parenteral nutrition (TPN) can prevent muscle atrophy – although supplemental TPN has not been shown to reduce mortality (Heyland 1998). The gut function of patients receiving TPN should be closely monitored to enable weaning onto enteral nutrition as soon as possible.

The problems of TPN include:

- gut atrophy – and so translocation of gut bacteria
- infection
- impaired neutrophil function (Schears & Deutschman 1997)
- lipid agglutination in capillaries (increased afterload)
- cost

TPN provides a medium for exogenous infection: warm, moist food remaining in place for up to 24 hours. The TPN catheter infection rates of 6 per cent compare unfavourably with jejunosotmy rates of 1.5 per cent (Schears & Deutschman 1997).

TPN is usually 50 per cent glucose with added nutrients. The addition of fat gives TPN its typically cream colour, diluting glucose content to about 10 per cent (Grimble *et al.* 1989). Infusing large volumes of 50 per cent glucose (together with increased circulating catecholamines) causes hyperglycaemia, usually necessitating insulin supplements with TPN. Fifty per cent glucose is strongly acidic (pH 3) and hyperosmolar, and so should be given through a large (central) vein; the success of peripheral TPN has been limited, and it is not widely used in ICU.

Nutritional assessment

Nutritional needs in critical illness should be carefully assessed to prevent knee-jerk reactions. Assessment may be undertaken by nurses or others, such as dieticians.

Simple measurements (**anthropometry**) include:

- height
- weight
- mid-upper-arm circumferences (low = overall weight loss)
- triceps skinfold thickness (low = significant loss of fat stores)
- mid-arm muscle circumference (= protein depletion)

As half the body fat stores are subcutaneous, measuring skinfold thickness (e.g. triceps) gives an indication of energy reserves (Say 1997); accuracy can be increased with callipers and serial measurements (Say 1997). Table 9.2 presents a nomogram; lower figures indicate malnutrition. However gross oedema and deceptive increases in body weight may mask muscle atrophy (Say 1997).

Table 9.2 A normal anthropometric chart

mid-upper-arm circumferences	
m	26–29 cm
f	26–28.5 cm
	(below = overall weight loss)
triceps skinfold thickness	
m	11–12.5 mm
f	16–16.5 mm
	(below = significant loss of fat stores)
mid-arm muscle circumference	
m	23–25 cm
f	20–23 cm
	(below = protein depletion)

Metabolic analysers (included in some ventilators) calculate energy expenditure from differentials between inspired and expired gases ('indirect calorimetry') (Adam & Osborne 1997). But metabolic analysers are expensive, and inaccurate with high oxygen concentrations, acidosis and haemofiltration (Adam & Osborne 1997).

Plasma albumin indicates protein synthesis (Say 1997), but hypoalbuminaemia in critically ill patients is multifactorial. Transferrin levels also indicate protein synthesis, but levels rise with iron deficiency (Say 1997), making results 'abnormal' with usual ICU haemoglobin levels of about 10 g/dl.

Urinalysis may identify abnormalities such as ketonuria (from fat metabolism, e.g. starvation, diabetes mellitus (Say 1997)). Periodic urinalysis is cheap, simple and quick, and so although the causes of abnormalities may be unclear, it provides a means both to detect problems and monitor progress.

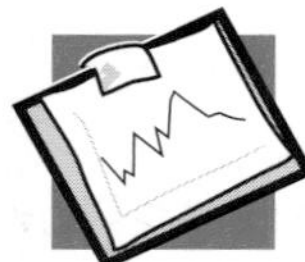

Implications for practice

- nutrition benefits from multidisciplinary team approaches; bedside nurses can usefully coordinate care
- enteral feeding is *usually* preferable
- if nasogastric feeding fails, lower gastrointestinal tubes should be considered
- feed regimes should be individually assessed
- feed regimes should be fully completed, benefits (and problems) being monitored
- diarrhoea is rarely caused by nasogastric feeding, so is not an indication to stop feeds

Summary

Feeding critically ill patients remains problematic, yet it is fundamental to their recovery. Nurses therefore have an important role in promoting and delivering nutrition.

Nutritional needs and benefits are often less obvious than those of other major systems, but this chapter has included various noninvasive ways to assess nutritional needs.

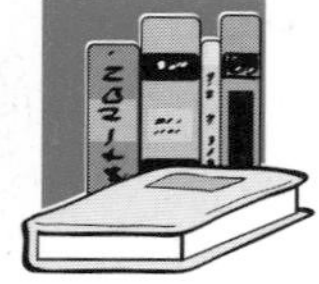

Further reading

Although much is written on nutrition, material does date quickly. Horwood (1990), despite its age, remains a useful overview. Verity (1996b) and Say (1997) offer more recent nursing perspectives, while Schears and Deutschman (1997) is a comprehensive medical article. Methany (1993) presents a rigorous literature review of nasogastric nutrition; Kennedy (1997) contains useful material on enteral feeding, although does overstate some aspects. Most ICU texts include a substantial chapter on nutrition.

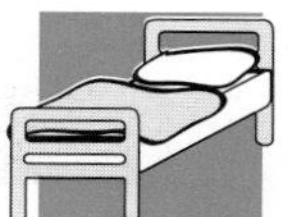

Clinical scenario

Sally Day is 35 years old, weighs approximately 60 kg, with an arm span of 1.65 m. She has recently been admitted to ICU following blunt trauma injury from a road traffic accident. Her injuries include fractures to lower ribs, pulmonary contusions, and she has a high index of suspicion for damaged spleen.

Sally is sedated, fully ventilated; pain management includes intravenous opiate. In order to reduce any inter-abdominal pressure on her potentially injured spleen, Sally's stomach was carefully emptied (decompression of stomach). Careful fluid management is necessary to avoid potential fluid overload.

Q.1 (a) Identify the appropriate methods/tools/approaches to assess effectively Sally's nutritional status and requirements in ICU.
(b) Calculate Sally's Body Mass Index (BMI) and Basal Metabolic Rate (BMR).
(c) Estimate Sally's energy requirements using her BMR and history of injuries.

Q.2 Analyse the benefits and risks of enteral and parental nutrition. How can the risks be minimised and Sally's energy requirements met (in relation to her injuries, fluid management, and metabolic response to injury and starvation).

Q.3 Select the most suitable and effective nutritional strategies to promote healing and recovery and which minimise starvation and other complications for Sally.

Chapter 10

Mouthcare

Contents

Fundamental knowledge

Oral anatomy
Composition of dental plaque

Introduction

Hygiene is a fundamental activity of living, yet information on mouthcare in ICU books or journals is sparse. What does exist is largely anecdotal residue from rituals (Hatton-Smith 1994); much research uses inadequate sample sizes: De Walt and Haines' much-cited 1969 study used one adult (Kite & Pearson 1995), while Nelsey's (1986) sample size was four patients, one being used for control. This makes evidence-based practice difficult. Yet oral ill-health has significant short-term and long-term effects. Oral hygiene facilitates

- comfort
- sensory balance
- prevention of infection.

Patients in ICU often develop dry mouths (xerostomia) from:

- absence of oral intake
- adverse effects of therapeutic drugs (e.g. morphine, diuretics, tranquillisers and antibiotics (Treloar 1995))
- sympathetic nervous system stimulation (reduces salivary secretion)
- poor salivary production (Marsh & Martin 1992)
- drying (convection) from mouths wedged open by oral endotracheal tubes

The moistening of patients' mouths provides comfort, but it also reduces the oral stasis which, together with immunosuppression, exposes them to potential oral infection. Plaque formation can occur rapidly; survivors of ICU may subsequently suffer tooth loss from plaque damage.

Oral hygiene also contributes to psychological comfort. The mouth is used to communicate (lip-reading is possible despite intubation, and following extubation, oral discomfort may make speech difficult). The mouth is also associated with intimate emotions (smiling, kissing); patients with, or thinking they have, dirty mouths or halitosis may feel psychologically isolated.

The provision of oral hygiene merely replaces activities ICU patients would normally perform for themselves, if able. Mouthcare should therefore

- maintain hygiene
- keep the oral cavity moist
- promote comfort
- protect from infection
- prevent trauma
- prevent dental decay.

This chapter reviews the current available specialist literature and applies material from other areas to ICU nursing. Oral anatomy is briefly revised, but readers should supplement any aspects they are not familiar with from anatomy texts.

Anatomy

Unlike all other major body systems, gut stimulation is counterproductive to 'fight or flight' responses: parasympathetic nerve stimulation accelerates gut functions, while sympathetic nerve stimulation decelerates them.

Saliva contributes both to digestion and immunity. Saliva contains:

- water (97–99.5 per cent)
- linguinal lipase, ptyalin/salivary amylase (digestive enzymes)
- mucins (lubricate food, protect oral mucosa)
- immunoglobulin A (immunity)
- lysozyme (immunity – note: not lysosome)
- lactoferrin (immunity)
- growth factor (promoting healing)
- proline-rich proteins (protecting tooth enamel)
- metabolic waste (urea, uric acid)

Saliva is primarily secreted from three pairs of extrinsic glands (outside the oral cavity), with the additional production by supplementary intrinsic glands throughout mouth (see Figure 10.1). Placing cotton wool rolls on the main salivary glands can remove excess saliva as effectively (and with less trauma) as endotracheal suction.

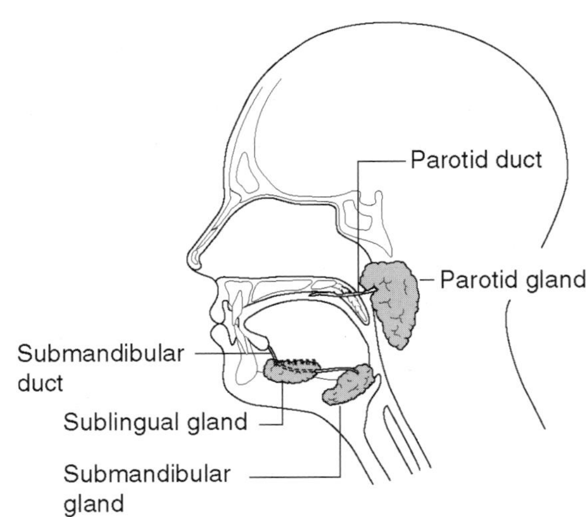

***Figure 10.1* The main anatomy of the oral (buccal) cavity showing salivary glands**

Saliva is produced in response to stimuli:

- oral pressoceptor stimulation (from anything in the mouth, including endotracheal tubes)
- oral chemoreceptor stimulation (especially acids)
- thoughts of food
- smelling food (in environment, on clothing)
- lower gut irritation (e.g. absence of enteral feeding, bacterial toxins)

Saliva is normally slightly acidic (pH 6.75–7.0 (Marieb 1995)); increased acidity (Treloar (1995) found mean salivary pH of 5.3 in ICU patients) increases dental demineralisation.

Sympathetic vasoconstriction and dehydration reduce salivary gland perfusion, making saliva viscous and mucin-rich (dry mouths are familiar from 'fight and flight' responses). Endogenous sympathetic stimulation from stress may be compounded by exogenous catecholamines (adrenaline/noradrenaline). Saliva production also decreases with age (most ICU patients are elderly).

Teeth have four layers:

- enamel (brittle, acellular, irreparable)
- dentin (bulk of tooth, mainly collagen)
- cementum (covering roots, mainly collagen)
- pulp (central part of tooth, mainly collagen; unlike other layers, contains blood vessels and nerves (Murray *et al* 1994))

Plaque

Plaque (sugar, bacteria and other debris) metabolises to acids, especially lactic acid. Plaque can contain 10^8–10^{11} bacteria per gram (Murray *et al* 1994). Gingival crevices are especially susceptible to plaque formation (Mallett & Bailey 1996). Accumulated plaque calcifies into calculus or tartar, disrupting seals between gingivae and teeth. Gingivitis (sore, red and bleeding gums) occurs within ten days of plaque formation (Kite & Pearson 1995).

Plaque is not water soluble, so that mouthwash solutions do little to remove plaque; antibacterial mouthwashes (e.g. chlorhexidine) can supplement, but not replace, brushing teeth (Murray *et al* 1994). Oral neglect enables bacteria to multiply around teeth and dissolve bone (peritonitis/periodontal disease). Perodontitis is the main cause of adult tooth loss (Marieb 1995) so that neglect in ICU can have rapid and enduring effects.

Infection

ICU patients' mouths can provide ideal environments for bacteria, viruses and fungi, due to

- being warm, moist and static

- saliva accumulation at the back of throats (supine positions, impaired gag/swallowing reflex)
- protein from blood and plaque
- destruction of normal flora by antibiotics
- immunosuppression (enabling growth of opportunistic organisms).

Infection is usually bacterial (Clarke 1993) – common organisms including *Staphylococcus aureus* and *Pseudomonas* sp. (Scannapieco *et al* 1992). Candidiasis, the most common fungal infection (susceptible to nystatin), can be recognised by white spots (Clarke 1993). Herpes simplex, the major oral virus (susceptible to aciclovir cream), creates sores and cysts around the mouth and lips (Clarke 1993).

Oral secretions accumulate rapidly when swallowing reflexes are impaired (experienced during almost any dental examination). Oral suction can remove much accumulated saliva, debris and microorganisms, but removal is almost inevitably incomplete. Microorganisms may bypass low-pressure endotracheal cuffs – Scannapieco *et al* (1992) found respiratory pathogens in 64 per cent of ICU patients, compared to 16 per cent of dental clinic patients; oral trauma (e.g. from suction) enables pathogens to enter the bloodstream. ICU nurses should therefore reassess oral health and hygiene regularly.

Oral decontamination (similar to selective digestive decontamination – see Chapter 15) may prevent spread from oral to respiratory infection. Pugin *et al* (1991) found that only 16 per cent of ICU patients given topical oropharyngeal antibiotics developed oral infections (78 per cent of the control group receiving placebos developed infection). Oral decontamination may reduce ICU morbidity, but the routine use of antibiotics is generally discouraged (House of Lords Select Committee on Science and Technology 1998).

Assessment

Oral assessment should include each aspect of the oral cavity:

- lips
- gums
- teeth
- tongue
- hard palette
- soft tissue
- salivary production
- evidence of any infection
- evidence of any cuts/purpura/blood

These should be assessed against risk factors from

- overall condition
- underlying pathology

- treatments (including effects of drugs)

Although assessment should be individualised to each patient, assessment tools can provide a useful structure. Holmes and Mountain (1993) found problems with three tools tested with oncology patients.

Jenkins (1989) adapted his assessment tool (Table 10.1) from the Norton (pressure sore) scale. This tool is potentially useful, but his article is not a research report of the tool's effectiveness, and the tool requires subjective evaluations (e.g. good/fair/poor/very poor oral condition).

Treloar (1995) presents useful criteria (salivary flow, plaque, gingiva, lip

Table 10.1 The Jenkins oral assessment tool

Patient's age	*Score*
15–29	4
30–49	3
50–69	2
70+	1
Normal oral condition	
good	4
fair	3
poor	2
very poor	1
Mastication ability	
full	4
slightly impaired	3
very limited	2
immobile	1
Nutritional state	
good	4
fair	3
poor	2
very poor	1
Airway	
normal	4
humidified oxygen	3
ET tube	2
open-mouth breathing	1

Source: Jenkins 1989

Notes: score 15 and above = 3 hourly care
12–14 = 2 hourly care
below 12 = hourly care
If the patient has:
1 large-dose antibiotic steroid therapy
2 diabetes mellitus
3 low Hb
4 immunosuppression
then the score of 1 should be subtracted from the previous 'at risk' calculator score.

colour, tongue colour, mucosa colour) used for evaluating oral health, but this checklist still requires subjective interpretation by nurses. Heals's (1993) assessment tool (designed for oncology) contains a similar list of useful cues; Heals also includes a scoring system, but the only composite evaluation is that patients scoring under 25 (out of 32) are 'at risk' – all ICU patients being at risk, Heals's assessment chart can provide useful cues for more detailed assessment, but would need further development before being suitable for use in ICUs.

Oral assessment necessitates viewing the oral cavity, so tongue depressors and torches are helpful (Jenkins 1989). Endotracheal tubes may obscure much of the cavity. Observations should be recorded. As part of universal precautions (see Chapter 40), protective gloves should be worn.

Lotions and potions

Many mouthcare solutions and other aids have been marketed, most with little support beyond custom and practice. Few remove or prevent plaque, or provide other significant benefits, and many leave unpleasant tastes (nurses can understand patients' experiences by tasting non-prescription products themselves).

Lemon-flavoured swabs (introduced to stimulate salivary production) can decalcify teeth (Crosby 1989).

Glycerine is hypertonic, so causes dehydration and reflex salivary gland exhaustion (Crosby 1989).

Insufficient dilution of chemicals such as *sodium bicarbonate* and *hydrogen peroxide* can cause mucosal burns (Tombes & Galluci 1993); even *chlorhexidine* rinse can alter oral flora and stain teeth black.

Although tap *water* may be used, immunocompromise often encourages ICU nurses to use sterile water; whether this is treating patients or staff is unclear.

Some mouthwashes are antibacterial: pharmacists can advise which solution is best for each patient.

Foam sticks can moisten mucosa between cleaning, but do not remove debris from surfaces or between teeth (Pritchard & Mallett 1992), and so plaque accumulation continues (Pearson 1996). As hard sticks cause oral trauma, they should be used carefully and (when possible) with good light.

Toothbrush

Toothbrushes (with or without toothpaste) remain the best way to clean patients' teeth, loosening debris trapped between teeth and removing plaque from tooth surfaces (Pritchard & Mallett 1992).

The technique reflects that of brushing one's own teeth: brush away from the gums to remove, rather than impact, plaque from gingival crevices. Manipulating toothbrushes in other people's mouths, especially when orally intubated, can be difficult; smallheaded multitufted toothbrushes, with soft, small, nylon heads and hollow-fibred bristles, are best for brushing the teeth of others (Pritchard & Mallett 1992; Jones 1998). Pritchard & Mallett

(1992) and Jones (1998) recommend the 'Bass' method: placing the toothbrush at 44° to the gingival margin, using very small vibratory movements so bristles reach subgingivally to collect and remove plaque. With trismus (limited mouth opening), an interspace toothbrush will remove plaque (although not clean between teeth) (Pritchard & Mallett 1992). Brushing once each day with 0.4 per cent fluoride gel is adequate if teeth are clean (Burglass 1995); choice of toothpaste is largely cosmetic, but patients may find the taste of their usual brand comforting. Gentle brushing of gums and tongue can also be useful with endentitious patients (Day 1993). Toothpaste should be removed with mouthwashes (Jenkins 1989) and gentle suction, as residual toothpaste can cause further drying of the mucosa.

Vigorous brushing may cause bleeding, especially if patients have coagulopathies (e.g. DIC); oral care should therefore be planned holistically.

Lips

Lips are highly vascular, with sensitive nerve endings, and are even more closely associated with communication (e.g. lip-reading) and intimacy (e.g. kissing) than the mouth. As lip mucosa is exposed, it can dry quickly. Lipcare can therefore prevent drying and cracking, while providing psychological comfort. White petroleum jelly is often used to keep lips moist.

Frequency

Two-hourly mouthcare rituals are unhelpful and time consuming. Dental decay from plaque and debris occurs after one day (Pritchard & Mallett 1992), and so care should be performed at least daily (Treloar 1995; Burglass 1995), but comfort (e.g. to prevent drying) and nursing accountability probably require more frequent care (at least once every shift to enable assessment); following assessment, mouthcare should be individualised (Jenkins 1989). The Jenkins tool (Table 10.1) can guide appropriate frequency of care.

Pressure sores

Any body surface area is susceptible to pressure sore development (see Chapter 12). Treloar's (1995) study of 16 ICU patients found most had multiple lip, tongue and mucosal lesions, while seven patients suffered severe dryness. Endotracheal tubes and tracheostomies place pressure on various tissues, including the mouth and nose. Sores are especially likely when tubes rest on gingival surfaces rather than teeth (Liwu 1990); sides of lips are particularly susceptible to sores. The loosening and moving of tapes and tubes relieves prolonged pressure (Clarke 1993).

Dentures

Intubation and impaired consciousness normally necessitates removal of any dentures, but property should be checked on admission so that dentures are not lost. Nursing records should include whether patients normally wear partial or complete dentures, and relevant care.

Like patients' own teeth, dentures are easily damaged, warping easily, particularly if left dry or cleaned in hot water (Clarke 1993). As dentures containing metal may corrode, Jones (1998) suggests that they should be immersed for just 20 minutes, although this contradicts recommendations (Crosby 1989; Clarke 1993) that they should be left soaking in cold water.

Room-temperature water is a medium for bacterial growth, and should be changed daily (Clarke 1993). If denture cleaners are available, these should be used; as toothpaste can damage denture surfaces (Clarke 1993), it should be avoided.

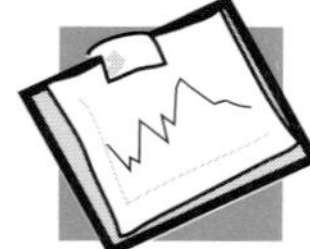

Implications for practice

- mouthcare should be individually assessed, rather than following routine/rituals
- toothbrushes (with or without toothpaste) are the best means for providing mouthcare
- toothpaste should be removed with oral suction
- mouthwashes or moist swabs can provide comfort, although are not on their own adequate for hygiene
- if antibacterial washes are needed, consult pharmacists
- find out whether patients wear dentures, recording where they are stored
- lubricate lips (e.g. with white petroleum jelly)

Summary

Mouthcare is too easily forgotten in the physiological crises of critical illness, but problems developing from their time in ICU can cause long-term or permanent oral/dental disease. The current paucity of material on mouthcare in ICUs makes evidence-based practice difficult.

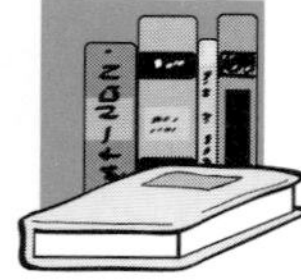

Further reading

Of the limited literature available, Day (1993), Kite and Pearson (1995), and Pearson (1996) are specifically related to ICU. Clarke (1993) and Jones (1998) provide useful articles from wider nursing perspectives; Jones (1998) includes summaries of many available mouthwashes, although often relies on potentially dated sources. *The Royal Marsden manual of clinical nursing procedures* gives practical and substantiated advice; the 3rd edition (Pritchard & Mallet 1992) is more useful for mouthcare than the 4th edition (Mallett & Bailey 1996).

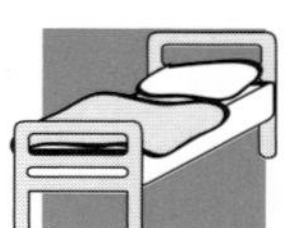

Clinical scenario

Pamela Merrell is 60 years old and employed as a television presenter. She was admitted to ICU three days previously after sustaining a closed head injury from tumbling down a flight of concrete steps at work.

She has been unconscious and invasively ventilated since admission. Computed tomographic scan revealed a large contused area to her frontal lobe leading to development of intracranial hypertension. Nursing interventions that could increase Pamela's intracranial pressure are necessarily restricted. Consequently she has had minimal oral hygiene care and her teeth have not been brushed for at least 84 hours.

Q.1 List the equipment needed to inspect and assess Pamela's oral status (gums, tongue, salivary glands, teeth, palate, lips, jaw).

Q.2 Review the oral assessment charts used in clinical practice:

- Identify Pamela's risk factors for developing oral complications (e.g. lesions or ulcers on tongue/palate/gums/lips, plaque erosions, gingivitis, infections).
- How may such complications impact on Pamela's recovery, consider effect on her physical, and psychosocial status?

Q.3 Evaluate documentation of oral assessment and care in your own clinical practice (e.g. charts, risk scores, care plans, standards).
Is documentation:

- systematic?
- research or evidence-based?
- effective at identifying at-risk patients?
- effective in guiding nursing care (e.g. frequency of interventions, choice of equipment, solutions etc.)?

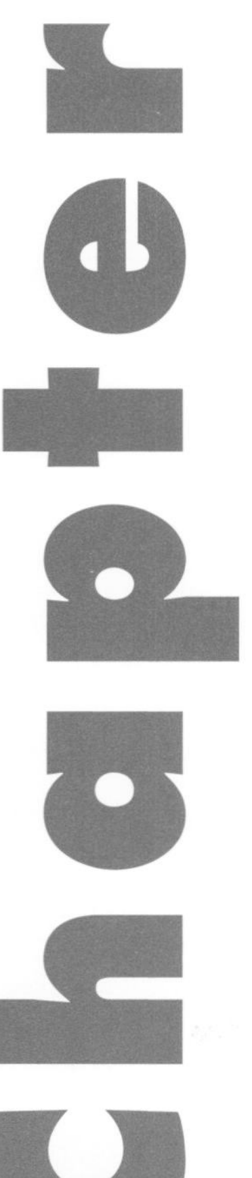

Chapter 11

Eyecare

Contents

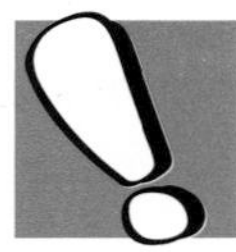

Fundamental knowledge

Anatomy – cornea, lens, tear production, blink reflex

Introduction

Patients are seldom admitted to ICU for ocular pathologies, but most ICU patients rely on nurses to maintain normal and pathophysiological hygiene needs, and should not suffer unnecessary complications from substandard care. This chapter considers reasons for and types of eyecare needed by most ICU patients, but does not discuss specialist ocular pathophysiologies.

Eyecare in ICUs often suffers from the vagaries of ritual, priorities and knowledge, and receives scant attention in the nursing literature, so that ICU nurses have little evidence beyond scattered anecdotes to guide practice. This chapter illustrates some of the risks ICU patients' eyes are exposed to, and discusses some approaches to care from the little specialist literature on this topic. However, suggestions necessarily remain tentative, substantial research being needed to develop evidence-based practice.

Eyecare is important for both physiological and psychological reasons. Eye contact helps communication; nurses may feel squeamish about touching eyes, but ocular abnormalities often provoke anxiety among patients and relatives. Vision is, for most people, the most used sense, and so visual deficits contribute significantly to sensory imbalance. Therefore, ICU nurses should evaluate:

- the eyecare performed
- visual appearance
- how care is described

While assessing and caring for a patient's eyes, nurses can also make neurological assessment of

- pupil size and reaction
- accommodation for near and long vision (assessed by placing a finger near the patient's nose – moving the finger away should cause pupils to diverge).

Ocular damage may invalidate any or all of these tests.

Ocular damage

The cornea, the outer surface of the eye, is vulnerable to trauma and lacerations (e.g. from pillows, endotracheal tapes). Blink reflexes and tear production, which normally protect and irrigate corneal surfaces, may be absent or weak (e.g. from paralysing agents; drugs such as atropine, antihistamines and paralysing agents also inhibit tear production).

The cornea and lens are avascular, absorbing oxygen and nutrients from aqueous humour. Thus corneal damage exposes deeper layers to infection. Avascularity also delays healing, often leaving opaque scar tissue. Ocular trauma may remain unrecognised until patients regain full consciousness, finding their vision permanently impaired.

Normal intraocular pressure is 12–20 mmHg (average 15 mmHg); impaired drainage of aqueous humour (e.g. from IPPV, tight ETT tapes, oedema, poor head alignment, prone positioning) may cause intraocular hypertension and ocular damage (including subconjunctival haemorrhage (Farrell & Wray 1993)). ICU patients are therefore at high risk of intraocular hypertension; head elevation (e.g. 30° if supine) assists venous drainage.

Incomplete eyelid closure (e.g. from periorbital/other oedema, paralysis) or loss of blink reflexes causes corneal drying, which can lead to corneal ulceration (Farrell & Wray 1993), an acutely painful condition.

Glasses and contact lenses are usually best removed (include in nursing records) for safety, although fully conscious patients often benefit from wearing them.

Infection

Fox (1989) suggests that most eye infections are caused by

- *Staphylococcus aureus*
- *Haemophilus influenzae*
- *Streptococcus* spp.

Milliken *et al.* (1988) report ocular infection in 7 per cent of paediatric ICU patients, but increased exposure to respiratory pathogens (Hilton *et al.* 1983; Farrell & Wray 1993) and reduced tear production probably place adults at greater risk. Eye infection from respiratory pathogens has necessitated corneal transplants with some patients (Ommeslag *et al.* 1987), and so simple infection control measures such as covering a patient's eyes during suction (Hilton *et al.* 1983) and keeping the disconnected ventilator tubing (Cobley *et al.* 1991) and used suction catheters away from the patient's eyes can significantly reduce eye infection.

If ocular infection is suspected, it should be reported and recorded; swabs may need to be taken and topical antibiotics prescribed.

Assessment

Although structured eye assessment tools are not generally used in ICUs, nurses can make effective assessment using

- existing documentation
- visual observation of patients
- knowledge of normal ocular anatomy
- verbal questions (to patients or family).

Cues to consider include:

- contact lenses/glasses
- abnormalities (e.g. eyelids, lashes, exophthalmus); are abnormalities unilateral/bilateral?
- periorbital oedema
- patient positioning (and venous drainage)
- muscle weakness ('droopy eye')
- eye closure – do lids cover cornea completely?
- do eyes look infected/inflamed?
- do eyes look sore ('redeye')?
- tear production (excessive/impaired)
- blink reflex (absent, impaired, slow)
- eye pain (flinching during eyecare/interventions)
- visual impairment (double, cloudy, difficulty focusing)
- how does the patient feel (e.g. are eyelids heavy?)

Closed questions are often easier for intubated patients to answer.

Unless patients have specific ocular disease, eyecare should

- maintain ocular health
- replace lost functions
- ensure comfort
- protect from trauma/infection

To perform eyecare

- patients should be nursed supine, with head titled down (Mallett & Bailey 1996) (this helps nurses to see what they are doing and retains solutions in the eyes);
- good light should be used (Mallett & Bailey 1996), but avoid shining it directly into the patients' eyes.

Frequency of eyecare has been guided by ritual and serendipity; Lloyd (1990) suggests that two-hourly is probably unnecessary and suggests four times a day, but without giving a rationale. Nursing care should be individually planned in response to nursing assessment and evaluation. Care to maintain hygiene and comfort will differ from the treatment of existing infections or damage.

Interventions

Individual nursing assessment should identify

- how moist/dry a patient's eyes are
- whether blink reflex is present/poor/absent
- whether eyelid closure is incomplete
- other factors (e.g. ambient room temperature/humidity)

and whether supplementary moisture is needed. Various solutions are marketed for eyecare; reliable and objective research is lacking, but *artificial tears* appear a logical replacement if tear production is dysfunctional. Artificial tears are not required routinely, although may be needed up to half-hourly (Lloyd 1990). They should be dropped into the outer side of the lower fornix or arch (see Figure 11.1), which is less sensitive than the cornea (Mallett & Bailey 1996); over-vigorous use of eyedrops on the cornea may realistically be compared to water torture. To minimise infection risk, solutions should be stored in a clean area and, if reusable, should be marked with date and time of opening.

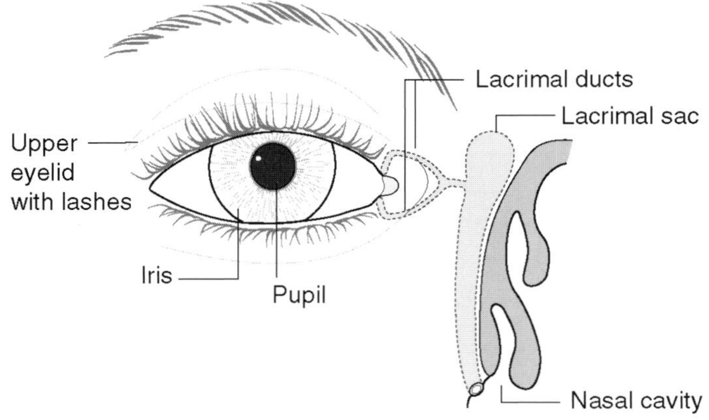

Figure 11.1 The external structure of the eye

Saline may soften crusts (Jamieson & McCall 1992), but also causes ocular irritation, increasing tear production twentyfold (Farrell & Wray 1993); it also causes tear fluid evaporation, aggravating corneal drying (Lloyd 1990). Saline swabs are safe when eyes are intact, but can sting if patients have corneal ulcerations. Excess moisture should be removed to prevent discomfort. Saline solutions can also be media for bacterial growth and so should be stored cleanly and changed frequently (at least once every shift).

Specialist eye hospitals use *cotton buds* rather than cotton wool, as detachment of fibres may cause corneal damage (Laight 1996). Nurses using cotton buds should take care that the sticks do not cause trauma.

Choice of external dressings should be partially guided by aesthetic considerations. Many people are particularly squeamish about eyes, and relatives may become especially anxious when eyes are covered; dressings that look like amateur improvisations for more sophisticated products may be functional but can cause psychological distress.

Geliperm®, an occlusive gel wound dressing, has been used to provide a barrier to infection and prevents corneal drying (Farrell & Wray 1993); it is nonadherent, and so removal does not cause trauma (oedematous eyes being especially vulnerable to slight trauma) (Farrell & Wray 1993). Being water-based, Geliperm® needs to be rehydrated (Farrell & Wray 1993) or replaced. Laight's (1996) small study suggests extending the standard recommendation for changes from 2–3 hours to 6–12 hours. There have been some anecdotal reports of eye infections, and so replacement may be safer (although more expensive) than rehydration. Eyecare is not included among the indications for Geliperm®; nor is it available on the NHS tariff (BNF 1998).

Tarsorrhaphy, stitching the eyelids together, is an effective, albeit barbaric, way to enable healing without exposing the cornea to drying or trauma from blink reflexes. Although this is sometimes useful for long-term patients, its practice cannot be supported for most ICU patients.

Implications for practice

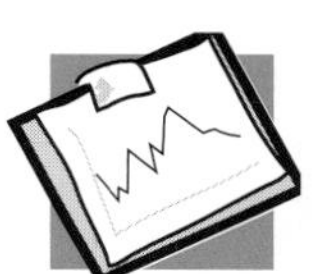

- plan individualised care on the basis of individualised assessment
- elevating patients' heads facilitates venous drainage, and so reduces oedema
- prone positioning predisposes to orbital (dependant) oedema formation; oedema can be reduced by elevating the bedhead by 10°, being careful to avoid uncomfortable head alignment
- eyecare solutions are potential media for infection and should be changed regularly (check unit/hospital policy; if not specified, change at least once each shift)
- exposed corneas are vulnerable to trauma and so if blink reflexes are weak or absent, nurses should ensure that patients eyes are closed and protected
- keep pillow edges, endotracheal tape and other equipment away from eyes

Summary

The high dependency of patients in ICU makes them vulnerable to harm. Normal ocular physiology and protective mechanisms are usually disordered by their underlying pathology and treatment. Yet eyecare is often given low priority by clinical nurses. For those nurses who do approach eyecare conscientiously, there is little reliable and substantiated literature to guide interventions, forcing them inevitably to rely on custom, practice, rituals and anecdotal support.

Like other fundamental aspects, for true holistic care to be realised greater emphasis needs to be placed on the importance of eyecare. Practice needs to be examined through more and more rigorous studies. Guidelines may be useful to help practitioners, but should not replace the need for individualised assessment, planning and delivery of care.

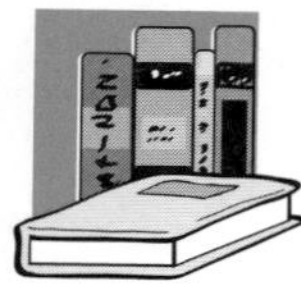

Further reading

Of the little ICU literature available on eyecare, the best articles are those by Farrell & Wray (1993) and Laight (1996). Lloyd (1990) is worth reading, but does make some questionable assumptions and statements. The *Royal Marsden NHS Trust manual of clinical nursing procedures* (Mallett & Bailey 1996) offers sound advice of practical aspects of eyecare.

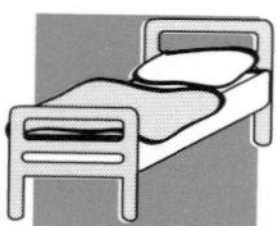

Clinical scenario

James Smith is 45 years old and works as an air traffic controller at London's Heathrow Airport. James is known to wear non-gas permeable contact lenses and has recently received treatment for conjunctivitis. James's admission to ICU was planned following his second (redo) mitral valve replacement. In his first 24 hours postoperatively, James is fully ventilated (on IPPV) and sedated with positive end expiratory pressure (PEEP) of 7.5 cmH_2O.

Q.1 List potential factors (patient's characteristics, treatments, drugs, etc.) which may cause eye complications (oedema, abrasions, pain) in ICU patients. Identify the potential risks associated with James.

Q.2 Analyse eyecare in clinical practice, both ocular assessment and nursing interventions. Are these:

- systematic in approach and documentation?
- knowledge and/or evidence-based?
- effective at identifying risk patients, and before complications occur?
- effective in guiding nursing care?

Q.3 James developed corneal ulceration from oedema and exposed cornea whilst ventilated. Consider how this affected his recovery in relation to his perceptions, vision, communication interactions and pain. Reflect on the legal, ethical and professional responsibilities towards James. (Had substandard practice or negligence occurred? If yes, who might be responsible?)

Chapter 12

Skincare

Contents

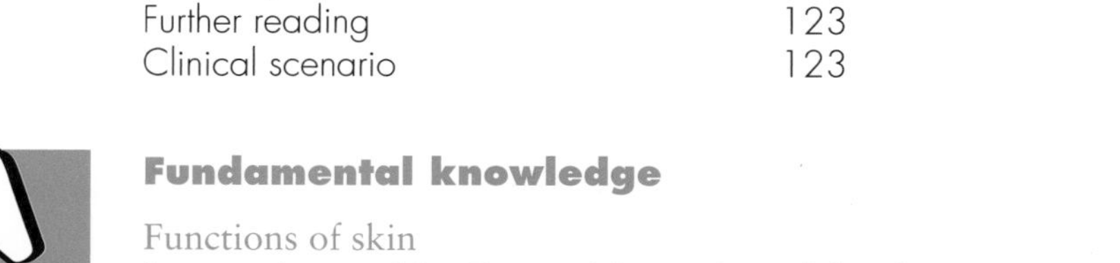

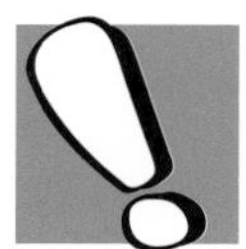

Fundamental knowledge

Functions of skin
Stages of wound healing and formation of decubitus ulcer

Introduction

Ten per cent of hospitalised patients develop pressure sores, and most occur in patients over 70 years old (Reid & Morison 1994a). The increased risk factors from critical illness and immobility place ICU patients at especial risk of skin breakdown.

Despite the high profile of wound and pressure area care, skincare remains problematic in ICUs with many patients developing sores. Traditionally, pressure sores were equated with bad nursing, and this created a culture of guilt and denial in nursing. Most ICU patients are exposed to high risk of skin breakdown from:

- prolonged peripheral hypoperfusion
- oedematous tissue
- anaerobic metabolism
- immunocompromise
- malnutrition

Injury can be through disease or treatments (e.g. surgical incision, invasive equipment). Since the skin is renewed every 28 days (Matlhoko 1994), healing is prolonged compared to most ICU admissions. The high ICU nurse–patient ratios should facilitate individualised assessment and care to prevent breakdown and minimise complications.

This chapter revises pressure sore development, identifies some assessment systems available, and describes some ways of preventing pressure sores. Emphasis remains on prevention, and so wound dressings are not discussed – the rapid changes in practice and availability of dressings makes their inclusion in this book impractical.

Much of the literature on skincare originates, or is sponsored/promoted by, people and companies with vested interests and so should be treated especially critically.

Necrotising fasciitis, a dermatological condition that can often prove fatal, is included here.

Pressure sores

A pressure sore is localised tissue necrosis (Reid & Morison 1994b). Forty per cent of American ICU patients develop pressure sores (Westrate & Bruining 1996); in the UK the incidence is probably higher due to the higher dependency of ICU patients here.

Waterlow (1995) suggests that pressure sores can be caused by both extrinsic factors:

- unrelieved pressure
- shearing
- friction

and intrinsic factors:

- age
- malnutrition
- dehydration
- incontinence
- medical condition
- medication.

The supply of tissue oxygen and nutrients and the removal of waste products of metabolism require capillary perfusion; initial damage causes cellular microtrauma (Lowthian 1997), and so supporting microcirculation and the provision of adequate nutrition are fundamental to pressure sore prevention. Capillary perfusion depends on various forces (see Chapter 33), including external pressure. The pressure needed to prevent capillary flow is called **capillary occlusion pressure.** Landis's 1930 study measured capillary pressures ranging from 21 to 48 mmHg (from 125 normotensive volunteers; mean 32 mmHg) (Lowthian 1997); however, ICU patients usually have systemic hypotension and so capillary pressures probably tend to be at the lower end of this range. Currently, measurement of patients' capillary pressures is impractical, but aids and equipment to prevent pressure sore development or progression should not exert continuous pressures above likely capillary occlusion pressures (20–25 mmHg – this is probably over-conservative, as the spread of pressure enables tolerance of higher pressures with deeper tissue (up to 35–40 mmHg in health), but until occlusion pressure can be safely measured, hypoperfusion of critical illness necessitates caution).

Shearing forces, pushing the walls of capillaries together by folding the skin over, increases the (blood) pressure needed to open capillaries (Matlhoko 1994).

Breakdown is quicker if the skin is excessively moist or dry. Urine, which may leak around urinary catheters, is a weak acid and so excoriates skin. Perspiration (e.g. from pyrexia) makes skin excessively moist and contains urea; faeces also includes acids (Lowery 1995) – many ICU patients have diarrhoea. 'Comfort' washes and hygiene therefore reduce risk factors. Similarly, lubricating dry skin (e.g. with aqueous cream) can prevent breakdown.

Skin over bony prominences (e.g. sacrum) is traditionally associated with pressure sores; prolonged supine positioning exposes ICU patients to the risk of sore development in these areas, but continuous bedrest also exposes ICU patients to prolonged pressure in other (less cited) areas:

- head (especially the back)
- ears
- lips/nose/mouth (around ETTs)
- beneath invasive equipment (e.g. hubs of arterial lines)
- skinfolds (e.g. breasts, abdomen)

Sores on the back of the head (Mihissin & Houghton 1995) may be hidden by hair and go unnoticed until blood is found on pillows; regular and active nursing assessment can enable early identification, and so treatment, of impending problems. Waterlow (1995) suggests that patients should be reassessed every day; critical illness may necessitate more frequent assessment.

In 1993 the Department of Health instructed that incidence of pressure sores in hospitals must be reduced by 5 per cent each year. This cumulative target, progressively more difficult to achieve, places pressure directly onto nursing staff, especially when ICU patients are increasingly sicker. Individual assessment of risk factors should therefore be fundamental to ICU nursing.

Assessment

Although there is no nationally recognised classification of pressure sores (Waterlow 1996), a 1992 consensus conference produced the 'Stirling' scale (Reid & Morison 1994a) (see Table 12.1), which provides a structure for initial assessment and nursing records (for subsequent comparison). Whichever classification system is used, all staff on the unit should be familiar with it (a wall poster is often helpful). However, classification only describes current problems; risk assessment and prevention requires an additional risk assessment tool. Unfortunately no existing scoring system fully meets ICU needs (Malone 1992). Tools relying on colour codes can also be difficult to use if black and white photocopies are made (copyright status should be checked before making photocopies).

Norton's pioneering work proved useful for many years, but was not designed for ICU and is now largely superseded by more sophisticated scoring systems. Gosnell's (1973) (modified Norton) scale is similarly oversimplistic for ICU. Barrett (1990) found the Douglas Pressure Sore Risk Calculator comprehensive and easy to use, but this again slightly modifies Norton, and has not been widely adopted in ICUs.

Waterlow (1985) is probably the most widely used scale in the UK, even if supporting literature is limited and unreliable (Bridel 1993; Edwards 1994). Birtwistle (1994) and Westrate and Bruining (1996) found it useful for ICU, but Sollars (1998) found it too insensitive; scores by different observers can be highly discrepant, especially if items rate 5 points.

A handful of assessment tools have been designed specifically for use in intensive care. Birty's tool (Birtwistle 1994) uses colour rather than numerical codes. Birtwistle's study (1994) found it easy to use and appropriate for critically ill patients; while visually clear and simple, the absence of a score necessitates incorporating the whole tool with each record in nursing documentation, and the tool does not appear to have been widely adopted.

Cubbin and Jackson's (1991) scale, developed specifically for ICU, was published following a pilot study on only five patients, with changes made between the second and third patient; reliability and validity were therefore inadequately tested. Hunt's (1993) substantive trial of this scale (100

Table 12.1 UK consensus classification of pressure sore severity ('Stirling scale')

Stage 0	No clinical evidence of a pressure sore 0.0 Normal appearance, intact skin 0.1 Healed with scarring 0.2 Tissue damage, but not assessed as a pressure sore	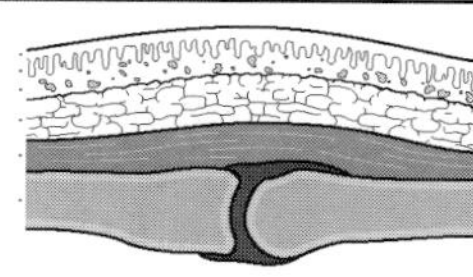
Stage 1	Discolouration of intact skin (light finger pressure applied to the site does not alter discoloration) 1.1 Non-blanchable erythema with increased local heat 1.2 Blue/purple/black discoloration or induration. The sore is at least Stage 1.	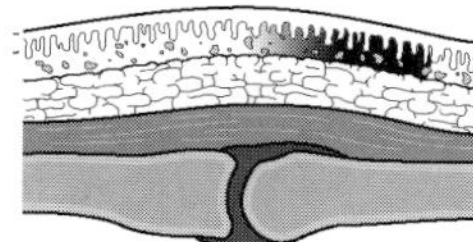
Stage 2	Partial-thickness skin loss or damage involving epidermis and/or dermis 2.1 Blister 2.2 Abrasion 2.3 Shallow ulcer, without undermining or adjacent tissue 2.4 Any of these with underlying blue/purple/black discoloration or induration. The sore is at least Stage 2.	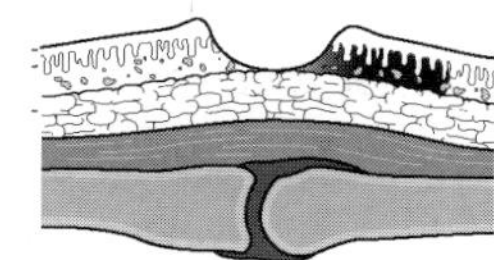
Stage 3	Full-thickness skin loss involving damage or necrosis of subcutaneous tissue but not extending to underlying bone, tendon or joint capsule 3.1 Crater, without undermining of adjacent tissue 3.2 Crater, with undermining of adjacent tissue 3.3 Sinus, the full extent of which is not certain 3.4 Full thickness skin loss but wound bed covered with necrotic tissue (hard or leathery black/brown tissue or softer yellow/cream/grey slough) which masks the true extent of tissue damage. The sore is at least Stage 3. Until debrided it is not possible to observe whether damage extends into muscle or involves damage to bone or supporting structures.	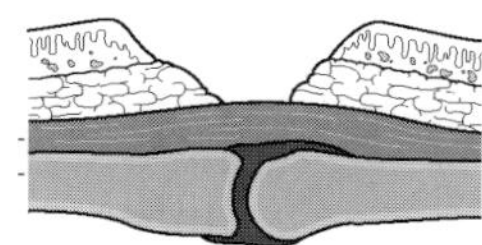
Stage 4	Full thickness skin loss with extensive destruction and tissue necrosis extending to underlying bone, tendon or joint capsule 4.1 Visible exposure of bone, tendon or capsule 4.2 Sinus assessed as extending to bone, tendon or capsule	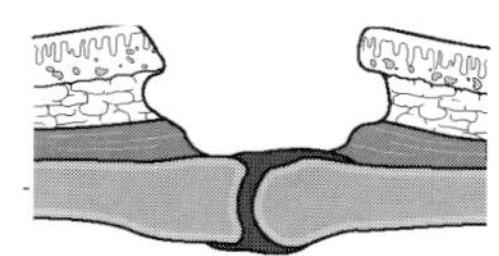

Third digit classification
for the nature of the wound bed

x.x0 Not applicable, intact skin
x.x1 Clean, with partial epithelialisation
x.x2 Clean, with or without granulation, but no obvious epithelialisation
x.x3 Soft slough, cream/yellow/green in colour
x.x4 Hard or leathery black/brown necrotic (dead/avascular) tissue

Fourth digit classification
for infective complications

x.xx0 No inflammation surrounding the wound bed
x.xx1 Inflammation surrounding the wound bed
x.xx2 Cellulitis bacteriologically confirmed

***Source*: Reid & Morison 1994a**

patients) found pressure sore calculation proved over-simplistic and unreliable for choosing therapeutic beds, and the weighting for inotropes needed revision, although using a scoring system helped raise staff awareness. Greater complexity may improve accuracy, but also discourage use. Like Waterlow's scale, Cubbin and Jackson's scale is an aid, not a substitute, for more detailed assessment. Lowery (1995) reports successfully adapting Cubbin and Jackson's scale (the 'Sunderland' scale); Sollars' (1998) single-patient study supports this adaptation. A revised version of Cubbin and Jackson's scale was published in 1999 (Jackson 1999).

A more sensitive scale has been developed for ICUs by Bateson *et al.* (1993). This was also published following a pilot study, although the sample size was 51 patients. While based on substantial research, its presentation appears (rather than is) unnecessarily complicated; the proposed 'next stage' for the scoring system does not appear to have been published yet, and the system has not been widely adopted.

Assessment is helped by using a scale. However, until a reliable scale for ICU use has been substantively validated, units should continue to use whichever scale they find most useful; this will usually be the one staff are most familiar with. Units dissatisfied with their current system should pilot other tools and consider adapting them through action research.

Prevention

Most intrinsic factors identified by Waterlow (1995) are either unalterable or the cause of ICU admission (although malnutrition and dehydration should be resolved). For all patients, pressure on skin can be decreased either by changing position or increasing the surface area over which pressure is spread. Two-hourly pressure area care owes more to ritual than logic; prevention strategies need to be individually planned following individual assessment of risk factors.

Many aids have been marketed; bedding includes:

- mattress overlays
- alternating pressure mattresses
- tilting beds
- fluidised beds

Booth (1993) lists many available mattresses, although others have been marketed since his article.

Mattress overlays and other static equipment are unsuitable for ICU (Waterlow 1995); although they help to spread pressure, low capillary occlusion pressures of ICU patients mean that ulceration is delayed rather than prevented. In addition, the lack of airflow from prolonged immobility allows the accumulation of perspiration.

Alternating pressure mattresses assist healing provided the capillary occlusion pressure remains below the minimum mattress inflation pressure. Some alternating pressure mattresses have static head areas to prevent seasickness; this exposes cranial skin to constant high pressures, and so checking for back-of-head sores should not be neglected.

Various *tilting* and turning beds have been developed for spinal injury units (Waterlow 1995). Kinetic therapy can assist ventilation (see Chapter 27), and also prevent pressure sores; it enables rotation through 124°, but hard mattresses and pressure from straps can often cause, rather than heal, sores (Dobson *et al.* 1993).

Fluidized silicone beds have proved popular in many units, although difficulties in maintaining upright positions are frequently identified by nurses. The beds are useful for patients with burns (Waterlow 1995) or large exposed wounds as they enable drainage of exudate; this can prevent the need for traumatic dressings.

Some aids are unhelpful or positively harmful. With the choice of commercial aids available, *improvised aids* are best avoided in view of the increasing levels of litigation and the professional individual accountability of nurses. For example, latex gloves filled with water can easily be overfilled (Waterlow 1995), thus exerting excessive (unmonitored) pressure on a single concave point and exposing patients' heels to greater pressure than if left on hospital mattresses.

Waterlow (1995) discourages use of powder for skin. Although *talc* dries perspiration and masks odours, so providing comfort and reducing the risk of breakdown from dampness, some patients are allergic to it. Talc is an aid to hygiene, not a substitute for pressure area care.

Waterlow recommends gel, head and elbow *pads* and 30° tilts for pillows (Waterlow 1995). High-risk ICU patients may gain little from such interventions, although anything reducing or delaying skin breakdown should be considered.

Changes in knowledge and products are rapid; just as many hospitals benefit from employing tissue viability nurses, ICUs can benefit from appointing a member of staff to specialise in tissue viability in order to:

- provide information for all unit staff
- apply information to the special needs and problems of ICU patients
- audit skincare
- link to wider resources (e.g. the hospital tissue viability nurse).

Cost

Pressure sores increase

- human suffering
- recovery time (1,000 kcal may be needed each day to replace exudate protein loss and promote healing)
- mortality
- financial costs (prolonged stay, additional treatments, litigation).

The much cited NHS costs of £200m per year (Waterlow 1985) will have escalated with inflation. Bateson *et al.* (1993) estimated cost of pressure sore management on a 14-bedded ICU and 8-bedded HDU to be £6,000 per month. The cost of treating just one severe pressure sore can be £40,000 (Waterlow 1995). But litigation costs can be higher: one ICU pressure sore resulted in an out-of-court settlement of £144,000 (Waterlow 1995), diverting significant funds from patient care. Tingle (1997a) cites costs ranging between £4,500 and £12,500 in recent cases where pressures sores contributed to mortality, but no records exist of nursing pressure area assessment.

Necrotising fasciitis

Necrotising fasciitis, an extension of cellulitis, is caused by aerobic and anaerobic soft tissue infection (Neal 1994). Although not a 'new' pathology, UK public concern followed 1994 media publicity of a 'killer bug' (Loudon 1994); progressively invasive and radical treatments, together with immunocompromise, make necrotising fasciitis a significant potential problem in ICUs.

Necrotising fasciitis usually follows minor trauma or surgery (Neal 1994), beginning as cellulitis unresponsive to antibiotics. Infection often progresses to septic inflammatory response syndrome (SIRS) and multiorgan dysfunction syndrome (MODS) (Roberts *et al.* 1985). Tissue necrosis causes gas production (hydrogen, methane, hydrogen sulphide, nitrogen) and putrid discharge (Neal 1994) – although purely streptococcal infections have no odour (Neal 1994). The smell (and grey colour) of rotting flesh, distressing enough for staff, will probably cause profound anxiety to patients and visitors. Air fresheners can help mask the smell, although chemicals should not be allowed to enter exposed wounds. Gross swelling of flesh (oedematous) may make patients almost unrecognisable so that visitors need to be carefully prepared.

Early stages of the disease are acutely painful (Neal 1994), but with progressive destruction of superficial nerve endings the later stages are often painless (Lipman 1997). Extensive infection often leaves residual deformity (Hinds & Watson 1996).

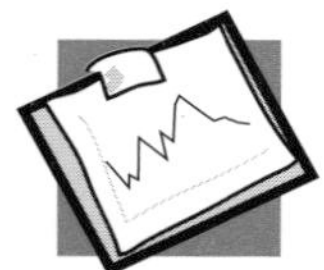

Implications for practice

- ICU patients can be at special risk of back-of-head pressure sores
- active nursing assessment of all skin surfaces and risk factors should be made at least once each day; assessment should identify any special aids needed
- no ideal assessment tool exists for ICU; units should use whichever tool they find useful, and may wish to adapt existing tools through action research
- improvised aids may cause harm, and so are usually best avoided

- pressure area aids should allow tissue perfusion, therefore pressures should be below capillary occlusion pressure (20–25 mmHg) for part of each cycle
- unit coordinators for tissue viability can offer many benefits

Summary

Skin has many functions; the cost of skin breakdown can be measured in mortality, humanitarian terms (morbidity), increased length of stay in ICU, increased financial costs and litigation.

Various scoring systems have been designed to assess skin integrity, but none are ideal for ICU, and the best system is only as good as the staff using it. Pressure sores continue to occur in ICU. The culture of guilt surrounding pressure sores is unhelpful to everyone; despite good nursing, sores will occur, and so nurses should assess and minimise risk factors in order to reduce the incidence.

Further reading

General nursing journals frequently carry articles on skincare; some journals specialise in the topic; regular library scans can identify new material.

Lowthian (1997) and Westrate & Bruining (1996) give useful ICU perspectives. Following up at least one article on the assessment scale used by your unit can identify its strengths and limitations. Waterlow (1995) is also worth reading, although it is now rather dated and also shows the expected bias for the author's own scale.

Occasional articles appear on necrotising fasciitis; Lipman (1997) is useful.

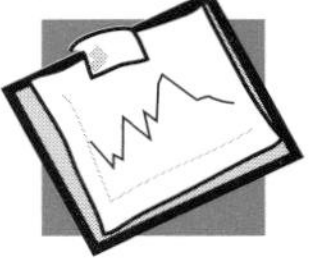

Clinical scenario

Gorgina Okra was admitted to intensive care following a cholecystectomy for postoperative respiratory management. She is 62 years old, of African ethnicity, weighs 90 kg and is 1.55 m tall. She has Type 2 diabetes and has not yet commenced an oral diet. She has an abdominal wound drain (T-tube) with large absorbent wound dressing, urinary catheter and oral endotracheal tube.

Q1. List Mrs Okra's intrinsic and extrinsic risk factors for developing pressure sore; include sources and likely sites.

Q2. Using some of the published or adapted pressure risk assessment tools with Mrs Okra, analyse her potential for developing skin damage. Which gives her the highest score risk?

Q3. Appraise the benefits and limitations of using a pressure relieving static mattress to those of a low air loss bed with Mrs Okra. Which would be best for her immediate care, longer-term recovery and prevention of skin pressure points? (Consider a broad range of factors such as patient comfort, costs, nurses preference for ease when delivering care, any weight restrictions, effects on systems physiologically, e.g. on hydration, skeletal support, posture, ventilation, etc.)

Chapter 13

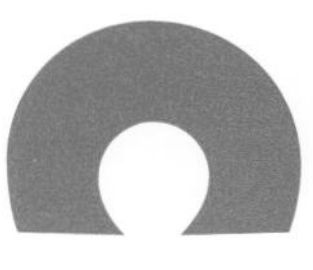
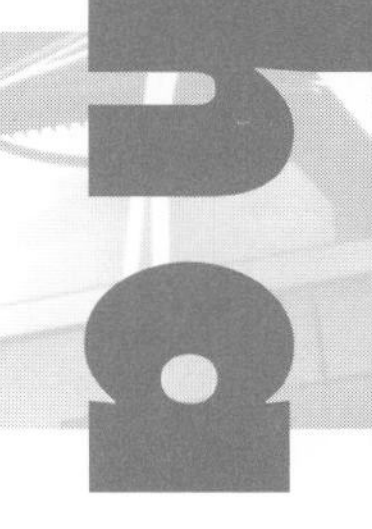
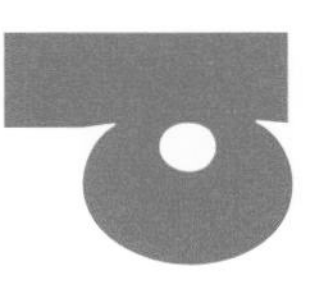
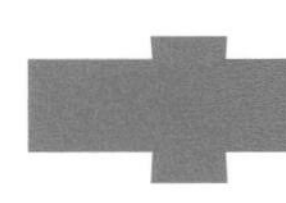
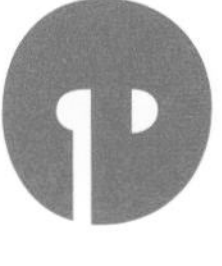

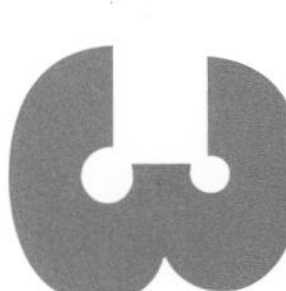

Paediatric admissions to adult ICUs

Fidelma Murphy

Contents

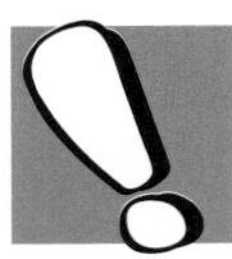

Fundamental knowledge

Specific anatomy and physiology of the child

Introduction

In 1993 the British Paediatric Association (BPA) report highlighted that substantial numbers of critically ill children were being cared for either in intensive care facilities designed for adults (one-fifth) or general ward areas. Although the BPA survey was not based on conclusive research evidence, it has been instrumental in commencing valuable debate regarding the need for efficient paediatric intensive care services within current NHS resources. There has been a wealth of guidance from both the clinical areas and policy makers; Department of Health (DoH 1997) recommendations indicate that designated general ICUs will continue to provide care for children requiring life support and that all general ICUs will need to initiate such care. To achieve optimal results for staff, child and family, adult intensive care nurses should develop their knowledge and become familiar with specific equipment associated with caring for critically ill children.

This chapter gives a brief overview of caring for children on adult ICUs, emphasis being placed on the psychological needs of children and their families. After describing the initial assessment, the effects of critical illness on major body systems are identified, and the implications for nursing care are drawn. The chapter includes the two most frequent paediatric pathophysiologies seen in adult ICUs: meningitis and acute upper airway obstruction.

Children are different

Caring for critically ill children requires nurses who are more familiar with nursing adults to adapt their skills and knowledge. Children differ from adults in several important ways: physically, psychologically and emotionally they are immature. Because of this many illnesses and their complications are more likely to occur in children. Immature respiratory and cardiovascular systems provide less reserve function so that children often deteriorate more rapidly. Children have higher metabolic rates, resulting in

- higher cardiac index
- greater gas exchange
- higher fluid intake per kilogram
- greater calorie intake per kilogram.

Although proportionately greater, absolute measures (e.g. cardiac output) are usually smaller, due to children being smaller than adults (Hazinski 1992).

Any nurse caring for critically ill children should recognise signs of organ dysfunction and failure, and respond appropriately when deterioration occurs.

Initial assessment

Hazinski (1992) emphasises the importance of every critical care nurse developing a system of determining the severity of each child's illness, extending the familiar **ABC of resuscitation** to seven points (Hazinski 1992):

- Airway
- Brain
- Circulation
- Drips/Drugs
- Electrolytes
- Fluids
- Gastrointestinal/genitourinary

Appearance

Skin colour and temperature may indicate cardiorespiratory distress; a pink colour must be consistent all over the child's body including mucous membranes, nail beds, palms of hands and soles of feet. Pale mucous membranes and mottled extremities may signify hypoxia. Poorly perfused extremities are cold to touch and have sluggish refill.

Responsiveness

Normal healthy infants make good eye contact, orientate to familiar faces and are visually attracted to bright colours. They should move all extremities spontaneously. Sick children become more irritable, making high pitched or weak cries. As illness progresses, all extremities may become flaccid and the child unresponsive.

Vital signs

Vital signs and respiratory effort should be evaluated at rest. Children's' pulse and respiratory rates normally increase during stress and decrease during sleep (Table 13.1); while this also occurs with adults, children's immature central nervous systems limit homeostatic controls, causing more exaggerated responses.

Table 13.1 **Normal parameters for a child at rest**

Age	*Pulse rate**	*Mean arterial pressure (mmHg)*	*Respiratory rate†*
<1 year	120–160	50–100	30–60
1–3 years	90–140	50–100	22–40
4–5 years	80–110	60–90	22–34
6–10 years	75–100	60–90	18–30
11–13 years	60–95	65–95	14–20

* beats/minute ;† breaths/minute

Psychosocial care

Paediatric nursing widely acknowledges the importance of treating the child not the illness (Platt report, DoH 1959). All patients have psychological and emotional needs, but the needs of the critically ill child differ from those of adults and recognition of this is paramount for the ICU nurse. Family, play, education and maintenance of routine become central considerations when nursing children.

Admission of a child to ICU causes extreme distress and is likely to throw the family unit into turmoil, necessitating nursing emphasis on integrating the needs of children and their families within holistic care. The way families respond to this disruption may drastically affect the sick child. In order to meet the needs of each family, these should be individually assessed by the nurse (Hazinski 1992).

When children are admitted to intensive care, family members often feel frustrated about not being able to contribute to the child's care and treatment. Allowing parents to remain with children and to help with care helps them to cope with this stressful situation, as well as providing the child with familiar and trusted people. Since parents know their children best, they should be allowed to participate in the care team; Cox (1992) emphasises the importance of partnership in care. Nurses can support families both by involving them in care and helping them to maintain home routine. As the family's confidence grows, they may wish to take over more aspects of the child's care.

Physical care

Critical illness often complicates various body systems. Although many of the effects on children are similar to those on adults, there are some important physiological differences. These are identified here.

Neurological

Evaluation of children's level of consciousness is based largely on alertness, response to environment and parents, level of activity and their cry. Neurological evaluation resembles that of an adult (see Chapter 22), but with infants some reflexes (e.g. **Babinski's sign**) remain. Management of sedation and muscle relaxants is discussed in Chapter 6.

Respiratory

Respiratory anatomy does not reach full maturity until approximately 8 years of age; after this the child is, in respiratory terms, considered an adult. The immature respiratory system differs not only in size and anatomical position but, with growth of the thorax, lung mechanisms are altered. Many anatomical differences affect respiratory care:

- Infants are obligatory nose breathers, with a longer epiglottis which may need to be lifted by a straight blade during intubation.
- Until puberty the cricoid ring is the narrowest part of the airway; being vulnerable to trauma and swelling; this limits endotracheal tube size.
- This cartilage acts as a physiological cuff and so uncuffed endotracheal tubes are used for children. Endotracheal tubes should allow a small leak while achieving adequate pulmonary inflation pressures.
- Mucous and oedema, which may have minimal affect on adult airways, often critically reduce airway radius and airflow in children. Paediatric artificial airways may quickly become obstructed by mucous, therefore humidification with an appropriate system is vital (Tibballs 1997).

Artificial ventilation for children is similar to adults, but with less margin for error (Betit *et al.* 1993). Children below 10 kg are usually ventilated with pressure control cycles; volume cycles are used for larger children. Pressure control ventilation reduces barotrauma in the immature lungs of smaller children and compensates for the airleak from uncuffed tubes.

Physiotherapy and appropriate positioning assists artificial ventilation. For infants, prone positioning does not interfere with diaphragmatic action (unlike supine positions). Nursing infants on alternate sides assists lung drainage. Unilateral lung disorders necessitate careful positioning: lying on the affected side helps to ventilate the good lung but decreases perfusion, improving overall oxygenation; positioning the affected lung uppermost helps drainage but impairs expansion, and so oxygenation. During physiotherapy the child is repositioned to assist lung drainage, possibly requiring additional oxygen during treatments (Robb 1995).

Endotracheal suctioning of adults and children is similar (see Chapter 5), but there are additional complications with children, requiring special considerations:

- correct size suction catheters
- suction pressures 7–13 kPa (50–100 mmHg)
- preoxygenation to prevent hypoxia
- during bagging, use of pressure monitors is advisable to prevent barotrauma
- limit manual inflation pressures to 10 cmH_2O above set peak pressures

Complications of endotracheal suction can include

- accidental extubation
- cilia damage (see Chapter 5)
- perforation of carina (rare)

Cardiovascular

Cardiac dysrhythmias and arrest are rare in children unless they have congenital abnormalities or are exposed to sustained hypoxia (e.g. respiratory distress/failure, shock). Limited respiratory reserves make children very sensitive to hypoxia. As with adults, persistent hypoxia causes metabolic acidosis and dysrhythmias (especially bradycardia); dysrhythmias reduce cardiac output, provoking cardiac arrest (Hazinski 1992).

As with adults, shock not responding to intravascular fluids and adequate oxygenation may require inotropic support. Inotropes are the same as those used for adults (see Chapter 34), but higher doses per kilogram may be needed and combinations of two or more are often used.

Fluid balance

Children's fluid requirements should always be individualised. Children have higher metabolic rates and greater insensible water loss than adults so that daily fluid requirement per kilogram (Table 13.2) is proportionally larger. Nurses should therefore consider the child's fluid balance and clinical condition when calculating children's fluid requirements. Fluid input includes all infusions, bolus drugs, flushes, transducer flushes and nutrition. Continuous transducer infusions deliver 3 ml/hour for each transducer when the pressure bag is inflated to 300 mmHg.

Table 13.2 Body weight daily maintenance formula

0–10 kg	100 ml/kg
11–20 kg	1,000 ml for first 10 kg + 50 ml/kg for kg 11–20
21–30 kg	1,500 ml for first 20 kg + 25 ml/kg for kg 21–30

Body surface area formula:
1500 ml/m^2 body surface area/day

Fluid challenges for hypovolaemia are given as a bolus of 10 ml/kg body weight, repeated as prescribed and indicated by clinical condition.

Electrolyte disturbances include hypoglycaemia, hypocalcaemia, hypo/hypernatraemia and hyperkalaemia (Hazinski 1992). As infants require high levels of glucose, drug infusions are ideally mixed in a glucose solution.

Normal urine output for children is 2 ml/kg body weight/hour below 2 years and 1 ml/kg/body weight/hour above 2 years. Total volume being small, a slight reduction is significant. If a catheter or collecting bag is not used, nappies should be weighed to maintain a correct fluid balance (1 g = approximately 1 ml water).

Differences of more than 4°C between core and peripheral temperature indicate inadequate perfusion, which may respond to a fluid challenge.

Immunological

Immaturity causes immunocompromise in the very young, making them especially prone to respiratory tract infections, meningitis and urinary tract infections. Infants and young children may show non-specific signs of infection, although temperature usually rises or falls significantly. Sepsis often causes:

- a reluctance to feed
- drowsiness
- vomiting
- failure to gain weight
- greyish pallor and an anxious look (Robb 1995)

Hygiene and care

Nurses should discuss and plan hygiene care with parents. Parents should be encouraged to continue their central role in the child's life, and be supported while they adjust to the ICU environment. Despite sedation, children may be aware of their parents' presence through sensory stimulation (touch, sound, smell).

Drugs and infusions

Drugs are given according to body weight (kg) so that actual doses may differ significantly between children. As nurses on general ICUs are more used to adult doses, and children have less reserve to tolerate drug errors than adults, nurses should check each dose carefully, using a paediatric formulary.

Common paediatric disorders admitted to ICU

Meningococcal disease

Meningococcal infection causes high childhood morbidity and mortality worldwide (Nadel *et al.* 1995). Before antibiotics were available, infection was fatal. Antibiotics have reduced mortality by 10–20 per cent. Children with moderate to severe meningococcal disease are usually admitted to ICU.

Meningococcal disease usually causes meningitis, but can also cause septicaemia. Meningococcal meningitis increases intracranial pressure, resulting in a range of neurological symptoms common to all forms of meningitis:

- high fever
- vomiting
- drowsiness
- headache
- stiff neck
- photophobia

- declining level of consciousness
- convulsions
- coma

With meningitis, circulatory failure is rare. A purpuric rash, or meningococci in blood or cerebrospinal fluid (CSF), will confirm the diagnosis of meningitis.

Meningococcal septicemia is less common but carries greater mortality. Features are similar to many febrile childhood illnesses, but the disease progresses rapidly. Clinical features include:

- poor peripheral perfusion – capillary refill more than three seconds
- increased toe/core gap
- tachycardia (see above for normal rates)
- cold, mottled peripheries
- oliguria/anuria
- tachypnoea
- cyanosis
- ultimately a low blood pressure (not a feature of shock in children until a preterminal stage)
- petechiae/purpuric rash

Treatment of meningococcal disease is supportive, with a third generation cephalosporin (e.g. cefotaxime, ceftriaxone) (Nadel *et al.* 1995). Meningococcal disease can rapidly become fatal; prompt specialist care in appropriate units can make the difference between survival and death. Children with meningococcal disease may require urgent transfer to paediatric intensive care.

Acute upper airway obstruction

This is a medical emergency, requiring immediate treatment. The airway must be secured while the cause of obstruction is being identified. Children with obstructed airways are usually otherwise fit and healthy so that the cause of obstruction will usually be completely reversible (Hillman & Bishop 1996). Upper airway obstruction is usually caused by:

- viral croup
- acute epiglottitis
- foreign body
- oedema

Croup is far more common than epiglottitis. Features of viral croup include:

- usually occurring at 3–6 months

- afebrile/mild fever
- stridor (especially when upset)
- hoarse cough
- upper respiratory tract infection for 2–3 days

Epiglottitis usually occurs in children aged between 2 and 6 years, but can occur at any age. Typically,

- the child sits upright, mouth open with drooling secretions
- history is less than 24 hours
- there is no cough.

However caused, upper airway obstruction results in stridor and tachypnoea; with exhaustion, children become bradycardic, cyanotic and bradypnoeic (Hillman & Bishop 1996). A clear airway should be established urgently in all severe cases.

Viral croup is treated with nebulised adrenaline 2–5 ml of 1:1000 solution every 1–2 hours. Antibiotics are indicated only if bacterial tracheitis is present. Steroids may be beneficial. To reduce cortical stimulation, children should be nursed in quiet, relaxed environments, and not upset.

Epiglottitis is diagnosed by clinical signs; children should not lie flat, and the enlarged epiglottis should only be examined for intubation. Blood cultures should be taken and antibiotics such as ampicillin or ceftriaxone should be commenced intravenously. The response to treatment tends to be rapid, possibly within 24 hours.

ICU admission may also be needed for other diseases involving organ dysfunction, such as convulsions, postoperative care and trauma. Critically ill children need a safe environment, with staff who are confident and competent in their care.

Implications for practice

- all nurses caring for critically ill children should keep updated in their knowledge and skills
- adult ICUs should provide specialist equipment to adequately care for children
- ICU nurses should adapt their skills to suit the needs of each child and their family
- nursing a child should include considering the whole family's needs
- environments should be suitably adapted for both the child and family

Summary

Caring for critically ill children requires ICU nurses to adapt existing skills. Many skills are transferable from adult nursing, but size and volumes of drugs and other treatments need special care. Parents and family are central to each child's care, and so ICU nurses should actively involve and include them in care.

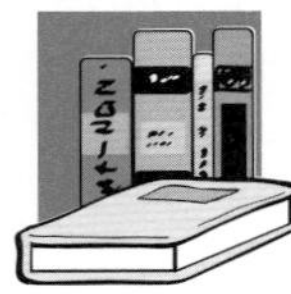

Further reading

Material about children frequently appears in ICU literature, but most is written from paediatric ICU perspectives; Robb (1995) is a useful article about nursing children in adult ICUs. Hazinski (1992) is a useful reference text.

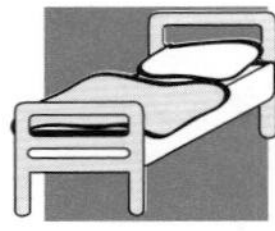

Clinical scenario

Rebecca Brooks, a 7-year-old, was transferred to adult ICU with acute breathing difficulties. Her mother and two older brothers aged 10 and 12 years accompany her. On admission Rebecca is self-ventilating with a respiratory rate of 46 breaths per minute, audible stridor and use of accessory muscle particularly on expiration, heart rate of 130/min and core temperature of 39.2°C.

Q.1 How should the bed area be prepared for Rebecca and her family? Specify resources needed (e.g. equipment, sizes, possible therapies and investigations, specialists).

Q.2 Humidified oxygen is administered via a facemask. Rebecca is very distressed and dislikes this therapy. Analyse various nursing strategies and other approaches which may promote her compliance with oxygen therapy (e.g. alternative O_2 administration equipment, drugs, restraints, involvement of mother and siblings, story telling, magical thinking).

Q.3 From the literature, review the expected developmental and behavioural milestones for a child of Rebecca's age. Consider the potential impact of the ICU environment on Rebecca and also that of her and her family's presence on other ICU patients.

Chapter 14

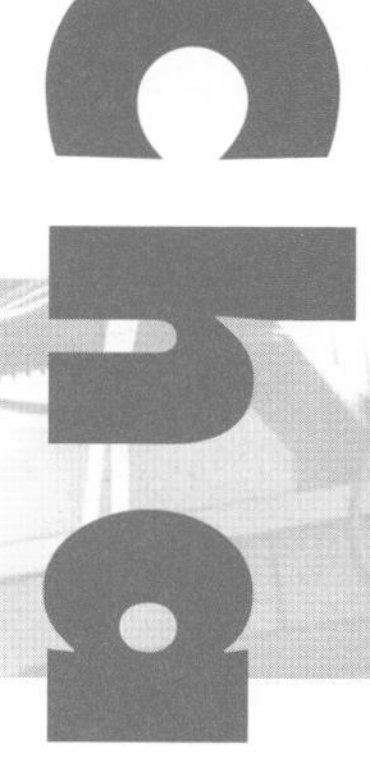

Older adults in ICU

Contents

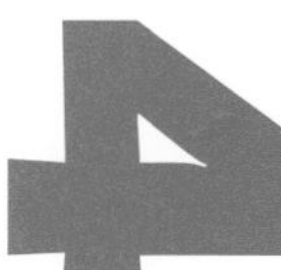

Introduction

Although the UK population is ageing, and about half of general ICU admissions are older adults (a number likely to grow), there is limited material about older people in specialist literature, making elders a potentially neglected majority; comparisons with quantity and quality of paediatric critical care literature against numbers of paediatric admissions to adult ICUs illustrate the relative neglect.

Being old is not a disease, and diseases suffered by older people are not unique to their cohorts. Physiological ageing, multiple pathology and polypharmacy often complicate their physical needs, while negative attitudes (by society, hospitals and staff) can mar their psychological care.

The speciality of caring for older people is often considered a 'Cinderella' service (lacking the money, glamour, rewards or career prospects of acute specialities such as ICU). This ignores significant contributions that nurses specialising in caring for older patients have made (e.g. primary nursing). Caring for older people requires special skills and knowledge; achieving quality care for critically ill older patients combines the knowledge of two specialities. ICUs should have RSCNs on duty whenever children are admitted (Fulbrook 1996a), but no similar expectation is made for nurse specialists qualified in caring for older people.

Most older people are healthy, but healthy people are not admitted to ICUs. This chapter outlines the effects of physiological ageing on major body systems before focusing on wider social and attitudinal issues. The International Council of Nurses' position statement on 'Nursing Care of the Elderly' (ICN 1991) advocates that nurses should help older people maintain independence, self-care and quality of life. Such aims can be easily lost in events of physiological crises and technological intervention.

Ageing

Ageing can be:

- chronological (number of years lived, e.g. over 65)
- sociological (role in society, e.g. retirement)
- physiological (physical function) (de Beauvoir 1970).

Chronological ageing is statistically simple and clear, and is adopted by much medical literature (especially quantitative research), but it is usually medically arbitrary, failing to recognise each person's uniqueness and individuality. Nurses should therefore approach each person as an individual, rather than as chronological stereotypes.

Physiological ageing is individual to each person, influenced by multiple factors such as gender, genetic inheritance, lifestyle and social class (Black *et al.* 1988). Ageing almost inevitably brings decline in function; but rates of decline vary between systems and individuals. *Reserve function* (the difference between actual level of function and minimum function needed for homeostasis) provides a barrier against disease; progressive reduction in reserve function increases likelihood of chronic disease in later years (e.g. diabetes mellitus). As reserve function of all systems (variably) declines, multiple pathology and effects become more likely (Kilner & Janes 1997); so reduced renal and hepatic function prolong metabolism (and so effect) of drugs and toxins.

Underlying chronic conditions (including chronic pain such as arthritis) are more common among older people. Arthritis may be visually apparent, but individual assessment may identify other needs, enabling nurses to avoid inflicting accidental pain.

Physiological effects

With age, *cardiovascular homeostasis* slows and baroreceptors become less sensitive (Rebenson-Piano 1989), impairing response to sudden hypotension.

Cross-linking of collagen fibres causes calcium deposit formation (Herbert 1991), reducing penetrability of arterial tunica to lipids (e.g. cholesterol) and increasing systemic vascular resistance (and hypertension) by about 1 per cent every year from the age of 40 (Herbert 1991). Lipid accumulation forms plaque, enabling platelet adhesion and aggregation within the arterial lumen (Todd 1997). Thrombi and emboli can cause ischaemia and major organ failure (cerebrovascular accidents, myocardial infarction, renal failure, pulmonary embolus). Myocardial collagen cross-linking limits ventricular filling, so reducing stroke volume. Most older patients in ICU have myocardial insufficiency from coronary artery disease (endemic in the UK).

Most *respiratory insufficiency* in older people is caused by ageing of airway tissue, chemical damage (especially smoking and environmental pollutants) and muscle atrophy. Average pulmonary function is halved between 30 and 90 years of age (Hough 1996); decreased expiratory recoil reduces vital capacity and lung compliance. Pulmonary circulation also suffers atherosclerosis, increases pulmonary artery pressures.

Older people are more frequently *malnourished* than younger people (Doyle 1990) due to factors such as poverty, poor mobility, maldentition, lack of facilities or constipation. Malnourishment may reduce plasma albumin by 10–20 per cent (Wingard *et al.* 1991) – leading to hypovolaemia and oedema – and cause immunocompromise and muscle weakness.

Gastrointestinal tract atrophy makes villi shorter and broader, reducing bowel fluid absorption (Herbert 1991).

Hepatic blood flow falls by nearly half (Wingard *et al.* 1991), causing decline in hepatic function; atrophy reduces storage capacity for nutrients (Herbert 1991) (glucose and trace elements – e.g. iron and vitamins). The liver is a major source of body heat, and so reduced hepatic function contributes to impaired thermoregulation.

Central nervous system degeneration progresses throughout life so that older patients are more likely to suffer:

- organic brain disease (e.g. dementia)
- acute confusion
- sensory impairment (vision, hearing, touch, taste, smell)
- cerebral thrombi/emboli
- toxaemia/uraemia (from renal/hepatic impairment) (Schwertz & Buschmann 1989).

Thus older people are more often labelled 'confused' than younger people. However, confusion may be caused by

- absence of sensory aids (glasses, hearing aid)
- hypoxia
- toxic metabolites
- alcohol (alcoholism is increasing among older people (Godard & Gask 1991)).

Therefore, apparent 'confusion' should be holistically assessed, and care planned to meet individual needs.

Reality orientation can provoke aggression (sensory imbalance); psychiatry has developed a range of alternative approaches, such as validation therapy (Feil 1993), that seeks to empower rather than control people, but most approaches rely on verbal responses, limiting their value for intubated, sedated patients.

Renal problems typically associated with ageing (e.g. incontinence, prostatic obstruction) are alleviated by catheterisation. Impaired renal function of most ICU patients is compounded by ageing: creatinine clearance declines about 6.5 ml per minute per decade after the age of 40 (Hudak *et al.* 1998).

As *skin ages*, epidermis flattens, with loss of papillae (Herbert 1991) so that epidermal and dermal layers peel apart more easily, causing pressure sores from sheering (see Chapter 12). Capillary loss reduces oxygen, nutrients and hydration; skin becomes dryer, more brittle and prone to tearing with delayed healing. Re-epithelialisation time doubles between 25 and 75 years of age. Most pressure sores occur in people over 70 years of age (Mihissin & Houghton 1995), hence the weighting for age on Waterlow and other assessment scales. Pressure area aids can reduce the incidence of pressure sores, but optimising endogenous factors (nutrition, perfusion) reduces risks. Reduced capillary perfusion impairs cutaneous drug absorption (e.g. GTN/fentanyl patches, 'essential' massage oils) and removal of metabolic waste (e.g. acidosis).

Muscular and skeletal atrophy contribute to weakness (which delays weaning from ventilation).

Critical care

Approximately half of all ICU patients are over 65 years old (Adelman *et al.* 1994); 18 per cent of all admissions are over 75 (Bodenham *et al.* 1994). As the numbers of over 75s peak in the next quarter century, the 'old old' (85+) will double, while the numbers of 'younger old' (65–75) will remain virtually static; since illness generally increases with age, the number of old patients admitted to ICU is likely to increase. This raises ethical questions:

- Should older patients be admitted to ICU?
- With limited resources, what proportion should be spent on older people?
- Can suffering caused by ICU admission be justified by outcome?
- Should older patients be treated differently?

Most studies on older ICU patients measure mortality (increasingly, to hospital discharge or later); whether old patients benefit from critical care, or whether consuming limited critical care resources for the old is justified, is debated, partly depending on different measures and viewpoints. Elpern *et al.* (1989) found mortality high and treatment costly among older patients receiving prolonged ventilation, and Ridley *et al.* (1990) found post-discharge survival poor, but Chalfin and Carlon (1990) found older patients used fewer resources and obtained better outcomes from ICU than younger patients. ICU mortality in the over-80s is about 35 per cent (Lakshmipathi *et al.* 1992; Ryan 1997b); this is in the upper range of overall ICU mortality and so reflects the conclusions of Kilner and Janes (1997) and many earlier studies (e.g. Heuser *et al.* (1992), Chelluri *et al.* (1993)) that age alone is a poor indicator for ICU admission and treatment.

Mortality is easily measured, but quality of life is a more valuable (if more subjective) measure of outcome. Mahul *et al.* (1991) found that most elderly survivors of ICU returned home to regain independent lifestyles. However, overt or covert admission criteria may prevent sicker elderly patients being admitted, so that comparison with younger (potentially sicker) cohorts of ICU patients can be misleading; Castillo-Lorente *et al.*'s (1997) Spanish study found that over-75s received less aggressive care and less frequent treatment than younger patients. Conflicting research and practice makes healthcare for the critically ill older adults into a covert lottery.

Ageism

'Ageism', the 'notion that people cease to be people … by virtue of having lived a specific number of years' (Comfort 1977: 35), leads to

- prejudice
- stereotyping
- negatives attitudes (Redfern 1991)

and may be overt (e.g. age limits for admission) or covert (e.g. attitudes).

Overt chronological age criteria, once commonplace in ICUs (Artinian *et al.* 1993), are now rare, but reluctance to refer or admit older people 'too sick' for ICU attention persists (Knaus 1987; Chalfin & Carlon 1990). Evidence-based medicine and predictive scoring (e.g. APACHE (Knaus *et al.* 1985)) can create covert ageism. (APACHE II adds points for chronological age to account for physiological ageing; as pathophysiologies are also scored separately, older people are scored differently from younger people with similar conditions.)

Like the Waterlow pressure sore scoring system, APACHE adds increments for age. Older people are likely to suffer from multiple pathology, but physiological deficits should have been identified in other scores and so APACHE scores of older people are disproportionately increased. APACHE II and the supposedly less ageist APACHE III (Knaus *et al.* 1991) retain age-related scores.

Maclean (1989) suggests that old people receive suboptimal critical care due to stereotyping by staff; applicability to UK ICUs today is debatable, but staff should beware of insidious prejudice, stereotyping or other negative attitudes (e.g. speaking loudly to all old people, rather than assessing whether they have any hearing deficit; adopting over-familiar language, such as addressing them as 'dear').

Today's elders grew up before the National Health Service existed, and so remember a very different society (and social values) – doctors (and nurses) then were presumed always to know best. Therefore, the beliefs and values of the older patients may differ significantly from those of the nurses caring for them – and different generational values may cause misunderstandings.

Bereavement, social mobility and physical immobility are more likely to leave older people isolated, depriving them of the social supports (families, friends) that younger people usually have; friends and family may treat the older person as a burden. Psychological isolation can become self-fulfilling, encouraging older people to adopt child-like dependent behaviour and/or appear confused.

Problems encountered by older people using hospital services can persist after leaving the department; specialised assessment forms for older people (e.g. Kingston and Hopwood 1994) can help discharge planning.

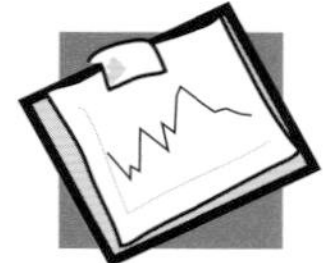

Implications for practice

- older patients already form about one-half of UK ICU admissions; numbers will probably increase, ICU nurses should actively consider needs and quality of care
- the function of all body systems declines with age; rate of decline varies between systems and individuals so that nursing care should be individualised and holistic

- in-service and post-registration education should include significant focus on nursing older people in ICUs
- ageism, insidious throughout society, can easily and insidiously influence care; reflecting on and evaluating nursing care (individually and in groups) can help to identify areas for development

Summary

Definitions of 'old' are arbitrary, but pragmatically many ICU admissions are 'old' – a potentially neglected majority. The paucity of literature on older patients in ICUs makes this one of the most neglected aspects on ICU nursing.

Although pathologies experienced by older people are largely those suffered by younger patients, multiple pathologies and system dysfunction make physiological needs of older patients complex; ICU admission can also threaten their psychological and social health. Nurses can humanise potentially threatening and ageist ICU environments to meet the needs of older patients.

Further reading

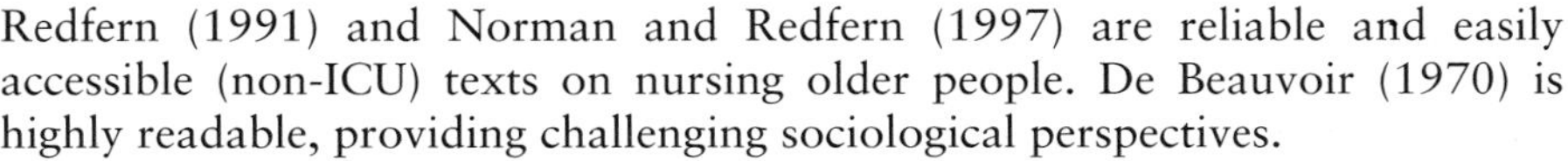

Redfern (1991) and Norman and Redfern (1997) are reliable and easily accessible (non-ICU) texts on nursing older people. De Beauvoir (1970) is highly readable, providing challenging sociological perspectives.

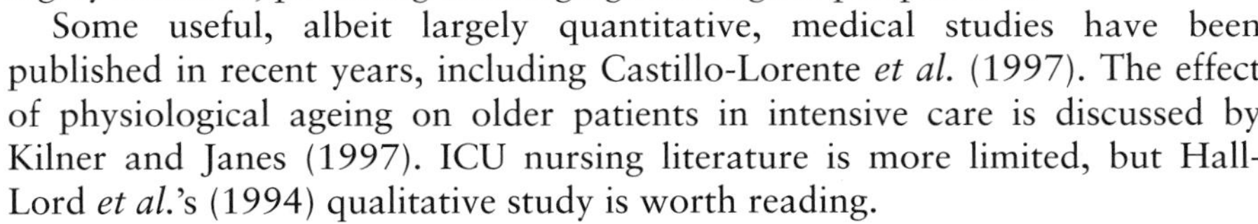

Some useful, albeit largely quantitative, medical studies have been published in recent years, including Castillo-Lorente *et al.* (1997). The effect of physiological ageing on older patients in intensive care is discussed by Kilner and Janes (1997). ICU nursing literature is more limited, but Hall-Lord *et al.*'s (1994) qualitative study is worth reading.

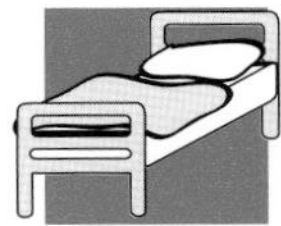

Clinical scenario

Frank Hobson is a very socially active and independent 84-year-old retired civil servant. He enjoys completing crossword puzzles and is a keen bridge player. Mr Hobson was admitted to ICU following elective repair of aortic aneurysm.

Q.1 List the expected normal parameters of an 84-year-old male for the range vital signs and investigations, e.g. BP, HR, ECG, CVP, respiratory rate, SaO_2, PO_2, CO_2, pH, etc. Note the main age-related physiological changes and how these are incorporated into planning postoperative care.

When conscious and extubated, Mr Hobson becomes very

disorientated and confused. His friends and family state this is not his normal behaviour and are concerned.

Q.2 Analyse possible causes of Mr Hobson's altered mental state (e.g. drugs, interventions, auditory, visual and short-term memory changes, ICU environment, other stimuli/factors).

Q.3 Evaluate the long-term survival of 84-year-old ICU patients following discharge from hospital. Formulate nursing strategies that the ICU nurse can use to:

(a) promote Mr Hobson's physical and mental recovery;
(b) prepare Mr Hobson and his family for discharge;
(c) enhance the quality of his life.

Chapter 15

Infection control

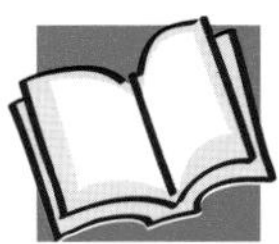

Contents

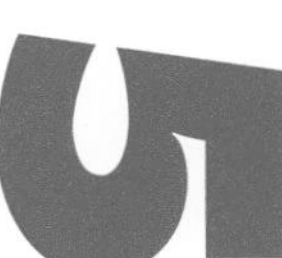

Introduction

ICU patients are particularly vulnerable to infection due to

- immunocompromise
- treatments
- contact
- invasive procedures/monitoring

Infection significantly increases

- mortality
- length of stay
- costs (human and financial)

Controlling infection has generated much research and debate, but fewer solutions.

This chapter identifies incidence, sources and effects of infection in ICUs, describes some prevalent bacteria (multiresistant *Staphylococcus aureus*, *Pseudomonas* sp.) and medical/nursing treatments, but emphasis is placed on prevention rather than treatment. Maintaining safe environments is fundamental to nursing: nurses can do much to reduce **nosocomial infection** rates in ICUs.

Colonies of organisms may be harmless ('commensals', e.g. skin, gut); 'infection' occurs only when hosts develop pathological responses to microorganisms. Destroying commensals enables opportunist organisms to replace them.

Immunocompromise and infection are often part of a complex pathological process; related material can be found in other chapters, especially chapters 9, 39 and 40.

Van Saene *et al.* (1993) suggest that ICU mortality is caused by

- underlying disease
- infection on admission
- ICU acquired infection.

Underlying disease (possibly due to infection) may cause ICU admission, but significant mortality results from admission. Patients with pre-existing infections need treatment and medical support, but this chapter focuses on ICU acquired infection and prevention.

Infection can be endogenous or exogenous. Endogenous infection (from organisms already harboured by patients) on ICUs usually occurs through the respiratory tract (e.g. ventilator associated pneumonia – VAP), but can also occur through skin and gut. Exogenous infection is usually through contact (staff, procedures, equipment), but can also be airborne.

Infection in intensive care units

Overall, nosocomial (hospital acquired infection – HAI) rates remain 8–10 per cent (Emmerson 1997), ICU rates being variable, but higher: Emmerson (1997) cites 60 per cent. Trilla's (1994) American study found that one-quarter of hospital infections occurred in ICUs, and that ICUs caused most hospital outbreaks of infection. Infection rates climb steeply after a few days on ICU, Alcock and Ledingham (1990) suggesting that four-fifths of ICU patients develop infection after five or more days – an ironic contrast to Nightingale's ([1859] 1980) suggestion that hospitals should do the sick no harm.

Most ICU patients are immunocompromised, whether from pathologies (e.g. hepatic failure, leukaemia, AIDS) or treatments (immunosuppressive drugs), making them susceptible to opportunistic infection from organisms colonising (but not necessarily infecting) healthier people. Each member of staff is a potential carrier of infection. Immunity develops with age and exposure to pathogens so that children are at greater risk of infection (e.g. adult leucocyte and T-lymphocyte levels are not reached until 2–3 years of age (Robb 1995)). Highly invasive equipment used with critically ill patients provides multiple entry sites for microorganisms so that benefits should be weighed against infection risks.

Nosocomial pneumonia is the main cause of ICU infection. ICU-acquired infection depends largely on whether airway reflexes are impaired on admission and whether artificial ventilation is used; most studies show high (if variable) infection rates: artificial ventilation increases pneumonia rates twentyfold (Crowe 1996), although Papazian *et al.* (1996) found no increase in mortality from ventilator-associated pneumonia.

Enteral tubes and infected feeds facilitate microorganisms entry into the gut, bypassing many nonspecific immune defences (e.g. gut acid/alkaline contrasts); infected parenteral nutrition and equipment facilitates entry directly into the bloodstream. Feeds standing for prolonged times at room temperature provide ideal media for bacterial growth. The fasting gut (parenteral/no nutrition) is a major mediator for infection.

EPIC (European Prevalence of Infection in Intensive Care)

The study by Vincent *et al.* (1995), 'European Prevalence of Infection in Intensive Care' (EPIC), is the most substantial study of ICU infection. Data from a single day (29 April 1992), together with patient outcome 30 days later, was collected from over 10,000 patients across 1,417 ICUs in 17 European countries. Applicability to individual nations will vary (e.g. UK ICU patients are sicker) and seasonal factors may have influenced results.

EPIC identified seven key risk factors predisposing to ICU infection:

- pulmonary artery catheters
- central lines

- stress ulcer prophylaxis
- urinary catheters
- mechanical ventilation
- trauma on admission
- length of stay

The study found that most ICUs mixed medical and surgical patients so that immunocompromised but uninfected surgical patients could be exposed to bacteria from medical patients admitted for treatment of infection.

Forty-five per cent of patients stayed over 5 days, with infection rates tripling after 3–4 days. Patients staying longer were usually sicker, but exposure to secondary infections compounded mortality. The report suggested that one-half of nosocomial infections were preventable, with risks increasing when units had more than eleven beds.

The two most prevalent organisms identified by EPIC were *Staphylococcus aureus* (30.1 per cent) and *Pseudomonas* sp. (32.1 per cent) (Rennie 1993b), both opportunistic infections.

Organisms

Bacteria are small, usually 1–2 micrometres in diameter, and a single bacterium will divide up to a million times within 6 hours (Wilson 1997). Gram positive or gram negative levels indicate whether bacteria retain crystal violet-iodine complex stain (Murray *et al.* 1994). Gram positive organisms, such as

Acinetobacter spp.
Enterobacter spp.
Escherichia coli
Klebsiella spp.
Proteus spp.
Pseudomonas spp.
Serratia spp.

are usually found in the community, are easily treated and so less problematic than gram negative (hospital) organisms, such as

- Staphylococci (including multiresistant *Staphylococcus aureus* – MRSA)
- Streptococci

although incidence of serious gram positive infections is increasing (Fagan 1995).

Damage to gram negative bacterial membranes (e.g. from complements and antibiotics) exposes lipid-A (Kimmings *et al.* 1994). Lipid-A

- induces fever
- initiates complement and coagulation cascades
- activates B-lymphocytes
- stimulates production of TNF_{α}, interleukin-1 and prostaglandins (Murray *et al.* 1994)

These damage endothelium, releasing vasoactive substances and enabling oedema formation (including pulmonary). Gram negative organisms cause 70 per cent of all cases of sepsis (Wardle 1996), while mortality from gram negative septicaemia is 40–70 per cent (Michie & Marley 1992).

Most *Staphylococcus aureus* remains methicillin sensitive (MSSA), but methicillin resistant *Staphylococcus aureus* (MRSA) causes more bacteraemia and sepsis (Humphreys & Duckworth 1997), increasing mortality twentyfold (Rello *et al.* 1994). There are over 170 strains of Staphylococci, mutations and variants making control problematic.

Duckworth (1990) cites a 1982 American study which found that MRSA caused nearly one-third of bacteraemias and nearly one-half of bacteraemic deaths. In this study, most MRSA outbreaks originated in ICUs (ICUs transfer patients to most hospital wards).

Skin colonisation (throat, groin, axillae) by Staphylococci is widespread (Murray *et al.* 1994) (30 per cent of the population) so that surgery, wounds, oral trauma (intubation, suction) and invasive treatment/monitoring provide access for infection. Using gloves significantly reduces nosocomial MRSA infection (Hartstein *et al.* 1995).

MRSA infection is difficult and expensive to treat. Chlorhexidine reduces surface colonisation, while most strains remain susceptible to vancomycin (Murray *et al.* 1994) and tiecoplanin, although recent emergence of epidemic strains of MRSA (EMRSA), especially strains 15 and 16, are more difficult to control (Cookson 1997).

Disposable aprons and theatre-style clothing can reduce carriage: Amyes and Thomson (1995) cite a Swedish finding that 20 per cent of staff were colonised, but 82 per cent of their clothes carried MRSA.

Most strains of *Pseudomonas* cannot survive human body temperatures, but *Pseudomonas aeruginosa* grows at body temperatures, tolerates 40–42°C (Murray *et al.* 1994), and survives until exposed to 58°C for one hour (Wilson 1985).

An opportunistic organism, skin colonisation occurs in only 2 per cent of healthy adults, but 38 per cent of hospitalised patients and 78 per cent of immunocompromised patients (Murray *et al.* 1994). It especially colonises moist environments (e.g. water humidifiers, washbasins) (Stewart & Beswick 1977). *Pseudomonas*, the most prevalent organism identified by EPIC, remains the single main cause of ventilator-associated pneumonia (Brewer *et al.* 1996; Crowe 1996).

Vancomycin-resistant enterococci (VRE) is increasingly prevalent (Molyneux & Chadwick 1997), and as vancomycin is used to treat many resistant microorganisms, this poses a major threat.

Fungi are a form of plant life. Fungal infection and mortality among critically ill patients are rising due to increasing immunosuppression (transplants, leukaemia, AIDS) (Richardson 1994). The most common fungal infection in ICUs is from the *Candida* spp. Amphotericin is the most widely used antifungal drug, although some fungi have developed resistance to this (Richardson 1994). Since ICU patients are especially susceptible to oral and skinfold fungal infection, maintaining hygiene significantly reduces infection rates.

Controlling infection

Infection-free environments remain unrealistic, but the spread of infection can be controlled. Endogenous infection requires

- a source
- means of transmission
- means of entry.

Removing one link breaks the chain of infection.

Family and friends rarely move between patients, but *staff* can easily transfer hospital (often resistant) pathogens between patients. Hygiene (especially handwashing) temporarily reduces numbers of skin-surface bacteria; particularly problematic pathogens may be targeted by specific treatments for staff (e.g. chlorhexidine to remove multiresistant *Staphylococcus aureus* – MRSA). The use of gloves and no-touch techniques significantly reduces cross-infection, but handwashing remains the simplest and most important way to reduce infection; minimising movement of staff between patients also reduces risks. While nurses need help for many aspects of care, the one-to-one nurse/patient ratio of most ICUs helps to limit the movement of nurses; other staff groups necessarily need to move between patients, especially sicker patients, so that nurses should discourage any unnecessary staff.

Movement of *equipment* between patients can also spread infection. Where dedicated equipment is not practical (e.g. portable X-ray machines, 12-lead ECG machines), nurses should encourage staff to ensure that any equipment touching patients is clean. Most equipment is used with the sickest, most susceptible, patients.

Airborne bacteria can also be transmitted through

- dust
- airborne skin scales
- droplets (e.g. from endotracheal suction – see Chapter 5)

Airborne infection can be reduced by

- recommended ICU bedspaces of 20 m^2 (Intensive Care Society 1992)
- hygiene

- planning higher-risk procedures at times of least disturbance
- careful disposal of linen (e.g. bringing linen skips/bags to bedsides and gently placing the side of the linen on which the patient has been lying inmost to minimise shedding of skin scales)
- air-flow systems

Handwashing remains the simplest, easiest, cheapest and most important way to reduce hospital-acquired infections (Doebbling *et al.* 1992), but is often inadequately or poorly performed and relegated to a 'basic' task which, because everyone should know, remains inadequately taught. Washing hands thoroughly between contact with different patients reduces cross-infection – 20–40 per cent of pathogens are transmitted through touch (Weinsten 1991); everyone entering an ICU should be reminded to wash their hands.

Taylor's (1978) classic study of nurses' handwashing techniques identified poor technique by qualified staff; student nurses fared better, possibly due to recent education or anxieties about their clinical assessment. Poor handwashing technique may be improved through continuing (in-service) education (Gould & Chamberlain 1994) and feedback (Mayer *et al.* 1986), although long-term benefits are limited (Mason 1991), necessitating frequent updating.

Taylor also found that while palms of hands were effectively cleaned when handwashing, thumbs, tips of fingers and backs of hands were poorly washed. Fingertips, the most likely part to touch patients, may harbour bacteria unless consciously washed – observing almost anyone washing their hands (in or outside hospital) supports Taylor's observation.

Hands should be dried thoroughly after washing; wet hands (and wet alcohol) provide ideal warm, moist environments for bacterial growth.

Each ICU bedspace should have its own washbasin (Hinds & Watson 1996) to

- facilitate handwashing
- isolate pathogens to patients' own washbasin.

Recontamination after handwashing can be reduced by

- elbow-operated taps
- disposable towels (not trailing in water)
- foot-operated pedal bins.

These should be accessible and maintained (tap levers blocked by other wall fittings, empty towel dispensers or broken pedal bins are counterproductive).

Chlorhexidine causes a greater reduction in skin surface bacteria than soap (Doebbling *et al.* 1992). Alcohol rubs are as effective as handwashing, provided the alcohol is allowed to dry (Heinz & Yakovich 1988).

Gowns/aprons reduce transmission of bacteria carried on staff clothing, while reminding staff to wash their hands (associations with 'gowning up') and discouraging unnecessary staff from visiting bed areas. Compared to theatre gowns, aprons worn on most ICUs leave significant areas exposed, some of which are likely to touch patients and bedding.

Some units adopt colour codes for each bedspace; by limiting staff having direct patient contact to those wearing the apron colour for the bedspace ensures that staff change aprons (and wash hands) between patients.

Ideally clean *uniforms* should be worn each shift, and not worn outside the unit. Infected clothing is both a medium for growth and a means of transfer. Inadequate hospital laundry supply or turnover and limited changing facilities at work encourages staff to wash uniforms at home. Hospital laundry washes of 71°C kill most microorganisms (Wilson 1997) (although not necessarily hepatitis B); while uniforms should withstand such temperatures, most casual clothing will not (see labels on clothing). Home washes are usually considerably cooler and domestic washing therefore seldom sterilises clothes. Hot-air dryers may also be extensively contaminated with bacteria (Bruton 1995). ICUs using theatre-style 'pyjamas suits' need adequate supplies to ensure all staff have clean uniforms each shift.

Staff from other areas in direct contact with patients should be encouraged to either change into unit clothing, or remove jackets and coats worn outside the unit (before washing their hands).

Everyone in direct patient contact is a potential source of infection. Critical illness necessitates contact with many staff, but *unnecessary staff* should be discouraged from visiting, and movement of staff between beds minimised. Conflicts with educational needs (particularly in teaching hospitals) need to be evaluated against risks to patients. Units should not be used as corridors between other parts of the hospital.

EPIC identified that one-quarter of units had *infection control nurses* (Rennie 1993b). Additionally, ICU staff linking or specialising in infection control can help raise awareness of colleagues, provide on-site information and education, and recognise issues and problems surrounding specialist practice.

Communication and teamwork between different multidisciplinary team members, including microbiologists and infection control teams, can proactively minimise infection risk; multidisciplinary audit should identify unit-specific issues; action research may develop solutions.

Inadequate staffing (quantity and quality) increases cross-infection (Hanson & Elston 1990). Busy staff are more likely to try and 'make time' through short-cuts (e.g. token handwashes, incompletely drying hands (Gould 1994a)). There should be adequate staff to meet each individual patient's requirements (RCN 1994); a 'runner' reduces need for other nurses to move between beds.

Many *invasive* procedures and treatments are unavoidable with critical illness, but each may introduce infection into immunocompromised patients. Nurses can usefully question whether some may be avoided: alternative routes for drugs may be possible (e.g. rectal metronidazole), and noninvasive monitoring (e.g. blood pressure) may suffice.

Central vein *cannulae* remain the major cause of nosocomial septicaemia (Randolph 1998), and so should be replaced whenever practical. Some IV drugs can only safely be given centrally (e.g. dopamine), and hypoperfusion may make peripheral routes ineffective, but peripheral lines remain underused in ICUs. Unused cannulae (peripheral or central) create unnecessary risks and should be removed.

Despite extensive research, time limits for replacing invasive equipment vary between equipment type, insertion site and researchers. Hospitals and units often provide evidence-based guidelines for replacement times, and manufacturers should state recommended times; staff extending manufacturers' times should consider their legal liability (see Chapter 45). Insertion dates of all invasive equipment should be recorded so that they can be changed promptly.

Gut translocation of bacteria occurs within hours of shock (Sagar *et al.* 1994) and is the main cause of endogenous infection (Alcock & Ledingham 1990). Improving gut perfusion with dopamine (McClelland 1993b) has proved disappointing; dobutamine may be more effective (Levy *et al.* 1997). Measuring intramucosal pH (pHi) indicates sepsis and mortality (Lavery & Clapham 1993), although benefits remain controversial. Selective digestive decontamination (SDD) can prevent pathogen colonisation by routine use of selective non-absorbable antibiotics, although heated debate continues around its value. A 1991 European Consensus conference decided not to recommend SDD for ICU use (Carlet 1992). SDD may fail to reduce mortality (McClelland 1993b), replacing gram negative organisms with gram positives (including *Staphylococcus aureus*) (Carlet 1992), although more recent reports appear favourable (Selective Decontamination of the Digestive Tract Trialists' Collaborative Group (1993); Baxby *et al.* (1996); Palomar *et al.* (1997); d'Amico *et al.* (1998)). SDD has not (yet) become widely established in UK practice. Enteral nutrition (see Chapter 9) remains the most effective way to enhance gut defences and reduce translocation of gut bacteria.

Isolation can halve nosocomial infection rates (Hanson & Elston 1990), but increase psychological stress (see Chapter 3) and delay discharge, thus exposing patients to prolonged risk of nosocomial infection (Teare & Barrett 1997).

Staff *screening* has recently generated heated debate in the *British Medical Journal*, Lessing *et al.* (1996) suggesting that the costs of screening programmes, together with negative financial and psychological effects on staff, make preventative screening programmes undesirable.

Infecting organisms are identified by *specimen* collection. Specimen contamination can occur from:

- skin surface bacteria (e.g. around cannula tips)
- storage at room temperature

If possible, collection is usually best delayed until laboratory hours. Specimen analysis incurs costs and usually requires medical approval; however vigilance by nurses often identifies signs of potential infection.

Treating infection

The *antibiotic* era has witnessed many microorganism mutations, creating resistance to successive generations of (increasingly expensive and toxic) antibiotics. Drug companies face escalating investment costs for products increasingly difficult to market, and potentially soon obsolete; Gould (1994b) reports that one-half of drug companies are stopping or seriously reducing antibiotic production. The Chief Medical Officer for Scotland has predicted that by 2020 healthcare will run out of antibiotics (cited by Amyes & Thomson 1995). Such statements may appear sensationalist, but they emphasise the need to reorientate from relying on drugs to preventing and controlling infection.

Antibiotics remain useful adjuncts to treatment, but will probably become progressively less effective. The inappropriate use of antibiotics has created more pathogenic, resistant organisms (Parke & Burden 1998), and so unnecessary use is actively discouraged (House of Lords Select Committee on Science and Technology 1998). Early onset pneumonia (from aspiration during trauma) is usually antibiotic-sensitive, but late onset pneumonia (ventilator-associated pneumonia) is usually resistant (Rello *et al.* 1994).

Monoclonal antibodies are cloned and genetically engineered human B-lymphocytes (Eburn 1993). Centoxin (HA-1A), a single-dose IgM antibody targeting endotoxin (Eburn 1993), was costly (£2,200 (Michie & Marley 1992)) and withdrawn in 1994, but more effective products will probably be licensed before long.

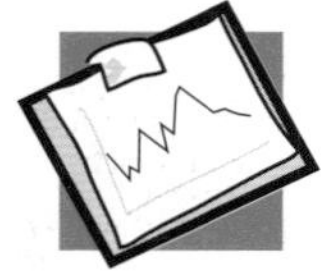

Implications for practice

- equipment (e.g. Heat Moisture Exchangers) should be changed according to manufacturers' instructions (normally daily); catheter mounts should be changed at the same time as humidifiers
- invasive techniques and disconnection of intravenous lines should, when possible, avoid times of dust disturbance (e.g. floor cleaning)
- strict asepsis must be observed when breaking any intravenous circuit or treating any open wound
- using prepacked intravenous additives (e.g. potassium) reduces contamination risks
- clothing worn outside ICUs should be removed before approaching patients
- adequate laundry facilities should be provided for staff to change uniforms daily

- handwashing should be carried out before and after each aspect of care, and before approaching and after leaving each bed area
- antiseptic hand cleansers should be available at each bed area
- all taps should have elbow-operated levers at elbow height; taps should not be turned on by hand
- towel dispensers should provide individual paper towels that will not drape in moist sink units
- hospital infection control nurses and other specialists should be actively involved in multidisciplinary teamwork
- colour coding bed areas (aprons, equipment) discourages inappropriate movement between bedspaces

Summary

Infection incurs high costs: in human life, in morbidity (quality of life for survivors) and financially. Antibiotics and other medical treatments can reduce morbidity and mortality, but preventing infection is humanly (and usually financially) preferable.

Handwashing remains the most important way to prevent infection. Hygiene is helped by adequate and appropriate facilities, including sufficient washbasins, aprons and unit guidelines and protocols. All multidisciplinary team members should be actively involved in making decisions, but nurses have an especially valuable role in coordinating and controlling each patient's environment.

Prevention can literally be 'life-saving'. Problems from infection are likely to escalate; continuing vigilance and care can minimise infection risks and the spread of microorganisms. The importance of nursing to infection control is emphasised through its inclusion in the *Standards of Care for Critical Care Nursing* (RCN 1994).

Further reading

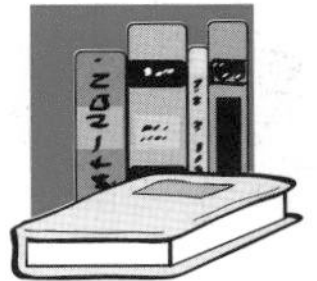

Articles on infection control frequently appear in specialist and general journals. EPIC provides valuable information on infection and its control in European ICUs; Vincent *et al.* (1995) is the main report, although Rennie (1993b) gives a succinct preliminary summary. Williamson and Spencer's (1997) review of ICU infection and Amyes and Thomson's (1995) article about crises of antibiotic resistance are also useful.

Taylor's (1978) classic article on handwashing is recommended; issues for nursing practice regularly appear in many general nursing journals.

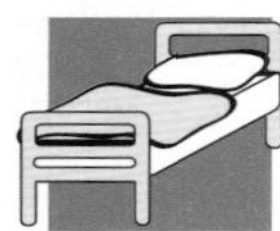

Clinical scenario

Catherine Welch is a 67-year-old with known chronic obstructive pulmonary disease (COPD). She was transferred from elderly care facilities with rapidly deteriorating respiratory function, copious mucopurulent sputum and atelectasis. On admission to ICU for non-invasive positive pressure ventilatory support, she was routinely screened for infection. The microbiological results indicate methicillin resistant *Staphylococcus aureus* (strain EMRSA-16) in her throat and *Streptococcus pneumonia* in her sputum. Catherine's previous respiratory tract infections had been treated with oral Amoxycillin (**beta lactam** class of antibiotics).

Q.1 Using the literature and the multidisciplinary team, describe the main features of these microorganisms:

(a) Are they viruses, protozoa, yeasts or moulds?
(b) Specify the usual modes of transmission for MRSA and *S. pneumonia*.
(c) Rank or rate likely 'vectors' for cross-transmission in ICU (e.g. pens, uniforms, hands).
(d) Discuss their pathogenicity (i.e. ability of microorganism to cause infection/disease).

Q.2 Catherine had these microorganisms as commensals. Examine her risk factors prior to ICU admission for developing pneumonia and MRSA infection.

Q.3 Management of Catherine's infection is focused on:

(a) containment (e.g. necessity of protective isolation versus universal protection in ICU, screening of staff/visitors/others);
(b) prevention of cross-transmission (exogenous, to other patients; endogenous, to her other body areas, minimising vectors);
(c) eradication (types of antibiotic/antiseptic, administration route, etc.).

Using published Infection Control Guidelines, local clinical practice guidelines and a holistic approach, design a nursing care plan for Catherine in ICU (integrating professional, psychosocial and physiological aspects).

Issues related to infection control are included in end-of-chapter scenarios in chapters 39 and 40.

Chapter 16

Ethics

Contents

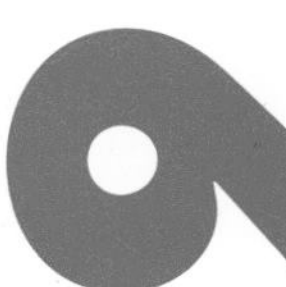

Introduction

The value of ethics for healthcare has been increasingly recognised: critical care often adds greater focus and poignancy to ethical dilemmas. Ethics raises questions rather than provides answers; dilemmas have more than one solution. To help ICU nurses understand the values underpinning care, this chapter explores ethical theory. Each person has values; some are formed or shared with peer groups, others are individual. Different values may cause conflict (for example, the care versus cure debate of Chapter 1). Active questioning enables evaluation of beliefs underpinning practice, helping nurses to understand others' perspectives, but solutions necessarily remain individual.

Increasing public expectations (and litigation) of healthcare, and changes within nursing (increased autonomy, responsibility and accountability) are reflected by greater emphasis on ethics in nursing education. A high public and media profile makes intensive care nursing a much-scrutinized area. This chapter provides a basis both for practice and for the remainder of this book; professional development can usefully be extended through discussion with colleagues and further study.

The UKCC represents and prescribes professional nursing values in the UK. It exists to represent and protect patients' interests, and has the statutory power to regulate who can practice as (qualified) nurses in the UK. Professional expectations (expected norms), clarified in UKCC publications – especially the Code of Conduct (UKCC 1992a) – should underlie all professional nursing practice in the UK. Most other nations have similar professional bodies and requirements.

This chapter describes the four main ethical principles identified by Beauchamp and Childress (1994):

- autonomy
- non-maleficence
- beneficence
- justice

and the three main ethical theories identified by Rumbold (1993):

- duty-based
- goal-based
- rights-based

Other authors may give different arrangements, wording or additional theories and principles. Ethical principles provide a framework with which to work through dilemmas, identifying what is harmful, what is good and what is just. Decisions may differ between individuals because individual morals (values and beliefs) influence decision-making processes. Ethical theories identify different sets of beliefs; understanding our own and others' sets of beliefs (values) helps towards the understanding of differences.

Some examples presented in this chapter include legal and professional perspectives; unlike ethics, these expectations can be enforced, and so nurses should consider their individual professional (and legal) accountability.

Ethics are guides to decision-making, and decisions are influenced by sources such as

- religion
- law
- society (and social values)
- peers
- individual values

If growth from novice to expert entails moving from following rules to initiation (Benner 1984), understanding sources of 'intuitive' decisions can substantiate accountable evidence-based practice.

Meanings of *ethics* and *morals* vary. The literal translation of both is 'norm' (Greek *ethos*, Latin *mores*), but they have different connotations. Many (but not all) people interpret 'ethics' as applying to groups (e.g. nursing ethics), whereas 'morals' imply individual and personal values; these are the interpretations followed in this text, but some texts use the terms interchangeably.

Time out 1

Using a dictionary, jot down the definitions of 'ethics' and 'morals'. Consider similarities and differences between definitions.

How close are these definitions to your own understanding of the terms?

Can ethics ever be immoral, or morals unethical? Why? Include professional ethics/morals in your consideration. National ethics/morals are supposedly represented by national law. So can laws be immoral/unethical? Why?

ICU: an ethical quagmire?

Ethical dilemmas in ICU are caused by:

- cost
- technology
- values

All nations face dilemmas between limited budgets and increasing healthcare costs and demand. Rationing resources is therefore inevitable. Financial *costs* in ICUs are especially high (see Chapter 50), and so cost/benefit analyses inevitably influence (some) decisions. Many staff are uncomfortable with applying economics to healthcare, but while decisions should never be made solely on economic grounds, finance cannot be ignored where resources remain finite. (For example, whether the ICU should invest in a new ventilator or monitoring equipment.) If economic decisions are not made by those delivering care, they will be made by others; therefore the involvement of nurses with economic decision-making (rationing) can promote patients' interests.

Intensive care nursing relies on *technology* to support and monitor physiological function. Breathing and heartbeat can be replaced by technology (causing redefinition of death as absence of brainstem function), but intervention may prolong dying rather than prolong life: Rachels (1986) draws a distinction between living and the physical process of being alive. Highly invasive technology exposes patients to risks: if not infected on admission, most ICU patients acquire infection within one week (see Chapter 15). Technology may be used inappropriately; no treatment, intervention or observation should become 'routine'.

Appropriateness of interventions may be influenced by quality of life. This much-used term is value-laden: what one person considers acceptable quality, another may not (e.g. Jehovah's witnesses may prefer death to receiving blood transfusions). Values vary between the extremes of preserving life at all costs, and always letting 'nature' take its course. Respecting others' values enables autonomy.

Ethical principles

Autonomy

Beauchamp and Childress (1994) suggest that each ethical principle is part of a continuum. Autonomy, the first principle, is usually interpreted as 'self-rule' – that is, making an informed free choice. How far anyone fully 'rules' themselves is questionable. Impaired consciousness, debility and treatments (e.g. intubation) severely limit the abilities of ICU patients to rule themselves – they are disempowered. The ICU staff control information, the patients' environment and even their basic physiological functions (including rest/sedation). Disempowerment can be (literally) fatal (Seligman 1975).

Health professionals often limit information to gain consent (Rumbold 1993); ICU staff often presume consent. Safety may necessitate some reflex behavioural responses being overruled (e.g. attempted self-extubation), but where possible informed (cognitive) decisions, however small, should be enabled.

Consent by relatives for mentally competent adults has no legal validity (Brazier 1992; Dimond 1995; Braithwaite 1996). Mental incompetence is different from inability to communicate, and very few ICU patients have legally appointed guardians, so that this is rarely an issue for ICU nurses.

Parents or guardians have the right to consent to treatment for children under 18 (Dimond 1995), but the 1989 Children's Act and civil law precedent of 'Gillick competence' emphasise rights of children to make their own informed decisions provided they have achieved sufficient maturity to fully understand what is proposed (Brazier 1992). So one relatively young child may (legally) make more profound decisions than an older child. If in doubt, nurses should seek help to clarify the rights and duties of all concerned (most hospitals have legal advisors).

The law assumes that healthcare staff will act in patients' best interests (Brazier 1992). Actions in patients' best interests may be condoned, but *nonconsensual touch* (including any nursing/medical intervention without valid consent) is technically assault. 'Best interests' may be unclear: since quality of life is subjective, values of patients and healthcare staff may differ and decisions made for an unconscious patient (advocacy) may not reflect that patient's best interest. The consent of relatives, while not legally binding, may provide an insight into the patient's wishes, while building goodwill between relatives and staff. However, the relatives' values may also differ, and extreme stress and guilt can result from believing they are making 'life or death' decisions.

Advance directives ('living wills') state patients' wishes for specific (stated) treatments to be withheld (e.g. ventilation). Although not (yet) legally binding in the UK, the House of Lords Select Committee on Medical Ethics and the British Medical Association (Robertson 1995) support the principle of advance directives.

Advance directives must necessarily anticipate scenarios where patients cannot express their wishes. They therefore provide a means for nurse advocacy (Cowe 1996). However the ability of most people to make informed decisions about hypothetical situations is questionable (Ryan 1996); most consultants oppose withdrawing treatment only on the basis of advance directives (Grubb *et al.* 1996). Patients' views may have changed since writing the document, especially if it is old (although this would not affect validity of a last will and testament). Nurses finding evidence of an advance directive (possibly through discussions with relatives) should alert unit managers and the multidisciplinary team.

Non-maleficence

Not doing harm has been fundamental to healthcare since the Hippocratic Oath, and restated in Nightingale's (1980 [1859]) *Notes on Nursing*, Roper *et al.*'s first (and presumably primary) activity of living (1996), and the *Code of Conduct* (UKCC 1992a). In law, proven harm is more culpable than failing to do good.

Healthcare exposes patients to potential *harm* (e.g. nosocomial infection). Benefits of invasive equipment may justify risks from infection; psychological dilemmas are often more complex. Healthcare workers may justify white lies or withholding truth and diagnoses as being in the patients' and families' best interests, while others may consider deliberate untruth or withholding information is unjustifiable (unethical).

If life is sacrosanct, then death is presumably the greatest possible harm; if death is preferable to continued suffering, then life support can be harmful. About one-quarter of ICU patients die on the unit; survivors often suffer temporary or permanent complications (physical disability or psychological distress). Harm (quality of life) is therefore individual and debatable; ICU patients unable to express their wishes are vulnerable to (unintentional) harm. Individual assessment of each patient can help nurses to understand what they would consider harmful; once identified, potential and existing harms (e.g. fear, anxiety, loss of dignity, humiliation) can be resolved or reduced, promoting the human/humane values discussed in Chapter 1.

Withdrawing, or not initiating, treatment is passive *euthanasia*, and occurs in up to 7 per cent of ICU admissions, resulting in 40–60 per cent of ICU deaths (Phelan 1995). Euthanasia ('good death') presumes life is no longer preferable to death and so treatment becomes harmful, 'mercy killing' (active euthanasia) or 'letting die' (passive euthanasia) becomes beneficent.

Active euthanasia is illegal (murder) in the UK (and in most countries). But doctors (or, implicitly, other healthcare workers) are not absolutely obliged to maintain life in hopeless cases (Bennett 1995), and so passive euthanasia (withholding treatment) may legally be practised: in such cases, patients die from their existing conditions, not by human actions (Bennett 1995).

But withdrawing/withholding treatment causes dilemmas. If life is sacrosanct, then euthanasia violates the sanctity of life. The acceptance of passive euthanasia may prove to be the 'slippery slope' to greater (involuntary) extermination (Randall 1997).

If the principle of withdrawing treatment is accepted, deciding what to withdraw can create dilemmas in practice: most ICUs will stop supplementary oxygen, inotropes and haemofiltration, but maintain ventilation. The Roman Catholic theology distinguishes ordinary from extraordinary interventions (Rachels 1986): ordinary interventions ('natural' or 'God-given') must be preserved, but extraordinary interventions (those created by humans, thus unnatural) may be withdrawn. Ventilators replace breathing, a natural function, and so may be 'ordinary', whereas drugs (e.g. inotropes) may not – although following the Karen Quinlan case in the USA, American courts were divided over whether ventilators were 'ordinary' (Rachels 1986). The distinction is often unclear. The House of Lords (1993) ruled that a nasogastric tube was 'extraordinary', and so removal from a patient in a persistent vegetative state (where brainstem function remains, but higher function is absent) would not lead to prosecution; the tube was removed, so that the patient effectively died of starvation. This – the apparent absurdity of nasogastric tubes being extraordinary while ventilators are ordinary – can make decisions difficult. Decisions should therefore be made by team consensus – and the individual team members have each to live with their own conscience.

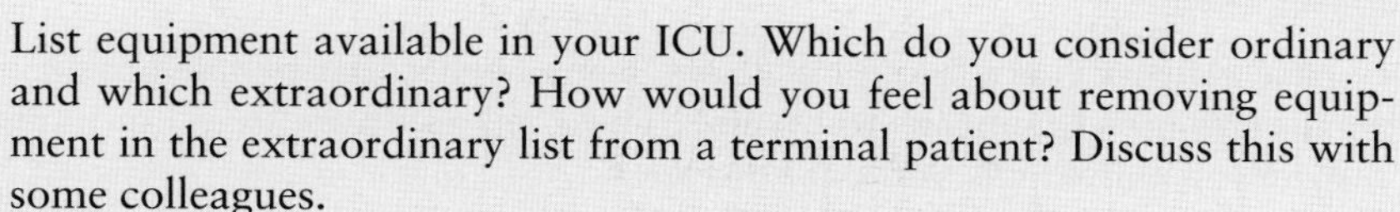

Time out 2

List equipment available in your ICU. Which do you consider ordinary and which extraordinary? How would you feel about removing equipment in the extraordinary list from a terminal patient? Discuss this with some colleagues.

Beneficence

Not doing harm can be extended to doing good. Beneficence underlies Clause 2 of the nurses' *Code of conduct* (UKCC 1992a), but deciding what is 'good' involves further value judgements (e.g. quality of life). Eudaemonistic (Smith 1980) and eupsychic (Maslow 1971) models of health identify what individuals enjoy with health; this conflicts with the biomedical model prevalent in ICUs. If patients' wishes can be ascertained, advocating for patients should be beneficent.

Harm and good can co-exist: the doctrine of *double effect*. If relieving pain is good, but killing is harmful, morphine can both do good (relieve pain) and harm (kill). Pope Pius XII ruled that actions (e.g. giving morphine) should be judged by primary and secondary intentions (Rachels 1986). If the primary intention is to relieve pain, then undesirable effects (death) may be acceptable; but giving morphine with the primary intention of hastening death is active euthanasia, which is a criminal offence in the UK.

Justice

Justice carries connotations of

- retribution/punishment
- fairness.

Denying treatment to one group of patients (e.g. cardiac surgery to current smokers) may be viewed as *punishment* for their deliberate actions, but limited resources necessitates rationing, which should attempt *fairness*. However, fairness is a subjective concept – those denied access usually consider injustice has been performed.

NHS *rationing* largely adopts the 'first come, first served' principle; private healthcare tends to ration by ability to pay. The Society of Critical Care Medicine's Ethics Committee (1994) states that obligations to existing ICU patients generally outweigh obligations to accept new patients, and so if ICU beds are unavailable, admissions may have to be refused, even if the patients refused admission have better potential quality or length of life, or better chances of survival from interventions, than the patients already on the unit. Hence, the nurses' duty of care may conflict with their own values about fairness.

Ethical theories

Duty

Duty-based theory (deontology) develops Kant's belief that people are an end in themselves, not the means to an end. These values are reflected in nursing by respect for individuals and duty of care.

These apparently laudable aims can create dilemmas:

- nursing is learnt though clinical practice, so patient care (means) is a learning experience (end) for the nurse
- nurses caring for two patients (e.g. covering breaks) may have to choose between two conflicting duties of care
- how far does (moral) duty of care extend? Refusing admission because beds are unavailable means denying care
- whether or not nurses who have not completed care (e.g. nursing records) when shifts end should work (usually overtime) to complete their duty of care

Goal

Goal-based (utilitarian, consequentialist) theory supports actions that achieve desired goals ('the end justifies the means'), following Jeremy Bentham's maxim of the greatest good for the greatest number. Rationing services can be justified if they do not meet the needs of the majority.

Problems with this theory include

- minority rights may be denied (e.g. should visiting by extended families be restricted in the interests of other patients?)
- potentially 'unethical/immoral' means may be used to achieve a laudable end (cf. placebos in Chapter 47)

Rights

Although the UK traditionally places less emphasis on rights than many other nations, *The Patient's Charter* (DoH 1991, 1995) (soon to be replaced by an NHS charter) reflects growing emphasis on rights. The right of one person necessarily imposes a duty on another person, and so nurse advocacy may be a consequential duty of patients' rights.

Problems with rights include

- conflict between rights of different people (should there be a Nurses' Charter?)
- rights stated in the Patients' Charter often prove elusive
- claiming to uphold others' rights (e.g. nurse advocacy) may be used for paternalistic or other ends

Implications for practice

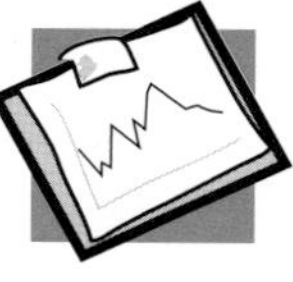

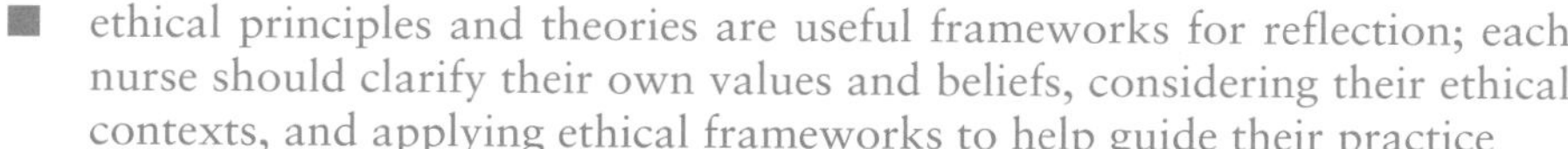

- ethical principles and theories are useful frameworks for reflection; each nurse should clarify their own values and beliefs, considering their ethical contexts, and applying ethical frameworks to help guide their practice
- ethical dilemmas seldom have absolute answers; ethics should help nurses justify their professional decisions, recognising that different ethical beliefs may result in differing conclusions
- advance directives are not (yet) legally enforceable in the UK; nurses should alert the multidisciplinary team to their existence, but decisions should be made by the whole team
- where appropriate, patient choice should be empowered
- when paternalistic decisions are necessary, they should be guided by patients' best interests
- practice raises various ethical dilemmas; informal discussion can be cathartic, while an ethical forum (preferably multidisciplinary) can diffuse conflict and contribute to professional (and unit) development

Summary

Ethics is about understanding values and justifying decision-making. The ethical principles and theories outlined in this chapter provide frameworks for considering dilemmas raised in later chapters or through practice. Various dilemmas have been briefly raised; each can be pursued through the wide range of texts and articles on ethics. But ethics should be used to guide practice, not stored on library shelves. Readers are therefore encouraged to consider and discuss ethical dilemmas with colleagues.

Further reading

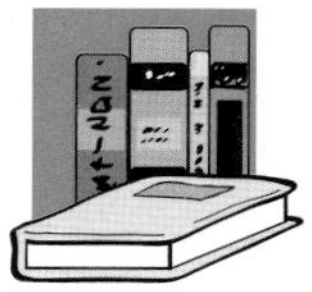

Beauchamp and Childress (1994) is a major biomedical text, much material being applicable to nursing. Downie and Calman (1994) develop profound and well-supported issues with especial emphasis on rights.

There are many nursing-specific texts; Rumbold (1999) is highly approachable, with clear, well-written discussion.

There are nursing and medical journals devoted to ethical issues, but other journals frequently include ethics. Purcell (1997) gives a particularly sensitive analysis of withdrawing treatment from a child, while Cook *et al.* (1995) identify disturbing differences between units.

Dimond (1995) remains the key text on nursing and the law.

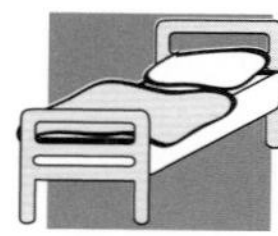

Clinical scenario

John is a 65-year-old business man and long-term ICU patient. He was admitted to ICU following cardiopulmonary resuscitation. Investigations revealed severe left ventricular failure, an ejection fraction of 20 per cent with very poor medical prognosis. In the sixth week of John's ICU stay he remains dependent on ventilatory support and inotropic drugs despite several attempts at weaning.

John communicates a wish to die and for all treatments to be discontinued.

Q.1 Identify the ethical principles involved in this case and any ethical conflicts (e.g. with John's autonomy, non-maleficence, consent, justice, resource distribution, Professional Code of Conduct).

Q.2 Who has the right to decide if treatment can be withdrawn and/or subsequent interventions withheld (e.g. commencing antibiotics, do-not-resuscitate orders)?

Q.3 Compare your ethical understanding and moral reasoning with that of other members of the multidisciplinary team (e.g. other grades, doctors), and legal department of your hospital.

Reflect on your own practice of delivering autonomous, patient-centred care. Consider effective strategies which facilitate patient involvement in the planning and delivery of care (e.g. specific sources of information, resources, interpersonal skills and values, training, attitudes).

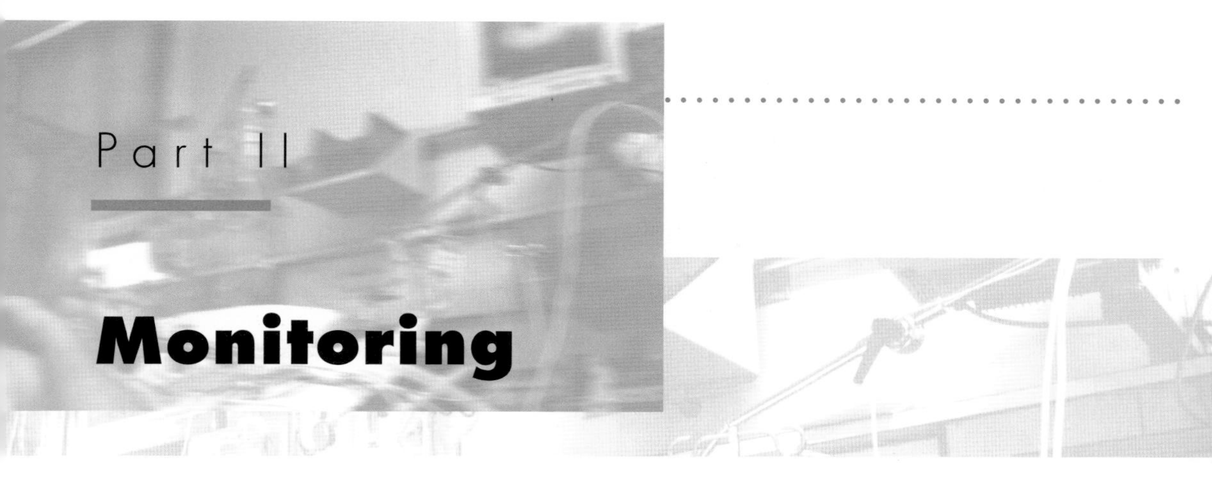

Part II

Monitoring

ICUs grew out of facilities for monitoring and treating respiratory and cardiac disorders; this section therefore focuses on aspects of monitoring more frequently used by nurses. Many additional forms of monitoring are used in ICU (e.g. chest X-rays), but this section restricts discussion to those likely to be used by nurses on general ICUs.

The first chapter describes various means of respiratory monitoring; additional aspects of ventilatory and airway monitoring were covered in Chapters 4 and 5. Carriage of gases, particularly the oxygen saturation curve and the relationship between arterial oxygen tensions and peripheral saturation of oxygen, is illustrated in Chapter 18; blood gas analysis is then explored in Chapter 19.

The chapter on haemodynamic monitoring focuses mainly on CVPs and cardiac output studies. Common dysrhythmias seen in ICU, together with usual treatments, are identified in Chapter 21. The final chapter describes neurological monitoring, with especial reference to intracranial pressure monitoring and treatment of intracranial hypertension.

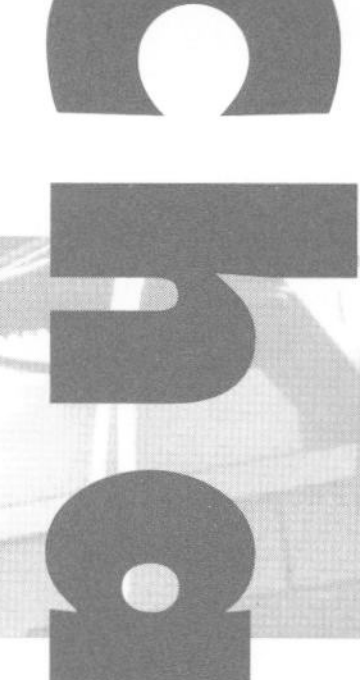

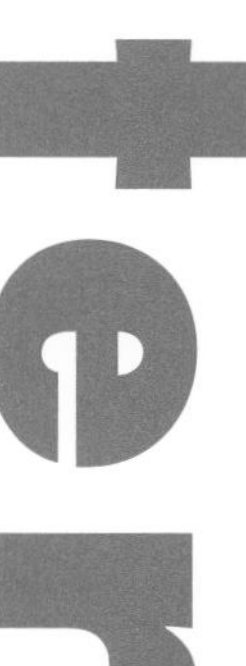

Respiratory monitoring

Contents

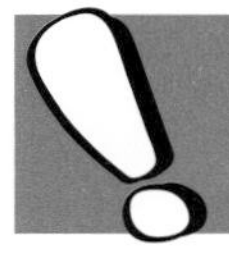

Fundamental knowledge

Haemoglobin carriage of oxygen (see Chapter 18)
Respiratory anatomy
Normal (negative) respiration

Introduction

Traditional nursing observations of respiratory rate and depth are extended in ICUs by visual and aural observation of ventilation. This chapter assumes familiarity with simpler respiratory observations (including spirometry); more frequently used ventilator settings are discussed in Chapter 4 and arterial blood gas analysis in Chapter 19. This chapter mainly describes technological monitoring used by nurses, especially pulse oximetry. Means used by other professions (e.g. chest X-rays, imaging, bronchoscopy) are not discussed.

Whatever means are used, all procedures should be explained to patients. The information gained should be interpreted holistically, focusing on patients rather than monitors, and trends rather than absolute figures. 'Acceptable' error margins for medical technology may be 5–10 per cent.

Burroughs and Hoffbrand (1990) found inaccurate nursing records from following previously charted observations rather than what is actually observed; nurses should have confidence in their observations, noting and reporting significant changes.

Visual

Observing patients' colour and appearance is fundamental to all areas of nursing; skin richly supplied with blood (lips, oral membranes, nail beds) gives the best visual indication of perfusion. Good light, preferably daylight, should be used when assessing skin colour; artificial light, especially fluorescent, can cause distortion. Cyanosis only occurs when haemoglobin desaturates to 5 g/dl (Takala 1997); such severe hypoxia is unsafe for clinical practice, especially as haemoglobin is usually maintained at 10 g/dl in ICU. Visual assessment is subjective, and may be complicated by skin tone. In the absence of reliable early visual signs, technology is needed to support respiratory monitoring.

Cough reflex (e.g. on suction) may be lost with deep unconsciousness, but most ICU patients have some (weakened) cough reflex. Coughs may be productive or unproductive. Possible sounds include: dry, hoarse, barking or whoops. Observations should be recorded.

Sputum should be observed for

- volume
- colour (e.g. black, white, pink)
- consistency (e.g. frothy, tenacious, watery)
- purulence
- haemoptysis

If specimens are required, these should be collected and sent when fresh. Observations (including frequency of suction) should be recorded.

Auscultation

Breath sounds are created by air turbulence, and so are limited to upper airways (Hough 1996). Sounds may be normal, abnormal, diminished or absent. Chest (and abdominal) sounds can be deceptive, and so should not be relied upon absolutely. Listening for air entry is used to assess:

- intubation (bilateral air entry)
- bronchial patency/bronchospasm
- secretions
- effect of suction (before and after)

The stethoscope diaphragm best transmits lung sounds (especially high pitches, such as wheezes; the bell is better for low pitches (e.g. heart sounds). Where possible, reduce external noise (e.g. silence alarms and suction). Note *pitch, intensity, quality* and *duration* of sounds, listening:

- anteriorly, posteriorly, laterally
- on both right and left
- at apices and bases
- during both inspiration and expiration
- over any dependent lung areas, where fluid and mucus tend to collect

Missing any areas (for example, because difficult to reach) makes assessment incomplete. Normal sounds are:

- vesicular: most lung fields, especially peripheries; continuous, low pitch and volume, like rustling wind, with short expiratory phase
- bronchovesicular: lung apices; medium pitched, louder than vesicular
- bronchial: trachea; high pitched, loud, short inspiration, like blowing through a tube

Abnormal sounds include:

- wheeze (rhonchi): from bronchospasm, continuous
- crackle (rales, crepitations): bubbling, from fluid, exudate or secretions; interrupted
- pleural rub: grating sound from (abnormal) friction between pleura

Sound may be absent with any obstruction (e.g. bronchial plug). Artefactual sounds may be caused by:

- clothing
- friction of stethoscope against equipment (e.g. cot sides)
- chest hair (crackles)

Breath waveform

Ventilator breaths should ideally

- maximise gas exchange
- minimise peak inflation pressure (barotrauma)
- use safe (nontoxic) oxygen concentrations.

Breath waveforms (available on most ventilators; see Figure 17.1) enable breath pattern adjustments to

- optimise delivery (e.g. peak inflation pressure, peak expiratory flow)
- reduce work of breathing
- facilitate weaning (Levy *et al.* 1995).

Each breath has three potential parts: inspiration, plateau and expiration. Inspiration affects, and is affected by, bronchial muscle stretch; thus patients with chronic obstructive pulmonary disease cannot fully dilate bronchi during short inspiratory time. Most gas exchange occurs during plateau (peak inflation pressure). Expiration is passive recoil; the short expiration time of muscle spasm (asthma) causes gas trapping (and distress).

Bedside monitors to measure work of breathing enable more accurate titration of pressure support (Banner *et al.* 1994).

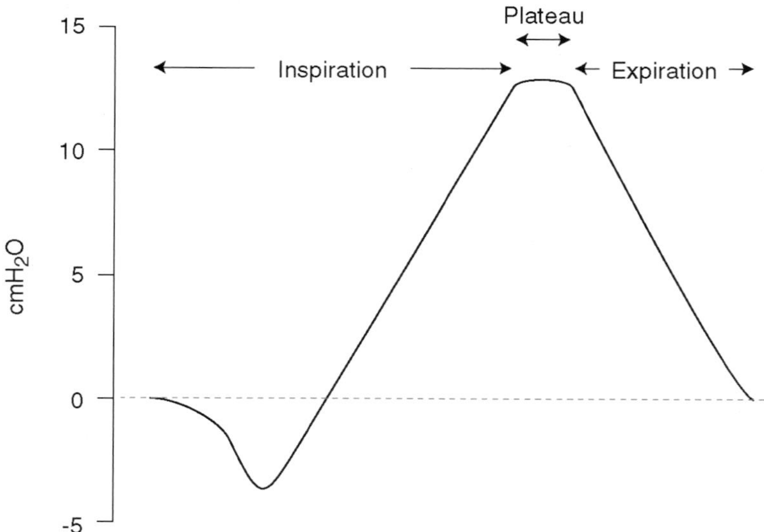

Figure 17.1 Normal (self-ventilating) breath waveform

Pulse oximetry

Pulse oximetry measures peripheral (capillary) saturation of haemoglobin by oxygen (SpO_2). Peripheral saturation is within 2 per cent of arterial blood gas saturations (Jones, A. 1995), and so differences of SpO_2 and SaO_2 are insignificant for practice.

Signals measure (usually) over five pulses (Harrahill 1991), causing slight delay when commencing monitoring. Arteriole emptying during diastole enables differentiation of infrared light absorption by bone, vein and skin pigmentation from absorption by blood. Blood only absorbs two per cent of total infrared light, so poor signal to noise ratios (= poor flow, 'noisy signal') frequently occur (Clutton-Brock 1997). 'Noise' may

- cause complete signal failure (i.e. no reading)
- underestimate SpO_2.

So oximetry becomes least reliable when most needed. Waveform display, rather than just a bar, usefully indicates vasoconstriction and vasodilation, and reliability of readings.

Oximetry is the most widely used means of respiratory monitoring, but limitations include

- *oxygen availability* to tissues and SpO_2 are not identical as
  - relationship between SaO_2 to PaO_2 is complex (oxygen dissociation curve – see Chapter 18)
  - reduced erythrocyte counts reduces oxygen carriage but not SaO_2.

  Thus *anaemia* is not detected by oximetry.
- *haemoglobinopathies*: although detecting problems with oxygen carriage, oximetry will not identify causes; laboratory analysis and other clinical signs remain necessary to fully assess respiratory pathophysiology.
- *carbon monoxide* levels above 3 per cent cause progressive over-reading (Jensen *et al.* 1998), SpO_2 often reading 100 per cent (Stoneham *et al.* 1994). Carboxyhaemoglobin is bright red, increasing infrared light absorption. Inhaled carbon monoxide affects readings four hours after a cigarette (Dobson 1993), so oximetry is unreliable if carbon monoxide poisoning is suspected.
- *hypercapnia*: oximetry does not measure carbon dioxide tensions; Davidson and Hosie (1993) report a postoperative self-ventilating patient with normal PaO_2, but arterial carbon dioxide tensions of 37.4 kPa, creating profound respiratory acidosis (base excess −21.2). Thus oximetry alone is unreliable with chronic obstructive pulmonary disease (Stoneham *et al.* 1994) or poor lung tidal volumes. The ICU use of oximetry to supplement other respiratory monitoring largely avoids this problem, but it should be remembered when introducing others to its use.

- *peripheral vasoconstriction*: oximetry relies on perfusion and pulse so that poor peripheral perfusion (e.g. sepsis/SIRS) causes 'noisy signals'.
- *dysrhythmias* impair perfusion, causing noisy signals.
- *shivering*: Stoneham *et al.* (1994) suggest that shivering can give poor readings, although Ralston *et al.* (1991) found shivering to have minimal effect.
- *bilirubin* may cause underestimate, depending on the type of bilirubin. Dobson (1993) and Coull (1992) warn about false readings; Stoneham *et al.* (1994) and Ralston *et al.* (1991) suggest that effect is negligible.
- *dark skin/dried blood/nail varnish* absorb light, causing significant under-readings (black/blue nail varnish can cause 3–5 per cent errors in SpO_2 (Wahr & Tremper 1996).
- *intravenous dyes* can affect light absorption, and so affect readings; half-lives of dyes indicate period for which readings may be unreliable following use.
- *external light* can overestimate SpO_2 (Stoneham *et al.* 1994), especially with fluorescent light and heat lamps (Ralston *et al.* 1991). Most finger probes include light shields, but ear probes may detect overhead lighting. Shields should be examined when purchasing oximeters.
- *low level accuracy*: accuracy below SpO_2 of 80 per cent is unproven, (manufacturers cannot ethically induce severe hypoxia in volunteers to calibrate machines (Webb *et al.* 1991)). However, if SpO_2 falls below 90 per cent, arterial blood gas analysis is advisable.

Oximetry probes can be very uncomfortable; by testing probes on yourself you can gauge what patients are experiencing. Uncomfortable probes may need more frequent changes of position, or replacement with less uncomfortable models. Heat may cause burns, especially with poorly perfused peripheries (frequent in ICU). Many units change probe positions every hour or two; some anecdotal reports suggest changing every half-hour. Changes should be individually assessed rather than ritualized, depending on

- heat from probes (assess by trying probes on yourself)
- perfusion
- visual observation of probe sites
- nursing records.

Transcutaneous gas analysis

Transcutaneous gas analysis is noninvasive, but more useful for neonates than adults, being affected by

- thickness (Gibbons 1997)
- poor capillary flow (Gibbons 1997).

This makes it unreliable with shock (Hinds & Watson 1996). Transcutaneous carbon dioxide tensions are higher than arterial, but do show useful trends (Rithalia *et al.* 1992).

Probes heat skin to 43°C (Hinds & Watson 1996), increasing skin permeability and blood flow while overriding autoregulated vasoconstriction (e.g. from pain, anxiety); this heat can cause burns and probes should be moved 3–6 hourly (Gibbons 1997).

Intra-arterial electrodes

Intra-arterial electrodes enable continuous gas tension monitoring, PiO_2 correlating well with arterial samples (PaO_2) (Abraham *et al.* 1996). However, large (20g) needles may occlude arteries, and brittle fibres may break when patients move (6 of 21 in Roupie *et al.*'s (1996) sample). Equipment is also costly. Intra-arterial monitoring has not (yet) established itself in ICU practice.

Capnography

Carbon dioxide is a waste product of metabolism, so monitoring carbon dioxide production indicates metabolism. Arterial carbon dioxide tensions are identified through blood gas analysis, but capnography (end-tidal carbon dioxide – $PECO_2/PETCO_2$) enables continuous noninvasive monitoring of expired levels (end-tidal approximates residual alveoli levels).

$PECO_2$ is normally 0.5 kPa below arterial tensions (Clutton-Brock 1997), but ratios between expired and mixed venous carbon dioxide diminish as dead space increases (V/Q mismatch); differentials of up to 3 kPa have been reported (Clutton-Brock 1997). Capnography does not hasten ventilatory weaning, and is unreliable when lung pathology is abnormal (most ICU patients), so its value is limited (Drew *et al.* 1998).

Implications for practice

- choice of modes for respiratory monitoring should meet clinical needs while minimising risks
- where appropriate, noninvasive or minimally invasive modes should be selected
- pulse oximetry provides continuous information without needing noninvasive equipment
- oxygen saturation (SpO_2) and partial pressure (PaO_2) have a non-linear relationship, shown by the oxygen dissociation curve
- capnography provides noninvasive information of metabolic function and carbon dioxide production, but discrepancies from venous tensions are increased with severe respiratory disease

- check effectiveness of ventilation by auscultation, blood gases, oximetry saturation
- ICU nurses should recognise different breath sounds; physiotherapists and other colleagues can help develop these skills
- whatever technology is used, information should be placed in context of the whole person (including visual observations)

Summary

Respiratory monitoring is fundamental to intensive care nursing and medicine. This chapter assumes familiarity with interpreting information gained from ventilators themselves, and so has focused on other modes. Oximetry, simple and noninvasive, is widely used in most areas of healthcare, although critical illness usually necessitates additional monitoring. Whatever means is used, observations can only be as reliable as those making and interpreting the observations. ICU nurses therefore should understand the physiology and mechanics of lung function and pathophysiology. Respiratory monitoring is therefore fundamental to care underlying many of the pathologies discussed in the third section of this book.

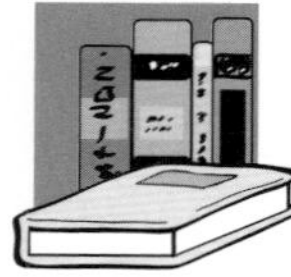

Further reading

Most texts describe widely used methods of monitoring; occasional articles appear on less commonly used modes, usually in medical journals. Physiotherapy literature, such as A. Jones (1995), is a useful source for information on auscultation; there are fewer recent nursing articles, but O'Hanlon-Nichols (1998) describes techniques. Much has been written on pulse oximetry; S. Jones (1995) and Jensen *et al.* (1998) being especially useful articles. Drew *et al.* (1998) usefully describe capnography and its limitations. Gibbons (1997) provides a recent nursing article on transcutaneous monitoring.

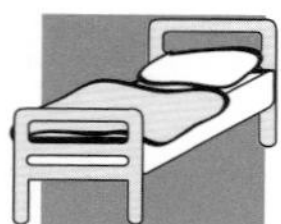

Clinical scenario

Michael Herschel is 39 years old and was admitted to ICU 20 days previously for invasive ventilation to support his deteriorating respiratory function. His initial diagnosis was *Pneumocystis carinii* pneumonia (PCP). His ventilatory support has been slowly weaned and he now receives inspired O_2 of 35 per cent, CPAP (+ 6 cmH_2O) during the day, augmented by nocturnal SIMV (with PS 15–18 cmH_2O, PEEP +4 cmH_2O, TV 500–600 ml, rate 20–25 min). He remains intubated via tracheotomy.

The most recent microbiological results of his sputum show presence of *Pseudomonas* and *Escherichia coli*. Three days ago skin swabs revealed Michael had become colonised with MRSA. His sputum on spontaneous coughing and aspiration is thick, mucopurulent, yellow-green and copious. On auscultation, vesicular breath sounds are diminished in apices, with crackles in both bases.

Michael has no arterial line for sampling blood gases, however his E_TCO_2 is 4.1 kPa and venous blood gas is:

pH: 7.44
PO_2 : 6.8 k Pa
PCO_2 : 4.7 kPa
H_2CO_3 : 23.3 mmol/l
BE: −0.2 mmol/l
SvO_2: 79%
SpO_2 : 96%

Q.1 Identify abnormalities in Michael's results and explain their relevance.
Q.2 What other investigations or monitoring can be used to assess Michael's respiratory function?
Q.3 Evaluate the nurse's role with respiratory monitoring in your own clinical practice area. Consider the range of monitoring approaches and specify which one nurses initiate/use, nurses role in interpreting and acting on results, troubleshooting, training, supervising use of monitoring equipment.

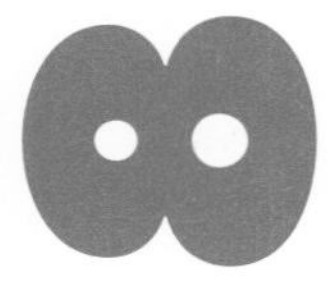

Chapter 18

Gas carriage

Contents

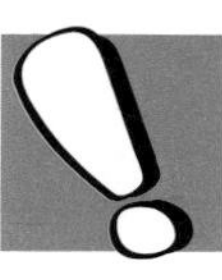

Fundamental knowledge

Pulmonary anatomy and physiology (including vasculature)
Normal respiration (including chemical + neurological control and mechanics of external respiration)
Dead space
Erythropoietin and erythropoiesis

Introduction

Studying physiology and pathology necessitates reductionism, but body systems function as parts of the whole body not in isolation. Cardiovascular and respiratory functions are particularly closely interdependent: delivering oxygen (and nutrients) to tissues while removing carbon dioxide (and other waste products) from the tissues. Respiration should achieve adequate tissue oxygenation, so that gas movement across the lung membranes forms external respiration, while gas movement between tissue cells and capillaries forms internal respiration.

This chapter explores internal respiration, identifying various factors that affect tissue perfusion and oxygenation. The structure of haemoglobin, and its effect on oxygen carriage and the oxygen saturation curve are identified. Carbon dioxide carriage and some haemoglobinopathies (methaemoglobin, sickle cell, thalassaemia) are also discussed.

The fraction of inspired oxygen (FiO_2) should be expressed as a decimal (or a fraction). Thus 100 per cent oxygen = FiO_2 of 1.0 (not 100).

Oxygen carriage

Oxygen is carried by blood in two ways:

- plasma (3 per cent)
- haemoglobin (97 per cent)

At normal (sea-level) atmospheric pressure 0.3 ml of oxygen is dissolved in every decilitre of blood (Green 1976), so that an average 5-litre circulation would contain $0.3 \times 10 \times 5 = 15$ ml oxygen. As cardiac output would need to be about 100 litres per minute to meet metabolic demands (Prencipe & Brenna, undated), oxygen carriage by plasma is normally insufficient to maintain life. When haemoglobin oxygen carriage is prevented (e.g. carbon monoxide poisoning), increasing atmospheric pressure (hyperbaric oxygen) will increase plasma carriage enabling therapeutic levels to be achieved. Oxygen tensions in plasma determine partial pressure (PO_2), the pressure gradient that enables transfer of oxygen to tissues.

Tissue oxygen supply is determined by:

- haemoglobin level
- oxygen saturation of haemoglobin
- oxygen dissociation
- perfusion pressure

This chapter focuses on the first two of these factors, although the effects of hypoperfusion should be remembered, especially as it so often complicates pathologies seen in ICUs.

Erythropoiesis occurs primarily in bone marrow. Adults have

approximately two litres of bone marrow. Erythrocyte production takes eight days, cells remaining functional for approximately 120 days, with 1 per cent of erythrocytes being replaced each day.

Renal or bone marrow disease reduces erythrocyte production, resulting in hypoplastic anaemia.

Haemoglobin

Haemoglobin combines haem (iron) and globin (polypeptide protein). Each haemoglobin molecule contains two pairs of polypeptides, making haemoglobin a large molecule (weighing about 64,450 Da (Ganong 1995)) and so above capillary permeability. Haemoglobin is therefore not normally lost into interstitial fluid (oedema) or urine.

An average 70 kg adult has about 900 grams of circulating haemoglobin, giving 'normal' levels of 14–18 g/dl for men and 12–16 g/dl for women (Rowswell 1997). Lower concentrations decrease viscosity, so aid perfusion: 10 g/dl being preferred with critically ill patients. Each hour, 0.3 g of haemoglobin is destroyed and synthesised, the average erythrocyte life being 120 days (Buswell 1996). Macrophages metabolise old erythrocytes, releasing iron (for further haemoglobin synthesis) and waste (excreted in bile).

Polypeptides of normal adult haemoglobin (HbA) consist of two alpha and two beta chains: $\alpha_2 + \beta_2$. The slight biochemical differences between alpha and beta chains are not significant for clinical nursing, but abnormalities of either chain can cause pathologies. Each erythrocyte contains approximately 640 million haemoglobin molecules (Hoffbrand & Pettit 1993).

Fetal haemoglobin (HbF) is similar to haemoglobin A, except that gamma chains replace beta chains and 2,3 DPG (diphosphoglycerate) concentrations are higher, increasing its affinity for oxygen. This facilitates the transfer of oxygen from maternal blood (HbA). Adult haemoglobin normally replaces fetal haemoglobin soon after birth, although the latter can (abnormally) persist throughout life, predisposing patients to tissue hypoxia. Other haemoglobinopathies are discussed later in this chapter.

One gram of haemoglobin can carry 1.34 ml oxygen. Haemoglobin levels of 10 g/dl with an average 5-litre circulating volume give a total body haemoglobin of $10 \times 5 \times 10 = 500$ grams. If fully saturated, this would carry 500×1.34 ml oxygen = 670 ml of oxygen (plasma carries only 15 ml oxygen).

If all four limbs of the molecule carry oxygen, the haemoglobin is described as fully (100 per cent) saturated. Saturation of total haemoglobin (not single molecules) can be measured through oximetry (e.g. pulse oximetry), 'normal' arterial (SaO_2) or capillary (peripheral – SpO_2) saturation being about 98 per cent.

While haemoglobin is an efficient transport mechanism for oxygen, usually only 20–25 per cent of available oxygen unloads, leaving normal venous saturations (SvO_2) of 70–75 per cent. This large venous reserve can provide oxygen without any increase in respiration rate or cardiac output so that, while SaO_2 indicates oxygen availability, the $SaO_2 - SvO_2$ gradient indicates tissue uptake (consumption) of oxygen, measured through cardiac output studies (see below).

Chemicals (e.g. prussic acid), can inhibit release of oxygen from haemoglobin. Prussic acid is found in cyanide, one of the degradation products of sodium nitroprusside.

Partial pressure of gases

Air contains approximately 21 per cent oxygen and 79 per cent nitrogen, with negligible amounts of other gases (carbon dioxide is 0.03 per cent of air content). Barometric, and so alveolar, pressure (at sea level) is 101.3 kPa (Green 1976). Total atmospheric pressure includes water vapour. At 37°C (i.e. normal alveolar temperature) water vapour exerts a constant pressure of 6.3 kPa (Green 1976), irrespective of total barometric pressure. Thus the partial pressure of each gas is determined by the difference between total barometric pressure and water pressure vapour percentage concentration of gas, which is then divided in proportion to percentage concentration of gases (see Table 18.1).

Table 18.1 Partial pressures of gases (approximate)

	Concentration in air (%)	*Pressure in air (kPa)*	*Pressure in alveoli (kPa)*[a]
water vapour		variable[b]	6.3
oxygen	21	21.27	13.3
carbon dioxide	0.03	0.03	5.3
nitrogen	79	80	76.4

Notes: a air warmed to 37ºC, hence constant water vapour
b depends on temperature

The remaining 95 kPa of sea-level pressure is divided proportionally between gases (see Table 18.1). Alveolar gas tensions are altered by rebreathing 'dead space' gas, relatively rich in carbon dioxide and poor in oxygen. Physiological adult dead space is about 150 ml; additional pathological dead space exists when alveoli are not perfused. With artificial ventilation, dead space begins at the inspiratory limb ('Y' connector) of ventilator tubing. Small breaths or large dead space lower alveolar partial pressure of oxygen.

Cellular respiration

The purpose of respiratory function is to supply tissue cells with sufficient oxygen to enable mitochondrial activity and remove carbon dioxide (a waste product of metabolism). Mitochondria are the powerhouses of the cell, so that their failure leads to cellular damage and eventual cell death. Currently, it is not practical to monitor mitochondrial respiration, and cruder parameters (e.g. arterial gas tensions) are measured instead. However, the end of respiratory function should be remembered when assessing intermediate parameters.

Partial pressures of oxygen progressively fall with further stages of internal respiration: capillary pressure of 6.8 kPa gives tissue pressure of 2.7 kPa and mitochondrial pressure of 0.13–1.3 kPa (facilitating gas diffusion, which depends on continuing pressure differentials). Similarly, carbon dioxide tensions increase. Relative differences in pressures create the concentration gradient that enables diffusion across capillary and cell membranes. However, a fall in alveolar partial pressure (from respiratory failure) reflects proportional reductions in tensions throughout the body, resulting in tissue hypoxia. Similarly, giving oxygen concentrations above 21 per cent increases alveolar tensions, reflected in proportional increases in tensions throughout the body. Alveolar carbon dioxide tensions vary with frequency and size of tidal volume, $PaCO_2$ and buffers (mainly HCO_3^-).

Oxygen dissociation curve

The complex relationship between partial pressures of arterial oxygen (PaO_2) and oxygen saturation of haemoglobin (SaO_2) are shown in the oxygen saturation curve (Figure 18.1), which determines oxygen dissociation. Transfer of gasses across capillary membranes is determined by differentials in partial pressure on either side of the membrane.

Oxygen content of arterial blood is the sum of the oxygen dissolved in plasma (PaO_2) and the oxygen carried by haemoglobin (SaO_2). Most oxygen is carried by haemoglobin, but oxygen in solution determines the partial pressure and, thus, tension of gas across the capillary membrane.

On the *plateau* of the curve (SaO_2 above 75 per cent) oxygen readily dissociates from haemoglobin, causing marked fluctuations in PaO_2 , and making oxygen saturation a relatively insensitive marker of oxygen content (e.g. patients receiving supplemental oxygen may have saturations nearing 100 per cent with excessively high PaO_2). Increasing SaO_2 above 90 per cent has little effect on oxygen delivery.

Below the 'venous point' (75 per cent saturation), oxygen saturation falls rapidly in relation to partial pressure. This is sometimes called the 'steep' part of the curve, where oxygen readily dissociates from haemoglobin to maintain the oxygen pressure gradient (PaO_2) (Hough 1996). Small reductions in partial pressure can therefore mask large reductions in saturation and, consequently, significant falls in total oxygen content and reserve.

The oxygen dissociation curve can be shifted to the right or left by various factors (see Table 18.2). A shift to right decreases affinity of haemoglobin for oxygen, causing increased unloading of oxygen, and so increasing tissue oxygenation. This occurs in order to meet increased demand for oxygen by hypoxic tissue; exercising muscles are hot, hypercarbic and need oxygen.

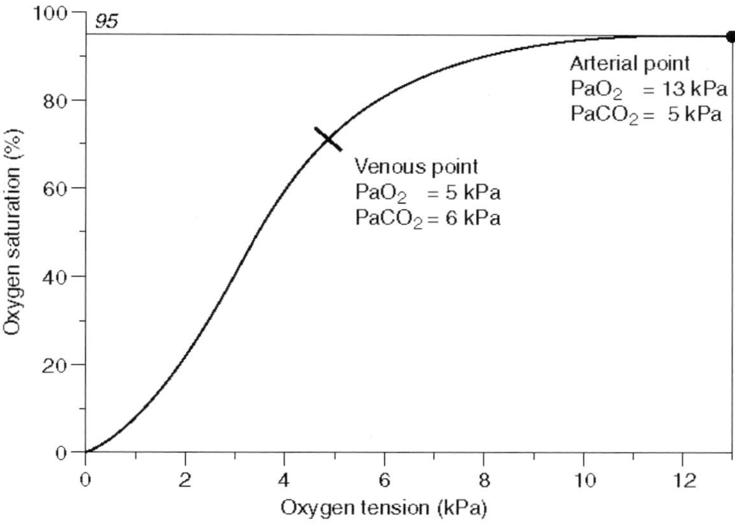

Figure 18.1 Oxygen dissociation curve

Conversely, a shift to left increases affinity of haemoglobin for oxygen, resulting in reduced tissue uptake; pink ears and noses on cold mornings are caused by haemoglobin retaining oxygen (Hough 1996).

Table 18.2 Factors causing shifts in the oxygen dissociation curve

SHIFT TO RIGHT caused by
high temperature
acidosis (pH)
high 2,3 DPG concentrations
endocrine disorders

SHIFT TO LEFT caused by
hypothermia
alkalosis
low 2,3 DPG
(some) haemoglobinopathies (e.g. HbF, methaemoglobin)
carbon monoxide

Intracellular changes in haemoglobin molecules are caused by:

- **Bohr effect:** increasing hydrogen and pCO_2 (acidosis) decreases oxyhaemoglobin saturation
- 2,3 DPG levels: these organic phosphates are highly charged anions in erythrocyte which bind to haemoglobin, reducing its affinity for oxygen

Oxygen toxicity

Inducing/mimicking critical illness in healthy volunteers for research is unethical. Since evidence for oxygen toxicity is largely derived from animal studies (humans can differ from animals) or critically ill patients (potential extraneous variables and small sample size), evidence remains contentious, but likely effects include

- pulmonary capillary cell swelling (Hinds & Watson 1996)
- interstitial oedema (Hinds & Watson 1996)
- damage to (surfactant-producing) type-1 alveolar cells (Hinds & Watson 1996)
- progressive decrease in lung compliance (Oh 1997)
- haemorrhagic interstitial + intra-alveolar oedema (Oh 1997)
- (eventual) pulmonary fibrosis (Oh 1997)
- mucociliary impairment, causing sputum retention (DiRusso *et al.* 1995)
- alveolar distension and atelectasis from nitrogen displacement
- substernal pain (Hinds & Watson 1996)

Exact mechanisms of oxygen toxicity remain unclear, but possible mechanisms include:

- production of superoxide anions (**free radicals**)
- overpowering of normal antioxidant defenses (e.g. vitamin E) by excessive concentrations of oxidants
- increased sympathetic activity (cf. inotropes)
- reduced surfactant
- antioxidant (vitamins E and C) deficiency
- hypermetabolism
- adrenocortical excess

Delivering high concentrations of oxygen therefore necessitates weighing dangers from tissue hypoxia against dangers from oxygen toxicity. There is no evidence to suggest that short periods of high concentrations are harmful, but length of 'safe' periods and levels at which toxicity begins remain contentious.

Ganong (1995) suggests that after eight hours oxygen concentrations above 80 per cent irritate respiratory passages, progressing to lung damage after 24 hours exposure. DiRusso *et al.* (1995) argues that oxygen concentrations of about 50 per cent for 24 hours or above 40 per cent for 72 hours, cause lung damage (DiRusso *et al.* 1995). Most literature falls between these two extremes; clinical signs of damage are rare with prolonged concentrations of 50 per cent oxygen, or 100 per cent for less than 24 hours (Oh 1997). Hyperbaric oxygen (100 per cent) accelerates damage in proportion to atmospheric pressures used (Ganong 1995).

Most intensivists limit prolonged (over 24 hours) oxygen exposure to 50–60 per cent whenever possible, meeting oxygen demand through adjusting other supports (e.g. PEEP, I:E ratio).

Brief hyperoxygenation (e.g. 100 per cent for 5 minutes before/after endotracheal suction) reduces risks of significant hypoxia (and anaerobic metabolism). However prolonged hyperoxygenation can cause toxic hyperoxia. Hyperoxia can be detected by blood gas analysis, but not pulse oximetry, due to the sigmoid relationship between SaO_2 and PaO_2 (the oxygen dissociation curve) (Hough 1996).

Carbon dioxide transport

This chapter concentrates on oxygen rather than carbon dioxide carriage, oxygen being vital for life, whereas carbon dioxide is a waste product of metabolism. Carbon dioxide carriage is also relatively more simple than the carriage of oxygen.

Metabolism produces 200 ml/minute of carbon dioxide. Normal blood concentrations vary between 48 ml per decilitre (arterial) to 52 ml/decilitre (venous) (Green 1976), a narrow pressure differential. Carbon dioxide is twenty times more soluble than oxygen, enabling rapid diffusion (and so removal) across capillaries (Hough 1996).

Carbon dioxide is carried by blood in three ways:

- plasma
- haemoglobin
- bicarbonate

PLASMA Carbon dioxide is approximately twenty times more soluble than oxygen, and so is readily carried in solution by plasma. Prencipe and Brenna (undated) suggest that 6.92 ml is carried in every decilitre, reflecting normal venous partial pressures. Volumes will be lower when partial pressure ($PaCO_2$) is lower. About one-tenth of carbon dioxide carriage is through plasma solution.

HAEMOGLOBIN About one-quarter of carbon dioxide is carried as carbaminoglobin. Carbon dioxide binds to globin, not haem, so unlike carbon monoxide does not displace oxygen.

BICARBONATE Most (approximately three-quarters) of carbon dioxide carriage occurs as a component of plasma bicarbonate (see Chapter 19):

$$CO_2 + H_2O \rightleftharpoons H_2CO_3 \rightleftharpoons HCO_3 + H^+$$

Diffusion of carbon dioxide occurs through simple tension gradients, uncomplicated by factors such as affinity of haemoglobin for oxygen. So the carbon dioxide dissociation curve is virtually linear (see Figure 18.2). Like the oxygen dissociation curve, carbon dioxide dissociation can move to the right or left. Rightward shifts (favouring dissociation of oxygen from haemoglobin) occur with raised levels concentrations of oxygen in blood.

Haemoglobinopathies

Critical illness is frequently complicated by haemoglobinopathies; four are described here.

METHAEMOGLOBIN This occurs when oxidation changes iron from a ferrous to a ferric state. This makes blood a dusky, cyanotic colour. Methaemoglobin shifts the oxygen dissociation curve leftwards, reducing oxygen availability for tissues. Oxidation can be caused by various drugs, including lignocaine, nitrates and metoclopramide (Adam & Osborne 1997) and nitric oxide. Methaemoglobin causes pulse oximetry readings of 85 per cent, regardless of arterial oxygen saturation (Wahr & Tremper 1996).

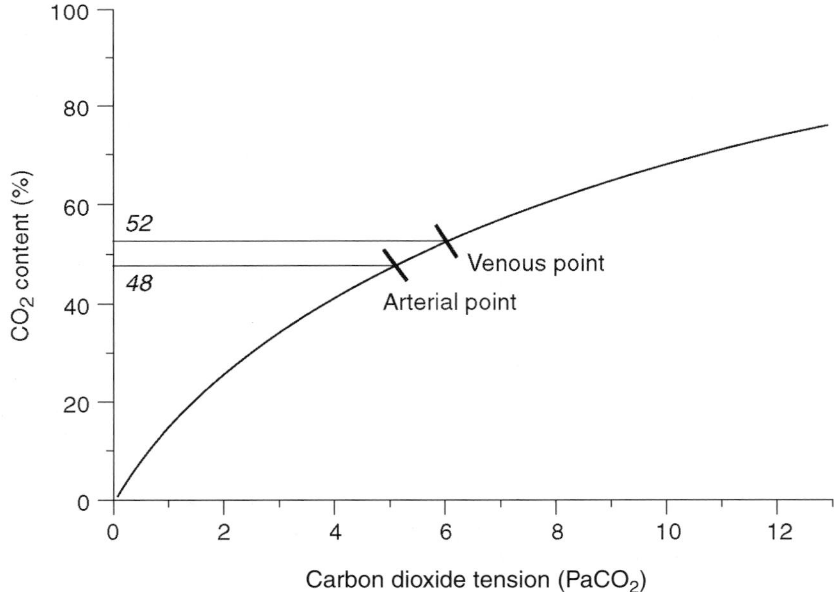

***Figure 18.2* Carbon dioxide dissociation curve**

CARBON MONOXIDE This has greater (200–250 times (Harper & Collee 1997)) affinity for haemoglobin than oxygen, thus preventing oxygen carriage. Ten per cent carboxyhaemoglobin (e.g. from smoking cigarettes) is generally asymptomatic, but 40 per cent carboxyhaemoglobin generally causes collapse and coma (Armstrong 1997). The half-life of carbon monoxide in air is 250 minutes; this time can be reduced by increasing oxygen concentration or atmospheric pressure (see Chapter 29).

THALASSAEMIA ('COOLEY'S ANAEMIA') This is caused by defective globin genes; the anaemia is classified as alpha or beta thalassaemia, depending on which gene is affected (Arya & Bellingham 1997). Thalassaemia may also be classified as major, intermedia or minor, depending on its severity. The genetic defect reduces erythrocyte life (Buswell 1996), thus reducing erythrocyte concentration below 2 million per cubic millimetre (Marieb 1995). The abnormal haemoglobin is also less able to release oxygen. Typically, people with thalassaemia have Mediterranean ancestry.

Since anaemia is caused by lack of erythrocytes, traditional treatment has been blood transfusion to increase haemoglobin concentration. However, frequent transfusion can cause iron overload (Buswell 1996), and so desferrioxamine (an iron chelator) helps to prevent hepatic failure. Splenectomies may be performed where erythrocyte destruction exceeds production, and younger patients may receive bone marrow transplant if a sibling or parent is HbA compatible.

SICKLE CELL (HBS) This is due to replacement of glutamic acid in beta chains by valine residue; with hypoxia, this abnormality causes chains to link together as stiff rods, changing erythrocytes from elliptical into sickle shapes. HbS cells have reduced life spans, causing chronic haemolytic anaemia. Sickle-shaped erythrocytes can occlude small capillaries, causing necrosis, infarction and ischaemic pain in tissue beyond occlusions. Deformed erythrocytes rupture, causing clotting and further obstruction. Cerebral and renal microcapillaries are at special risk; small peripheral blood vessels often cause intense pain.

Sickle genes cause erythrocytes infected by malarial parasites to adhere to capillary walls, denying parasites the potassium they need to survive. Sickle cells provide protection from malaria (Marieb 1995), and so this mutation has flourished in the malarial belt. However people with sickle cell disease now live worldwide (4 million in total, 6,000 in the UK (Fuggle *et al.* 1996)).

Sickle cell crises may occur with any hypoxic stressor, such as exercise, altitude, surgery, anaesthetic gases or critical illness. Crisis carries a significant mortality, so that although people with both haemoglobin chromosomes (HbS, HbS) are most at risk, people with sickle cell trait (HbS, HbA) can sickle with extreme hypoxia. Those at risk should be safeguarded by optimising oxygen (e.g. pre-oxygenating with endotracheal suction).

Crisis management focuses on providing:

- analgesia
- oxygen
- fluids
- blood (exchange) transfusion

Sickle crisis pain is intense, requiring strong analgesia. Traditionally, pethidine was used, although poor absorption and tolerance reduce benefits below the usually cited two hours, so morphine is increasingly used (Thomas & Westerdale 1997). Despite anecdotal concerns about addiction and feigning crises to obtain opiates, benefits from analgesia to those in crisis far outweigh risks from drug abuse (see Chapter 7).

The delivery of oxygen to ischaemic tissues relieves ischaemic pain and prevents further damage (although *reperfusion injury* may damage tissue – see Chapter 26). Giving intravenous fluids to increase blood volume and reduce viscosity, while optimising alveolar oxygen, favours oxygen delivery. Exchange blood transfusion reduces circulating HbS cells in favour of HbA.

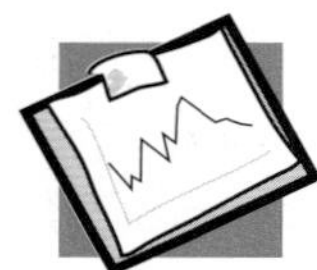

Implications for practice

- most blood gas samples and observations of continuous monitoring are recorded by nurses, and so ICU nurses should interpret samples, reporting unexpected abnormalities
- pulse oximetry can valuably supplement other observations, but cannot detect hypercarbia, and can be affected by extraneous factors
- SaO_2 measures plasma oxygen, whereas PaO_2 measures oxyhaemoglobin; ICU nurses should understand how oxygen dissociation affects these observations

Summary

Oxygen is primarily carried by haemoglobin, plasma carriage being normally insignificant. The complex dissociation of oxygen has been discussed in this chapter; the dissociation curve will be referred to in some later chapters to help nurses apply its principles to bedside care. Haemoglobinopathies will also affect oxygen carriage. Although carbon dioxide is carried through three mechanisms, its dissociation is relatively linear and simple.

Blood gas analysis is widely used to assess both respiratory and metabolic function. Non-invasive and continuous display technology may replace intermittent arterial sampling, but components measured are likely to remain, and so have been described. Nurses can valuably develop their skills with blood gas analysis by working through samples from practice, remembering to apply information within the context of the whole patient.

Useful contacts

The Sickle Cell Society: 54 Station Road, London, NW10 4UA; 0208–961 7795 or 4006
OSCAR (Organisation for Sickle Cell Research): Tiverton Sickle Cell Community Centre, Tiverton Road, London, N15 6RT; 0207–274 5999
UK Thalassaemia Society: 19 The Broadway, London; 0208–882 0011

Further reading

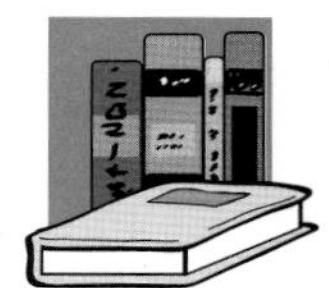

Blood gas analysis is described in most ICU textbooks and worthwhile anatomy texts. Although old, Green (1976) gives much useful information about carriage of gases. Articles on haemoglobinopathies appear periodically in nursing journals (Thomas & Westerdale 1997); further information can be obtained from the support groups mentioned above.

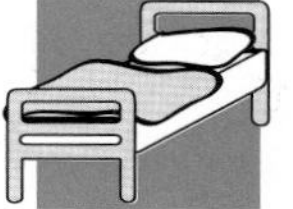

Clinical scenario

Julie Panks, who is 36 years old, was admitted to ICU unconscious from taking aspirin overdose the previous day. Her plasma salicylate level is 890 mg/l. She has sickle cell trait and Hb of 9.2 g/dl and core temperature on admission was 36.5°C

Arterial blood gas analysis revealed:

	On admission to ICU	*6 hours later*	*12 hours later*
pH	7.25	7.21	7.32
PaO_2 (KPa)	9.32	12.4	13.5
$PaCO_2$ (KPa)	8.10	6.24	5.85
HCO_3 (mmol/l)	21.2	17.4	19.7
BE	1.9	−8.6	−4.7
Lactate (mmol/l)	1.5	4.5	3.2

Q.1 Using the Oxygen Dissociation Curve (Figure 18.1) calculate Julie's percentage of O_2 saturation of haemoglobin (SaO_2) for each of the three arterial blood gas results (plot the position of her PaO_2 incorporating Julie's Hb, temperature and other arterial blood gas values)

Q.2 Explain any shifts in the oxygen dissociation curve and haemoglobin's affinity for O_2 at Julie's cellular (tissue) and alveolar membrane. How does the level of carbon dioxide in blood affect oxygen transport?

Q.3 Review alternative assessment approaches that can be used by nurses to monitor effectiveness of oxygen transport to Julie's tissues (consider and specify types of visual observation, laboratory investigations, assessing for complications associated with Hb*S*).

Chapter 19

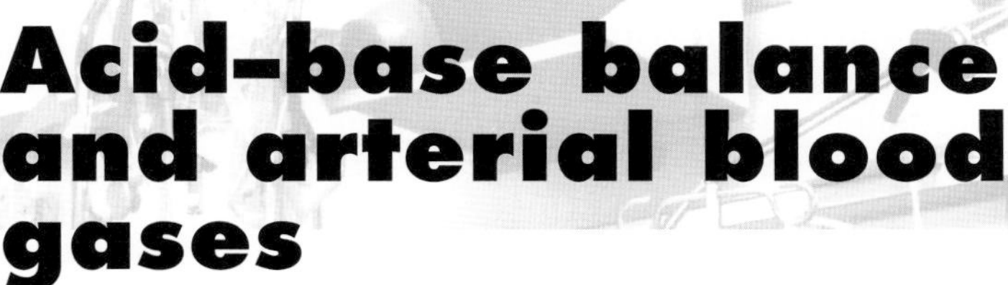

Acid–base balance and arterial blood gases

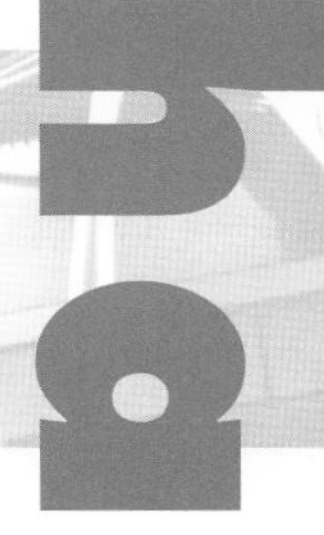

Contents

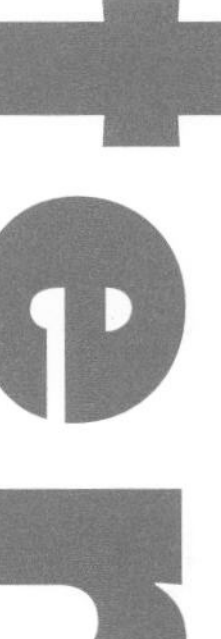

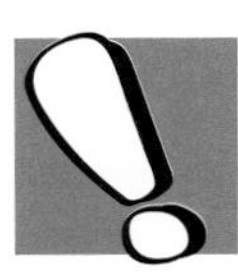

Fundamental knowledge

Cellular metabolism, oxygen consumption and carbon dioxide production

Introduction

Nurses are introduced to arterial blood gas analysis early in their ICU careers, and so parts of this chapter provide a revision of applied, rather than pure, biochemistry; in addition, controversies not always identified through orientation programmes are also raised.

This chapter begins with a discussion of acid–base balance, goes on to suggest briefly good practice for taking arterial blood gas samples, and then discusses other results commonly found in blood gas analysis. Like many other aspects of practice, the technology for blood gas analysis varies, as does the data used between units. Using sample printouts from your unit may be helpful.

The standard UK use of kPa is followed here (in the USA, mmHg is most frequently used). The conversion of scales is: 1 kPa × 7.5 approximately equals 1 mmHg.

Acid–base definitions

An acid is a substance capable of providing hydrogen ions; a base is capable of accepting hydrogen ions. Acidity is determined by amount of free hydrogen ions, not the total number of hydrogen ions; hydrogen ions can bind (associate) to negative ions (anions), such as bicarbonate (HCO_3^-). Therefore, a strong acid (e.g. hydrochloric) is highly dissociated, releasing many hydrogen ions, whereas a weak acid has few free hydrogen ions. Similarly strong bases (alkali) absorb many free hydrogen ions. Acid–base balance, therefore, is the power of hydrogen ions (pH) measured in moles per litre ('power' used in the mathematical sense, for the negative logarithm). The power of hydrogen ions can be controlled (balanced) either through *buffering* or exchange. Hydrogen is a positively charged ion (cation) which can be buffered by negatively charged ions (anion) such as bicarbonate. Hydrogen may move into another body compartment, either through pressure gradient differentials or in exchange for similarly charged ions. The only other significant cations in the human body are sodium and potassium, while the only significant anions are chloride and bicarbonate.

pH measurement

Hydrogen ion concentrations in body fluids are about one million times less than concentrations of other ions (Hornbein 1994). Blood contains about 0.00004 mmol (or 40 nanomoles, nmol) of hydrogen per litre (cf. plasma sodium concentration is about 140 mmol/l). Despite these very small concentrations, hydrogen ions are highly reactive, with small changes in concentration creating significant changes in enzyme activity (Hornbein 1994) and oxygen carriage (the Bohr effect – see Chapter 18). With plasma concentrations being so small, ions are measured by a negative logarithm.

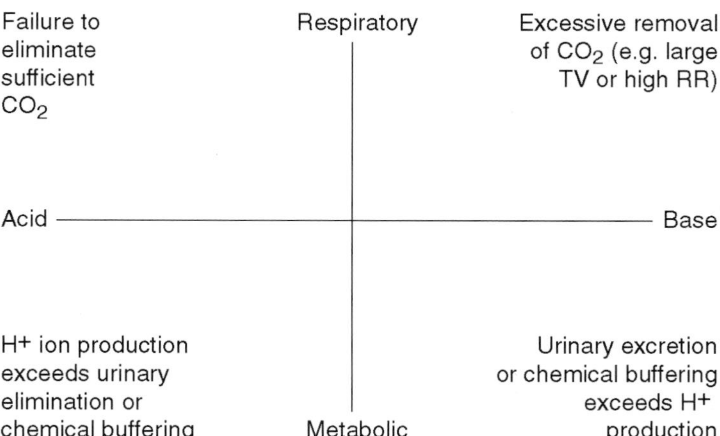

Figure 19.1 The origin of acid–base imbalance

Logarithms are ways to cope with large numbers. Thus, the log to the base 10 represents multiples of 10 by a power:

$10^1 = 10$
$10^2 = 10 \times 10 = 100$
$10^3 = 100 \times 10 = 1000$
$10^4 = 1000 \times 10 = 10{,}000$

Increasing one figure in the power represents a tenfold increase in the actual number. Bacterial concentrations are often expressed using the log to the base 10. Negative logarithms use the same principle to manage very small numbers, so that:

$10^{-1} = 0.1$
$10^{-2} = 0.01$

Normal plasma concentrations of 0.00004 mmol/l can be rewritten as pH 7.4. While the pH scale enables concentrations of huge ranges within confined limits of 0–14 (absolute acid to absolute alkaline), small alterations in pH can significantly alter hydrogen ion concentrations. Doubling or halving acid concentrations alters pH by 0.3:

pH 7.7 = 20 nmol/l H^+
pH 7.4 = 40 nmol/l H^+
pH 7.1 = 80 nmol/l H^+
pH 6.8 = 160 nmol/l H^+

The chemical pH scale ranges from 0–14 so that pH 7.0 is chemically neutral. The homeostatic pH of human blood is 7.4, and so blood pH of 7.4 is physiologically neutral (although chemically alkalotic). With homeostasis, arterial pH maintains a bicarbonate to carbon dioxide ratio of 20:1 (Prencipe & Brenna, undated). Because minute concentrations of hydrogen ions have such profound effects, blood pH needs to be maintained within very narrow ranges – usually given as 7.36–7.44. Blood below this range is therefore termed 'acidotic', even though chemically it remains alkaline until reaching a pH of 7.0.

Hydrogen ion exchange relies on partial pressure gradients. Metabolism produces about 40–80 nmol of hydrogen each day (Marshall 1995), creating a concentration gradient between intracellular (highest) levels and plasma. Normal interstitial pH is 7.33–7.43 (Sherwin 1996) (more acidic than plasma), so that venous blood pH is lower than arterial.

Although chemically useful, extremes of human life have narrow pH ranges: Marieb (1995) cites 7.0–7.8 (although Selby and James (1995) report a rare survival with pH 6.4). Arterial pH below 7.0 usually leads to coma and death, while levels above 7.8 overstimulate the nervous system, causing convulsions and respiratory arrest. Homeostasis, therefore, aims to maintain levels within physiological levels of about 7.35–7.45. Acid–base balance is controlled through three mechanisms:

- respiratory
- renal
- chemical buffering

Respiratory control

In the lungs, carbonic acid, being unstable, dissociates into water and carbon dioxide:

$$H_2CO_3 \rightleftharpoons H_2O + CO_2$$

Thus, partial pressure of carbon dioxide in plasma indicates carbonic acid level, and carbon dioxide is therefore considered a potential acid (lacking hydrogen ions, it is not really an acid). Hence, *respiratory acidosis* is failure to remove sufficient carbon dioxide (i.e. high pCO_2); *respiratory alkalosis* is excessive removal of carbon dioxide (i.e. low pCO_2).

The body produces 15,000–20,000 mmol of carbon dioxide each day (Coleman & Houston 1998). Hypercapnia stimulates medullary chemoreceptors, thus stimulating the respiratory centre to increase rate and depth of breaths, which removes essential components of carbonic acid. Although respiration cannot remove hydrogen ions, it can inhibit carbonic acid formation, so restoring homeostasis.

Respiratory acidosis is caused either by lung disease (impairing carbon dioxide exchange) or hypoventilation. Respiratory alkalosis is caused by hyperventilation (high rate, tidal/minute volume).

Respiratory response to acidosis occurs within three minutes of imbalance, exerting up to double the effect of combined chemical buffers (Marieb 1995). Doubling or halving alveolar ventilation can move pH by 0.2, but alveolar ventilation can increase fifteenfold or fall to nothing (Marieb 1995), which could return a life-threatening pH of 7.0, to 7.2 or 7.3 in 3–12 minutes (Guyton & Hall 1997).

Metabolic balance

Metabolic balance is more complex. Acids are produced through

- metabolism (e.g. Krebs cycle)
- secretion (e.g. gastric)

removed through the

- kidneys

and buffered by

- chemicals

Bases (bicarbonate) are

- produced
- reabsorbed (renally)

and sometimes

- ingested/infused (e.g. antacids)

Metabolic acidosis is failure to remove/buffer sufficient hydrogen (H^+) ions as a result of:

- excessive H^+ production (e.g. shock, MI)
- renal failure
- insufficient buffers

Metabolic alkalosis is excessive removal/buffering of hydrogen (H^+) ions or excessive production/absorption of bases as a result of:

- polyuria
- hypokalaemia (so excess H^+ in urine)

- gastric acid loss (e.g. excessive nasogastric drainage, vomiting, diarrhoea)
- excessive buffers (e.g. colonic reabsorption from constipation)

Lactic acidosis is sometimes divided between type A (with clinical evidence of hypoperfusion) and type B (where hypoperfusion is not clinically identifiable) (Mizock & Falk 1992); these terms, which are found in some medical texts, have little significance for nursing acidotic patients.

Renal control

The kidneys actively contribute to acid–base balance in two ways:

- hydrogen ion excretion
- chemical buffering (producing and reabsorbing filtered bicarbonate and phosphate)

and passively remove water (the remaining product of carbonic acid dissociation following respiratory removal of carbon dioxide).

Although respiration controls carbonic acid, hydrogen ions can only be removed from the body by the kidneys, where they are actively exchanged for other cations, primarily sodium. Since potassium competes with hydrogen for sodium exchange, hyperkalaemia competes with acidosis for clearance of excess cations.

The normal renal excretion of hydrogen ions is 30–70 mmol each day (Raftery 1997), although levels can reach 300 mmol per day within 7–10 days (Worthley 1997). This enables metabolic (renal) compensation for prolonged respiratory acidosis (e.g. respiratory failure). Hydrogen is excreted in urine as an ammonium ion (NH_4^+) (Worthley 1997) and phosphate (HPO_4^-); urinalysis can measure urinary pH (normally 5.0), but remembering the relationship between small shifts in pH and large shifts in (effects of) hydrogen ion loss above, dipstick urinalysis pH is a relatively insensitive marker.

Tubular selective reabsorption preserves most bicarbonate ions; the kidney also generates bicarbonate ions, so that renal failure can cause potentially profound metabolic acidoses.

Chemical buffers respond rapidly, within seconds, balancing hydrogen ions by binding acids to bases, but do not eliminate acids from the body. Thus hydrogen ions remain, with the potential for later rebound imbalances. The three main chemical buffers in blood are bicarbonate, phosphate and plasma proteins.

Bicarbonate is the major chemical buffer of extracellular fluid, responsible for one-half of all chemical buffering (Coleman & Houston 1998). Hydrogen ions are essential to produce bicarbonate (HCO_3^-). Bicarbonate combines with hydrogen to produce carbonic acid:

$$HCO_3^- + H^+ = H_2CO_3$$

Carbonic acid, the main acid in blood, is weak, readily dissociating into carbon dioxide and water (see Chapter 18). Therefore high serum bicarbonate can result in hypercarbia; carbon dioxide diffusing into intracellular fluid and across the blood–brain barrier may lead to intracellular acidosis and respiratory acidosis, although supporting evidence for these theories is lacking (Deakin 1997).

Bicarbonate, being an anion, couples with a cation, such as sodium to produce sodium bicarbonate ($NaHCO_3$). Bicarbonate is reabsorbed and produced by the kidneys, and so bicarbonate mediation of acid–base balance relies on normal renal function (Coleman & Houston 1998). The body produces about 20,000 mmol of carbonic acid each day (Prencipe & Brenna, undated), making this a very efficient medium for acid–base balance.

Phosphate has similar but more efficient effects to bicarbonate. Plasma phosphate concentrations are low, but phosphate is the main urinary and interstitial buffer.

Plasma and intracellular proteins: most chemical buffering occurs intracellularly. Histidine (in haemoglobin) is the main chemical buffer among plasma proteins, dissociating more readily from oxygen-poor haemoglobin.

Acidosis

Acidosis (blood pH below 7.35) may be caused by respiratory or metabolic failure (or both):

- respiratory = failure to excrete sufficient carbon dioxide (= high pCO_2)
- metabolic = failure to excrete/buffer sufficient H^+ ions (= negative base excess below 2; HCO_3 is usually low)

However caused, acidosis has various detrimental effects. The respiratory centre is driven by hypercapnia, acidaemia or hypoxia, and so normal or slightly raised carbon dioxide levels are needed to create the respiratory drive for weaning, while acidaemia shifts the oxygen dissociation curve to the right, favouring unloading of oxygen from haemoglobin; but hypercapnia may create unwanted respiratory drive before weaning is appropriate. Acidosis has a negative effect on cardiac and other muscle conduction, and affects enzyme activity. It may activate tumour necrosis factor and macrophages (Bakker 1996), aggravating SIRS and other critical pathologies.

Bicarbonate infusions (to reverse acidosis) can cause many problems; this is summarised by Mizock and Falk (1992):

- leftward shift of dissociation curve from alkalinisation (theoretically) impairs oxygen dissociation
- potential hyperosmolality/congestive cardiac failure from high sodium load
- metabolic alkalosis if infusion volume is excessive
- electrolyte imbalance (hypokalaemia, hypocalcaemia) impairing myocardial function
- reflex vasodilation and hypotension
- stimulation of glycolysis, producing further carbon dioxide and metabolic acidosis
- myocardial depression

Bicarbonate infusions are now usually given later (e.g. pH below 7.2) and limited to 50 mmol aliquots, after which pH should be rechecked.

Acidosis is a symptom, not a disease; underlying pathologies should remain the focus of treatment. Oxygen delivery to peripheries should be optimised, without increasing cell metabolism; the use of large amounts of vasodilators and volume expanders to achieve this will probably necessitate cardiac output studies and monitoring.

Tonometry

Gastric (intramucosal) pH (pHi) is a good indicator of acidaemia, due to high blood flow to the gut (Fiddian-Green 1995; Bakker 1996). However, intramucosal bicarbonate may give a poor reflection of arterial levels, especially in hypoperfused patients (Gomersall & Oh 1997). While tonometry has become a useful indicator of septic inflammatory response syndrome, multiorgan dysfunction syndrome, and so ICU mortality (Maynard *et al.* 1993), wider use is largely prevented both by its expense and the time it takes to obtain a reading (20 minutes) (Adam & Osborne 1997). With prolonged severe pathological processes, tonometry has some value, but it is not currently widely used for routine monitoring of acidaemia.

Blood gas samples

Various user errors can occur when sampling arterial blood. Syringes using wet heparin (whether prepared in-house or purchased commercially) may cause *dilutional inaccuracies*; syringe lumens should be coated with heparin, then excess expelled, leaving only enough heparin to fill the hub of the syringe (Gosling 1995; Beaumont 1997) – 0.1 ml of heparin is adequate for a 2 ml blood sample (Hinds & Watson 1996). If over one-tenth of the sample is heparin, carbon dioxide and bicarbonate readings will be significantly reduced (Hutchison *et al.* 1983) affecting various other derived measurements. Dilution probably has little effect on oxygen tensions (Hinds & Watson 1996). Beaumont (1997) suggests that standard (wet) heparin is unsuitable for haemoglobin, electrolytes, glucose or lactate measurement, and that electrolyte-balanced wet heparin is unsuitable for haemoglobin, co-oximetry, glucose, lactate or magnesium measurements. Additionally, sodium heparin or calcium heparin may affect electrolyte levels: sodium or calcium by addition, and other electrolytes by dilution.

Sufficient fluid should be withdrawn from arterial lines to prevent *dilution from saline* flush. Preusser *et al.* (1989) found that samples were accurate provided 2 ml had previously been discarded; although length of arterial lines varies, lumen content is small enough for this normally to be a negligible variable.

With infants and very small children, fluid drawn to clear lines is usually returned afterwards to prevent progressive *anaemia*; with adults, dangers from loss of such small volumes of blood are outweighed by infection and other risks from returning discarded blood.

Applying *negative pressure* may cause frothing (Szaflarski 1996), and so minimal aspiration should be used (Beaumont 1997); arterial samples normally fill passively from blood pressure. Air in samples causes spuriously low readings, and so should be expelled (Szaflarski 1996); samples should be covered (with hubs, not fingers) to prevent atmospheric gas exchange.

Delay in analysing increases inaccuracies from continuing erythrocyte and leucocyte metabolism (potassium and carbon dioxide levels increase, pH and oxygen tensions fall (Gosling 1995)). Room temperature samples should be analysed within 10 minutes (Biswas *et al.* 1982); samples stored in ice should be tested within 60 minutes (Clutton-Brock 1997); fridge temperatures (usually 4°C) are not a substitute for ice (Biswas *et al.* 1982).

Erythrocyte sedimentation affects haemoglobin, pH, and carbon dioxide results so that samples should be mixed continuously, using a thumb roll, not vigorous shaking (which causes haemolysis).

Currently, continuous gas analysis has too many complications for widespread clinical use (see Chapter 17). However, the future may well bring gas analysis into the realm of effective continuous measurement, removing or reducing the need for aspiration sampling.

Reading samples

Different analysers provide various measurements, in varying sequences. 'Normal' values differ between texts, substantial variations may occur between different samples (Sasse *et al.* 1994), and machine error can cause artefactual differences; as with almost any clinical measurement, trends are more important than absolute figures.

TEMPERATURE Blood gas analysers can measure samples at a range of temperatures. Temperature affects dissociation of gases, as seen when samples are re-analysed at different temperatures. If no specific temperature is selected, analysers use a default setting of 37°C. Carbon dioxide levels will affect pH, so that altering temperature will affect PaO_2, $PaCO_2$, pH, base excess and HCO_3^-. To individualise results to patients, many units analyse samples at monitored temperature, although some units measure all samples at a standard 37°C. There is debate about whether analysing samples by patient temperatures is beneficial.

Patient temperature is not constant between different sites (see Chapter 8); comparisons between different sites is much debated, although pulmonary artery temperature is recognised as the 'gold standard' temperature. Thus, when pulmonary artery temperature is available, this will normally be the 'core' temperature used for blood gas analysis, but on removal of pulmonary artery catheters, 'core' temperature must be measured at another site. As a result, possible changes in blood gas tensions may arise not from any physiological change in the patient, but because a means of monitoring has been removed.

Beliefs that reheating (from hypothermia) caused acidosis led to a vogue for correcting temperature; but reheating acidosis does not appear to be problematic, and so the value of temperature correction is questionable (Prencipe & Brenna, undated). Debate over whether to correct for temperature has created two theories: pH-stat (correcting to patient temperature) and alpha-stat (seeking a pH of 7.4 with all samples analysed at 37°C) (Hornbein 1994). Studies on cold-blooded animals first suggested that temperature of gas was less significant that previously thought (Hornbein 1994); subsequent studies in both dogs and humans found ventricular fibrillation occurred less often when alpha-stat treatments were used (Hornbein 1994), although inevitably there are some (albeit fewer) studies supporting pH-stat approaches.

The balance of evidence currently seems to favour non-correction for temperature, although as gas measurements are used to follow trends rather than absolutes, consistency between staff is probably more important than differences between either approach. Units should therefore identify which approach they wish to follow and ensure that all staff, including occasional (agency/bank) staff, follow one approach.

Hb Haemoglobin analysis may be inaccurate if samples are not fully mixed, and so syringes should be agitated constantly until analysed (Beaumont 1997). Most ICU patients have high erythrocyte sedimentation rate (ESR), which hastens the separation of blood from plasma.

pH This measures overall acidity or alkalinity of blood; it does not differentiate between respiratory and metabolic components. If electrodes are contaminated by proteins, results will be erroneous (Hinds & Watson 1996). Normal pH may be taken as 7.35–7.45 (see above).

$PaCO_2$ Normal arterial carbon dioxide tensions are 4.5–6.0 kPa (Cornock 1996). Carbon dioxide is a potential acid (see above), and so high carbon dioxide tension (high $PaCO_2$) indicates respiratory acidosis, while low carbon dioxide tension indicates respiratory alkalosis.

Since carbon dioxide is more soluble than oxygen (see Chapter 18), normocapnia may exist despite hypoxia (for example, with pulmonary oedema). However, with gas trapping and hyperventilation, high alveolar carbon dioxide concentrations inhibit clearance, so predisposing to hypercapnia.

PaO_2 Normal oxygen tensions are 11.5–13.5 kPa (Cornock 1996); however, alveolar arterial gradients (A-a) increase with age: in youth, A-a gradient is normally 2 kPa, but in old age may reach 3.3 kPa (Hillman 1997), reducing the 'normal' level of oxygen in older people (the majority of ICU patients).

PaO_2 measures only the partial pressure of oxygen in plasma, but only about 3 per cent of arterial oxygen is carried by plasma, the majority (97 per cent) being carried by haemoglobin (see Chapter 18). While gas dissociation across haemoglobin cell membrane will enable some indication of total oxygen from PaO_2, *oxygen content* (derived from both PaO_2 and oxygen saturation) is the sum of both oxygen in solution and oxyhaemoglobin.

HCO_3^- Normal bicarbonate levels are 22–28 mmol/l (Cornock 1996). Being the main chemical buffer of extracellular fluid, low bicarbonate levels indicate metabolic acidosis, while high levels indicate metabolic alkalosis.

Although primarily a metabolic figure, respiratory function affects bicarbonate levels:

$$CO_2 + H_2O \rightleftharpoons H_2CO_3 \rightleftharpoons HCO_3^- + H^+$$

(carbon dioxide + water forms carbonic acid, which dissociates to bicarbonate and a hydrogen radical)

Hypercapnia from respiratory failure contributes, therefore, to raised bicarbonate levels. Computer calculation enables the removal of the respiratory component to provide an (estimated) purely metabolic figure, the *standardised bicarbonate* (SBC). As bicarbonate is used to assess metabolic function, it is logical to use SBC rather than HCO_3^- figures. With normal blood gases, differences will be minimal, but with deranged gases, there can be significant differences. Readers are advised to note and consider the differences between these two figures on samples taken, discussing them with unit staff.

BASE EXCESS This indicates numbers of moles of acid or base needed to return 1 litre of blood to a pH of 7.4 (provided pCO_2 remains constant at 5.3 kPa), and so it measures acid–base balance, but from a metabolic perspective. Base excess therefore complements and affects pH.

Unlike pH, base excess uses a linear scale and so is easier to understand. Neutral is zero, positive base excess is too much base (alkaline, thus metabolic alkalosis), and negative base excess is insufficient alkaline (thus metabolic acidosis). Normal base excess is ±2 (Cornock 1996), although faint or absent minus signs may need to be inferred by readers from other measurements (if bicarbonate levels are low, then base excess must be negative).

Base excess is calculated from bicarbonate levels, and so although base excess is taken as a metabolic figure, respiratory effects of carbon dioxide on bicarbonate similarly affect base excess measurements. As with bicarbonate measurement, computerised standardisation (Standardised Base Excess – SBE) enables a more accurate calculation of metabolic components.

SATURATION This indicates haemoglobin saturation by oxygen of arterial blood. Saturation indicates the percentage saturation of haemoglobin, but oxygen carried will also depend on the amount of haemoglobin; the complex relationship between saturation and PaO_2 is illustrated by the oxygen dissociation curve (see Chapter 18), so that oximetry should be read in conjunction with Hb levels. Falsely high levels can be caused by carbon monoxide, which makes blood bright red. Bedside oximetry has reduced the frequency with which blood gas samples need to be taken.

Compensation

Homeostasis aims to achieve a pH of 7.4. Overall pH of blood is the balance between respiratory and metabolic function (see Figure 19.1). Acidosis or alkalosis from one quadrant will, with time and effective homeostatic mechanisms, compensate for excess in another to maintain a 'neutral' blood pH of 7.4.

When analysing a sample, therefore, first identify whether compensation is occurring (if carbon dioxide and SBE are deranged, is pH normal?). If compensation is occurring, then identify whether respiratory function is compensating for metabolic acidosis/alkalosis, or vice versa. This will usually need to be analysed in the context of knowledge about the patient's pathological condition: for example, respiratory failure causes respiratory acidosis, while renal failure causes metabolic acidosis. Respiratory compensation occurs quickly (within a few minutes), but metabolic compensation can take hours or days to occur. Hence, metabolic compensation will only occur in response to prolonged respiratory complications.

If pH is not returned to normal limits, compensatory mechanisms have failed. If pH is life-threatening and compensatory mechanisms cannot be adequately mimicked (e.g. through artificial ventilation), then exogenous bases or acids may need to be given. In practice, sodium bicarbonate is sometimes given (in small aliquots), but exogenous acid is rarely given. Life-threatening acidosis is more common than life-threatening alkalosis.

Even with critical illness, compensatory mechanisms are often safer than exogenous intervention.

Implications for practice

- units should consider and clarify through unit policy whether to adopt pH-stat or alpha-stat approaches on blood gas analysis, and so whether samples should be analysed at patient temperature or at a standard 37°C
- standardised bicarbonate and base excess levels should be used rather than HCO_3^- and BE figures
- for teaching/learning purposes, readers should re-analyse samples at differing temperatures
- exogenous chemical compensation for acidosis or alkalosis is not normally indicated, unless imbalances are life-threatening

Summary

Blood gas analysis remains one of the most valuable methods of monitoring respiratory and metabolic function; most ICU nurses will be familiar with taking and interpreting samples. However, interpreting examples is open to more controversies and assumptions than staff new to ICUs may be made aware of.

This chapter has suggested 'normal' values, although there are slight variations between authors. However, as with almost any measurement, trends are more important than absolute figures. Despite their name, blood gas samples are used to monitor both respiratory and metabolic function; this chapter has therefore offered detailed discussion of acid–base balance.

Further reading

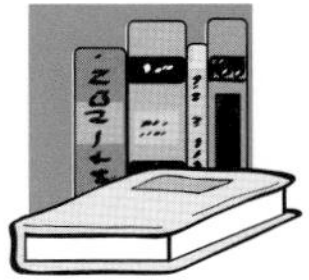

Chapters on acid–base balance may be found in many physiology, ICU and clinical chemistry/biochemistry texts. Occasional articles appear in nursing and medical texts; Coleman and Houston (1998) outline acid–base balance, while Szaflarski (1996) gives a comprehensive overview of potential errors from arterial blood gas sampling.

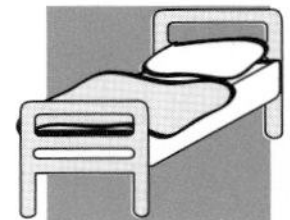

Clinical scenario

Julie Panks (see Clinical scenario, Chapter 18), who is 36 years old, was admitted to ICU unconscious from taking an aspirin overdose the previous day. Her plasma salicylate level is 890 mg/l. She has sickle cell trait and Hb of 9.2 g/dl, and core temperature on admission was 36.5°C.

For arterial blood gas analysis see the table on p. 187.

Q.1 Identify the acid–base status of Julie's three blood gases (acidosis, alkalosis, respiratory, metabolic, compensated or uncompensated). Discuss reasons for abnormalities and changes over time.

Q.2 Analyse the cause of Julie's acid–base disturbance; review how she may respond physiologically. Consider the effect on other organs/systems and how the ICU nurse assesses, anticipates and minimises any potentially adverse effects.

Q.3 The first blood gas was taken during Julie's admission by a new member of staff who could not recall how much time elapsed between aspirating and analysing sample. Review potential sources and direction of analytical errors (e.g. air bubbles in blood sample can falsely increase PO_2) which can occur with this first blood gas measurement.

Chapter 20

Haemodynamic monitoring

Contents

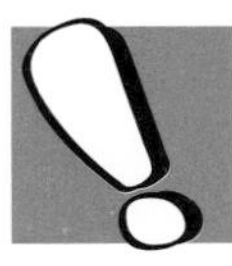

Fundamental knowledge

Experience of using invasive monitoring (including 'zeroing')
Cardiac physiology – atria, ventricles, valves
Cardiac cycle: systole, diastole
How breathing affects venous return
V/Q mismatch
Oxygen dissociation (see Chapter 18)

Introduction

Haemodynamic monitoring is central to ICU care. This chapter describes more frequently used modes, with some noninvasive options, to extend knowledge rather than develop psychomotor skills.

Cardiovascular and respiratory function is interrelated, and so although another chapter discusses respiratory monitoring, this chapter includes monitoring internal respiration (e.g. VO_2, DO_2), normally included in 'cardiac output studies'.

Electrocardiography (ECG) is discussed in Chapter 21.

Formulae are not included, as microchip technology has replaced the need for nurses to calculate them.

Invasive equipment increases infection risks (see Chapter 15); risks increase with more invasive equipment (usually used on sicker, so more immunocompromised, patients). Aseptic technique and infection control are especially important, therefore, with all invasive equipment. All monitoring equipment is diagnostic rather than therapeutic, and should be removed once risks outweigh benefits, or maximum time limits are reached.

'Normal' figures are cited here as a guide, but many figures assume an 'average' 70-kg patient; trends are more important than absolute figures. Consistency between measurements (and measurers) is therefore as important as accurate technique.

Arterial blood pressure

This is the pressure exerted on arterial walls and so affects perfusion and oxygen/nutrient supply to, and waste removal from, tissues. Pressure is determined by *flow* and *resistance*.

Flow is affected by driving force (cardiac output) and viscosity, while resistance (afterload) is determined by vascular (arteriole) and interstitial resistance (e.g. oedema). Small (capillary) vessels are especially susceptible to poor flow from high viscosity. Pressure progressively alters throughout the cardiovascular system; distal measurement (e.g. pedal arterial lines) may overestimate central pressure by nearly one-third (Runciman & Ludbrook 1996).

Systolic pressure, maximum perfusion pressure, is momentary; perfusion continues, variably, throughout the pulse, so mean arterial pressure (MAP) more accurately indicates perfusion. MAP (calculated and displayed by most monitors) is:

$$(\text{systolic} - \text{diastolic})/3 + \text{diastolic}$$

Pulse pressure, the pressure created by each pulse (systolic minus diastolic), indicates vessel response to pulse. Poor artery wall compliance (e.g. atherosclerosis) creates wide pulse pressures (Campbell 1997). Narrow pulse pressures indicate hypovolaemia.

Left ventricular myocardial oxygen supply can only occur when coronary artery pressure exceeds left ventricular pressure (diastole), and so tachycardia (reduced diastolic time) reduces myocardial oxygen supply while increasing demand.

Reduced diastolic pressure is caused by either hypovolaemia or vasodilation.

Detecting hypo- or hypertension identifies a symptom, rather than cause, of problems, and so additional haemodynamic information is usually needed in ICUs.

Noninvasive blood pressure measurement

Auscultation of sphygmomanometer blood pressure usually reveals five ('Korotkoff') sounds:

- I (first sound heard, sharp thud) = systolic pressure
- II (soft, tapping, intermittent)
- III (loud)
- IV (low, muffled, continuous; start = 1st diastole)
- V (disappears, although may not occur, e.g. with aortic regurgitation; it is close to IV; start = 2nd diastole)

Inaccuracy of cuff pressure measurement may occur from:

- equipment malfunction (sphygmomanometers should be regularly recalibrated)
- wrong cuff size (bladder width should be 40 per cent of arm circumference (Bridges & Middleton 1997); small cuffs give falsely high readings (Runcimann & Ludbrook 1996))
- height differences between sphygmomanometers and heart level (compare raising or lowering arterial transducers)

Sphygmomanometer pressure monitoring provides adequate information for most hospitalised patients, but greater frequency and accuracy is usually needed in ICUs. Automated noninvasive pressure monitors (e.g. Dynamap®) can measure bloodflow-induced oscillation on arterial walls. Most machines overestimate low pressures and underestimate high pressures (Gomersall & Oh 1997) so that they are least useful when most needed. However, noninvasive monitoring avoids dangers from arterial cannulation.

Cuff inflation pressures of noninvasive monitors can be high and uncomfortable and should be adjusted to give safe, but not excessive, margins between each patient's systolic and cuff inflation pressure. Nurses should check inflation pressure, trying cuffs on themselves to realise what their patients will be subjected to.

Arterial tonometry displays beat-to-beat waveforms and digital readings of pressure. Reflecting principles of intra-arterial monitoring, this is potentially useful, but not yet reliable enough to replace invasive monitoring (Windsor 1998).

Intra-arterial measurement

Direct (invasive) arterial pressure monitoring (see Figure 20.1) provides

- continuous measurement
- greater accuracy (intra-arterial measurements are usually 5–20 mmHg above noninvasive pressure measurements (Coad 1996))
- visual display

Left ventricular contraction (systole) causes a surge in pressure, displayed by the upstroke on traces. Rapid upstrokes with sharply defined apexes indicate good left ventricular contractility (Windsor 1998). Upstrokes are normally uninterrupted, but resistance (e.g. aortic stenosis) can cause **anacrotic notches.**

When left ventricular contraction ends (and pressure begins to fall) the aortic valve closes, causing a momentary surge in aortic root pressure (**dicrotic notch**). Reduced afterload from vasodilation (e.g. SIRS) widens anacrotic and dicrotic notches (Windsor 1998).

Arterial 'swing' indicates hypovolaemia (Adam & Osborne 1997) and so can monitor response to fluid challenge (Windsor 1998). Measuring the area under the curve represents stroke volume (Windsor 1998), although is less accurate than thermodilution estimation (Gomersall & Oh 1997).

Potential problems with intra-arterial measurement include:

- infection
- occlusion
- disconnection
- air emboli
- user error

Cold and blanched/cyanosed peripheries indicate arterial occlusion, although unsymptomatic thromboses may occur in 70 per cent of patients (Windsor 1998).

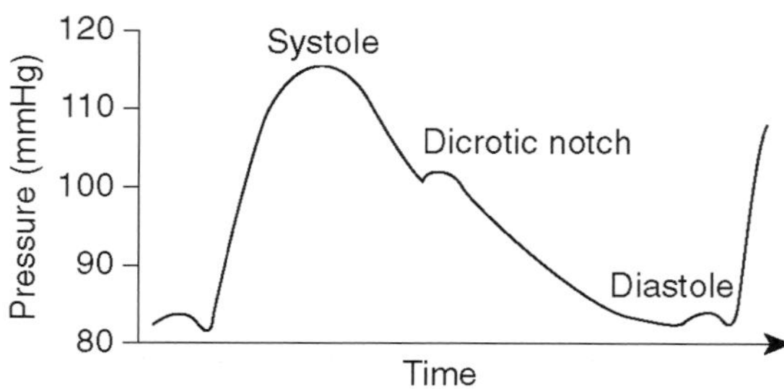

Figure 20.1 Intra-arterial pressure trace

Disconnection, or significant oozing around arterial cannulae, can cause rapid blood loss. Arterial cannulae should (if possible) be easily visible.

Various user errors can occur, including

- transducer level (should be at heart level; small changes in height cause large errors in measurement)
- patency should be maintained with continuous infusion (normally at 300 mmHg) with isotonic crystalloid
- drugs should not be given through arterial lines (bolus concentrations can be toxic) and so lines and all connections/taps should be clearly labelled/identified (e.g. using red bungs).

Central venous pressure

Palpating jugular venous pressure indicates venous return to the heart, and so is a right heart function, but it can be very misleading (Windsor 1998), thus invasive central venous pressure (CVP) measurement is often essential for fluid and cardiac management. CVP is right atrial *filling pressure* or *preload*. Normally about 65 per cent of blood volume is in the veins; inadequate return necessarily makes cardiac output (arterial pressure) inadequate. Central venous pressure results from

- vascular tone (e.g. endogenous/exogenous vasodilators, valves in veins)
- 'pumps' (thoracic from breathing, skeletal muscle from movement)
- blood volume (e.g. hypovolaemia)
- right heart and pulmonary vascular function (e.g. cardiac failure)
- intrathoracic pressure (positive pressure ventilation, PEEP)

Central venous pressure is also *right atrial pressure* (RAP). During diastole, right atrial pressure becomes *right ventricular end diastolic pressure* (RVEDP), and so

$$CVP = RAP = RVEDP$$

Most nursing texts use CVP, but alternative terms may be found elsewhere.

Low CVP usually indicates loss of fluids (e.g. haemorrhage, excessive diuresis, excessive extravasation). High CVP is more complex, but likely causes are:

- hypervolaemia (e.g. excessive fluid infusion)
- cardiac failure (e.g. right ventricular failure, pulmonary embolism, mitral valve failure/regurgitation, tamponade)
- lumen occlusion/obstruction (e.g. cannula against vein wall; thrombus)
- high blood viscosity (rare, but possible following massive blood transfusion)

- artefact (e.g. viscous drugs remaining in transduced line)

If causes of high pressure are not obvious, nurses should seek advice.

Measuring CVP

Central venous pressure is usually measured supine from midaxilla (*phlebostatic axis*: intersection of lines from midsternal fourth intercostal space and midaxilla, see Figure 20.2) and recorded in millimetres of mercury. Normal supine midaxillary measurement is between 0 and +8 mmHg (mean +4 mmHg) (Tinker & Jones 1986); marking the measurement site on skin or fixing transducers to one position helps to maintain consistency between measurements. Monitor traces (or column of water) should show 'respiratory swing' as intrathoracic pressure alternates:

- rising with positive pressure ventilator breaths (increased intrathoracic pressure)
- falling with self-ventilating breaths (negative pressure)

Ideally, pressure should be measured between breaths.

Some centres measure from the sternal notch, although this does not absolutely reflect right atrial level.

Transducers should be 'zeroed' to the chosen site (open port from the monitor to air, and calibrate monitor to zero).

If patients cannot tolerate supine positions, a semi-recumbent (or other) measurement will still indicate trends provided the positions are consistent (e.g. same angle) between readings. Different positions should be clearly recorded (e.g. on observation charts).

If transducer monitoring is not available, manometers can measure CVP. Mercury is neurotoxic and so manometers use isotonic fluids (e.g. 5% dextrose). Readings are therefore in centimetres of water (cmH_2O) rather than millimetres of mercury (mmHg). The two scales are numerically similar: 1 mmHg is approximately 1.36 cmH_2O (Guyton & Hall 1997). This difference is insignificant with low pressures, but accumulates with higher pressures.

Dangers

Inserting central lines can puncture any surrounding tissue (lung puncture = pneumothorax, veins, myocardium). Although insertion is not currently a nursing role, nurses may assist or be present, and so should observe for dangers (ECG, airway pressures and CVP trace/flow) and report concerns. Position should (normally) be checked by X-ray before use, and lines secured with stitches.

Once inserted, problems include:

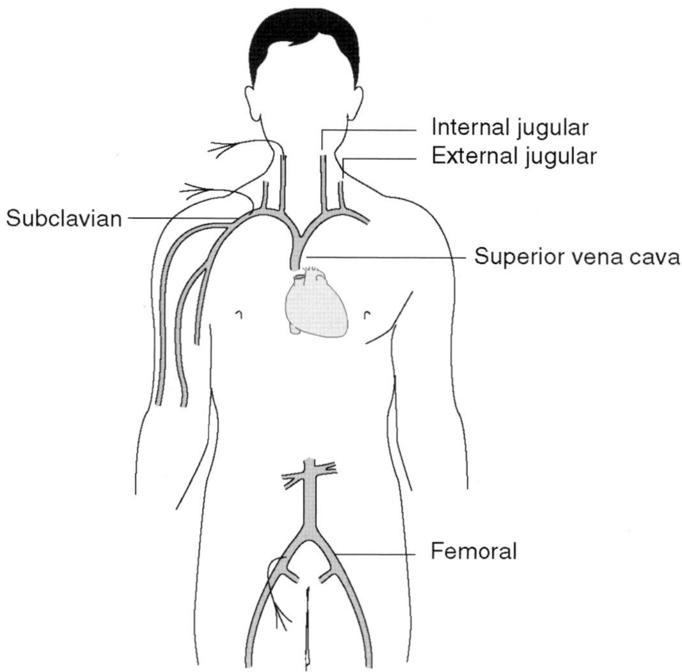

Figure 20.2 **Central venous cannulae**

INFECTION This is usually from skin commensals, occurring in 7–16 per cent of patients (Kaye & Smith 1988). Rates increase with

- femoral cannulae
- additional connections (e.g. three-way taps, so these should be kept to a minimum).

DYSRHYTHMIAS These can have many causes, including catheter displacement into ventricles (direct mechanical myocardial irritation). ECGs should be continuously monitored, and any unexplained dysrhythmias reported and recorded.

DRUGS These may need to be given centrally because

- peripheral blood flow provides insufficient dilution (hypotonic, hypertonic, too acidic, too alkaline; e.g. dopamine)
- peripheral flow is poor/absent (shock).

Drugs given centrally can have rapid effects, so patients should be closely monitored during and after administration. Residual particles of drugs in lines may precipitate with subsequent drugs (frusemide precipitates with many drugs) so that nurses should observe lines during drug administration, and flush lines through thoroughly afterwards and between drugs.

FLUID OVERLOAD This can occur through rapid flow; volumetric pumps should prevent this danger, although should be checked regularly (usually hourly) in case they malfunction.

THROMBOSIS Serious central vein thrombosis occurs in 4–35 per cent of patients with central lines (Kaye & Smith 1988); stasis (kinked catheters, poor flow) makes thrombosis more likely.

Obstructed flow may be due to thrombi or extravasation, and so fluid/drugs should not be forced through (which may dislodge emboli or force fluid into interstitial spaces). Dysfunctional cannulae should be reported, recorded and (usually) removed.

AIR EMBOLI Below 10–20 ml these rarely cause significant problems (Hudak *et al.* 1998), but larger volumes may cause pulmonary emboli and death. Negative intrathoracic pressure (self-ventilating) entrains air, resulting in larger volumes. Central lines should, whenever possible, be readily visible and checked regularly, especially with self-ventilating patients. Nurses should regularly check all connections are secure (with leur locks). Central lines should be removed with patients positioned head-down so that any accidental air emboli rise to pedal rather than cerebral circulation. Self-ventilating patients should breathe out and hold their breath during removal so that intrathoracic pressure equates with atmospheric pressure.

Pulmonary artery catheterisation

In health, blood volume returning to the right atrium will reach the left atrium, so central venous pressure indicates left ventricular filling. But cardiac failure can create unpredictable discrepancies. Cardiac output studies give clearer indications of left heart function.

Pulmonary artery (Swan Ganz) catheters (PAC; sometimes called *pulmonary artery flotation catheters* (PAFC), see Figure 20.3) provide direct information and (through thermodilution) calculated measurements. Noninvasive alternatives are also available. 'Swan Ganz' refers to original producers, so is avoided here.

Pulmonary artery catheters are diagnostic, and may guide therapy (e.g. inotropes) (Mimoz *et al.* 1994), but are not in themselves therapeutic. They share all the complications of central lines, and additional problems include:

- increased dysrhythmias (catheters are intracardiac, and cold bolus injectate irritates myocardium; this is especially likely on removal)
- valve damage

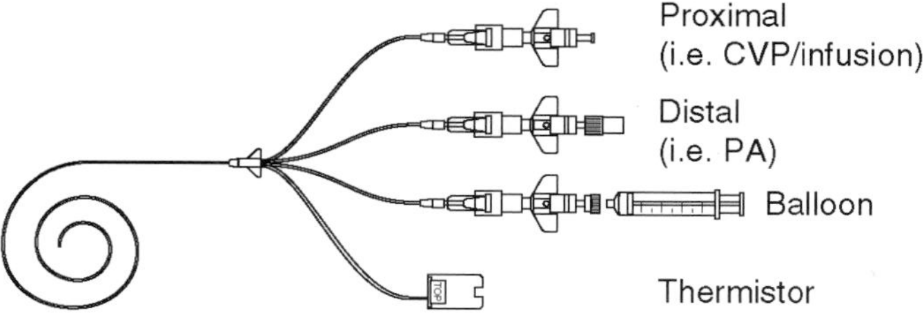

Figure 20.3 A pulmonary artery (flotation) catheter

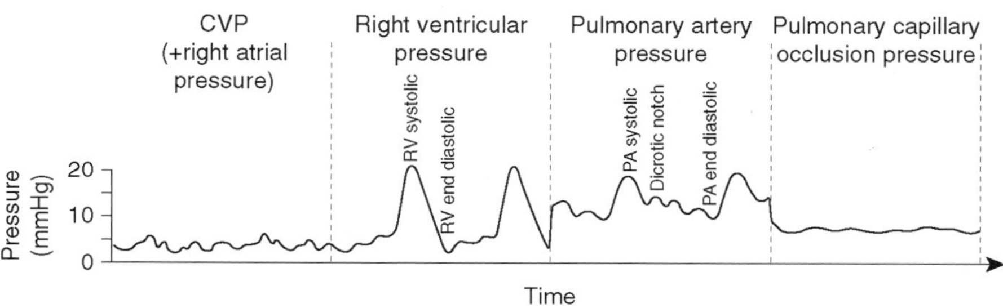

Figure 20.4 Pressure traces seen as a pulmonary artery catheter passes from the vena cava to the pulmonary artery

- pulmonary vascular occlusion
- emboli enter nearer pulmonary, coronary and cerebral arteries (pulmonary infarction incidence = 0.1–5.6 per cent)
- knotting of catheter is rare, but forcible removal can damage heart valves or other tissue – if removal is difficult, stop and request a chest X-ray

Catheters should be removed if no longer needed, and within times stated by manufacturers (usually 72 hours).

Thermodilution catheters are inserted like central lines (usually subclavian or internal jugular), but proceed through the right atrium and right ventricle into the pulmonary vasculature, where they 'float'. During insertion, right ventricular pressure may be measured; once inserted, *pulmonary artery pressures* are displayed (see Figure 20.4).

Pulmonary vasculature is more compliant than systemic vessels so that pulmonary pressures are lower (see Table 20.1). Many ICU patients have pulmonary hypertension (e.g. ARDS). Low pulmonary artery pressure despite high CVP indicates right heart failure (e.g. mitral valve regurgitation).

Table 20.1 Normal intracardiac pressures

central venous	0 to +8 mmHg (right atrial level)
right ventricle	0 to +8 mmHg diastolic
	+15 to +30 mmHg systolic
pulmonary capillary wedge pressure	+5 to +15 mmHg
left atrium	+4 to +12 mmHg
left ventricle	+4 to +12 mmHg diastolic
	+90 to +140 mmHg systolic
aorta	+90 to +140 mmHg systolic
	+60 to +90 mmHg diastolic
	+70 to +105 mmHg mean

Pulmonary artery catheters usually have balloon tips enabling *pulmonary capillary wedge pressure* (PCWP) measurement. This can also be called pulmonary capillary occlusion pressure (PCOP), pulmonary artery wedge/occlusion pressure (PAWP/PACP – although the pulmonary artery itself should NOT be wedged), or 'wedge pressure', and indicates left atrial filling pressure, just as CVP is right atrial filling pressure.

To measure PCWP, balloons should be inflated with 1–2 ml of air (sets normally include dedicated syringes); if occlusion occurs with less than 1 ml, the balloon is wedged in a very small capillary, which will not accurately reflect left atrial function. If 2 ml does not cause occlusion the balloon may have burst (= air embolus) or it may be in a large vessel (e.g. pulmonary artery); the problem should be reported before attempting further inflation.

Wedge pressure should be read once trace stops falling. Respiration (intrathoracic pressure) causes a slight waveform; ideally end expiration pressure should be measured. Following readings, the balloon should be deflated: continued occlusion causes distal ischaemia and infarction.

Cardiac output studies

This section describes direct and derived thermodilution measurements, with commonly used abbreviations. Measurements of tissue resistance and internal respiration, although not strictly speaking 'cardiac output', are included. Noninvasive modes are discussed separately, although implications of parameters measured is unchanged. Potent therapies (e.g. noradrenaline) are often prescribed according to cardiac output studies so that accurate measurements are especially important; nurses should remember their individual accountability for their actions and, if unsure of any aspects or results, seek advice. Most statistics are derived and so erroneous techniques may cause cumulative inaccuracies.

Injecting bolus (5–10 ml, depending on calibration) crystalloid and measuring temperature changes enables the estimation of stroke volume. Cold injectate (e.g. fluid run through ice) creates higher signal-to-noise ratio and so should be more accurate, but differences from room-temperature injectate are slight (Gardner 1995), especially as trends are more important than absolute figures.

Three readings are usually made. These should be taken at the same part of the respiratory cycle (normally end-expiration). Measurements differing more than 10 per cent from other readings, or displaying uneven traces, should be considered inaccurate, and discounted.

Thermal filaments in the right atrium can provide continuous cardiac output measurement; readings are slightly higher than thermodilution measurement, but acceptable (Boldt *et al.* 1994; Jakobsen 1995), with the bonus of continuous information.

cardiac output (CO)
normal: 4–8 l/min (Coombs 1993)
Cardiac reserve can increase output fivefold. Critical illness usually increases demand, and so most ICU patients have pathologically high cardiac outputs; (positive) inotropes also increase output. Myocardial dysfunction, myocardial depressant factor and other mediators may inhibit output.

cardiac index (CI)
normal: 2.5–4.2 l/min/m^2 (Coombs 1993)
'Normal' 4–8 litre cardiac output assumes an 'average' weight of 70 kg. Indexing output to body surface area (m^2) makes figures comparable between different (non-average) patients. Due to differences in both cardiac output and body surface area, children's cardiac index is high and decreases with age.

stroke volume (SV)
normal: 60–120 ml (Coombs 1993)
Stroke volume (with heart rate) determines cardiac output, so HR × SV = CO. Stroke volume relies on adequate preload and muscle contractility, if stroke volume is poor, preload (CVP/PCWP) should be optimised, then inotropes given.

stroke volume index (SVI)
normal: 35–70 ml/beat/m^2 (Fitzpatrick & Donnelly 1997)
Like cardiac output, stroke volume can be indexed: stroke volume index (SVI) or stroke index (SI).

left cardiac work (LCW)
left cardiac work index (LCWI)
normal LCWI: 3.4–4.2 kg·m/m^2 (Coombs 1993)

Using inotropes increases left ventricular work (and myocardial oxygen demand); but cardiac and/or pulmonary disease often simultaneously reduces supply, exposing ICU patients with little cardiac reserve to increased risk of infarction. Measuring left ventricular work enables calculation of muscle strength (contractility) and more careful titration of therapies.

left ventricular stroke work (LVSW)
left ventricular stroke work index (LVSWI)
normal LVSWI: 50–60 gm·m/m^2 (Coombs 1993)

Left ventricular contractility has the same relation to cardiac work that stroke volume bears to cardiac output/index.

right cardiac work (RCW)
right cardiac work index (RCWI)
right ventricular stroke work (RVSW)
right ventricular stroke work index (RVSWI)
normal RCW: 0.54–0.66 km·m/m^2 (Coombs 1993)
RVSWI: 7.9–9.7 gm·m/m^2 (Coombs 1993)
Measuring right ventricular function similarly enables finer management with right heart failure.

systemic vascular resistance (SVR)
normal: 900–1600 dyn/sec/cm^5 (Coombs 1993)
Systemic vascular resistance (SVR; afterload) is a major determinant of blood pressure; gross vasodilation (e.g. SIRS) reduces SVR, so causes peripheral pooling and hypotension. Noninvasive signs of peripheral pooling include:

- central hypotension
- warm/'flushed' extremities
- rapid capillary refill (within 3 seconds of blanching)
- metabolic acidosis

Cardiac output studies provide more precise estimation of SVR, enabling safer use of vasodilators (e.g. sodium nitroprusside – SNP) or vasoconstrictors (e.g. noradrenaline).

pulmonary vascular resistance (PVR)
normal: 20–120 dyn/sec/cm^5 (Coombs 1993)
Pulmonary hypertension may be caused by ARDS, pulmonary oedema, pulmonary embolism and other pathologies.

mixed venous saturation (SvO_2)
normal: 75 per cent (Coombs 1993)
Mixed venous saturation is measured by a light source in the catheter tip; pulmonary artery blood 'mixes' both superior and inferior vena cava blood, indicating total systemic oxygen consumption (blood samples from distal ports of pulmonary artery catheters can supply mixed venous saturation if fibre-optic sources are unavailable).

Tissue oxygen supply depends on

- cardiac output

- haemoglobin concentration
- arterial saturation
- oxygen dissociation (curve)

Mixed venous oxygen levels should therefore be interpreted against these factors.

Mixed venous oxygen shows the balance between oxygen supply and demand (Cathelyn 1998); in health, approximately one quarter of available oxygen is consumed. Higher figures indicate failure by tissue cells to utilise available oxygen; lower figures suggest increased oxygen demand and/or reduced oxygen supply.

Mixed venous oxygen levels of 50 per cent indicate compromised tissue oxygen supply so that metabolic acidosis and hypoxic damage are likely (Jakobsen 1995). Below 30 per cent, oxygen supply is insufficient to meet demand (Gomersall & Oh 1997).

delivery of oxygen (DO_2)
delivery of oxygen index (DO_2I)
normal: DO_2 900–1100 ml/min
DO_2I 520–720 ml/min/m^2 (Fitzpatrick & Donnelly 1997)

Delivery of oxygen to tissues (with consumption of oxygen by tissues) is the ultimate goal of respiratory management. Delivery can be indexed by body surface area (m^2).

consumption of oxygen (VO_2)
consumption of oxygen index (VO_2I)
Normal: VO_2 200–290 ml/min
VO_2I 100–180 ml/min/m^2 (Fitzpatrick & Donnelly 1997)
Oxygen delivery has little value unless tissues extract it. Anaerobic metabolism creates 'oxygen debt', the primary event and major determinant of organ failure and outcome (Shoemaker *et al.* 1988). Therefore DO_2 should be compared with VO_2.

Calculation of oxygen consumption through cardiac output studies indicates global oxygen uptake; monitoring specific systems (e.g. jugular bulb saturation, hepatic saturation, gastric tonometry) enables identification of regional variations. Relating regional figures to global uptake enables identification of local metabolic demands (e.g. hyperdynamic myocardium, fitting brain).

oxygen extraction ratio (OER)
Normal: 0.22–0.30 (Fitzpatrick & Donnelly 1997)
Combining oxygen delivery and oxygen consumption shows the proportion of oxygen extracted by tissues; OER therefore indicates shunting at tissue level.

Noninvasive approaches

The value of invasive haemodynamic monitoring (especially pulmonary artery catheters) remains controversial, but noninvasive alternatives for measuring cardiac output are increasingly reliable, often providing real-time information (enabling earlier intervention) (Asensio *et al.* 1996), although information may be more limited (e.g. unavailability of mixed venous oxygen saturation).

FINGER BLOOD PRESSURE WAVEFORM This can usefully show cardiac output trends to supplement periodic invasive measurement, but inaccuracy rates (nearly a quarter of measurements) (Hirschl *et al.* 1997) make this unreliable for replacement.

THORACIC ELECTRICAL BIOIMPEDANCE This measures changes in thoracic electrical conductivity with external electrodes, provides continuous information without risks from invasive monitoring (Shoemaker *et al.* 1998). Correlation with thermodilution measurements and clinical reliability are debated: Haller *et al.* (1995) found correlation poor, while Thangathurai *et al.* (1997) reported favourably. Readings can be unreliable with:

- dysrhythmias (especially bundle branch blocks and tachycardias above 150)
- myocardial infarction
- metal (e.g. sternotomy wires)
- sweating
- body fluid (e.g. pulmonary oedema, pleural effusions)

AORTIC DOPPLER This uses echo imaging to assess blood flow turbulence. Single measurements can take half an hour, and are affected by:

- anaemia
- breast tissue
- emphysema

Ideally all measurements should be performed by a single experienced operator, but this is often impractical.

TRANSOESOPHAGEAL DOPPLER This uses similar equipment placed inside the oesophagus; being near the aorta, this resolves many problems of aortic doppler measurement. Accuracy is within 2.9 per cent of thermodilution (Tibby *et al.* 1997) with most measurements being underestimates (Hinds & Watson 1996). Waveform display indicates hypovolaemia and response to inotropes (Tibby *et al.* 1997). Problems include

- discomfort (thus only suitable for sedated and ventilated patients (Hinds & Watson 1996));
- potential oesophageal trauma (Valtier *et al.* 1998), especially if varices are present.

Transtracheal probes at the distal end of endotracheal tubes can provide similar measurements with easier access, although preliminary reports often (40 per cent) show poor quality signals (Tibby *et al.* 1997).

Implications for practice

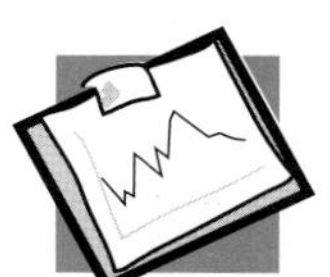

- haemodynamic monitoring can provide useful diagnostic information, but is not inherently therapeutic; decisions to use equipment should evaluate benefits against risks
- information may enhance patient care, but nursing should focus on the person rather than the machine
- needs to prioritise time may preclude taking observations in favour of more urgent tasks
- any equipment may introduce infection; more invasive equipment increases infection risk, so use should be aseptic
- noninvasive modes are preferable if they are available and reliable
- trends are more significant than absolute figures
- nurses should minimise discomfort from equipment wherever possible, providing prescribed analgesia and sedation where necessary and explaining equipment and procedures to allay anxiety
- no observation should be 'routine'; nurses should only perform observations if information may be used, and should consider carefully before delegating tasks to anyone unable to interpret information

Summary

Heamodynamic monitoring necessarily forms a major aspect of intensive care nursing; this chapter has described most methods currently used, with main complications. All modes, especially invasive ones, have complications and so should only be used as long as benefits outweigh problems. Nurses should actively assess and, where possible, initiate appropriate monitoring, and remember their individual accountability when using equipment (e.g. cannulae should be removed within prescribed times). Information gained should be actively used for patient treatment, and so where necessary should be reported and recorded.

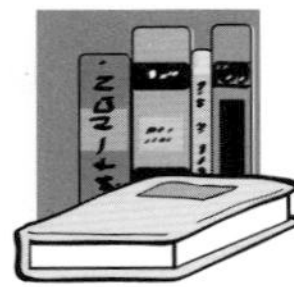

Further reading

Most textbooks include an overview of haemodynamic monitoring; Coombs's (1993) article offers useful nursing perspectives. Draper (1987) provides a thorough review of arterial cuff pressure measurement, while Campbell (1997) gives useful descriptions of arterial pressure waveform monitoring. Shoemaker's interest in invasive cardiac monitoring has been increasingly replaced by noninvasive modes (see Shoemaker *et al.* 1998).

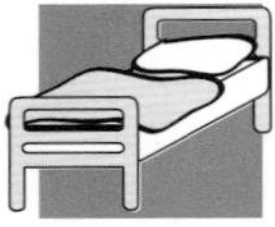

Clinical scenario

Mrs Rita Goodwin, 56 years old, is admitted with severe chest pain and her ECG shows sinus rhythm and an anterior wall MI. She is self-ventilating and conscious. Her vital signs include:

BP 85/60 mmHg (MAP 68–70 mmHg)
HR 125 beats/min
CVP 11mmHg
CO 3.0 l/min
CI 1.8 l/min/m^2
PAP 30/14 mmHg (mean PAP = 19 mmHg)
PCWP 12 mmHg
Echocardiogram reveals LV ejection fraction of 45 per cent

Mrs Goodwin has no previous cardiac history, she is 165 m (5 ft 6 in) tall and weighs 63 kg (139 lb), giving a body surface area of 1.7 m^2.

Q.1 Mrs Goodwin has a pulmonary artery catheter inserted at the bedside. Describe the nurse's role in assisting with the PAC insertion and preparing Mrs Goodwin for procedure; note the main potential complications likely to arise during insertion.

Q.2 Compare Mrs Goodwin's vital signs to normal parameters, consider the implications of abnormal results and calculate her derived values for:

(a) Stroke volume (SV)
(b) Systemic vascular resistance (SVR)
(c) Pulmonary vascular resistance (PVR).

From these numerical values, what results would you expect for Mrs Goodwin's peripheral perfusion and respiratory status (e.g. warm, cool, dilated, constricted, dyspneoa, tachypneoa, congested)?

Q.3 Consider the clinical implications of Mrs Goodwin's haemodynamic values. Formulate a care plan which includes rationale for choice of prescribed drug therapies aimed at reducing afterload, preload and myocardial oxygen consumption, increasing cardiac output and peripheral perfusion, whilst preventing further ischaemia.

(Note: Calculations for Q.2 can be verified in the Answers section at the end of the book.)

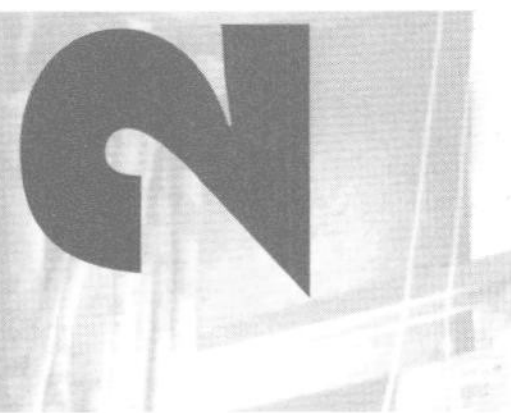

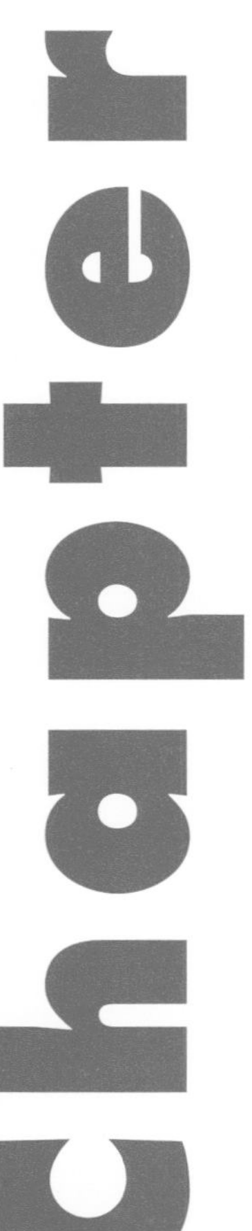

Chapter 21

ECGs and dysrhythmias

Contents

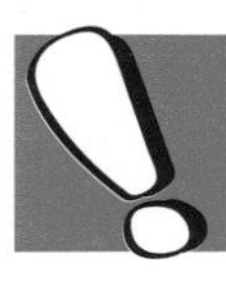

Fundamental knowledge

Myocardial physiology: automaticity, conductivity, rhythmicity
Normal limb electrode placement
Normal cardiac conduction (SA node, AV node, Bundle of His, Purkinje fibres)
Physiology of normal sinus rhythm
Current Resuscitation Council Guidelines
Experience of using continuous ECG monitoring and taking 12-lead ECGs

Introduction

In this chapter, basic principles of electrocardiograms (ECGs) are revised, providing reference for future use; although sinus rhythm is not revised, action potential is described. Frequently encountered dysrhythmias are also described following the normal conduction pathway.

The etymologically more accurate term 'dysrhythmia' is used rather than the common term 'arrhythmia', since, except for asystole, rhythms are problematic rather than absent. Texts from outside the UK may use different names for drugs (e.g. lidocaine = lignocaine; epinephrine = adrenaline).

ICU nurses should be able to identify dysrhythmias. Cardiac rhythm affects blood pressure:

$$\text{blood pressure} = \text{heart rate} \times \text{stroke volume} \times \text{systemic vascular resistance}$$

Atrioventricular dyssychrony (almost all dysrhythmias) causes loss of 'atrial kick', reducing stroke volume by one-fifth (Cohn & Gilroy-Doohan 1996).

Underlying causes (e.g. hypokalaemia) of dysrhythmias should be resolved; few asymptomatic dysrhythmias necessitate treatment. Common symptoms (e.g. pain, dyspnoea syncope) could remain unrecognised in semiconscious ventilated patients, and so nurses should actively assess effects of dysrhythmias. Some specific drugs and treatments are identified with each dysrhythmia discussed; other drugs may be seen in practice, and users should consult data sheets or pharmacopaedias for detailed information on drugs. Common problems and approaches include:

conduction:

- bradycardic dysrhythmias may need chronotropes (e.g. atropine)
- tachycardic dysrhythmias are often caused by overexcitability of conduction pathways
- atrial excitability can be reduced with digoxin (cardiac glycoside). Ventricular conduction may be blocked with:
  - β-blockers (esmolol, sotalol, propanolol), which inhibit beta receptors (see Chapter 34)
  - calcium antagonists (amiodarone, verapamil) which increase refractory periods of action potentials may be used to slow ventricular conduction. Verapamil should not be given after β-blockers (BNF 1998) or digoxin.
  - lignocaine (rhythm stabiliser)

thrombi may form with poor flow (e.g. atrial stasis), so anticoagulants are often used

poor cardiac output may necessitate inotropes; however these increase myocardial oxygen consumption, and so are usually monitored through cardiac output studies (see Chapter 20)

If drugs fail, cardioversion or pacing (temporary or permanent) may be used.

Vagal stimulation (e.g. carotid massage, orbital pressure) may temporarily reduce, but rarely resolves, tachycardia; however, it buys time for further treatment. Nurses choosing to use it should check local guidelines, remembering that the Scope of Professional Practice (UKCC 1992b) requires nurses to ensure that they each have sufficient knowledge for practice. Vagal stimulation is unreliable, imprecise, and not recommended.

Monitors are neither an end in themselves, nor a substitute for observing patients, but rather a means to providing information which should be evaluated in context of the whole person.

Basic principles of electrocardiography

An ECG is a graph of myocardial electrical activity representing three-dimensional events in a two-dimensional graph. This section summarises the basic principles for revision.

- ECG graph paper, unlike standard mathematical graph paper has only 25 (5 × 5) small squares in each large square
- each small square is 1 mm
- the horizontal axis represents time
- ECGs are normally recorded at 25 mm every second
- at 25 mm/s, one large square = 0.2 seconds, one small square = 0.04 seconds
- the vertical axis represents voltage; a calibration square (normally 1 cm = 1 mv = 2 large squares) should appear at the beginning or end of ECGs
- normal sinus rhythm (Figure 21.1) is labelled PQRST:
    - P = atrial **depolarisation**
    - QRS = ventricular depolarisation
    - T = ventricular **repolarisation**
- SA node innervation is both sympathetic (cardiac nerve) and parasympathetic (vagus nerve)
- electrical conduction is normally rapidly followed by related muscle contraction (but see EMD below)
- limb electrodes are normally colour-coded:
    - red = right arm
    - yellow = left arm
    - black/green = left leg
- electrical 'pictures' remain unchanged anywhere along the appropriate limb, or on a line between the limb joint and heart and so electrodes may be placed anywhere along the picture line

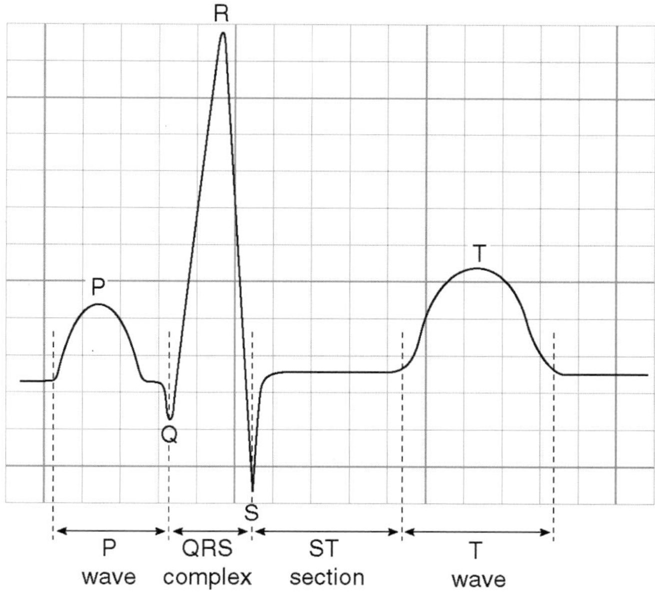

Figure 21.1 Normal sinus rhythm

- limb leads examine electrical activity along a vertical plane (see Figure 21.2a, p. 224; electrodes RA, LA and LL form 'Einthoven's triangle')
  - lead I = right arm to left arm (bipolar)
  - lead II = right arm to left leg (bipolar)
  - lead III = left arm to left leg (bipolar)
  - aVR = augmented Vector Right (arm; unipolar)
  - aVL = augmented Vector Left (arm; unipolar)
  - aVF = augmented Vector Foot (left leg; unipolar)
- Chest leads examine electrical activity along a horizontal plane, from right atrium, through right ventricle, septum, left ventricle, to left atrium (Figure 21.2b, p. 224):
  - C(or V)$_1$: 4th intercostal space, to right of (patient's) sternum
  - C_2: 4th intercostal space, left of sternum
  - C_3: between C_2 and C_4
  - C_4: 5th intercostal space, midclavicular line
  - C_5: between C_4 and C_6
  - C_6: 5th intercostal space, mid-axilla

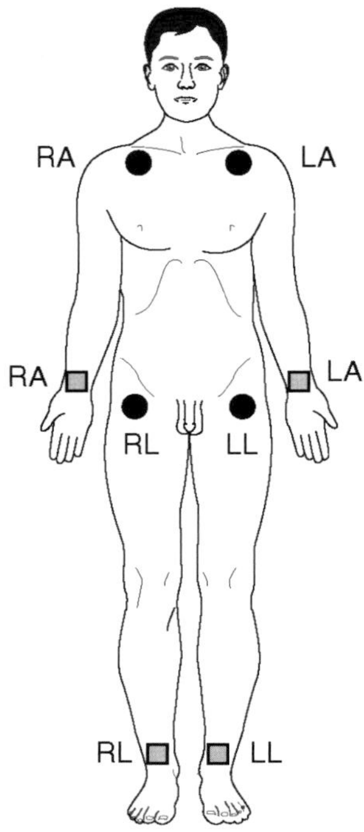

Figure 21.2a **Electrode placement: limb lead placement**

NB: breast tissue (fat is a poor conductor), wounds or invasive equipment may necessitate slight approximations.

Modified chest leads (MCL) enable one chest lead to be shown when only 3- or 5-lead ECG (continuous monitors) are available; thus placing a positive

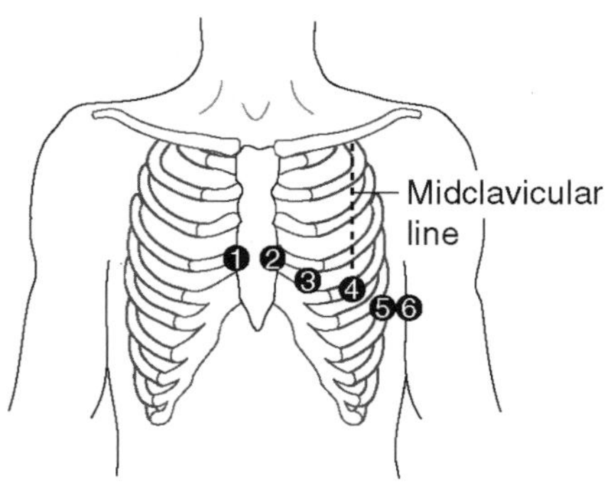

Figure 21.2b **Electrode placement: chest lead placement**

Table 21.1 Reading the ECG

Are the electrodes correctly placed (red = right arm; yellow = left arm; green/black = left leg)?
Is there a clear baseline (isoelectric line)?
Can P waves be seen?
Are the P waves within 2 small squares?
Are the P waves positive?
Is there one P wave before every QRS?
Is the PR interval 3–5 small squares?
Is the QRS positive?
Is the QRS within 3 small squares?
Does the isoelectric line return between the S and the T?
Is the T wave positive?
Is the T wave contained within four small squares?
Is the R–R interval regular?

electrode on the C_1 position shows MCL_1, with further MCL positions corresponding to other chest lead numbers (see Table 21.1).

- Normal ECG values:

  - P wave = 0.08 seconds (2 small squares)
  - PR interval = 0.12–0.2 seconds (3–5 small squares)
  - Q wave absence is not pathological; if present, it should take less than 0.04 seconds (1 small square)
  - QRS = 0.06–0.12 seconds (1.5–3 small squares)
  - T wave = 0.16 seconds (4 small squares)
  - QT = 0.32–0.4 seconds (8–10 small squares)

The same point should always be used for measurement; in practice, it is usually easier to measure from the start of each part (e.g. measure PR from beginning of P wave to beginning of next R wave).

Action potential

Ion exchange between intracellular and extracellular fluid creates transmembrane imbalances, enabling muscular (electrical) activity, hence action potential (Figure 21.3). All body muscles create action potentials. When electrical activity is absent, resting sinoatrial potential is about −90 millivolts (mv). The three main ions involved with action potential are

- sodium
- potassium
- calcium

Extracellular concentrations of about 140 mmol/litre of sodium and 4.0 mmol/litre of potassium are reversed in intracellular fluid; resting cell

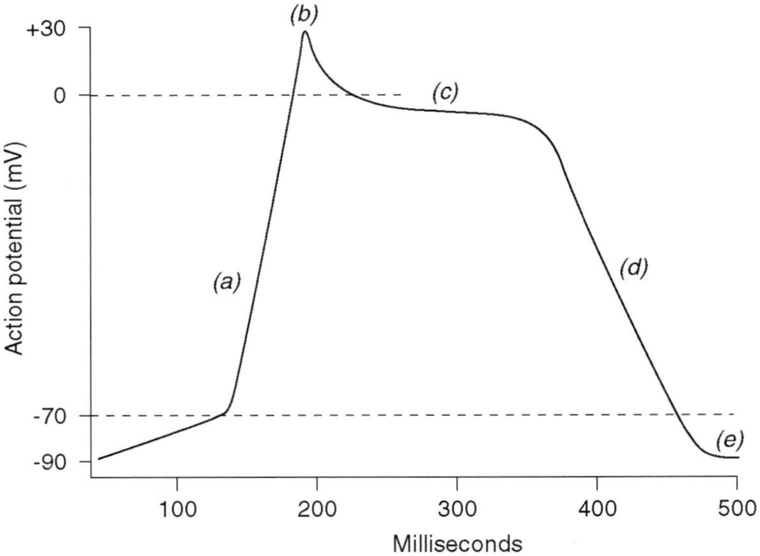

Figure 21.3 Action potential of a single cardiac muscle fibre

Note: (a) rapid depolarisation: influx via fast sodium channel (phase 0)
(b) fast calcium channel open (phase 1)
(c) plateau: slow calcium channel open (phase 2)
(d) rapid depolarisation: potassium channel open (phase 3)
(e) resting phase (phase 4)

membranes being more permeable to potassium than other ions, potassium leaks slowly (and passively) from intracellular into extracellular fluid. Action potential changes along conduction pathways to 'overpacing' lower pacemakers.

Ion movement (electrical charge) forms the action potential. This lasts only milliseconds before resting charge of −90 mv (repolarisation) is restored.

Action potential of pacemaker cells (sinoatrial node, atrioventricular node and conducting fibres) differs from other myocytes, reflecting the *automaticity* of pacemaker cells.

Action potential is divided into *phases*, numbered 0–4 (see Figure 21.3).

PHASE 0 (upstroke) occurs when the *fast sodium* opens, allowing rapid influx of extracelluar sodium ions into sodium-poor intracellular fluid. Rapid depolarisation occurs.

PHASE 1 (spike) is when the *fast* or transient *calcium* opens briefly, allowing calcium influx; this phase gives action potential graphs their characteristic peak

PHASE 2 is the 'plateau' (or absolute refractory period); the *slow* or long lasting *calcium* channel opens, calcium influx continuing for 300–400 milliseconds. This prevents cardiac muscle responding to further stimulus, thus ensuring coordinated contraction. Plateau time influences contractile strength of muscle fibres (which determines stroke volume). Hypercalcaemia increases contractility; calcium antagonists can reduce excitability. Hypocalcaemia (e.g. tetany) impairs contractility; calcium is protein-bound, so hypoalbuminaemia may cause hypocalcaemia (with dysrhythmias).

PHASE 3 is when the *potassium* channel opens, allowing potassium efflux and rapid repolarisation.

PHASE 4 is the 'resting' phase; slow potassium leakage from intracellular fluid makes the intracellular charge more negative than the surrounding fluid, eventually triggering a further cycle. Catecholamines increase depolarisation (increase duration of phase 4) in pacemaker cells, hence causing tachycardia. Vagal stimulation (mediated through acetylcholine) slows depolarisation (decreases slope in phase 4) of pacemaker cells, causing bradycardia.

Atrial/junctional dysrhythmias

Sinus arrhythmia

This occurs when inspiration increases intrathoracic pressure sufficiently to cause parasympathetic (vagal) stimulation, slowing sinoatrial rate; on expiration, the faster rate is restored. Variations between complexes (e.g. R–R interval) exceed 0.16 seconds (Lessig & Lessig 1998), but rate usually remains only 4–6 beats every minute apart. It occurs mainly in children and younger people; high ventilator tidal volumes may cause sinus arrhythmia. Unless problematic (rare), it should not be treated.

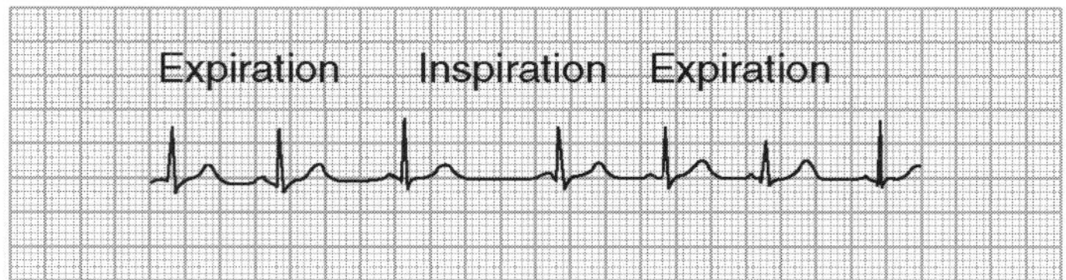

***Figure 21.4* Sinus arrhythmia**

Sinus bradycardia

Although any sinus rate below 60 beats/min is technically sinus bradycardia, most adults remain asymptomatic with higher bradycardic rates (increased ventricular filling compensating for reduced rate to restore cardiac output), only developing significant problems when rates fall towards 40 beats/min. Increased ventricular filling can over-distend ventricles.

Sinus bradycardia may be caused by:

- excessive parasympathetic stimulation (e.g. metoclopramide, severe pain/anxiety)
- conduction delays (ischaemic/infarcted myocardium)
- hypoxia
- hypothermia
- raised intracranial pressures
- CNS depressants
- antihypertensives
- β-blockers
- calcium antagonists
- digoxin
- some endocrine disorders (e.g. myxoedema, Addison's disease)

Children are especially susceptible to hypoxic bradycardia due to

- intrinsically higher rates
- less physiological reserve
- immature myocytes (until about 4 years old) usually respond with asystole rather than fibrillation.

Bradycardic children should be given oxygen urgently (unless there are other obvious causes for bradycardia).

TREATMENT Sinus bradycardia is only treated if symptomatic (e.g. syncope, dyspnoea, hypotension, chest pain). Obvious causes should be removed, so that oxygen should be optimised (on avoiding oxygen toxicity, see Chapter 18).

Drugs include

- anticholinergics (atropine) block parasympathetic stimulation
- sympathetic stimulants (adrenaline, isoprenaline).

Severe refractory sinus bradycardia may necessitate pacing (temporary or permanent).

Sinus tachycardia

Tachycardia is any rate over 100 contractions/minute. Young children often have intrinsic (normal) rates exceeding 100 contractions/minute. Sinus tachycardia is the most frequently encountered dysrhythmia in adult ICUs, due both to homeostatic compensation for oxygen supply–demand imbalances and chronotropic effects of drugs (e.g. adrenaline). Tachycardia reduces ventricular filling, so reducing stroke volume, but cardiac output may be maintained or increased due to increased numbers of contractions. Cardiac output is usually adequate with rates below 180 beats/min (bpm) provided venous return remains adequate, although rates above 140 bpm are usually treated.

Tachycardia reduces diastolic time, and so reduces coronary artery filling time and left ventricular muscle oxygen supply, while increasing left ventricular workload and myocardial oxygen demand.

TREATMENT See supraventricular tachycardia.

Supraventricular tachycardia

This severely compromises both cardiac output (rates of 160–250 (Cohn & Gilroy-Doohan 1996)) and myocardial oxygenation, usually necessitating treatment.

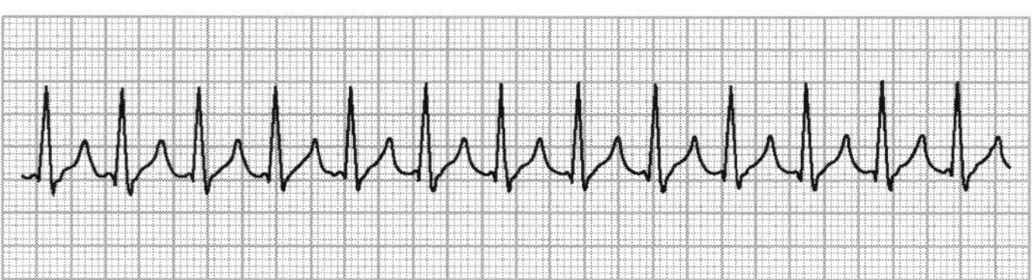

Figure 21.5 **Supraventricular tachycardia**

TREATMENT Drugs used include:

- calcium antagonists
- disopyramide
- adenosine
- β-blockers
- digoxin
- sedatives (central nervous system depressants)

If drugs fail, cardioversion may reverse supraventricular tachycardia (Cohn & Gilroy-Doohan 1996).

Sick sinus syndrome (i.e. sinoatrial node sickness)

This causes bradycardia and escape rhythms, with intermittent recovery and relapse of sinus function.

TREATMENT If problems persist, pacing can replace sinoatrial function.

Ectopics

Ectopic foci may be

- atrial
- junctional
- ventricular

Impulses may be

premature (before expected impulses) or
escape (expected complexes are absent, failing to overpace lower and slower foci, so ectopic impulses 'escape').

Premature complexes may suppress underlying rhythms; escape rhythms are inherently slower than underlying sinus rhythm. Ectopics often result from

- damaged conduction pathways (infarction, oedema, hypoxia)
- drugs/stimulants
- electrolyte imbalance (especially hypokalaemia; also calcium, magnesium)
- acidosis

TREATMENT Occasional ectopics rarely need treating, but persistent ectopics reduce cardiac output. Underlying causes should be treated.

Drugs used vary with ectopic type and cause (see below).

Atrial ectopics

These are premature electrical beats initiated in the atrial muscle outside the sinoatrial node. They may be idiopathic or due to atrial stretch (e.g. chronic pulmonary disease, valve disease, MI). Conduction and succeeding QRS complexes may be normal, but P waves may be abnormal or hidden in preceding T waves. Treatment is usually initiated when there are more than six atrial ectopics per minute.

TREATMENT Atrial ectopics rarely require treatment; if problematic, useful drugs include:

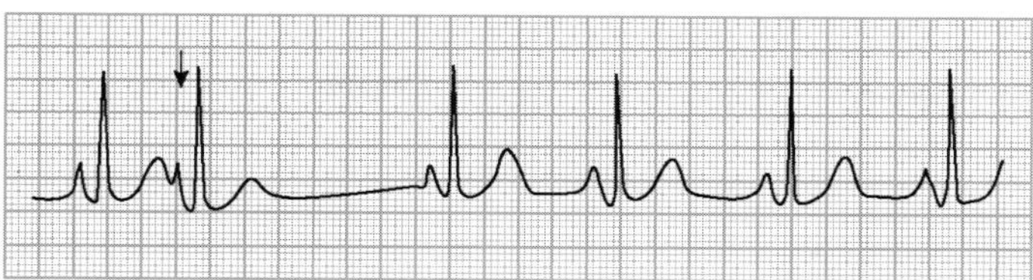

Figure 21.6 Atrial ectopics

- digoxin
- calcium antagonists

Atrial fibrillation (AF)

The commonest dysrhythmia (Lip & Beevers 1995), it originates from multiple atrial foci causing erratic, uncoordinated atrial muscle contraction ('quivering') (Figure 21.7). P waves are absent, but 'quivering' may cause 'f' waves (Cohn & Gilroy-Doohan 1996) – fine, but visible, waves, suggesting some coordinated conduction and so good prognosis. Alternatively ECG baselines may appear straight, indicating absence of group conduction and poor prognosis. Increasing ECG size may reveal f waves. The abbreviation 'AF' should not be confused with *atrial flutter*, a different, and usually more sinister, dysrhythmia.

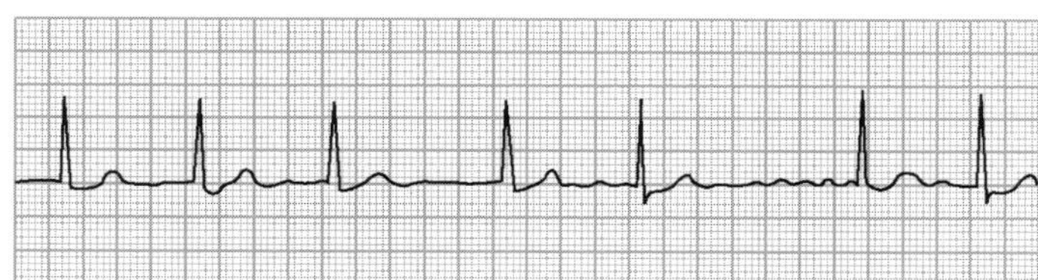

Figure 21.7 Atrial fibrillation

Atrial quivering is rapid, but relatively few atrial impulses reach the atrioventricular node. Provided ventricular pathways are intact, conduction from the AV node is normal (normal QRS complexes and T waves). Ventricular response may be fast ('fast AF'), normal or slow ('slow AF'), but is usually irregularly irregular and potentially volatile.

Asymptomatic atrial fibrillation ('controlled AF') with near-normal ventricular response may not need treatment, although often causes emboli (Lip & Beevers 1995). Symptomatic AF may significantly reduce cardiac output (e.g. 10–20 per cent), causing pain, dyspnoea and hypotension.

TREATMENT Digoxin (negative inotrope) remains the best drug for uncontrolled AF; other drugs used include:

- β-blockers
- anticoagulants

Persistent atrial fibrillation may be treated by cardioversion.

Atrial flutter

This is caused by macro re-entry circuits in the atrium (Creamer & Rowlands 1996), creating regular, but rapid, atrial impulses, P waves having distinctive saw tooth shapes (F waves). T waves are often buried in F waves (Cohn & Gilroy-Doohan 1996). Ectopic foci near atrioventricular node invert the F wave. Atrial rate is often 300 (Creamer & Rowlands 1996), with regular atrioventricular block (usually 2:1). Increased atrioventricular conduction can cause palpitations, dyspnoea and potentially life-threatening tachycardias.

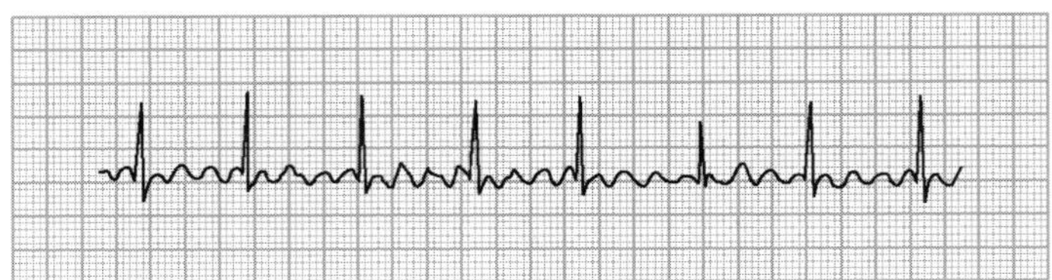

Figure 21.8 **Atrial flutter**

TREATMENT Cardioversion remains the main treatment; if cardioversion fails, drugs may block conduction or reduce atrial rates:

- calcium blockers
- digoxin
- β-blockers
- anticoagulants

Wolff–Parkinson–White syndrome

This is caused by abnormal atrioventricular conduction pathways (usually the Bundle of Kent) enabling re-entry of atrial impulses ('circus' movement). This widens bases of QRS complexes ('delta' waves) and shortens PR intervals (Shih *et al.* 1996). Rapid atrial rates are normally blocked, so ventricular response remains normal, but any reduction in block causes supraventricular tachycardia.

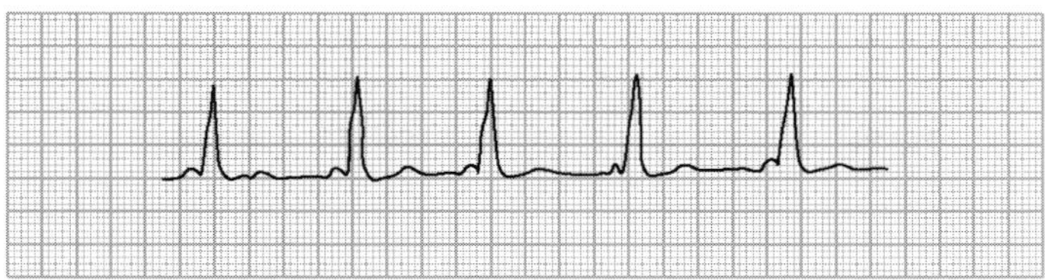

Figure 21.9 Wolff–Parkinson–White syndrome

TREATMENT The most useful drug is Amiodarone; drugs to avoid include verapamil (which increases ventricular response so may cause AF (BNF 1998)) and digoxin (which prolongs atrioventricular node block, so increasing aberrant P-wave conduction (Adam & Osborne 1997)).

Cardioversion may restore stability, but curing the underlying problem necessitates ablation of aberrant pathways. Ablation may be surgical (open heart surgery using normothermic bypass) or through coronary catheterisation (using DC shock or radio-frequency energy) (Shih *et al.* 1996). Catheterisation and surgery share similar success rates, but catheterisation reduces length of stay, trauma and cost (Shih *et al.* 1996).

A similar syndrome, Lown–Ganong–Levine syndrome, is caused by partial or total bypassing of atrioventricular node conduction, causing short PR interval (without the delta waves seen in Wolff–Parkinson–White). Treatments include antidysrhythmics, β-blockers, ablation and pacing.

Junctional rhythm

Sometimes called 'nodal', this describes impulses originating in the atrioventricular junction (AV node and surrounding area). Pacemaker rates slow as conduction pathways progress ('lower is slower'); higher impulses normally overpace, lower impulses only escaping when higher impulses are absent. Intrinsic junctional rate is usually 40–60, although acceleration can occur (Cohn & Gilroy-Doohan 1996).

Irritation (oedema, mechanical – e.g. intraventricular catheters) may cause junctional ectopics. Oedema from cardiac surgery often causes transient junctional rhythms (hence epicardial pacing wires).

Retrograde atrial conduction inverts P waves in positive ECG leads (I, II, III, aVL) (Cohn & Gilroy-Doohan 1996), which may occur before, during or after QRS complexes (depending on the pacemaker site).

TREATMENT Junctional rates are often sufficient to support life, but should be closely monitored. If bradycardia becomes symptomatic, treat as above (atropine, adrenaline, pacing).

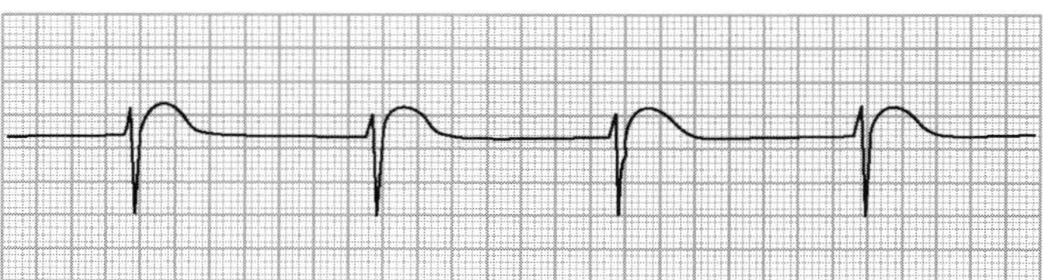

Figure 21.10 Nodal/junctional rhythm

Blocks

Any conduction pathway may be blocked by:

- infarction
- oedema
- ischaemia

If oedema or ischaemia resolve, blocks usually disappear. Infarction usually causes permanent block.

First degree block

This is delayed atrioventricular node conduction, and prolongs PR intervals beyond 0.2 seconds (5 small squares). Despite delay, every impulse is conducted so that a QRS complex follows each P wave. Delayed conduction may be caused by digoxin toxicity, β-blockers, or AV node infarction/ischaemia. First degree block can cause bradycardia, but is usually asymptomatic.

TREATMENT Provided asymptomatic, only close monitoring is necessary. If bradycardia is problematic, chronotropic (e.g. atropine) or other drugs may be needed.

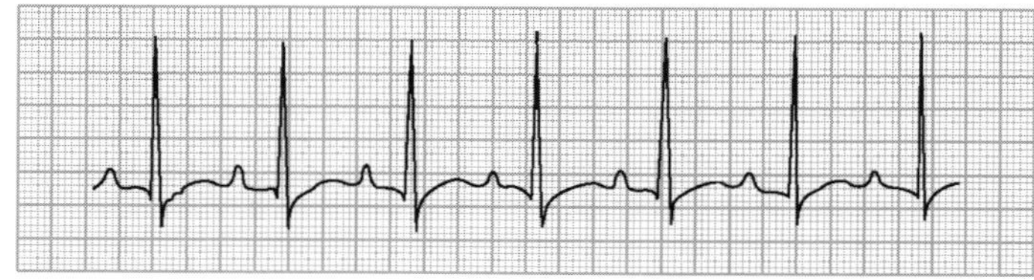

Figure 21.11 First degree block

Second degree block (or incomplete heart block)

This occurs when only some P waves are conducted, usually causing slow ventricular rates. There are two types of second degree block:

- Type 1 (Figure 21.12): progressive lengthening of PR intervals until an atrial impulse is unconducted (P without a QRS complex), caused by impaired atrioventricular node conduction.
- Type 2 (Figure 21.13): regular ratio between conducted and unconducted P waves (e.g. 2:1), caused by impaired intraventricular conduction (so more serious than type 1).

Formerly type 1 was named Mobitz type 1 or Wenkebach phenomenon; type 2 was called Mobitz type 2; these names, although technically obsolete, still persist in practice.

TREATMENT Oxygen should be optimised. Drugs used include:

- atropine
- isoprenaline (when unresponsive to atropine)

If symptoms persist pacing may be needed.

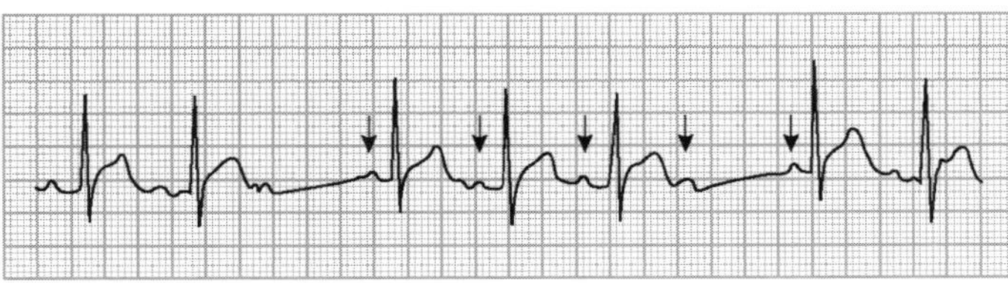

Figure 21.12 **Second degree block (type 1)**

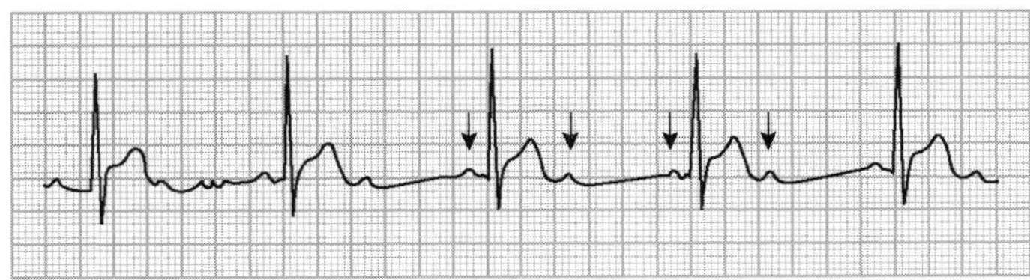

Figure 21.13 **Second degree block (type 2)**

Third degree block

This is a complete heart block that causes complete atrioventricular dissociation (Figure 21.14). Regular P-waves may occur, but are unrelated to QRS complexes; some P-waves may be 'lost' in QRS. Ventricular cells becoming the pacemaker, QRS complexes widen, and may invert (depending on focal site). Intrinsic ventricular rates are slow (about 40 beats every minute); cardiac output is severely impaired, causing hypotension.

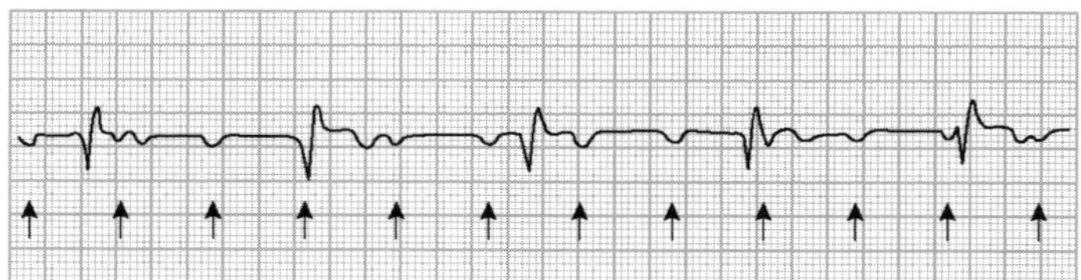

Figure 21.14 Third degree block

TREATMENT Unless transient, pacing is almost invariably needed. In the interim, oxygen should be optimised and isoprenaline may be used. Persistent block usually necessitates permanent pacing.

Bundle branch block

This is delayed partial intraventricular conduction (Figure 21.15). The Bundle of His divides into left and right branch bundles, the left branch further dividing between anterior and posterior fascicles. Conduction continues through intact pathways, the first QRS complex being followed by contraction of unaffected myocardium. The block prevents complete conduction, so impulses spread (more slowly) through muscle fibres to circumvent blocks, causing a second ventricular impulse (QRS, followed by contraction), creating characteristic M or W shapes on ECGs.

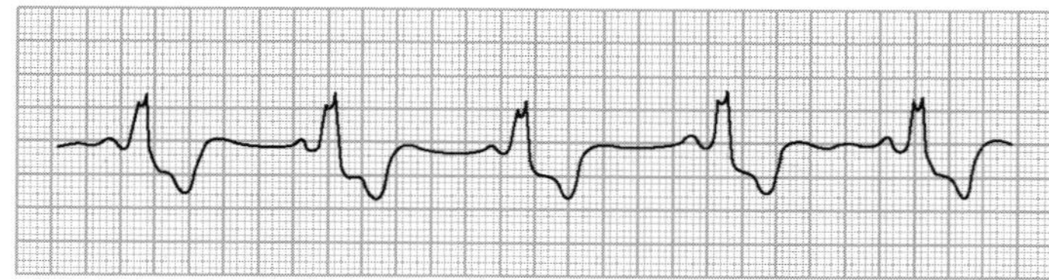

Figure 21.15 Bundle branch block

Although seen on limb leads, differentiation of right from left bundle block is clearest on chest leads. Left bundle branch block causes a W in early leads, and an M in late leads; right bundle branch block reverses this picture (mnemonics: MaRRoW and WiLLiaM).

Ventricular dysrhythmias

Ventricular ectopics

These originate from ventricular foci outside normal conduction pathways, and so lack P waves and are conducted (slowly) from muscle fibre to muscle fibre. Taking longer, this creates their characteristically wide (usually more than 2.5 small squares) and bizarre shape on ECGs (Figure 21.16). Ectopics originating near the ventricular apex are conducted downwards, giving positive complexes; those originating near the base have retrograde conduction through ventricular muscle, giving negative complexes. T waves are in the opposite direction to QRS waves.

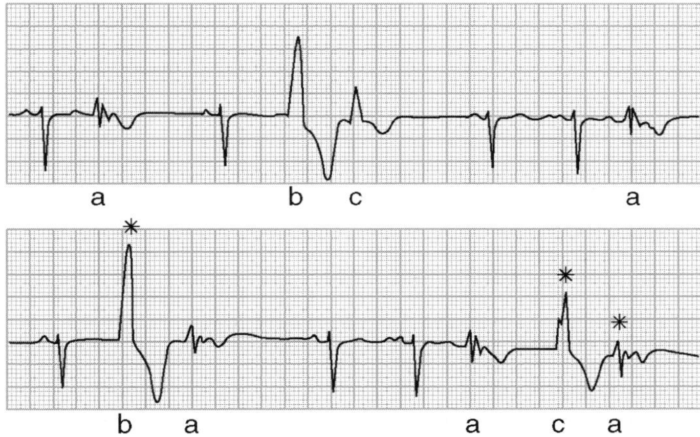

Figure 21.16 **Multifocal ventricular ectopics**

Shapes of ventricular ectopics vary, but all are wide and bizarre. Complexes from a single focus ('unifocal') look alike; ectopics with different shapes originate from different foci ('multifocal'). A sequence of three or more ectopics is sometimes called a *salvo*.

Ventricular ectopics may be premature or escape. Premature ectopics result from irritation to a focus, often from:

- electrolyte imbalance (especially potassium – both hypo- and hyperkalaemia)

- hypoxia/ischaemia (including MI)
- acidosis
- invasive equipment (e.g. central line, pulmonary artery catheter).

Escape ectopics occur with blocked or lost conduction.

Many ICU patients have occasional ectopics; although it is worth noting that infrequent ectopics are not usually treated. Treatment is usually initiated if it is

- persistent (more than six ectopics every minute)
- bigeminy/trigeminy
- multifocal
- occurring in vulnerable phases of electrical impulse conduction (R on T).

TREATMENT Electrolyte (especially potassium) balances should be restored; frequency and types of ectopics should be recorded. Premature ventricular ectopics may be reversed by overpacing (Hillel & Thys 1994).

Bigeminy and trigeminy

These are sinister extensions of ventricular ectopics, occurring regularly (Figure 21.17). Bigeminy is one ventricular ectopic every other complex; trigeminy is one ventricular ectopic every third complex. Ectopics are unifocal, usually from hypoxia or digoxin toxicity.

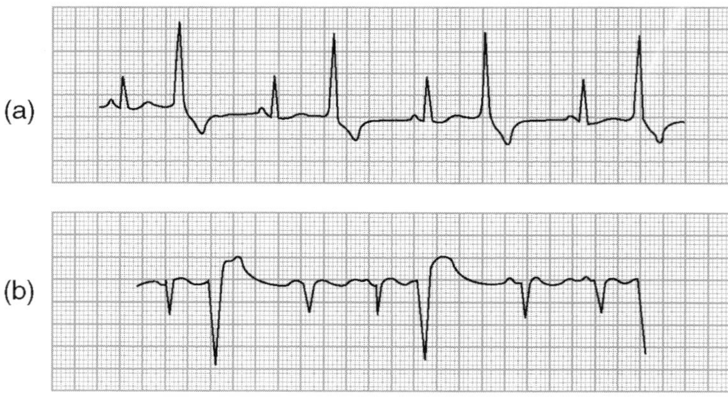

Figure 21.17 **Bigeminy and trigeminy ectopics**

TREATMENT Drug treatments include:

- disopyramide
- lignocaine

Ventricular tachycardia

This is a regular rhythm with unifocal rapid impulses (Figure 21.18) originating from an ectopic focus in ventricular muscle, usually caused by ischaemia (Thompson & Webster 1997). Rates vary from 100–250 (Cohn & Gilroy-Doohan 1996), usually nearer the upper end of this range. Inadequate ventricular filling time causes very poor stroke volumes and systemic hypotension; significantly increased myocardial workload with inadequate oxygen supply rapidly aggravates myocardial ischaemia, with imminent cardiac arrest. Prolonged ventricular tachycardia often progresses to ventricular fibrillation.

TREATMENT If pulseless, ventricular tachycardia is an arrest situation requiring urgent defibrillation. Unless patients are asymptomatic, help should be summoned urgently ('crash' call). Current resuscitation guidelines should be followed. If pulse is absent adrenaline is given. If myocardial depressants (e.g. lignocaine) have been used, defibrillation threshold may be increased, necessitating higher voltage.

Use of precordial thumps remains controversial; they may convert ventricular tachycardia into less easily treated rhythms. The 1997 resuscitation policy includes a single precordial thump 'if appropriate' for witnessed arrests between basic life support and attaching the defibrillator. With conscious patients, coughing can mimic thumps.

If asymptomatic, patients should be closely observed, and the doctor informed. Asymptomatic VT rarely persists, either reverting or progressing after a few minutes.

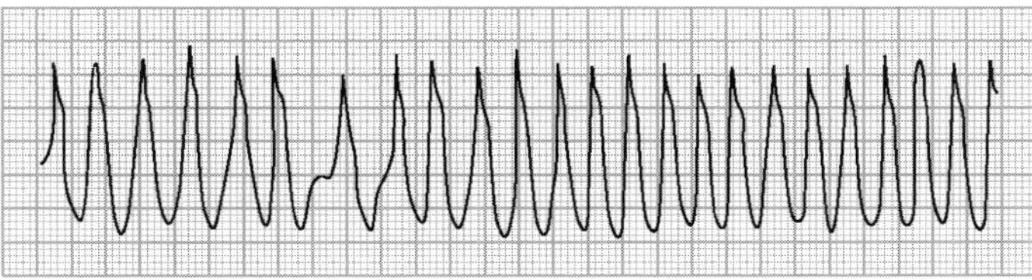

Figure 21.18 **Ventricular tachycardia**

TREATMENT Underlying causes (e.g. hypokalaemia, hypoxia, digoxin toxicity) should be resolved. Drugs include:

- calcium antagonists
- lignocaine

Temporary pacemakers can be inserted to overpace VT. Implantable defibrillators may be inserted for long-term management.

Torsades de pointes

This is a rare type of multifocal ventricular tachycardia that causes ECG traces to twist around isoelectric baselines (Figure 21.19). Rates are often 200–250. If prolonged or untreated it leads to ventricular fibrillation.

Torsades de pointes may be caused by drugs (e.g. quinidine, amiodarone), profound electrolyte imbalance (Creamer & Rowlands 1996) (especially hypokalaemia, hypomagnesaemia), subarachnoid haemorrhage, myocardial infarction, angina, bradycardia and sinoatrial block.

TREATMENT Electrolyte imbalances or underlying causes should be treated. Drugs include:

- magnesium (Tzivoni *et al.* 1988)
- antidysrhythmics (e.g. lignocaine)

If drugs fail, temporary atrial or ventricular pacing or cardiopulmonary resuscitation may be necessary.

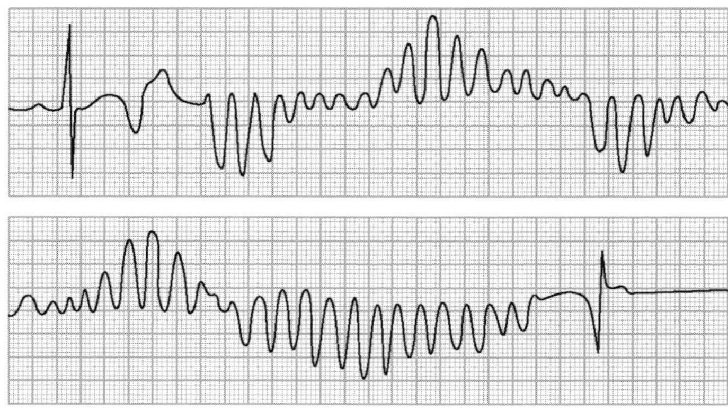

Figure 21.19 Torsades de pointes

Ventricular fibrillation (VF)

This is a lethal dysrhythmia (Figure 21.20). Patients will be unconscious, with absent or poor pulse and blood pressure. VF may be coarse or fine; fine ventricular fibrillation may appear like asystole, so increasing gain on ECGs shows whether 'f' waves are present. Like atrial fibrillation, ventricular fibrillation is totally irregular, with no significant cardiac output.

TREATMENT Ventricular fibrillation is an arrest situation, treated in a similar way to ventricular tachycardia, following current Resuscitation Council (1997) guidelines.

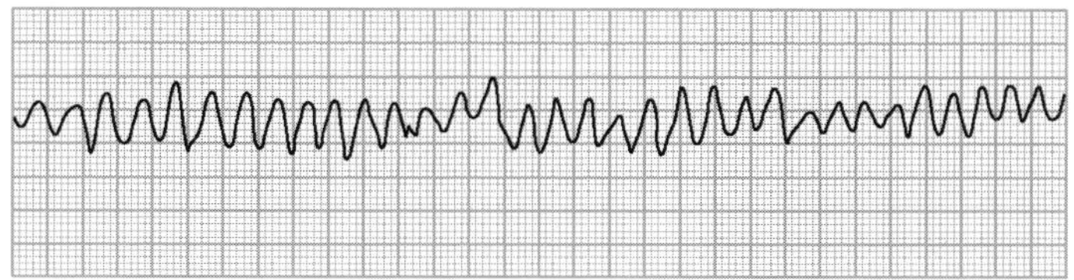

Figure 21.20 **Ventricular fibrillation**

Asystole

This is literally absence of systole and appears as an uninterrupted isoelectric line, although progression from dysrhythmias to asystole may persist for considerable time ('dying' heart), with occasional (usually ventricular) irregular complexes.

Absence of any cardiac function is an arrest situation, but few patients survive asystole. Before initiating arrest calls, staff should take ten seconds to assess patients (pulse, ECG) (Resuscitation Council 1997): absence of complexes on ECGs may be caused by

- disconnection
- failed electrodes (e.g. drying of gel)
- fine VF

If the patient appears moribund, electrodes are intact and increased gain on ECGs (see below) still shows asystole, then initiate cardiac massage and an arrest call.

TREATMENT The Resuscitation Council (1997) guidelines emphasise the need for cardiac massage to maintain effective circulation. Defibrillation is not recommended for asystole (there is no rhythm to defibrillate, and shocks interrupt cardiac massage). Drugs include:

- adrenaline (1 mg)
- atropine (3 mg)

If P waves are present, external or transvenous pacing may be used. Intubation prevents aspiration and enables ventilation.

Electromechanical dissociation

This is caused by dissociation between electrics (ECG) and mechanics (muscle contraction) of myocardium (dyssynchrony between ECG and arterial blood pressure traces and absence of palpable pulse). ECG traces are usually abnormal, often showing tachycardia and with low amplitude complexes.

Causes of electromechanical dissociation can be summarised as '4Hs and 4Ts':

- Hypoxia
- Hypovolaemia
- Hyper/hypokalaemia and metabolic disorders (e.g. from drug overdose/intoxication and electrolyte imbalances)
- Hypothermia
- Tension pneumothorax
- Tamponade
- Toxic/therapeutic disturbances (drug overdose/intoxication)
- Thrombolytic/mechanical obstruction (e.g. PE, MI)

Causes are often obvious from patients' histories.

TREATMENT Electromechanical dissociation (EMD) is an arrest situation. An arrest call should be initiated and the Resuscitation Council guidelines followed, with especial focus on correcting and treating underlying causes.

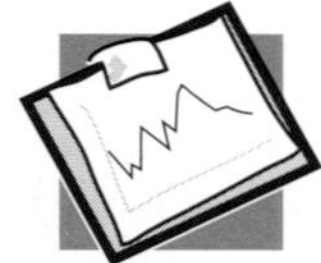

Implications for practice

- explain procedures, including 'routine' ECGs taken from unconscious patients
- information from ECGs should be interpreted in the context of the whole person; the patient is more important than the machine
- choose words carefully: 'electricity' and 'heart' may cause fears, which intubated, unconscious patients are unable to verbalise
- adhesive electrodes are potentially uncomfortable to remove, particularly if stuck to body hair, and so shave area first before applying electrodes
- if leaving 12-lead ECG electrodes in place, consider patient comfort and staff convenience in terms of patient esteem (unused electrodes on chests and arms can be undignified for patients and frightening for relatives)

- most ICU monitors are safely wall-mounted; if using portable monitors, ensure they will not fall or be knocked onto patients or other people
- posters of current Resuscitation Council guidelines should be displayed on units in easily visible areas for staff caring for patients
- nurses should know current Resuscitation Council guidelines, where emergency drugs and equipment are stored and how to summon help urgently
- nurses should attend regular updates of basic life support skills

Summary

Recording ECGs is only justified if the benefits to patients outweigh the burdens. Critical illness exposes ICU patients to various symptomatic dysrhythmias, and so ICU patients are usually continuously monitored; ICU nurses should therefore be able to recognise common dysrhythmias and initiate appropriate action. ICU staff should already be familiar with basic electrocardiography, and so this chapter has discussed dysrhythmias most likely to be seen in ICUs, together with standard treatments. Staff should be familiar with current Resuscitation Council guidelines.

Further reading

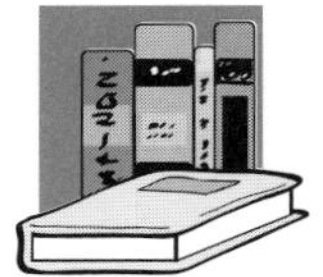

Current Resuscitation Council (UK) guidelines should be familiar and available. Woodrow (1998) provides a revision of basic ECG interpretation, but readers will probably need more advanced texts. Hampton (1997a) provides a useful overview, with supplementary detail in Hampton (1997b); readers already possessing other ECG books which they find useful are advised to continue using them. Most ICU textbooks contain reliable overviews of electrocardiography which can be extended through specialist texts or study days.

Clinical scenario

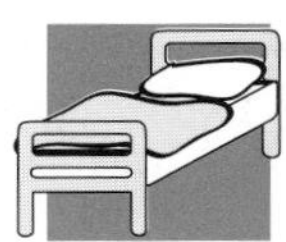

Q.1 Describe how you would perform a 12-lead ECG on an ICU patient who is awake? Include how you would explain procedure, position patient and apply electrodes to ensure an accurate and optimal ECG tracing.

Q.2 For continuous bedside ECG monitoring in an ICU, which lead (e.g. 1, II, III, aVF, aVR, MCL1) is usually chosen for waveform analysis? Justify your choice in relation to cardiac physiology and note expected waveform pattern.

Q.3 Reflect on situations where an external carotid massage has been performed for tachycardia. Appraise desired effects, limitations, safety issues and nurse accountability. What other strategies can be used to reduce life-threatening tachycardia in emergency situations?

Chapter 22

Neurological monitoring and intracranial hypertension

Contents

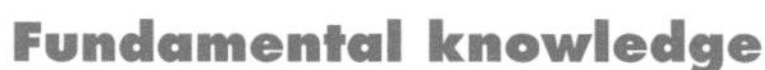

Fundamental knowledge

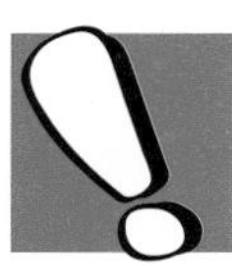

Intracranial anatomy
Cerebral autoregulation and the effect of hypo-/hypercapnia on cerebral arteries
Brain stem tests, 12 cranial nerves and physiology of vital centres
Cranial blood supply, circle of Willis

Introduction

While some ICUs specialise in neurosurgery or neuromedicine, most others receive patients with head injuries and pathologies. Raised intracranial pressure (ICP) can complicate many conditions (e.g. meningitis, hepatic failure). Since most ICU patients suffer neurological dysfunction, which may remain undetected but prolongs weaning (Kelly & Matthay 1993), the assessment and monitoring of neurological function is important for all ICU patients.

The Glasgow Coma Scale is a familiar neurological assessment tool; although discussed briefly, this chapter focuses on invasive (more precise) monitoring, such as intracranial pressure monitoring, traditionally largely confined to specialist neurosurgical units (Odell 1996), but increasingly being used by other ICUs. The value of various invasive modes remains debatable; this chapter reviews means and implications of invasive neurological monitoring, with especial emphasis on intracranial pressure monitoring.

Intracranial physiology

Average total adult intracranial volume is 1.7 litres: 150 ml blood, 150 ml cerebrospinal fluid (CSF), 1,400 ml brain tissue (Hickey 1997a). The skull is rigid and filled to capacity with essentially noncompressible contents (the *Monro-Kellie hypothesis*) so that increasing one component necessarily compresses others. Normal adult intracranial pressure averages 0–15 mmHg (Germon *et al.* 1994), being lower (3–7 mmHg) in young children (Chitnavis & Polkey 1998); pressure is not constant throughout the intracranium (Hickey 1997a).

Displacing blood or CSF into the spinal cord allows initial compensation (*compliance*) for increased volume (intracranial bleed, obstruction of CSF drainage, oedema) so that transient, even if very high, pressures are tolerated (e.g. coughing, straining, sneezing); but once compliance is exhausted, increased volume inevitably progressively increases ICP (see Figure 22.1).

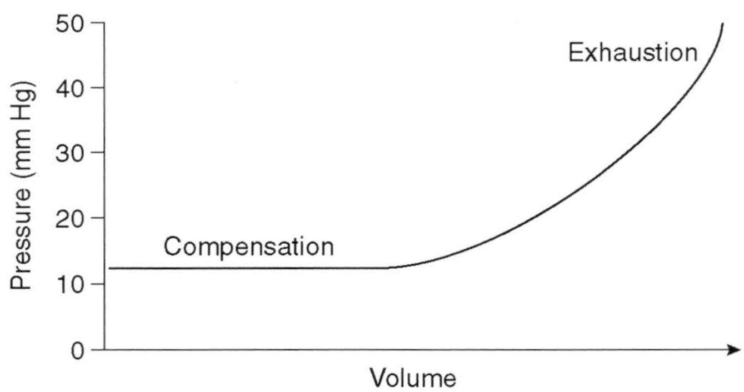

Figure 22.1 Intracranial pressure/volume curve

Sustained intracranial pressures of 20–30 mmHg may cause mechanical tissue injury (Hanley 1997). Cerebral autoregulation fails when ICP exceeds 40 mmHg (Hickey 1997a). Sustained intracranial pressure over 60 mmHg causes ischaemic brain damage and is usually fatal (Hudak *et al.* 1998). Progressive cellular damage (see Chapter 23) causes:

- release of vasoactive chemicals (e.g. histamine, *serotonin*)
- hyperkalaemia
- intracellular oedema and cell death
- increased capillary permeability, reducing colloid osmotic pressure

creating a vicious cycle of intracranial hypertension and tissue injury (see Figure 22.2).

Head injury

Each year 3 per cent of the UK population are admitted to hospital with head injuries (Addy *et al.* 1996); prehospital mortality remains high, but improved rescue increasingly means that more severe cases are reaching ICUs.

A head injury, together with the resulting intracranial hypertension, cause widespread neurological dysfunction, including

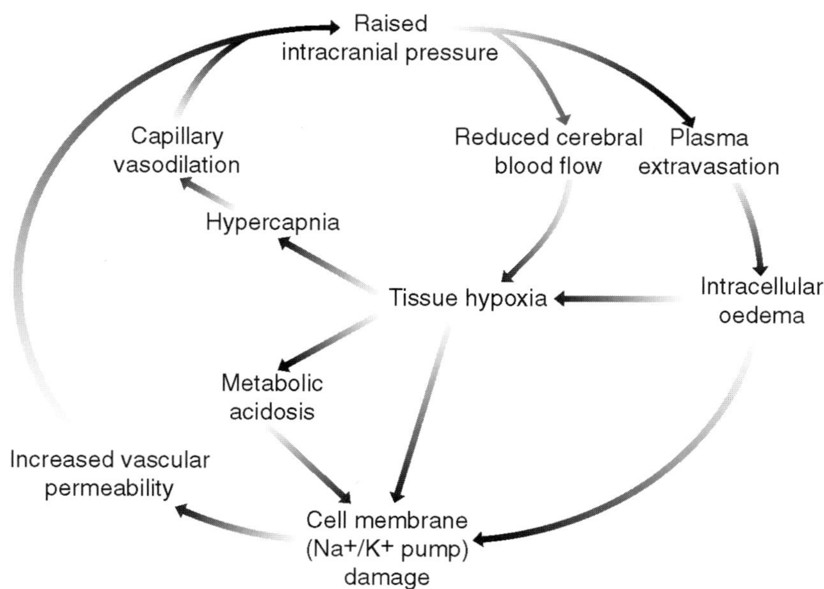

Figure 22.2 Intracranial hypertension and tissue injury: a vicious circle

- fitting
- thermoregulation.

While primary intracranial damage is usually irreversible, secondary damage from ischaemia and hypoxia can be treated or prevented (Odell 1996; Matta & Menon 1997); if untreated, further mechanical damage from cerebral depression is likely, potentially progressing to (fatal) *tentorial herniation* ('coning' – brain stem tissue forced through the foramen magnum into spinal cord, causing spinal cord compression).

Fits increase cerebral oxygen consumption and so should be promptly treated by:

- ensuring safety and privacy
- antiepileptics
- ventilation/oxygen
- removal of saliva/vomit
- reassuring family

Fits should be observed, timed and recorded.

Cerebral blood flow

The brain relies on glucose metabolism for energy and has little reserve so that unperfused tissues rapidly die. Although cerebral blood flow does not necessarily correlate with cerebral perfusion pressure (Cruz *et al.* 1995), cerebral perfusion pressure (CPP) can be readily calculated, being the difference between mean arterial pressure (MAP) and intracranial pressure:

$$CPP = MAP - ICP$$

Many monitors include facilities to directly measure CPP, although systemic mean arterial pressure may differ from mean cerebral arterial pressure. Cerebral oxygenation is also influenced by oxygen carriage (e.g. hypoxia, anaemia); therefore, management of intracranial hypertension should consider total trends and factors affecting cerebral demand and supply, rather than focusing on single measurements or parameters.

In health, mean arterial pressure significantly exceeds ICP, giving normal cerebral perfusion pressures of 70–100 mmHg (Hickey 1997a), but systemic hypotension makes perfusion pressure lower for many ICU patients (Germon *et al.* 1994). Since CPP below 50 mmHg often causes secondary ischaemic injury (Germon *et al.* 1994), perfusion pressure should be maintained at 70 mmHg (Hickey 1997a), which may necessitate inotropic support to increase mean arterial pressure. Excessive CPP can disrupt the blood–brain barrier and aggravate cerebral oedema.

Cerebral oedema

Cerebral oedema may be

- interstitial
- intracellular
- vasogenic

Interstitial and intracellular oedema formation is discussed in Chapter 33. Most cerebral oedema is vasogenic: blood–brain barrier disruption increases capillary permeability, causing fluid and protein leak. As cell damage progresses, fluid and electrolyte imbalances frequently occur (Parobek & Alaimo 1996). Steroid treatment (e.g. dexamethsone) to prevent vasogenic oedema remains controversial with little evidence of effectiveness against other causes of intracranial hypertension (Hickey 1997a).

Cushing's response triad (hypertension, bradycardia, abnormal respiratory pattern) indicates brainstem dysfunction and loss of compliance (Hickey 1997a); artificial ventilation and other therapeutic interventions may mask symptoms.

Neurological assessment

With neonates, an estimation of intracranial pressure can be gained by palpating the fontanelles; although giving only limited information, this is a useful, noninvasive way of assessment. After closure of the second fontanelle (between 9 and 18 months) measurement necessitates greater invasiveness so that benefits from information gained have to be assessed against risks of each procedure.

Price (1996) suggests that assessment needs to be continuous; while limiting intracranial pressure does improve outcome, and continuous measurement may be a useful adjunct to management, it remains unclear whether patients treated empirically fare any worse than those whose ICP is monitored (Chitnavis & Polkey 1998). The pursuit of information may reassure staff, but does not necessarily benefit every patient.

Methods of neurological assessment vary between units and patients. Whichever method is chosen, it should be understood by staff and beneficial to patients. Neurological assessment should account for effects from drugs (sedatives and paralysing agents, remembering metabolism may be delayed with renal/hepatic failure).

Glasgow Coma Scale (GCS)

Two-fifths of those losing consciousness following head injuries develop raised intracranial pressure (Odell 1996), and so monitoring consciousness is a relatively simple, noninvasive way to detect those most at risk from raised intracranial pressure.

The Glasgow Coma Scale is a 14-point (later modified to 15 points) assessment scale to monitor level of consciousness by patient responses (eye, verbal, motor). Scores are often added to suggest:

- severe impairment (coma) = 3–8
- moderate impairment = 9–12
- mild impairment = 13

However, equality of scores between the three groups of responses is untested, and so responses may be best recorded individually (as eye, verbal and motor, e.g. E2, V3, M4) (Watson *et al.* 1992). Pupil size is also usually added to Glasgow Coma Scale charts.

Advantages of the GCS include

- its relative simplicity;
- there is no need for special equipment;
- it is widely used and so most staff are familiar with its design;
- it is a good predictor of outcome.

However,

- it is poor at monitoring changes in levels of consciousness (Segatore & Way 1992), which limits its value for ICU, and,
- it is particularly unreliable in middle range scores (Segatore & Way 1992).

Ellis and Cavanagh (1992) found pupil size and motor weakness assessment varied between ICU staff, concluding that inexperienced users were more likely to make errors; however, Juarez and Lyons (1995) found GCS measurements consistent between observers.

Response is assessed using stimulation, usually to pain (central or peripheral). Central stimuli (e.g. suborbital pressure) assess arousal (consciousness), and so should be assessed before peripheral response to painful stimuli. There are three central stimuli (Shah 1999):

- trapezium squeeze (pinching trapezius muscle, between head and shoulders)
- suborbital pressure (running a finger along the bony ridge at the top of the eye)
- sternal rub (grinding the sternum with knuckles)

Peripheral stimuli (e.g. nail bed pressure) should only be used when patients are unresponsive to central stimuli (spinal injury may prevent higher transmission of peripheral stimuli). Peripheral stimuli should cause guarding or defensive movements ('best motor response'), indicating level of awareness. Such stimuli may conflict with therapeutic benefits from rest (to minimise

ICP). While vigorous pain stimuli are essential for isolated observations with major implications (e.g. brain stem death tests), most nurses are understandably reluctant to inflict regular strong pain stimuli.

Over one-half of ICUs in the UK do not routinely use ICP monitoring with patients whose Glasgow Coma Score is below 8 (Jeevaratnam & Menon 1996). Where specialised equipment is unavailable, pupil response and GCS provide readily available and familiar means of assessment. However, neurological crises may be rapid, secondary damage occurring before intermittent measurement (e.g. Glasgow Coma Scale) detects deterioration (Price 1998). Frequency of GCS monitoring varies from between every 15 to 20 minutes to once each shift or day. Frequency should be individualised to the patients' needs, weighing anticipated risks between observations against unnecessary stimulation and infliction of pain, but Price (1996) concludes that the GCS alone is sufficient for monitoring intubated, ventilated and sedated patients following head injury.

Cerebral function monitoring

The electroencephalogram (EEG) has long been used to assess neurological function, but its use is limited on ICUs due both to the impracticality of continuously monitoring multiple (usually 16) traces and the lack of any standard EEG pattern for anaesthesia (Stanski 1994). Although *Cerebral Function Monitors* (CFM) using single/double lead EEG channels proved disappointing for monitoring depth of sedation, the addition of analysers (Cerebral Function Analysing Monitor – CFAM) can identify pattern changes from different sedative drugs (Shelley & Wang 1992), and is used in some ICUs.

Near infrared spectroscopy

Near infrared spectroscopy (NIRS) is similar to mixed venous saturation monitoring; infrared light transmitted through the skull provides noninvasive, continuous trends of cerebral oxygenated and deoxygenated haemoglobin (Menon 1997). Healthy adult saturations should be about 70 per cent (Mead *et al.* 1995). However, since knowledge about transmission and reflection of near infrared light through brain structures is limited, Germon *et al.* (1994) suggest that this method needs further testing before clinical use. Subdural haematomas or air can reduce readings (Price 1998). Currently, infrared spectroscopy has been used more widely with neonates than with adults (Menon 1997).

Jugular venous bulb saturation

Jugular vein catheterisation (like a CVP catheter with oximeter) enables oxygen saturation and content measurement; on X-ray, the tip should rest at the border of the first cervical spine (March 1994). Probes can also be introduced through ICP microtransducer burr holes (Kiening *et al.* 1996). As with mixed venous saturation, jugular bulb saturation (SjO_2) indicates global cerebral oxygen delivery, but cannot detect regional ischaemia (Feldman & Robertson 1997). Cerebral oxygen consumption is normally 35–40 per cent of available oxygen so that normal SjO_2 is 60–65 per cent (March 1994); changes in SjO_2 reflect changes in cerebral metabolic rate and cerebral blood flow. High SjO_2 indicates

- increased cerebral blood flow
- reduced oxygen extraction
- hyperventilation (respiratory alkalosis; leftward shunt of oxygen dissociation curve increasing affinity of haemoglobin for oxygen (Sikes & Segal 1994))

Levels below 54 per cent suggest cerebral hypoperfusion; below 40 per cent indicate global cerebral ischaemia (Dearden 1991). Approximately one-half of desaturation episodes are artificial, often due to low light intensity (Sikes & Segal 1994).

ICP measurement

Catheters for measuring intracranial pressure (ICP) may be fluid-filled (like arterial pressure monitoring systems) or solid (fibre-optic devices). Fluid-filled devices may be passed intraventricularly, or through bolts. The choice of catheters therefore depends on:

- level of accuracy required
- likely duration of monitoring
- infection risk
- equipment available.

Intraventricular catheters with ventriculostomy (burr hole) provide the gold standard for intracranial pressure monitoring (Menon 1997).

Bolts usually measure subdural pressure (Sutcliffe 1997) and, by not penetrating the ventricle, the risk of meningitis is reduced (Hickman *et al.* 1990), although traces tend to be damp and unreliable (Waldmann & Thyveetil 1998).

Advancing catheters into the non-dominant hemisphere reduces potential damage (Hanley 1997). Infection risks with intraventricular catheters remain low for 72 hours, then rise significantly (Sutcliffe 1997) but variably (0.2–27 per cent (Hanley 1997)). Since infection means meningitis, the risk–benefit analysis should guide the choice and duration of intraventricular measurement. Infection risk is highest with fluid-filled systems (Price 1998) and so, as with other invasive equipment, maintaining closed circuits reduces infection (Hickman *et al.* 1990).

ICP is measured at the Foramen of Monro (see Figure 22.3), the duct joining the lateral and third ventricles, in alignment with the middle of the ear (Nikas 1998)). Monitoring equipment may be tested by applying momentary jugular venous pressure, which should cause ICP to rise briskly ('Quekenstedt test') (Chitnavis & Polkey 1998). Although both systolic and diastolic pressures are measured, normally mean pressure is the value recorded; all figures above refer to mean pressures.

Fibre-optic catheters produce a pulse and trend waveform (Hall 1997); initially more reliable than bolts (Bruder *et al.* 1995), after five days drifting makes readings unreliable (Waldmann & Thyveetil 1998), although the extent of reported drifts vary (Chitnavis & Polkey 1998). Once inserted, recalibration is not possible (Chitnavis & Polkey 1998).

Fibre-optic systems do not introduce fluid, and so infection rates are low (Chitnavis & Polkey 1998). They may safely be used for up to three days (Hickman *et al.* 1990; Chitnavis & Polkey 1998), and possibly longer (Hall 1997), although manufacturers' recommendations should not be exceeded without reliable evidence. Glass fibres are fragile and break easily (Chitnavis & Polkey 1998) – sheaths can protect patients from harm.

Fibre optics normally include a drainage channel, to relieve raised intracranial pressure. Once positioned, marking their location with permanent ink will help to identify any catheter migration (Hall 1997).

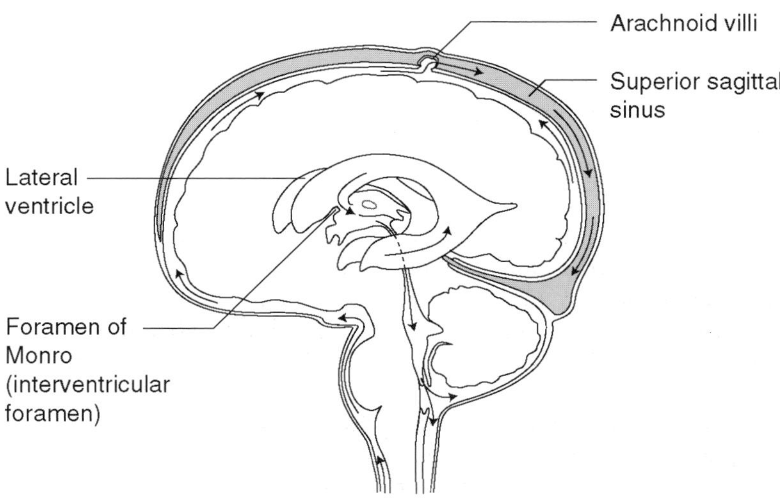

Figure 22.3 Cross section of the cranium, showing the Foramen of Monro

Pulse waveform

Cardiac pulse waves reach cranial circulation via the choroid plexus. Broadly similar to arterial waveforms, but with lower amplitude (Hall 1997), the waveform has three peaks (Hickey 1997a) (see Figure 22.4):

- P1: *percussion wave*: sharp peak, fairly constant amplitude; reflect pulse of arteries and choroid plexus
- P2: *tidal wave*: shape and amplitude more variable, ends on dicrotic notch; indicates cerebral compliance (Germon *et al.* 1994)
- P3: *dicrotic wave*: immediately follows the dicrotic notch

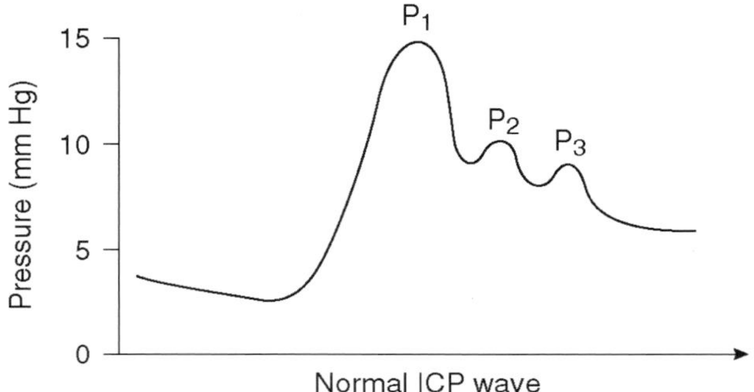

Figure 22.4 Normal intracranial pressure waveform

Lundberg classified three patterns of waveforms, labelled A, B and C (Chitnavis & Polkey 1998), but their clinical value is questionable (Germon *et al.* 1994) and so they are not included here.

Nursing intracranial pressure considerations

Nursing responsibilities combine the technical roles of monitoring and regulating treatments with the holistic, person-centred care fundamental to nursing.

Care of patients with raised intracranial pressure includes awareness of factors that might aggravate intracranial hypertension. While some common aspects are identified below, responses of different patients are individual so that nurses should always observe their patients to assess responses to each intervention (Odell 1996).

Anything stimulating arousal (e.g. alarms, loud noises) is a potential stressor that may increase intracranial pressure; allowing rest between interventions can limit negative effects. Chudley (1994) recommends spacing each intervention by at least ten minutes, although this may need to be balanced against enabling adequate rest periods (see Chapter 3). The primary aim of care is to prevent aggravating intracranial hypertension; therefore, numbers and extent of interventions should normally be minimised. Rising (1993) found that only suctioning, turning and bed bathing caused transient increases in pressure; other interventions had no significant effects.

Intrathoracic pressure

Obstruction to venous drainage causes vascular engorgement, provoking oedema formation and intracranial hypertension. Venous drainage is impaired by any rise in intrathoracic pressure (Odell 1996), such as:

- positive pressure ventilation
- PEEP
- manual hyperventilation (bagging)
- coughing and straining (valsalva manoeuvre)
- tight ET tapes
- awkward neck alignment
- cervical collars

Ventilatory management

Meeting cerebral needs while minimising adverse effects is a delicate balance. Historically, intracranial hypertension was treated by hyperventilation, hypocapnia causing vasoconstriction, so reducing intracranial hypertension.

Hyperventilation may provoke secondary injury, and so should only be used where it will prove beneficial and can be closely monitored (Gerraci & Gerraci 1996). It may be useful for rapid reduction of ICP during crises (Hickey 1997a), but $PaCO_2$ is now normally maintained at the lower end of normal ranges, around 4.5 kPa (Hall 1997).

Respiratory alkalosis may compensate for metabolic acidosis, but it

- reduces oxygen dissociation from haemoglobin (see Chapter 18);
- causes vasoconstriction, reducing cerebral blood flow and perfusion pressure;
- increases hydrostatic pressure, so causing oedema formation (Hinds & Watson 1996);
- causes anaerobic metabolism (= metabolic acidosis);
- lowers the seizure threshold (Winkelman 1995).

Patients with intracranial hypertension are often sedated and ventilated for 5–7 days following injury (Odell 1996). If paralysing agents are used to prevent stimulation, nurses should ensure patients are adequately sedated beneath paralysis, both for humanitarian reasons and because stress from being paralysed but not sedated will aggravate hypertension (see Chapter 6). Peripheral nerve stimulation may indicate depth of paralysis, but not sedation. Weaning commences once intracranial pressure is stable and below 20 mmHg (Odell 1996).

Use of PEEP with intracranial hypertension remains controversial; PEEP above 10 cmH_2O was traditionally thought to accentuate intracranial hypertension (Robb 1997), but McGuire *et al.* (1997) suggest that PEEP is safe provided it remains below ICP.

Suction

Endotracheal suction, necessary to remove excessive secretions, will provoke intracranial transient hypertension (Brucia & Rudy 1996; Rising 1993). Thus, suction should be planned following a risk–benefit analysis. Chudley (1994) suggests that suction is safe provided ICP is below 20 mmHg and CPP is above 50 mmHg. Bolus analgesia and sedation before suction can prevent dangerous hypertension (Hall 1997).

As cerebral hypoxia is already likely to be present, patients with raised intracranial pressure should always be preoxygenated (100% oxygen) before suction. Brief hyperinflation (for one minute) before endotracheal suction reduces suction-induced rises in ICP while maintaining CPP – although its value for neuroprotection, especially in ischaemic areas, is unclear (Kerr *et al.* 1997). Dangers progressively increase with the number of passes, and so Chudley (1994) recommends at least ten seconds rest between each pass, with at least two minutes rest after suctioning. Although rarely used in practice, Chudley (1994) recommends giving intratracheal lignocaine beforehand.

Positioning

Like most ICU patients, these patients are at risk of developing pressure sores. However, pressure area care interventions should be planned against risks from stimulation. Aggressive manual handling can significantly increase intracranial pressure.

Any positions impeding jugular venous drainage, such as head rotation (Hudak *et al.* 1998), knee flexion (angles over 30°) (March *et al.* 1990), or tight endotracheal tapes (Lockhart-Wood 1996) should be avoided; neutral alignment should be maintained (e.g. turning by log-rolling). Slight head elevation encourages venous drainage, so reducing intracranial hypertension. Some literature recommends a maximum 30° head tilt (e.g. Lockhart-Wood 1996)), but most emphasise the need for individual assessment (Chudley 1994; Simmons 1997) based on parameters such as intracranial and cerebral perfusion pressures. Patients should be positioned to minimise risk from falls, furniture or equipment. Pressure on bone flaps should normally be avoided.

Patients with raised intracranial pressure are often hypersensitive to environmental stimuli, developing photophobia. Unless otherwise indicated, it is generally kinder to reduce light levels to the minimum necessary.

Hyperthermia

Hypothalamic damage often causes hyperthermia. Hyperthermia increases metabolic rate, so increasing

- reduces intracranial blood flow
- intracranial pressure (each extra degree centigrade increases cerebral blood flow by 6 per cent (Hickey 1997a)
- cerebral oxygen consumption

in already hypoxic tissue; antipyretic drugs (e.g. aspirin) will therefore provide cerebral protection.

Glucose

Hyperglycaemia and hypoglycaemia can occur. Hyperglycaemia increases osmotic pressure, so provoking ischaemia; hypoglycaemia deprives neurones of fuel. Blood sugars should therefore be kept within normal levels and glucose (e.g. 5 per cent) infusions avoided (North & Reilly 1994).

Drugs

Drug therapy aims to both reverse the pathology and prevent complications. Drugs used therefore include:

analgesia: for comfort and to reduce agitation which would increase intracranial pressure

sedative agents: while sedation both provides comfort and reduces intracranial pressure, it makes pupil assessment unreliable (Price 1998). As thiopentone is negatively inotrope, reducing cerebral perfusion pressure and increasing intracellular acidosis (Price 1992), its use remains controversial (Hall 1997). Propofol reduces intracranial hypertension through systemic hypotension, but may reduce cerebral perfusion pressure (Hall 1997) and so is usually avoided. Mirski *et al.* (1995) review sedation for neurological pathologies.

neuromuscular blockade: to prevent stimulation from movement

antiepileptic drugs (e.g. phenytoin): as raised intracranial pressure is likely to provoke fitting. Phenytoin or other antiepileptic drugs are often prescribed.

Fluid management

Cerebral oedema, responsible for most complications of intracranial hypertension, is aggravated by movement of intravascular proteins into intracellular fluid. The resulting rise in intracellular osmotic pressure can be effectively countered with osmotic diuretics. With repeated doses, osmotic diuretics may cross the blood–brain barrier, reversing osmotic pressures to draw further plasma into extravascular spaces (Adam & Osborne 1997).

Twenty per cent mannitol has replaced earlier osmotic diuretics (Allen & Ward 1998). Its effect begins within 15 to 30 minutes and can last for up to six hours (Allen & Ward 1998). Transfer of water from intracellular to intravascular compartments may cause hyperkalaemia, while reduced renal water reabsorption may cause hypernatraemia (Wingard *et al.* 1991). Being hypertonic, mannitol should be given into a central (or large) vein.

Frusemide, a loop diuretic, inhibits CSF production (Winkelman 1995) and so may prevent further hypertension, but concurrent administration with mannitol is no longer recommended (Hudak *et al.* 1998).

One per cent of patients with head injuries develop diabetes insipidus (Matta & Menon 1997) from direct pituitary pressure/damage. While easily detected, fluid replacement to prevent total body dehydration (to keep serum osmolarity below 320 mmol/l) must be incorporated with fluid management to treat intracranial hypertension. Oedema can be reduced with colloids (Schell *et al.* 1992) and mild hypernatraemia (140–150 mmol/l).

Fluid resuscitation should replace loss without aggravating problems. Hypovolaemia (e.g. dehydration from diuretics/diabetes insipidus) triggers cerebral vasospasm, but hypervolaemia, especially with crystalloids, may increase oedema. Fluid replacement should be limited to 3 litres/day, with no more than 1 litre being crystalloid (Smith 1994).

Nasogastric tubes could herniate through existing fractures into brain tissue, and so until base of skull fractures have been definitively excluded, oral rather than nasal tubes should be used.

Syndrome of inappropriate antidiuretic hormone (SIADH)

When atrial blood flow/volume increases, vagal signals from stretch receptors in the right and left atria inhibit antidiuretic hormone (ADH) release. This negative feedback control is impaired by increased intrathoracic pressure (positive pressure ventilation), so many ICU patients develop SAIDH.

Additional pituitary gland control can be disrupted by head injury, central nervous system infection, intracranial hypertension and other factors. ADH release, despite absence of hyperosmolality or hypervolaemia, causes

- inappropriate fluid retention
- dilutional anaemia (causing tissue hypoxia and so metabolic acidosis)
- hyponatraemia (serum levels fall towards 120 (Parobek & Alaimo 1996) provoking nausea, muscle irritability, fits and coma)
- electrolyte dilution (hypocalcaemia and hypokalaemia provoke dysrhythmias)
- oedema
- oliguria and concentrated urine

SIADH is treated with hypertonic saline, but, once precipitating factors are removed, it usually takes 3–5 days to resolve (Parobek & Alaimo 1996).

Family support

Presence of anyone can cause stress or provide reassurance/relaxation. Studies of how conversation affects intracranial pressure remain inconclusive; familiar voices, such as family, may reduce anxiety (Odell 1996), but more studies suggest they have no significant effect (Treloar *et al.* 1991; Schinner *et al.* 1995). This may reflect differing interpersonal dynamics. Where visitors do cause undue distress, nurses may need to intervene to enable patients to rest, but visits that provide therapeutic benefits should be encouraged. Good nursing documentation can be a valuable means to communicate the effects of visitors.

While the prime duty of nurses is to their patients, care of relatives is an important, albeit secondary, nursing role. Relatives usually appreciate being given appropriate information. They also need adequate rest themselves; they may feel obliged to stay by the bedside, exhausting both themselves and the patient; thus, planning care with the next-of-kin can prove beneficial to all. Providing somewhere to stay and access to catering facilities can greatly reduce the stress experienced by relatives.

Implications for practice

- trends are more important than isolated observations
- nearly all units receive patients with head injuries, and so need some means to assess and monitor neurological status
- where specialised neurological monitoring is unavailable, intracranial pressure can be assessed using
    - Glasgow Coma Scale (with pupil responses)
    - spinal reflexes
    - blood tests (glucose, electrolytes, gases)
    - mean arterial pressure
- the Glasgow Coma Scale is familiar, but can necessitate infliction of pain; significant discrepancies can occur between different observers
- when raised ICP is suspected, care should be planned to minimise irritation (e.g. endotracheal suction, quiet environment)
- invasive methods increase risks of infection, especially meningitis
- NIROS holds future promise as noninvasive technology, but needs further development at present
- SjO_2 monitoring is potentially undervalued
- ICP should be 0–10 mmHg, but transient rises above this level are insignificant
- ICP waveforms are of limited use

- CPP offers more comprehensive indications of cerebral function than ICP alone
- continuous display is valuable for evaluating effects of all aspects of care
- patient care should be viewed holistically, so observations should be related to their overall effect

Summary

Intracranial hypertension can occur in many ICU patients; monitoring neurological status (outside neurological ICUs) often relies on the Glasgow Coma Scale, which assesses level of consciousness rather than cerebral perfusion. More invasive methods of assessment inevitably incur greater risks, but may provide more useful information to guide treatment. As with monitoring any aspect of patient care, benefits and burdens of each approach should be individualised to the patient, and justified by the extent to which they usefully guide treatments and the care given.

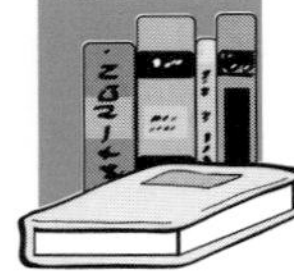

Further reading

Menon (1997) offers a useful overview of neurological monitoring, while Odell (1996) offers a comprehensive nursing perspective. Watson *et al.* (1992) and Shah (1999) review the Glasgow Coma Scale; Ellis and Cavanagh's (1992) critique of its reliability raises many valid concerns, although it should be read critically. Feldman and Robertson (1997) describe jugular venous oxygen saturation monitoring. Germon *et al.* (1994) have been influential in developing near infrared spectroscopy. North and Reilly (1994) offer a reasonable overview of intracranial pressure and monitoring, which can be usefully supplemented by Hickman *et al.* (1990). Nurses should consider the effects of their activities on intracranial pressure; Rising (1993) and Price (1998) give useful overviews of potential problems.

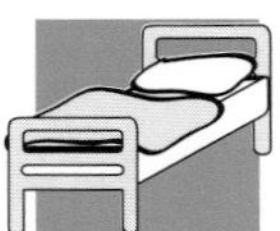

Clinical scenario

Mark Rhodes, a previously fit and healthy 20-year-old full-time student, who plays rugby for his university was admitted to ICU unconscious. At a party following a successful rugby game, Mark fell out of a second-floor window and sustained a head injury with fractured right elbow and pelvis. A head CT scan revealed diffuse cerebral oedema with no signs of haematoma. Mark's fractures were stabilised and intracranial pressure monitoring was initiated. He was invasively ventilated, sedated with midazolam and fentanyl infusions with pancuronium administered to promote muscle relaxation.

Mark's initial results include:

Glasgow Coma Scale (GCS)	4
Intracranial Pressure (ICP)	20 mmHg
BP	90/60 mmHg (mean BP 70 mmHg)
HR	115 bpm
CVP	2 mmHg
Central temperature	38.8°C
Blood sugar	16.5 mmols/l

Q.1 Explain why the GCS is used in Mark's neurological assessment. What does his score represent? How is its accuracy ensured? How often should it be performed, and by whom? Specify the most appropriate type and location of painful stimuli for Mark.

Q.2 Calculate Mark's Cerebral Perfusion Pressure (CPP = MAP − ICP) and explore its physiological implications (i.e. to cerebral perfusion and autoregulation; effect on other body systems, especially those controlled by the autonomic nervous system). What is the likely cause and significance of his temperature and blood sugar results?

Q.3 The aim of care in first 24 hours is to keep Mark's CPP > 70 mmHg by increasing MAP and reducing ICP. Formulate a holistic nursing care plan which incorporates:

(a) medically prescribed treatments, as well as
(b) specific nursing strategies aimed at restoring ICP and CPP to normal range and minimising secondary brain damage
(c) care related to invasive ICP monitoring.

Part III

Pathophysiology and treatments

This section includes some of the more common pathologies and treatments seen in general ICUs, together with some specialist aspects to encourage further development.

Since most pathophysiological processes originate at cellular level, Chapter 23 gives an overview of cellular pathology. Multiple, often interacting, pathology creates complex links between the pathologies and treatments discussed in this section, but chapters are then grouped largely by systems and treatments, starting with those more obviously related to cellular pathology: myocardial infarction, shock, multiorgan dysfunction syndrome and acute respiratory distress syndrome. These chapters do include some discussion of treatments, but further treatments are discussed in the next group of chapters: nitric oxide, alternative modes of ventilation and cardiac surgery.

Two frequent complications of critical illness are discussed next: disseminated intravascular coagulation and acute renal failure. Further treatments are then discussed: fluid management, (positive) inotropes and haemofiltration.

Chapters 36–39 discuss pathologies of other systems: gastrointestinal bleeds focuses on oesophageal varices and gastric ulcers; pancreatitis can necessitate urgent ICU admission; Guillain–Barre syndrome, critical illness neuropathy and autonomic dysreflexia are discussed in the chapter on neurological pathologies; most ICU patients suffer a degree of liver failure, even if it is seldom the primary diagnosis. Chapter 40 then discusses immunodeficiency, with particular reference to HIV and AIDS.

The final chapters in this section explore other problems that cause ICU admission, including a chapter on ecstasy overdoses illustrating the problems caused by amphetamines. Obstetric (usually post-natal) admissions are discussed in Chapter 42. Issues surrounding transplantation (donors and recipients) are discussed in Chapter 43; care of patients following graft surgery is covered in the chapter on hepatic transplants.

The complex interaction between systems necessitates holistic care, and so cross-references are given to other chapters; the reductionist presentation of each chapter is designed to assist easy reference by readers wishing to find out more about each pathophysiological process.

Chapter 23

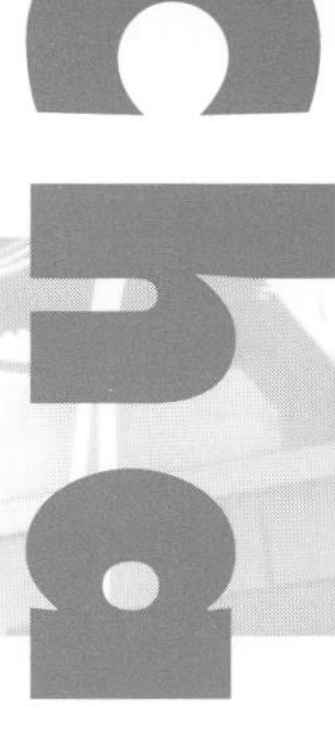

Cellular pathology

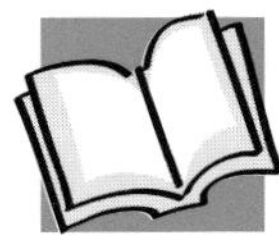

Contents

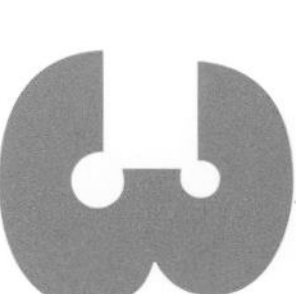

Introduction

Focus on visible macrophysiology (systems and organs) has increasingly been replaced by recognition that disease processes originate primarily at microphysiological levels; organ/system failure is more a symptom of widespread cell failure. This chapter therefore outlines pathological mechanisms underlying most critical illnesses; hence its placement before discussion on more familiar macrodisease processes. Cellular pathology, although significant in all critical illnesses, is inextricably linked to systemic inflammatory response syndrome (SIRS, see Chapter 25) and multiorgan dysfunction syndrome (MODS, see Chapter 26).

Recent growth in the understanding of microphysiological and microbiological processes necessitates selection of key aspects. Much remains to be discovered, clarified or proven; knowledge growth can rapidly outdate material covered in even relatively recent courses and texts. This chapter therefore begins with a brief revision of cell physiology; if unfamiliar, this should be supplemented from anatomy texts. The importance of cellular pathology in most diseases is reflected in the many references to this chapter in later ones; readers may find sections in this chapter useful as reference points for later use.

Cell membrane

Cell membranes (see Figure 23.1) are about 7–8 nm thick (Marieb 1995), constructed primarily from phospholipid, interspersed with cholesterol (which stabilises lipid membrane), glycolipid, protein and glycoprotein (Nowak & Handford 1996). Structural changes of these components allow selective movement of substances (e.g. electrolytes) across semipermeable membranes (Nowak & Handford 1996).

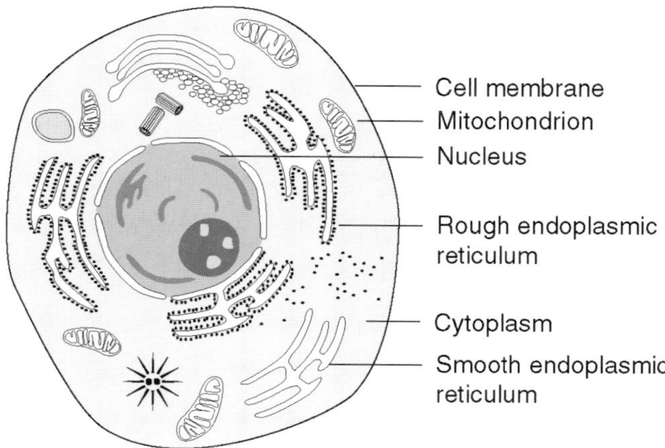

Figure 23.1 The main components of a typical human cell

Intracellular sodium and potassium concentrations (K^+ = *c*. 140 mmol/l; Na^+ = *c*. 4 mmol/l, reversing extracellular fluid concentrations) are maintained by the *sodium–potassium pump* in cell membranes. The movement of electrolytes across the membrane creates the *action potential* (see Chapter 21) needed for muscle movement: potassium leak during the resting phase of action potential creates a negative intracellular charge (−20 to −200 millivolts), causing influx of positively charged ions.

Water diffuses passively (from sodium's osmotic pull). Cell membrane damage allows potassium efflux, causing potential hyperkalaemia. Other active pumps (e.g. chloride, glucose) in cell membranes similarly prevent loss of intracellular chemicals.

Sugar (for cellular energy production) influx is facilitated by insulin, hence hyperglycaemia, but lack of energy when insulin production or function is impaired.

Cell membranes, therefore, maintain intracellular homeostasis; damage to the cell membrane disrupts cell function, with extensive damage resulting in organ dysfunction.

Mitochondria

Mitochondria:

- generate energy (mainly from glucose, via Kreb's cycle), stored as adenosine triphosphate (ATP)
- control cytoplasm calcium levels.

Glycolysis converts glucose into two pyruvic acid molecules, releasing four ATP (energy) molecules. The pyruvic acid molecules then enter the mitochondria, where normally further reactions with oxygen would form further ATP molecules (hence glucose being a very efficient source of energy). However, with anaerobic metabolism most intracellular pyruvic acid is converted to lactic acid, which then diffuses out of cells creating metabolic acidosis.

In aerobic conditions each gram of glucose produces 38 ATP molecules, but in anaerobic conditions only two ATP molecules are produced (Hinwood 1993); anaerobic metabolism also produces 2 mmol of lactic acid from every 1 mmol of glucose (Nunn 1996). Thus metabolism during hypoperfusion (shock, pressure sores) is inefficient, causing accumulation of toxic waste (acids and carbon dioxide) which enter capillary circulation causing metabolic acidosis.

Cell damage

Nowak and Handford (1996) identify three mechanisms for cell damage:

- deficiency (e.g. hypoperfusion, diabetic ketoacidosis)

- intoxication (e.g. viruses, bacteria, drugs/chemicals, toxic metabolites/free radicals)
- trauma (e.g. hypothermia, hyperthermia, radiation)

One mechanism often triggers another, causing cumulative cell injury. Hypoxic cells (especially endothelial) release various cytotoxic and vasoactive mediators (histamine, serotonin, kinins). Progressive equilibrium between intracellular and extracellular ions impairs action potential generation. The accumulation of intracellular fatty deposits accelerates cell damage and rupture, with the kidneys, heart and liver being especially susceptible (e.g. fatty liver).

Lysosome (released from damaged cytoplasm; NB not lysozyme) and cell debris trigger various autodestructive mechanisms:

- myocardial depression
- coronary vasoconstriction
- conversion of inactive kinins to (vasodilatory) bradykinin
- activate coagulation mechanisms (provoking DIC)

Lysosome is most effective in acidotic environments (especially pH 5.0 (Marieb 1995)), so that profound acidosis from critical illness and ischaemic tissue favours lysosomal autodestruction.

Tissue tolerance to hypoxia varies; central nervous system neurons have high metabolic rates, relying on glucose for energy and can only tolerate a few minutes of ischaemia (hence cardiopulmonary resuscitation times); renal and hepatic cells can tolerate an hour's ischaemia at normal body temperature (enabling safe isolation for most surgical procedures); hypothermia reduces metabolic rate, and so extends ischaemic toleration time (hence use of hypothermia for cardiac surgery).

Microcirculation

Most critical pathologies are fuelled by hypoperfusion from microcirculatory collapse (see Chapter 25). Vasoactive mediators (part of normal homeostasis) relax smooth muscle in arterioles, but venules remain constricted; the resulting pressure gradient forces plasma into interstitial spaces (oedema). Resulting haemoconcentration increases blood viscosity, which further reduces perfusion (see Chapter 18) and encourages thrombi formation.

Mediators are middle-sized molecules (20–30 kDa), small enough to extravase through leaky membranes:

- **cytokines** released by leucocytes (TNFα, interleukins)
- histamine
- arachidonic acid metabolites (**leukotrienes**, prostaglandins, thromboxane A, **eicosanoids**)
- endorphins

- nitric oxide
- complement cascade

Most mediators remain active for only a few microseconds, and so plasma concentrations may show only peripheral overspill (Williamson & Spencer 1997), and measuring early levels does not indicate the likely severity of an illness (Donnelly *et al.* 1994). Although a brief overview is given below, most have similar interdependent effects (proinflammatory, procoagulopathic and cytotoxic) causing progressive multiorgan dysfunction.

Neutrophil activation provokes oxygen-derived free radicals and protease production; oxygen radicals are discussed in Chapter 18.

Cytokines

Cytokines are chemical mediators of immunity which enhance inflammatory responses.

Tumour necrosis factor alpha (TNFα, also called cachectin) is released by activated macrophages in response to gram negative organisms. The first mediator to peak (Abbas *et al.* 1994), it initiates the cytokine cascade of SIRS and MODS (Tracey & Cerami 1993). TNFα stimulates growth of new surface receptors (adhesion molecules) on vascular endothelial cells, enabling leucocyte adhesion, accumulation and phagocytosis (Abbas *et al.* 1994), but causing intravascular thrombosis, occlusion and impaired perfusion (Barnett & Cosslett 1998) (accelerating leucopenia, thrombocytopenia and DIC). TNFα is a negative inotrope (Wardle 1997). Circulating levels and production of TNFα is reduced by chlorpromazine (Jansen *et al.* 1998).

Interleukins are a diverse group of chemicals, with various effects. They appear to cause various autoimmune disorders: meningitis, systemic lupus erythematosus, malaria, rheumatoid arthritis, Crohn's disease, cystic fibrosis, asthma, multiple sclerosis, atheroma, Alzheimer's (Grimble 1994). Interleukins 1, 6 and 8 are major mediators of critical illnesses.

Interleukin 1 (IL-1), released following TNFα activation, is a major mediator of inflammation, activating T-lymphocytes, endothelial cells and macrophages. It also induces

- fever
- sleep
- ACTH release
- **chemotaxis**
- leucocytosis (causing bone marrow depression)

IL-1 alone does not cause tissue damage, but accelerates TNFα-initiated damage. Interleukin 1 triggers the release of other mediators (e.g. prostaglandins, thromboxane A_2) and leukotriene formation (Wardle 1997).

Interleukin 6 (IL-6, also called β_2-interferon) follows TNFα and interleukin 1 production; it is antiviral, stimulating hepatocyte synthesis of plasma proteins (e.g. fibrinogen) to acute phase proteins (Abbas *et al.* 1994). It is also anti-inflammatory, inhibiting TNFα and other proinflammatory mediators (Wheeler & Bernard 1999).

Interleukin 8 levels are significantly raised during sepsis, but are low in cases of MODS where no infection is identified (Marty *et al.* 1994). Neutrophil lung injury is primarily mediated through interleukin 8 (Marty *et al.* 1994).

Platelet activating factor

In the early stages of shock, platelets release this mediator which

- increases vascular permeability
- increases smooth muscle contraction (arteriolarconstriction)
- activates neutrophils
- activates platelet surface adherence (accelerating hypercoaguable states)

Myocardial depressant factor

Released by the pancreas and spleen following lysosomal damage to cell proteins (e.g. pancreatitis, multiorgan pathologies such as SIRS and MODS), myocardial depressant factor is negatively inotropic.

Acute phase proteins

Infection initiates the early release of proteins, including *fibrinogen*, *alpha-1 protinase inhibitor*, *C-reactive protein* and *serum amyloid associated protein* (Nowak & Handford 1996) to assist phagocytosis.

Prostaglandins

These are potent vasoactive substances; **prostacyclin** (PGI_2 or epoprostenol), prostaglandins E_1 (PGE_1) and prostaglandins E_2 (PGE_2) cause vasodilation, further reducing systemic vascular resistance and aggravating coagulopathies (prostacyclin is used exogenously for anticoagulation). Prostaglandin E_1 is used therapeutically to reduce platelet adhesion and decrease systemic vascular resistance, so improving tissue perfusion (Appel *et al.* 1991).

Complement

Activated by endotoxaemia, the complement combination (C5b, 6, 7, 8, 9) forms a Membrane Attack Complex, part of antigen–antibody reactions to foreign proteins (especially gram negative bacteria). It also encourages migration to and activation of leucocytes in infected tissue. With systemic pathologies, such as shock, increased vascular permeability (C5), inappropriate neutrophil activation and gross fluid shifts complicate, rather than resolve, progression.

Endorphins

Endorphins (e.g. enkephalin, β-endorphin, dinorphin) are endogenous neural opiates which, like exogenous opiates, cause central nervous system depression.

Radicals

Any biochemical reaction can release *free radicals* (e.g. microorganism lysis by neutrophils, Krebs cycle). Free radicals are molecules with one or more unpaired electrons in their outer orbit, which makes them inherently unstable, reacting readily with other molecules to pair the free electron. The reaction of two **radicals** eliminates both, but reactions between radicals and non-radicals produces a further radical. Reactivity is indiscriminate, so that although their lifespan lasts only microseconds, chain reactions may be thousands of events long (Davidson & Boom 1995) causing the autocatalysis underlying most critical illnesses.

Oxygen radicals are particularly destructive, with oxidation modifying proteins (Hipkiss 1989), including cell membrane phospholipid. Free oxygen radicals are released with hyperoxia (Davidson & Boom 1995), so that prolonged high FiO_2 (above 0.5–0.6, see Chapter 18) accelerates oxidation.

Vitamin E (the main intracellular chain-*breaking* antioxidant (Davidson & Boom 1995)) can reduce mortality from ARDS (Deby *et al.* 1995). Other antioxidants include

- vitamin C
- intracellular glutathione (Davidson & Boom 1995)
- cytosolic superoxide dismutase (SOD) (which includes zinc) and other enzymes.

Hypoxic vascular epithelium releases endogenous *nitric oxide* (see Chapter 28); widespread tissue hypoxia (shock) therefore causes widespread nitric oxide release and systemic vasodilation.

Cells surviving initial injury exist in grossly disordered internal environments; anaerobic metabolism causes peripheral accumulation of metabolic acids, free radicals, oxidative enzymes (e.g. xanthine oxidase), and other toxic chemicals. *Reperfusion injury* can result from toxic products being flushed into the central cardiovascular system during recovery, potentially causing secondary (reperfusion) damage.

Calcification

Necrosis leads to microscopic calcium deposits; accumulation through persistent injury causes progressive tissue damage and rigidity, especially in renal, pulmonary, cardiovascular and gastric cells (Nowak & Handford 1996).

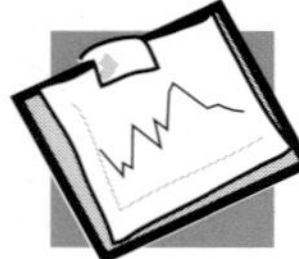

Implications for practice

- most critical pathologies originate at microcellular rather than macrosystem level; understanding these processes enables nurses to understand the pathologies and treatments covered in many of the other chapters (e.g. pressure sores, oxygen toxicity, fluid and electrolyte balance)
- microcirculatory resuscitation requires
  - perfusion
  - nutrition
  - ventilation
- high FiO_2 (above 0.5–0.6) is potentially toxic, and so should not be used for more than a few hours
- reperfusion injury can cause secondary damage, so that recovery requires close observation of effects (e.g. dysrhythmias) and prompt intervention

Summary

Most critical illnesses originate and progress at cellular level; macroscopic symptoms are accumulations of microscopic problems. Treatments should therefore focus on underlying mechanisms of disease rather than more easily observed effects. Understanding these microscopic mechanisms enables nurses to monitor and assess effects of treatments.

Abnormal figures (e.g. disordered arterial blood gases) may be tolerated to assist cell recovery (e.g. permissive hypercapnia: see Chapter 27).

This chapter has outlined the main mechanisms of cell dysfunction as a basis for understanding pathophysiologies described in the remainder of this section.

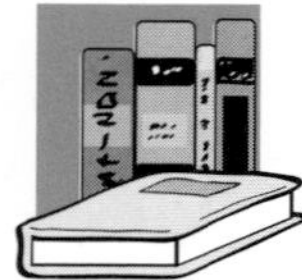

Further reading

Revision of normal cell physiology from a recent and appropriate anatomy text, such as Marieb (1995) or Guyton and Hall (1997), can provide a useful basis for understanding pathophysiology; Abbas *et al.* (1994) provide a more detailed account of pathophysiology. Mechanisms of key pathological processes can be complex, but some recent specialist articles usefully describe aspects such as free radicals (Davidson & Boom 1995) and treatments (Wardle 1997).

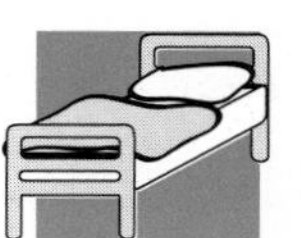

Clinical scenario

Robert Green, an 18-year-old with a history of poorly controlled asthma, is admitted to ICU following a respiratory arrest. On endotracheal suction his sputum is thick mucopurulant and arterial blood gases indicate hypoxia, hypercapnia and severe respiratory acidosis.

His blood results include abnormalities in differential white blood cell count:

WBC 13.3 × 10^{-9}/l
Platelets 177 × 10^{-9}/l
Neutrophils 11.7 × 10^{-9}/l
Eosinophils 0.8 × 10^{-9}/l
Basinophils 0.6 × 10^{-9}/l
Monocytes 0.7 × 10^{-9}/l
Lymphocytes 0.5 × 10^{-9}/l

Q.1 Draw and label a diagram of the typical eucaryotic cell. Include structures (and make brief notes on their functions) such as nucleus, cytoplasm, cytoskeleton, microtubules, endoplasmic reticulum, Golgi complex, ribosomes, mitochondria, lysosmomes, cell surface (or surface membrane) with its various structures and components (e.g. desmosomes, tight junctions, gap junctions, antibody response and hormone binding sites).

Q.2 Analyse Robert's WBC differential result; does it indicate inflammatory response or infection? (For example, consider functions of each cell type, cells which increase in response to bacteria, have digestive function and/or respond to allergens or toxins.)

Q.3 Robert develops systemic hypotension and pulmonary oedema. Review the cellular processes which caused this from his acute asthmatic attack (e.g. effect of hypoxia and hypercarbia on cellular function, cellular ATP production, cell membrane potential, mediators triggered, function and systemic effects of these mediators, causes of capillary permeability, role of basinophils, implications of associated histamine release).

Normal reference ranges:

WBC 4–11 × 10^{-9}/l
Platelets 150–400 × 10^{-9}/l
Neutrophils 1.5–7 × 10^{-9}/l
Eosinophils 0.04–0.4 × 10^{-9}/l
Basinophils 0.0–0.1 × 10^{-9}/l
Monocytes 0.2–1.0 × 10^{-9}/l
Lymphocytes 1.5–4 × 10^{-9}/l

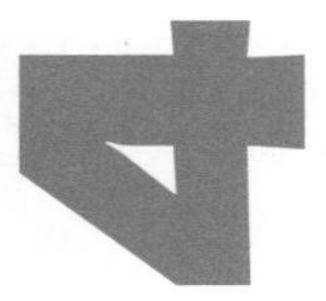

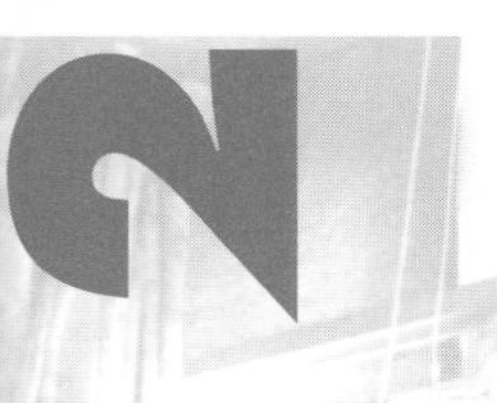

Chapter 24

Acute myocardial infarction

Contents

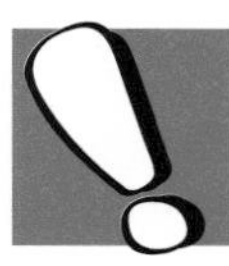

Fundamental knowledge

Coronary arteries: structure and location
Coagulation cascade and thromboxane A_2
Renin–angiotensin mechanism

Introduction

Myocardial infarction (MI) remains the leading cause of death in Western industrialised societies, despite decreases in prehospital and in-hospital mortality. In the UK, 300,000 MIs occur each year (Adam and Osborne 1997), causing over 500 deaths each day (Francome & Marks 1996), 25–30 per cent of all deaths (Adam & Osborne 1997). Despite *Health of the Nation* targets (DoH 1992), UK mortality rates from coronary heart disease remain among the highest in the world (Tunstall-Pedroe *et al.* 1994).

Cardiac disease may persist for years; when myocardial oxygen supply becomes inadequate, the myocardium infarcts. Symptoms (e.g. angina) are rapid (often less than 30 minutes before infarction), and survivors often suffer residual cardiac disease.

Patients with uncomplicated MIs are usually best cared for in specialist coronary care units (CCUs), away from the intense stressors of ICUs, but any ICU patient may suffer MI and not all hospitals have CCU facilities; where other pathologies complicate cardiac disease, ICU admission may be needed.

Rapid development of symptoms and relative speed of recovery make health promotion more readily achievable with patients and their families following MI than many other ICU patients. This chapter identifies the underlying pathophysiology and treatments (especially thrombolysis).

Myocardial oxygen supply

Five per cent of cardiac output enters the two coronary arteries (*right* and *left*) from the aorta. The left artery divides into the *left anterior descending* and *circumflex* (see Figure 24.1). At rest, myocardium normally extracts 70–80 per cent of available oxygen (Ganong 1995). Having more mitochondria than skeletal muscle, the myocardium relies on aerobic respiration (Clancy & McVicar 1995). This leaves little leeway for oxygen debt.

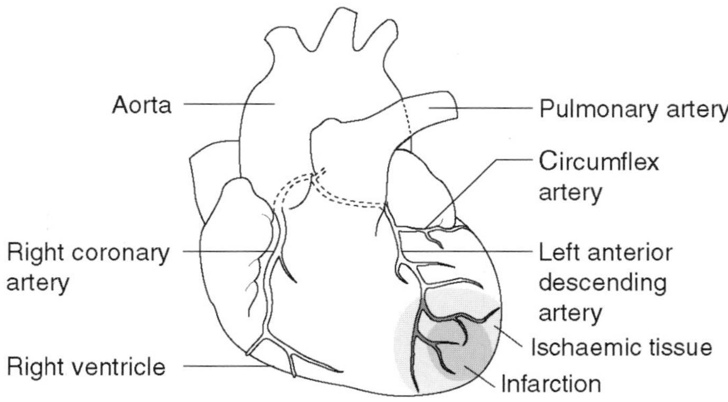

Figure 24.1 Coronary arteries, with inferior myocardial infarction

When myocardial oxygen demand exceeds supply, ischaemia results. Ischaemia is transient; if reversed (reducing oxygen demand, increasing oxygen supply, or both), the myocardium recovers; unreversed ischaemia will progress to infarction.

Coronary artery disease begins in childhood and is well advanced in many by the age of 30 (Herbert 1991); symptoms usually only occur when coronary arteries are three-quarters occluded (Carleton & Boldt 1992). This leaves little physiological reserve between the onset of symptoms and ischaemic tissue death. Forty-three per cent of people with coronary artery disease do not suffer angina.

About one-half of acute myocardial infarctions are due to occlusion of the left anterior descending artery, with a significant minority caused by right coronary artery perfusion, circumflex artery occlusion being a far less frequent cause of infarctions (Rowlands 1996a).

Atherosclerosis

Most MIs in Western societies are caused by atherosclerosis (Osguthorpe 1995). The *tunica intima* becomes penetrable to lipids, especially cholesterol and low density lipoproteins, altering the integrity of vasculature (Todd 1997); as fats, fibrin, cholesterol and calcium are deposited (Wilson 1983), lipids are covered by fibrous caps of tissue from proliferating cells in the *intima* (Todd 1997) which enables platelet adhesion to prominences in arterial walls (Wilson 1983). Nitric oxide, an endogenous vasodilator that enables coronary arteries to meet increased demand, is only released from intact endothelium (Todd 1997). Thus atheroma both occludes flow and causes failure of vasodilatory mechanisms.

MIs usually occur when three-quarters of the lumen is obstructed (Ganong 1995), but fissuring of atheromatous plaques can precipitate sudden crises. When obstruction causes ischaemia but is not extreme enough to provoke infarction, ischaemic myocardium, like other muscle, experiences cramp (angina). The severe pain of angina is both a warning of impending infarction and a sympathetic agonist. As sympathetic stimulation causes coronary vasoconstriction, pain accentuates ischaemia. Therefore prompt and sufficient analgesia is both a humanitarian and physiological necessity.

Weston (1996) suggests myocyte death depends upon work load (oxygen demand), prior episodes of ischaemia and collateral flow.

Collateral circulation

Like most body systems, the cardiovascular system is dynamic, changing to meet physiological needs. With progressive obliteration of flow, arteries can develop collateral circulation to bypass obstructions. Collateral vessels are small, weak and tortuous, offering temporary relief rather than permanent solutions, although they may limit infarct size.

Oestrogen production during reproductive years protects women from atherosclerosis, making men under 55 up to four times more likely to suffer from coronary artery disease than women (Lessig & Lessig 1998). Thus, although overall MI mortality rates are similar for men and women, women sufferers are usually older, with a higher incidence of known congestive heart failure and hypertension (Herlitz *et al.* 1997). However, the earlier development of coronary artery disease in men also means earlier development of collateral circulation; the sudden reduction in oestrogen levels during and following menopause exposes women to rapid atherosclerosis (Sloane *et al.* 1981; Walling *et al.* 1988) without the reserve from significant collateral circulation, making mortality-to-survival ratios higher among older women than among men of the same age.

Pathology

Up to one-quarter of MIs are asymptomatic (silent) (Thompson & Webster 1992). Before the ischaemic muscle dies, contraction ceases, prolonging the interval before irreversible damage (Ganong 1995); this interval provides an important window for treatment, especially for thrombolysis.

Left ventricle pressure far exceeds pressure in the other chambers; left ventricular ischaemia occurs if aortic pressure is lower than left ventricular pressure, making inferior MIs most likely.

Reperfusion of any ischaemic tissue releases vasoactive substances, many prolonging pathological processes (see Chapter 23). The uncontrolled release of oxygen free radicals and cytokines causes myocardial stunning (deBono 1992; Grech *et al.* 1995). Recovery of any injured tissue can be complicated by reperfusion injury; fortunately cardiac function is normally monitored so thoroughly that the early detection and resolution of problems is more likely than with most tissues.

Alcohol

Recent media publicity about positive cardiac benefits from alcohol have encouraged public misconceptions, providing excuses for further alcohol abuse. Current evidence is inconclusive, but it suggests that mild drinking (1–6 drinks each week) may reduce mortality (Francome & Marks 1996) – revastoral (in red wine) or salicylic acid (the main ingredient of aspirin) may be the effective agents (Francome & Marks 1996). Alcohol consumption may be under-reported, so that nurses can usefully provide patients and families with information to discourage excessive consumption.

Circadian rhythm

Most MIs occur between 6 a.m. and 10 a.m. (Todd 1997), plaque fissuring and thrombosis being provoked by

- vasoconstriction and tachycardia from increased endogenous catecholamine release following the early morning ebb
- sheering stress on coronary stenoses from vasoconstriction
- increased platelet stickiness in early morning
- increased blood viscosity (Todd 1997)

Although Todd (1997) suggests that getting up late only delays this physiological cascade of problems, vigorous early morning stimulation (e.g. 6 a.m. bed baths) is best avoided with all ICU patients.

Cardiac enzymes

Injured cells release enzymes. Identifying and measuring levels of enzymes enables diagnosis of which cells are damaged. The most useful cardiac enzymes are creatine kinase (CK) – formerly called creatine phosphokinase (CPK) – and lactate dehydrogenase (LDH), the myocardium containing higher concentrations than other organs (Ganong 1995). However, falsely positive results occur in 15 per cent of tests.

CREATINE KINASE This is the first cardiac enzyme to rise, levels peaking in about 24 hours, but returning to normal (under 130 IU/l) within 2–4 days. It is also released from the brain and skeletal muscle, and so serum levels are raised by intramuscular injections, surgery and any other bleeding/bruising (Wilson 1983). The release of creatine kinase by other muscles can lead to false diagnosis.

There are three isoenzymes which can be used to differentiate the origin of the enzyme (Adam & Osborne 1997): MM (skeletal muscle), MB (heart), BB (brain). CK-MB concentrates of more than 5 per cent of total CK indicate myocardial necrosis (Lessig & Lessig 1998). However, small quantities of CK-MB are found elsewhere (such as the diaphragm and small intestines) (Hockings & Donovan 1997). Two subforms of CK-MB have been identified: CK-MB_1 found in plasma, and CK-MB_2 in tissues (Hudak *et al.* 1998).

ASPARTATE AMINOTRANSFERASE (AST) Formally called serum glutamic oxaloacetic transaminase – SGOT), this is now rarely used. It rises within 8–12 hours, peaks in 18–36 hours, and returns to normal (5–30 IU/l) within 3–4 days (Thompson & Webster 1997). It is also released by renal, cerebral and hepatic damage (Wilson 1983). There are no cardiac-specific isoenzymes (Thompson & Webster 1997).

LACTATE DEHYDROGENASE (LDH) This peaks between 48 and 72 hours (Nowak & Handford 1994) and remains elevated for 5–14 days (Wilson 1983). It is also found with other tissue and erythrocyte damage (e.g. haemolysed samples) (Wilson 1983). There are five isoenzymes: LDH^1 is primarily cardiac, so that levels over 40 per cent and an increase in LDH^1:LDH^2 ratio indicates myocardial infarction (Thompson & Webster 1997).

TROPONIN T This is undetectable unless myocardial infarction has occurred (Banerjee *et al.* 1997), but can be detected within 4–6 hours of infarction (Albarran 1998), peaking in 10–24 hours, and can remain elevated for several weeks (Hudak *et al.* 1998).

Angiography

Angiography can confirm a diagnosis of coronary thrombi, and can be used to dilate coronary vessels (see Chapter 30), which may increasingly replace traditional surgical approaches of coronary artery bypass grafting (see Chapter 30).

Treatments

Analgesia

MIs cause severe 'crushing' pain, and so strong analgesia is needed; morphine has proved effective over many years. Angina may also be caused by coronary artery spasm, and so nitrates can usefully dilate coronary arteries and reduce preload.

Although a link between myocardial infarction and severe pain have long been established, O'Connor's (1995) pilot study found that nurses underestimate pain in 23–46 per cent of cases, while Gaston-Johansson *et al.* (1991) found that less than one-half of the patients in their study received morphine. They also found that men received less morphine than women.

Pain also has a high emotional component (Gaston-Johansson *et al.* 1991) so that anxiety will complicate the physiological causes of pain. Popular connotations of the heart make many patients fear cardiac disease more than disease of any other organ.

Drugs

Other drugs often used following MI include aspirin, β-blockers, ACE inhibitors, amiodarone, magnesium, calcium antagonists, lipid-lowering drugs, heparin and thrombolytics.

ASPIRIN Doses of less than 100 mg inhibit thromboxane A2, so preventing platelet aggregation; larger doses block the enzyme cyclo-oxygenase, which inhibits prostacyclin (Galvani *et al.* 1996). Giving aspirin with streptokinase can give a 3.7–1.8 per cent reduction in reinfarction (ISIS-2 1988). Unfortunately the optimum dose is unclear; deBono (1990) and McDonald (1997) suggest 150 mg; ISIS-2 recommended 160 mg, but this strength is not routinely available in the UK; Galvani *et al.* (1996) recommend 160–325 mg; Todd (1997) suggests that one 300-mg tablet can have an effect lasting 4–7 days. Some patients, who have been told to take one aspirin tablet a day and do not recognise the difference between tablet strengths, take one 300-mg tablet each day. Like colleagues elsewhere, ICU nurses should ensure that patients and significant others understand the prescribed dose.

Aspirin (and other platelet inhibitors) may offer most cardiac protection when taken in the evening, ensuring maximum effectiveness when platelets are stickiest.

NITRATES These (e.g. isosorbide mono-/di- nitrate, glyceryl trintrate) relieve angina. Isosorbide dinitrate can be given sublingually, enabling ready access and quick absorption.

ACE INHIBITORS These inhibit angiotensin converting enzyme (ACE), the hypertensive agonist released by renin. Inhibiting this enzyme therefore prevents hypertension. Angiotensin converting enzyme is a group of substances rather than a single enzyme, and so hypertension may persist despite ACE inhibitors (Kaufman 1997). Since ACE inhibitors may provoke hypoglycaemia (Herings *et al.* 1995), blood sugars should be checked.

MAGNESIUM Once fairly widely used following myocardial infarction, magnesium has largely been abandoned since ISIS-4 found it non-beneficial (ISIS-4 1995). It is still used for reperfusion dysrhythmias.

HEPARIN This is sometimes given with thrombolytics, but ISIS-3 (1992) showed no significant difference between streptokinase, APSAC, TPA, or their use with or without heparin, so that the use of heparin remains controversial (Galvani *et al.* 1996). Heparin increases the risk of CVAs (Weston 1996). It may be given long term to reduce reocclusion (Weston 1996), and Hockings and Donovan (1997) recommended heparin for 6–12 hours following thrombolysis.

A recent revival of interest in hirudin (leech extract), a thrombin inhibitor which, unlike heparin, is not neutralised by activated platelets, has proved disappointing; one trial was stopped due to adverse outcomes (Galvani *et al.* 1996).

Thrombolysis

Thrombolytics are best given within six hours (and preferably earlier) following infarction, although later use (e.g. 12 hours) still reduces mortality (LATE Study Group 1993). Nearly one-third of patients receiving thrombolytics suffer reocclusion within three months (Weston 1996).

STRETOPKINASE The cheapest thrombolytic drug, this is widely used in the UK. It activates plasminogen into plasmin (Ganong 1995), causing lysis for 12–24 hours. It is usually given with aspirin but not heparin (Weston 1996), which would increase risk of CVAs.

Being a streptococcal product, it can cause anaphylaxis; this is rare with first doses as antibodies develop after 4 days, but subsequent doses may be problematic, and so repeat doses should be avoided after 4 days (Kynman 1997). Due to possible anaphylaxis, patients should be given information sheets informing them (and other healthcare workers) when second doses may be safely given. Unfortunately, repeat times are disputed:

- Thompson (1990): avoid second doses between one week and 6 months;
- McDonald (1997): a one-year interval between doses;
- Hockings and Donovan (1997) cite 1996 Task Force of the European Society of Cardiology: two years;
- Kynman (1997): antibodies may survive for between 4 and 54 months; re-administration may prove ineffective and cause a fatal delay in giving other drugs that might be more effective. Therefore Kynman argues that second doses of streptokinase should never be given.

Hospitals may have local policies or guidelines for when/if repeat streptokinase may be given (often five years), but nurses should also be guided by evidence-based practice.

Anaphylaxis may occur with any second dose, so that hydrocortisone, antihistamines and adrenaline should be readily available whenever streptokinase is given. The antidote for streptokinase is tranexamic acid.

Previously called tissue plasminogen activator (t-PA) or recombinant tissue plasminogen activator (rt-PA), *alteplase* is an endogenous vascular epithelium enzyme which activates plasminogen bound to fibrin; this should limit systemic effects (Ganong 1995), but bleeding complications are similar to streptokinase (Hockings & Donovan 1997).

Reperfusion initially is more rapid than streptokinase (62 per cent at 90 minutes, compared with 31 per cent for streptokinase), but by 24 hours reperfusion rates are comparable (Weston 1996). Quicker reperfusion should salvage more myocardium, but this is unsupported by trials (Weston 1996). Its short half-life enables cannulation within half-an-hour after administration (Thompson 1990). As it is genetically engineered, alteplase is much more expensive than streptokinase, and this limits its use. Practice with thrombolytics varies. The GUSTO (1993) trial identified greater reductions in mortality with alteplase than streptokinase (both given with heparin). Weston (1996) suggests that alteplase is primarily used for younger patients within 4 hours of anterior MIs. Alteplase may be used if repeat doses of streptokinase are contraindicated (Weston 1996; McDonald 1997), such as following heparin.

Anisolylated plasminogen streptokinase activator complex (APSAC) is refined streptokinase, requiring only a single bolus dose (Thompson 1990). It does provide more sustained thrombolytic effects (Why 1994), but other than being a single bolus dose, offers no advantages over streptokinase and is more expensive (Hockings & Donovan 1997), and so is not in standard use in the UK (Weston 1996).

UROKINASE This is similar to streptokinase (Hockings & Donovan 1997) and is more costly, so little used (Why 1994) except for ocular thrombolysis and arteriovenous shunts (BNF 1998).

Although thrombolysis has reduced complications during recovery, *following thrombolysis* nurses should observe for:

- allergic reaction/hypotension
- haemorrhage

Revascularisation dysrhythmias (especially ventricular) are common but usually benign, one-half of all patients experiencing a degree of left ventricular failure (Thompson 1990); reperfusion injury may progress to ventricular fibrillation, and 5 per cent of patients develop cardiogenic shock (Thompson 1990.). The risk of major haemorrhage following thrombolysis is small (less than 5 per cent), but triples if patients have had previous vascular/cardiac procedures (deBono 1990), and so intramuscular injections should be avoided with all patients.

Rest

Rest, with bedrest for 48 hours (Hockings & Donovan 1997), promotes recovery. Rest and adequate sleep (quality as well as quantity) promote physical and psychological healing (see Chapter 3): planned care should include minimal interventions overnight and rest periods during the day, with active assessment of benefits. Relaxation and other stress-reduction techniques (e.g. guided imagery, biofeedback) may also be beneficial.

Prognosis

Within the first weeks, up to one-tenth of patients suffer a second infarction (Hockings & Donovan 1997), while only one-tenth recover without further complications (Nowak & Handford 1994). One-half of those patients surviving their first MI die or suffer a further ischaemic event within three years (Flapan 1994).

In the immediate post-MI period, newly infarcted myocardium is surrounded by oedematous, ischaemic tissue, causing the volatile ECG changes occurring following infarction. Oedema may subside, enabling reperfusion and recovery, or progress to further infarction.

Patients and families are often receptive to health information following MI. The British Heart Foundation produces a range of useful booklets that are available in most hospitals.

Implications for practice

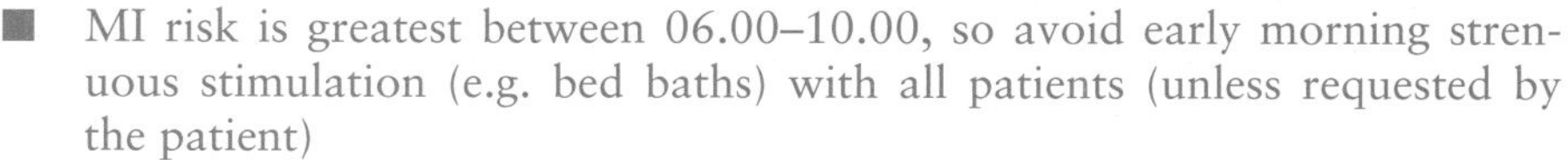

- MI risk is greatest between 06.00–10.00, so avoid early morning strenuous stimulation (e.g. bed baths) with all patients (unless requested by the patient)

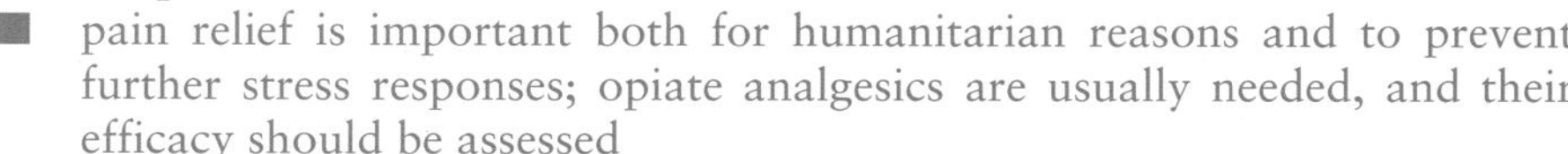

- pain relief is important both for humanitarian reasons and to prevent further stress responses; opiate analgesics are usually needed, and their efficacy should be assessed
- rest is important for healing; it should be actively planned, and its effectiveness assessed
- ICU nurses should be aware of local protocols/policies relating to thrombolytic therapies
- before giving streptokinase, nurses should ascertain whether their patient has previously been given a dose, and if so, when
- following MI, reperfusion dysrhythmias will occur, especially ventricular dysrhythmias; patients should be closely monitored as a minority will progress to severe left ventricular failure and cardiogenic shock
- health promotion for patients and families, an important role for all nurses (DoH 1998a), is often more easily achieved in relation to cardiac disease than many other pathologies encountered in ICU

Summary

Recent reductions in incidence of MIs in the UK are disappointing both in relation to *Health of the Nation* targets and reductions in most other countries. However, in-hospital prognosis following MIs is improving, partly from effective use of thrombolytic therapy. The incidence of patients with uncomplicated myocardial infarctions being admitted to ICUs will vary, depending on other hospital services (e.g. availability of CCUs), but usually ICU admission will be when MIs complicate other pathologies or progress to prolonged cardiac failure.

Nursing care of patients with myocardial infarctions should focus on prevention and close monitoring of further complications.

Further reading

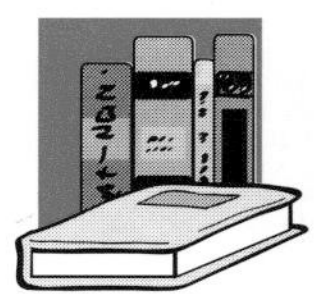

Readers should balance medical and nursing sources. Of medical sources, the reports of major international trials are especially useful; of these, ISIS-2 (1988) is particularly comprehensive and has been especially influential. Medical material can usefully be supplemented by whatever current textbooks readers have access to. Weston (1996) offers a useful overview of thrombolytics. Articles frequently appear in the nursing press. Todd (1997) is an especially valuable addition to the literature.

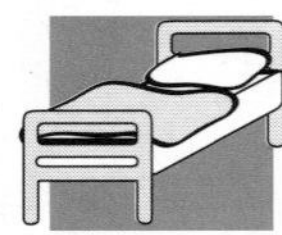

Clinical scenario

Howard Gray is a 52-year-old insurance broker with a history of angina. He was admitted to ICU 4 hours after he had woken up in the early morning with 'crushing' chest pains, unrelieved by sublingual nitro-glycerine, and with worsening dyspneoa.

His ECG shows wide Q waves (area of necrosis) in leads V_2–V_6, and ST elevation (area of injury) in leads I, aVL and V_2–V_6, with ST depression in II, III and aVF, no T wave inversion (peripheral area of ischaemia) noted.

HR 128 beats/min; BP 80/45 mmHg (MAP 57 mmHg)

Serum enzyme results on admission are:

Creatine kinase (CK)	50 IU/l
Aspartate aminotransferase (AST)	60 IU/l
Lactate dehydrogenase (LDH)	normal

Q.1 Using a diagram of the surface of the heart and Mr Gray's ECG changes, identify which part of his myocardium is damaged and note the main coronary arteries that supply this area.

Q.2 Mr Gray is given thombolytic therapy of streptokinase. Review your role in administering and monitoring the effectiveness of this therapy (note frequency and type of investigation/assessment, identification of potential adverse effects).

Q.3 Evaluate the advice, information and follow up services offered to patients like Mr Gray by your clinical practice area. What role does the ICU nurse have in relation to health promotion, advice and cardiac rehabilitation post-MI?

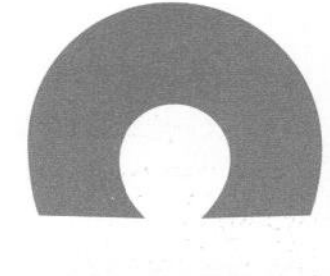

Chapter 25

Shock

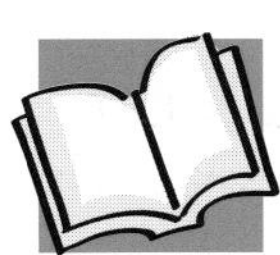

Contents

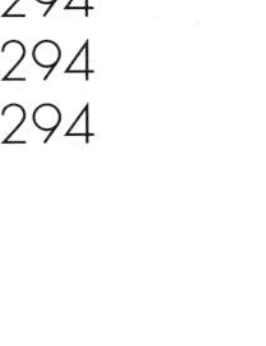

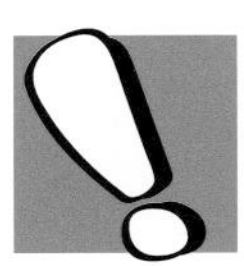

Fundamental knowledge

Cellular pathology (see also Chapter 23)
Pericardial anatomy
Baroreceptors and chemoreceptors
Renin–angiotensin–aldosterone cascade
Normal inflammatory responses (increased capillary permeability, leucocyte migration, vasoactive mediators release)

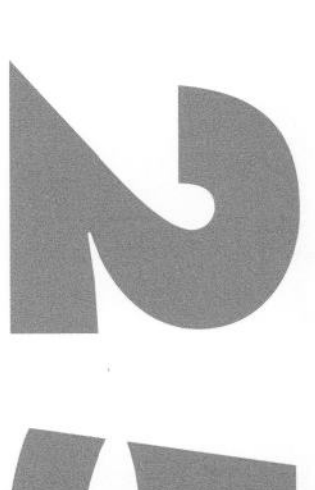

Introduction

Traditional labels of shock, by causal mechanisms, have some value: resolving the cause should relieve problems. However caused, shock impairs tissue oxygen delivery, and causes microcirculatory maldistribution and metabolic complications (Shoemaker & Beez 1996), with life-threatening cellular hypoxia progressing to whole system dysfunction. Urgent microcirculatory resuscitation is needed to prevent the complications of shock.

Perfusion pressure (mean arterial pressure) is the sum of:

- total capacity of blood vessels
- total blood volume
- local factors (e.g. resistance)

The first part of this chapter describes the effects of shock on major systems, and then identifies traditional classifications:

- hypovolaemic
- cardiogenic
- neurogenic/spinal
- anaphylactic
- obstructive
- toxic shock syndrome
- septic (SIRS)

Shock in ICU patients is usually caused by systemic inflammatory response syndrome (SIRS), which is described later in this chapter. Prolonged hypoperfusion damages tissues, with shock becoming irreversible once reperfusion is unachievable.

System failure

CARDIOVASCULAR In health, hypoperfusion causes baroreceptors and chemoreceptors to initiate endogenous catecholamine (primarily adrenaline) release and sympathetic nervous system responses. Blood pressure is the sum of heart rate, stroke volume and systemic vascular resistance ($BP = HR \times SV \times SVR$); adrenaline increases all factors, so restoring blood (perfusion) pressure. Renal hypotension causes renin release, increasing systemic pressure via the renin–angiotensin–aldosterone cascade.

Complex pathologies (most ICU patients) complicate this mechanism with endogenous cardioinhibitory and vasodilatory mediators (e.g. TNFα, IL-1, endorphins, myocardial depressant factor – see Chapter 23). Cellular dysfunction aggravates electrolyte imbalances (especially hypercalcaemia and hyperkalaemia), impairing cardiac conduction, so causing dysrhythmias.

RESPIRATORY Pulmonary hypoperfusion increases pathological dead space and V/Q mismatch. Anaerobic metabolism and metabolic acidosis (from systemic hypoperfusion) stimulates tachypnoea. Severe shock, therefore, increases the work of breathing without improving tissue oxygenation (Wheeler & Bernard 1999). Hypoxic lung tissue can progress to ARDS (once called 'shock lung').

METABOLIC Hypotension and hypoperfusion trigger the release of various hormones:

- antidiuretic hormone (ADH, from the pituitary gland)
- cortisol (from adrenal glands)
- aldosterone (renin cascade)

This increases sodium and water retention, increasing intravascular volume, so providing short-term compensation. However, prolonged hypoperfusion, reduced colloid osmotic pressure and increased vascular permeability from critical illnesses cause excessive fluid shifts into interstitial spaces, resulting in oedema and raised interstitial pressure (causing further resistance to perfusion), without sustaining perfusion pressure.

Anaerobic metabolism accelerates metabolic acidosis, and hypoxia damages cell walls, causing inappropriate movement of ions across cell membranes (see Chapter 23).

Hyperglycaemia may occur from

- cortisol
- growth hormone
- catecholamines

Inhibited glucose transport into cells impairs intracellular energy production, compounding cell (then organ) failure (see Chapter 23).

RENAL Prolonged renal ischaemia (pre-renal failure) causes acute tubular necrosis (see Chapter 32), which increases toxic levels of active metabolites (e.g. urea contributes to confusion/coma).

HEPATIC Hypoperfusion often causes deranged liver function. The liver has many functions (metabolic, digestive, immune, homeostatic), and so hepatic dysfunction causes many problems, including coagulopathies and immunocompromise.

Classifications of shock

HYPOVOLAEMIC (HAEMORRHAGIC) SHOCK This may be caused by

- acute haemorrhage (trauma, surgery, gastrointestinal bleeding)
- other excessive fluid loss (e.g. diabetic ketoacidosis).

SIRS is effectively hypovolaemic shock, but is described separately.

Hypovolaemic shock occurs once compensatory mechanisms (e.g. catecholamine release) fail; most people tolerate losses of 15–30 per cent of blood volume (Kerber 1995), although tolerance reduces with age (most ICU patients are elderly).

When compensation fails, venous return falls (low CVP), inevitably reducing stroke volume. Compensatory tachycardia may restore blood pressure, but increased myocardial oxygen consumption can cause ischaemia, dysrhythmias and infarction.

CARDIOGENIC SHOCK This is caused by cardiac failure, usually from myocardial infarction, but it may also be caused by

- tamponade
- myocardial stunning
- mitral regurgitation
- congenital defects

and other problems.

Cardiogenic shock follows extensive left ventricular damage. Compensatory tachycardia may increase myocardial oxygen supply, but it also increases consumption. Damage to over 70 per cent of the left ventricle is rapidly fatal (Hinds & Watson 1996).

Treatment attempts to increase systemic perfusion pressure while limiting myocardial hypoxia. Artificial ventilation and removing the work of breathing with paralysing agents (Nimmo & Nimmo 1993) optimises tissue oxygen availability. Inotropes may be necessary to increase cardiac output, but will aggravate myocardial ischaemia (Nimmo & Nimmo 1993). Intra-aortic balloon pumps can augment coronary artery and cerebral perfusion, while revascularisation (PTCA or CABG – see Chapter 30) improves survival (Visser & Purday 1998).

Mortality from cardiogenic shock varies between 30 and 90 per cent, survival being lower with aggressive treatment (Califf & Bengston 1994). Survivors often develop congestive cardiac failure, necessitating cardiac surgery.

NEUROGENIC/SPINAL SHOCK This is caused by the interruption of autonomic sympathetic control from central nervous system injury or oedema. The autonomic nervous system controls systemic vascular resistance (SVR), and so interruption causes inappropriate smooth muscle relaxation (vasodilation) and excessive peripheral pooling of blood. Since this large increase in blood vessel capacity is not being matched by increased volume, central pressure (and perfusion) falls. Bradycardia from excessive and uncountered vagal tone further reduces blood pressure.

Failure of autonomic response makes inotropes ineffective, but volume replacement may compensate for increased blood vessel capacity. Unresponsive sudden hypotension usually indicates a stroke; with a critically ill patient this often proves terminal so that medical assistance should be summoned urgently.

ANAPHYLACTIC SHOCK This is caused by histamine release. Histamine is released following an antigen–antibody reaction and is a potent systemic vasodilator, greatly increasing total blood vessel capacity. Being part of specific immunity, it is released on a second or subsequent exposure to antigens. 'Second doses' of drugs are the most likely time for anaphylaxis to occur, but 'first doses' may not be danger-free – previous exposure to antigens (e.g. drugs) may be unrecorded.

Anaphylactic shock can be an emergency, and is treated with adrenaline to restore circulating blood pressure and antihistamines (steroids). Volume expanders, oxygen and other system supports may be needed.

OBSTRUCTIVE SHOCK This is caused by any obstruction to the central blood flow:

- raised intrathoracic pressure (from positive pressure ventilation, manual hyperinflation, PEEP)
- obstructed intrapulmonary flow (ARDS, pulmonary emboli, pneumo/haemothorax)
- tamponade.

TAMPONADE This is direct continuous compression of the heart, usually caused by pericardial haemorrhage; accumulation forces myocardium inward, reducing intraventricular space and stroke volume.

Tamponade can be slow or quick. Slow bleeding (usually spontaneous) may be tolerated until 2 litres accumulate (Cockroft 1997); rapid tamponade (usually from cardiac surgery or trauma) is an emergency, usually causing imminent cardiac arrest once compensatory tachycardia and vasoconstriction fail. Tamponade should be suspected whenever sudden and large increases in CVP are accompanied by falling blood pressure, or cardiac drainage stops suddenly. These signs may be absent or masked by hypovolaemia; other indications include:

- dysrhythmias and low voltage ECG trace
- **pulsus parodoxus**
- muffled (apex) heart sounds
- mediastinal widening (on X-ray),
- pericardial fluid accumulation (shown by echocardiography)

Rapid tamponade seldom allows time for such diagnostic tests, requiring removal of pericardial fluid. A 16-FG ('spinal', 'cardiac') needle is inserted into the pericardiac sac by a doctor. Blood is then aspirated, needles usually remaining (capped off) in case further blood accumulates. Blood clots cannot be aspirated through spinal needles, but once coagulation begins, bleeding has probably ceased.

Following pericardial tap, patients should be closely monitored for further accumulation (ECG, CVP, drainage).

TOXIC SHOCK SYNDROME This is caused by a strain of *Staphylococcus aureus* (Willis 1997). This syndrome became widely recognised following its link to tampon use. Its incidence declined once tampon manufacturers removed the causative chemicals. There are now about 40 UK cases each year (Willis 1997), usually caused by poor hygiene, tampon (mis)use, and surgical wound infection (Hinds & Watson 1996).

Systemic inflammatory response syndrome (SIRS)

Definition

Until a 1991 consensus conference this was more usually called 'septic shock'. Sepsis will cause shock, but infection is only one of many triggers for the syndrome (ACCP/SCCM 1992), and may be absent when 'septic' pictures are caused by conditions such as pancreatitis and burns. The consensus conference therefore adopted the term *systemic inflammatory response syndrome* (SIRS) to define a host response to various severe clinical insults. The term sepsis should only be used once specific microorganisms are identified.

The consensus conference criteria for SIRS are:

- temperature above 38°C or below 36°C
- heart rate above 90 beats/min
- respiratory rate above 20/min or $PaCO_2$ below 4.3 kPa
- leucocyte count above 12,000 cells/mm^2, below 4,000, or containing over 10 per cent immature neutrophils (Bone *et al.* 1992)

The term '*septic* inflammatory response syndrome' rather than *systemic* may be encountered; in practice, there is little difference between them; 'systemic' is used here, as inflammatory responses occur throughout the cardiovascular system. This gross extension of normal homeostasis causes, rather than results from, the problem.

Sepsis

Sepsis rates increased by 137 per cent between 1984–94 (Bone 1994), largely due to escalating risks from:

- increasingly invasive techniques
- improved survival from simpler pathologies increasing immunocompromise
- ageing populations (immunity is impaired with age)
- greater use of immunosuppressive therapy (including steroids)
- more resistant organisms.

Only about one-half of patients with sepsis develop SIRS (Kulkarni & Webster 1996).

Mortality

The 1909 mortality rate from sepsis of 41 per cent remains essentially unchanged today (Ellis 1995), a stark (if alarmist) reminder of the problems and limits facing medicine. Overall mortality rates of 10–20 per cent for sepsis (Curzen & Evans 1996) increase to 50 per cent in ICUs (Groenveld & Thijs 1991), and so simple infection control measures (see Chapter 15) can literally be life saving.

Pathology

Bacteria initiate sepsis, but shock is a problem of inflammatory response rather than bacterial invasion so that treatment should limit excessive inflammatory responses (Deitch 1995).

Cell membrane damage (from microorganisms and inflammation) release vasoactive mediators (e.g. TNFα, IL-1,6,8 – see Chapter 23). As inflammation becomes systemic, inflammatory responses throughout the body cause

- total body vasodilation
- grossly increased intravascular space
- increased capillary permeability

with extravasation of plasma into tissues, oedema formation, hypovolaemia, hypoperfusion and generalised tissue hypoxia. Many chemical mediators also depress myocardial function, further reducing systemic blood pressure.

SIRS has two distinct stages, often called 'hot' and 'cold':

STAGE 1 ('HOT') TNFα, the first mediator to peak (Deitch 1995), is pyrogenic, causing the fever typically associated with this stage. Arachidonic acid, released from lipoproteins by TNFα, causes further pyrogen release (PGE_2, thromboxane A_2) (Wheeler & Bernard 1999). The net effects are:

- increased heart rate and cardiac output
    - increasing cardiac workload
    - increasing myocardial oxygen consumption

- decreased vascular resistance
  - impairing perfusion
  - causing tissue hypoxia
- oedema formation
  - causing shunting
- cell damage

STAGE 2 ('COLD') Progressive plasma extravasation accelerates hypovolaemia. Ischaemia increases gut permeability (Doig *et al.* 1998), facilitating translocation of gut bacteria (commensals or pathogens), escalating sepsis.

Local vasoconstrictive mediators unsuccessfully attempt to compensate, making peripheries cold and cyanosed. Myocardial ischaemia and dysfunction reduce cardiac output so that, despite increased SVR, profound hypotension and hypoperfusion persist.

Hypoalbuminaemia occurs due to:

- proteinuria
- hepatic impairment
- inhibition of albumin synthesis by TNFα and interleukin 1 (IL-1) (Kulkarni & Webster 1996)

Hypoalbuminaemia reduces colloid osmotic pressure (see Chapter 33), causing further extravasation and hypotension.

Treatments

However caused, shock results in tissue hypoperfusion. Where possible, causes are identified and treated and systems supported. Fluid management remains central to cardiovascular support. Some novel, and other, therapies for treating shock are discussed. Monoclonal antibodies (not currently available) are discussed in Chapter 15.

With SIRS, increased vascular permeability and low colloid osmotic pressure cause inappropriate fluid shifts. *Fluid resuscitation* with colloids (see Chapter 33) should therefore restore colloid osmotic and perfusion pressures, without compounding interstitial oedema.

Serum albumin is the main endogenous determinant of colloid osmotic pressure. Exogenous albumin only temporarily increases serum albumin, so that endogenous production (through adequate nutrition) should be promoted.

Shock creates a syndrome of microcirculatory hypoperfusion. Shoemaker and Beez (1996) suggest that mortality correlates with oxygen debt, and so treatment to reverse oxygen debt improves survival prospects. Oxygen debt, the difference between oxygen demand and oxygen delivery, cannot be measured directly, but Shoemaker *et al.* (1993) recommend *supranormal treatments*:

- cardiac index above 5.5 l/min/mm^2
- blood volume 500 ml above normal
- DO_2 above 1,000 l/min/m^2
- so driving supranormal VO_2 (190 ml/min/m^2)

These would be achieved by:

- giving colloids
- inotropes (e.g. dobutamine)
- vasodilators/vasopressors (to control afterload)

Supranormal treatment is increasingly questioned; Brazzi *et al.* (1997) consider this approach inappropriate for most ICU patients.

Plasmapheresis (see Chapter 35) can remove small solutes such as TNFα (Molnar & Shearer 1998), but clearance of cell-bound mediators is limited.

Phospholipidase is activated by endotoxin, which then triggers the platelet activating factor (Clarke 1997). Inhibiting phospholipidase can break this cascade. *Phosphodiasterase A_2 inhibitors* are effective in animal studies, but the precise effects in humans remains unknown (Clarke 1997) and ethical problems surrounding research (volunteers cannot be given SIRS) necessarily limit clinical studies.

Implications for practice

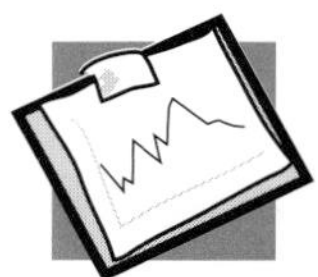

- severe shock necessitates close haemodynamic monitoring and observation
- where possible, underlying causes of shock should be removed (e.g. fluid resuscitation)
- nurses should question whether benefits from invasive equipment (e.g. monitoring) justify infection risks
- shock with ICU patients causes prolonged complications; management should focus on long-term effects, and so benefits may not be seen for a number of shifts
- colloids will be needed for fluid resuscitation when capillary permeability is increased (e.g. SIRS); although prescription is a medical role, nurses should contribute to multidisciplinary discussion
- sudden shock may be caused by tamponade, especially following cardiac surgery; nurses identifying signs of tamponade should attempt to restore patency of drains; if this does not resolve the problem, urgent medical help should be sought
- gut ischaemia increases problems from translocation of gut bacteria; enteral feeding should be encouraged/maintained whenever possible
- most ICU patients are immunosupressed; good infection control significantly reduces risks of sepsis

Summary

This chapter describes traditional classifications of shock by pathology with special emphasis on SIRS, the main cause of shock in ICU. Where precipitating causes cannot be removed, system support can make the difference between recovery and progression to MODS (see Chapter 26).

Close monitoring and observation by ICU nurses, with an understanding of the probable mechanisms of shock, enables prompt treatment; nurses have an especially valuable preventative role in promoting infection control and nutrition.

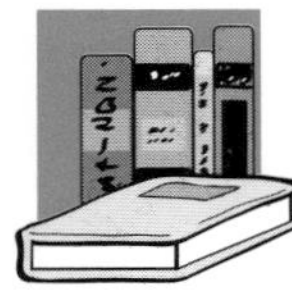

Further reading

Many texts cite consensus definitions of SIRS and discuss the syndrome; Bone's (1992, 1994, 1996) work is useful, although articles by the Consensus team have also appeared in a number of major medical journals (e.g. ACCP/SCCM (1992)).

Reviews of particular types of shock, such as Visser and Purday's (1998) article on cardiogenic shock, appear periodically. Kulkarni and Webster (1996) and Wheeler and Bernard (1999) review septic shock. Molnar and Shearer (1998) review plasmapheresis removal of mediators.

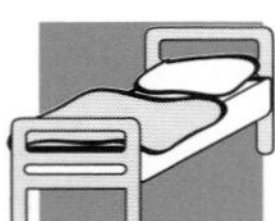

Clinical scenario

Brian Geller is a 62-year-old man, who was originally admitted to hospital with severe abdominal pain from ruptured gastric and duodenal ulcers. He admits to smoking more than 20 cigarettes and drinking over half a bottle of spirits per day. Surgery was performed and Mr Geller was recovering when he developed a chest infection. Despite antibiotic therapy his physical condition deteriorated, he became confused and was transferred to ICU.
Vital signs on ICU admission included:

Temperature	38.8°C (and flushed looking)
Heart rate	105 beats/min (with bounding pulses)
BP	90/45 mmHg
Respiratory rate	35/min
Hb	9.5 g/dl
WBC	$38{,}000 \times 10^{-9}$/l
Platelets	$75{,}000 \times 10^{-9}$/l

Ultrasound revealed a large collection of pus in Mr Geller's abdomen.

Q.1 From the signs and condition described above, identify the most likely classification of shock for Mr Geller. What other investigations might confirm this?

Q.2 Outline the invasive procedures and monitoring equipment required to fully assess Mr Geller's condition (hypoperfusion of organs and microcirculation).

Q.3 Mr Geller becomes oedematous with a systemic vascular resistance (SVR) of 360 dynes/sec/cm^{-5}. Review treatment goals and justify choice of:

Invasive ventilation (mode, rates, volumes, etc.)
Temperature management (antipyretics, antimicrobials, cooling methods if appropriate)
Volume replacement therapies (specify type of fluids)
Inotropic and vasopressor therapies (type and dose)
Immune/inflammatory response management (e.g. type of nutrition, prostaglandin therapy, anti-endotoxin monoclonal antibody therapy)

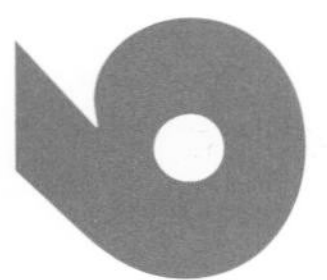
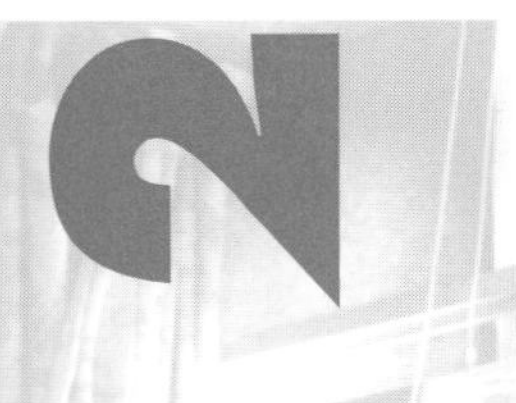
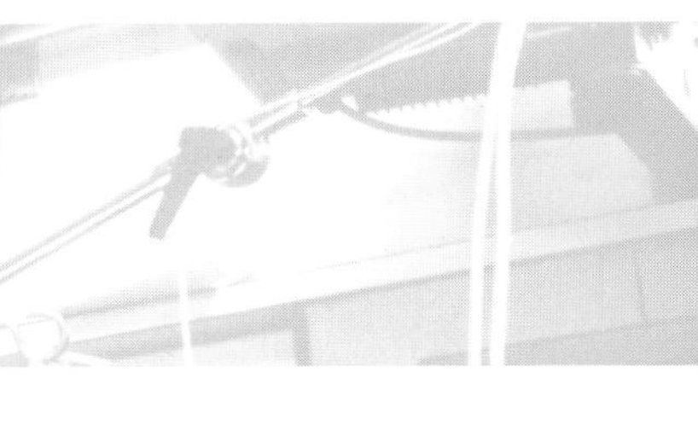

Chapter 26

Multiorgan dysfunction syndrome

Contents

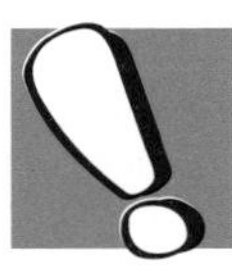

Fundamental knowledge

Cellular pathology (see also Chapter 23)
Systemic inflammatory response syndrome (see also Chapter 25)

Introduction

Previous chapters have discussed failure of individual organs and various syndromes that may necessitate or complicate ICU admission; this brief chapter discusses a frequent end result of progressive deterioration: multi-organ dysfunction syndrome (MODS). As its name suggests, this syndrome involves dysfunction of two or more organs. Other terms used to describe this syndrome include multiorgan failure (MOF).

The syndrome is largely a creation of the success of intensive care: within living memory single failure of a major organ was usually terminal. MODS is one of the main causes of ICU mortality (Beal & Cerra 1994); Tan and Oh (1997b: 733) call MODS the 'raison d'être of an ICU'. MODS therefore results in high mortality, and emotional and financial costs for patients and healthcare.

The treatment and support of each organ and system follow those described in previous chapters, and so are not repeated here. Instead, this chapter provides a synthesis of progressive pathology, prognosis and issues specific to the syndrome as a whole, rather than the individual parts discussed elsewhere. Mechanisms of reperfusion injury, which can complicate recovery, are discussed.

The syndrome extends problems originating at cellular level, complex interactions of mediators creating a range of (sometimes contradictory) effects.

MODS can be used to describe two-organ failure; more often, it is used where all major systems are failing. Lack of consensus about both terms and interpretation hinders comparison; for example, prognosis is considerably better for failure of two rather than four major organs.

Pathology

Being a progression of single organ/system pathology, MODS represents a vicious downward spiral of ischaemic complications, usually following infection, especially from translocation of gut bacteria (Crouser & Dorinsky 1994; Davidson & Boom 1995).

However caused, gross ischaemia causes hypoxia, anaerobic metabolism and failure of most or all organs. Sommers (1998) suggests that half the cases of MODS are caused by inadequate early resuscitation; although aggressive (colloid) fluid replacement in the early stages of shock may prevent progress to MODS, impaired left ventricular contractility limits the benefits from fluid resuscitation (Tan & Oh 1997b).

Failure of organs reflects damage at cellular level. Cytokines (especially tumour necrosis factor and interleukin 1) trigger hyperglycaemia and extreme protein catabolism ('autocannibalism') (Beal & Cerra 1994). As mitochondria develop abnormalities, energy production is severely impaired (Tan & Oh 1997b), leading to cell failure. Widespread cell failure impairs healing, exposing patients to further nosocomial infection (Tan & Oh 1997b).

The sequence of organ failure varies, but often starts with respiratory failure, a major cause of ICU admission. The liver, being especially rich in xanthine oxidase (Davidson & Boom 1995), is particularly prone to ischaemic damage. Low-grade liver failure is often under-recognised in ICUs (see Chapter 39) so that symptoms such as coagulopathies (including DIC), hypofibrinogenaemia and hypoalbuminaemia may not be noticed until progression to later stages. Cardiac and coronary artery disease are endemic in Western society; many patients admitted to ICUs have underlying cardiac failure. Mediators released during critical illness provoke cardiovascular failure. Systemic hypotension and hypoperfusion leads to hepatic and respiratory failure and renal failure, often (but not always) in that order.

Treatment

MODS is a late complication of various pathologies, and so treatments for underlying pathologies are likely to be maintained and intensified. There is no single treatment for MODS, but system support is attempted around each problem. A problem facing all systems is microcirculatory hypoperfusion, and so tissue perfusion should be optimised, assessing needs though cardiac output study monitoring and resuscitating with (colloid) fluids to achieve desired delivery and consumption of oxygen at tissue level (DO_2, VO_2). The lack of support for Shoemaker's use of supranormal treatments is discussed in Chapter 25.

Infection often causes MODS, but MODS also aggravates immunocompromise. This vicious circle makes infection control particularly important. MODS usually necessitates highly invasive monitoring and treatments, which provides access for further microorganisms.

Infection rates from central lines are far higher than from peripheral lines; sicker patients have more central lines, and so the risk to critically ill patients may not reflect the much cited sevenfold from peripheral versus ninetyfold from central lines. However, the transfer of drugs that can be given peripherally may enable removal of a central line, or the removal of an unused peripheral line, which may significantly reduce infection risks.

Plasmapheresis (see Chapters 25, 35) may remove circulating mediators. Critically ill patients have low antioxidant levels (especially vitamins C and E) (Davidson & Boom 1995). Giving vitamin E, the most important intracellular chain-breaking antioxidant (Davidson & Boom 1995), appears particularly beneficial. Other antioxidants that may prove useful include intracellular glutathione (Davidson & Boom 1995) and enzymes such as cytosolic superoxide dismutase (which includes zinc, long used for skin healing).

Reperfusion injury

Apparent recovery often leads to subsequent reversal. Reperfusion of ischaemic tissues which have survived through anaerobic metabolism flushes toxic oxygen metabolites and radicals into the cardiovascular system. These can trigger a further cascade of vasoactive and other endogenous chemicals (see Chapter 23). Apparent recovery can therefore be reversed with one or more vital organs failing for a second time. Reperfusion injury is a complication of thrombolysis (from cardioinhibitory mediators), but cerebral tissue is also particularly susceptible (survivors of MODS frequently suffer neurological damage and impaired function).

Prognosis

Failure of each vital organ carries significant mortality; mortality from MODS increases with the numbers of organs involved (Marshall 1995) – failure of all four major organs (lungs, heart, liver, kidneys) being almost invariably fatal (Sommers 1998). Overall mortality from MODS has remained 70–80 per cent for twenty years (Sommers 1998), although increasing severity of pathologies treated should be remembered.

Implications for practice

- multiorgan dysfunction syndrome is the result of pathological processes initiated at cellular level causing systemic inflammatory responses
- many ICU patients develop MODS, and so ICU monitoring and care of all patients should detect early signs of progressive organ failure; this is facilitated by holistic, rather than reductionist, care planning
- mortality rates from MODS remain very high, but early intervention to support failing systems (especially microcirculatory resuscitation) can improve survival
- maintaining high standards of fundamental aspects of care, especially infection control, can reduce incidence and severity
- apparent recovery may be confounded by reperfusion injury, and so close monitoring of vital signs should continue after initial recovery
- mortality reflects the number of major organs failing; multidisciplinary teams should consider whether prognosis justifies continued treatment (is death being prolonged?); nurses should be actively involved in team decisions

Summary

Multiorgan dysfunction complicates many ICU admissions, incurring high human and financial costs. High incidence and paucity of curative (rather than supportive) treatments has encouraged a search for novel solutions. Such is the need that possible solutions are sometimes pursued with little (or even adverse) benefit. This chapter illustrates how progression from single to multiorgan failure remains the greatest challenge facing intensive care.

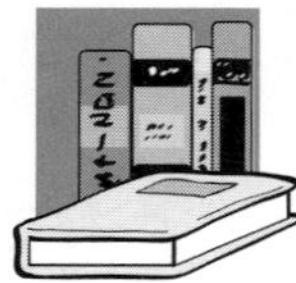

Further reading

The most recent medical texts include sections on MODS; Beal and Cerra (1994) provides a comprehensive overview.

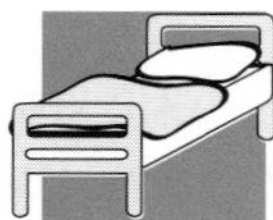

Clinical scenario

Brian Geller, a 62-year-old gentleman, was originally admitted to hospital with severe abdominal pain from ruptured gastric and duodenal ulcers. Surgery was performed and Mr Geller was recovering when he developed a chest infection, his physical condition deteriorated, he became confused and was transferred to ICU in a shocked state (see Chapter 25, Clinical scenario). By day 2 on ICU, he is ventilated and continuous venovenous haemofiltration (CVVH) has been commenced.

Q.1 Identify the various endogenous mediators of inflammation (cytokines and eicosanoids) and the symptoms associated with tumour necrosis factor-alpha (TNFα) seen in Mr Geller.

Mr Geller has multiple cannulation sites for haemodynamic monitoring, CVVH and the administration of drugs. He is intubated, has a urinary catheter *in situ*, and an abdominal wound with one drain.

Q.2 Evaluate Mr Geller's risk factors for secondary sources of infection and all possible exposures to microorganisms. Critically analyse how these may be minimised by nurses (e.g. risk assessment, IV policies, frequency of line changes, dressings, hand washing, enteral nutrition, skin care, etc.)

Q.3 Review survival rates of patients with multiorgan dysfunction syndrome (MODS) in your own clinical practice area. Estimate the average length of ICU days, acute hospital stay and typical morbidity for these survivors. Reflect on how the ICU nurse can prepare patients recovering from MODS for rehabilitation and discharge.

For answers to Q.1, see the Answers section at the end of the book.

Chapter 27

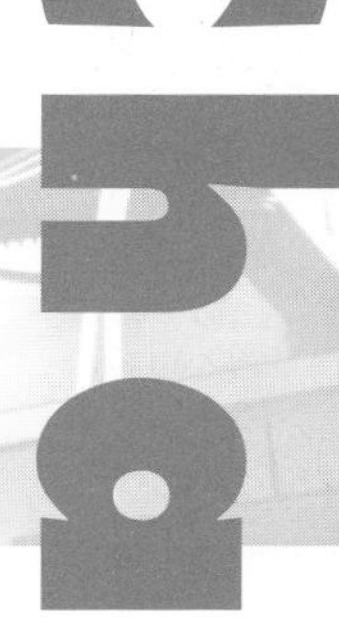

Acute respiratory distress syndrome (ARDS)

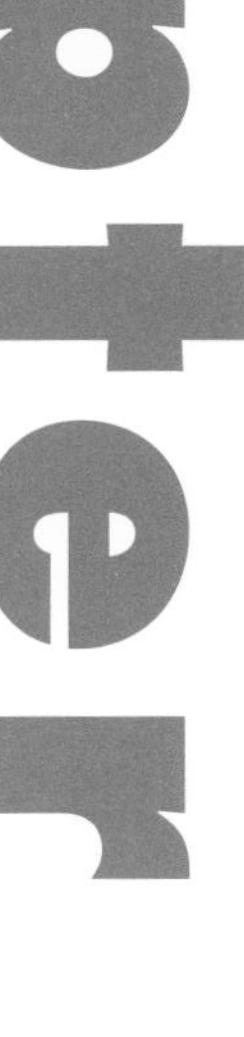

Contents

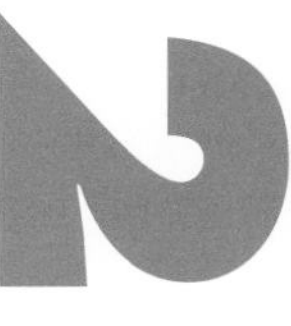

Fundamental knowledge

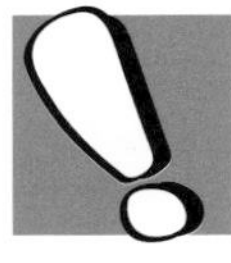

Respiratory anatomy and physiology: alveoli, pulmonary blood flow

V/Q mismatch; pulmonary shunting

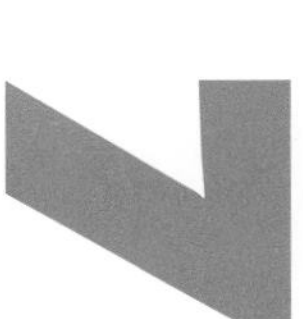

Introduction

Each year 1,000–1,500 people in the UK develop acute respiratory distress syndrome (ARDS) (Sair & Evans 1995), most needing artificial ventilation. This chapter concentrates on pathophysiology and medical interventions and treatments. As much nursing time is devoted to assisting doctors (monitoring, giving prescribed treatments), nurses need to understand pathology and treatments. The psychological needs of ICU patients and families may be increased from prolonged stay and poor prognosis. Death is usually caused by multiorgan dysfunction syndrome (MODS) or haemodynamic instability rather than respiratory failure, but mortality remains high, many victims being young.

Once called 'Adult Respiratory Distress Syndrome' (ARDS) because of apparent similarities to (Infant) Respiratory Distress Syndrome (IRDS or RDS), pathology and treatment of each are different. IRDS is simply lack of surfactant production from immature lung tissue in premature babies, and so easily treated by exogenous surfactant. However, ARDS became increasingly diagnosed in children.

A 1992 consensus conference modified terminology to *Acute* Respiratory Distress Syndrome (Bernard *et al.* 1994a, 1994b). The consensus definition is:

- acute injury to the lung with a PaO_2/FiO_2 ratio below 200 mmHg or < 27 kPa, regardless of PEEP
- bilateral chest infiltrates on X-ray
- pulmonary capillary wedge pressure below 18 mmHg. Increasingly, ARDS has been recognised as the pulmonary manifestation of wider inflammatory pathology (e.g. SIRS). Inflammation causes:
  - release of mediators
  - pulmonary oedema (not cardiogenic, hence wedge pressure criterion)
  - V/Q mismatch (poor perfusion, poor ventilation)

Surfactant, produced by type II pneumocytes, is a phospholipid compound that reduces alveolar surface tension. Pneumocyte damage impairs surfactant production (DiRusso *et al.* 1995). Alveoli being inherently unstable and prone to atelectasis, surfactant lack causes high intra-alveolar pressures and barotrauma, accelerating alveolar collapse and pulmonary oedema formation.

Early/exudative stage

ARDS is often described in two stages. Terminology again varies, and in practice these two stages are part of a continuum rather than distinct entities; but descriptions are clinically useful to understand disease progression.

The early or exudative stage, which begins as endothelial injury causes progressive pulmonary capillary permeability, results in

- interstitial and alveolar oedema (DiRusso *et al.* 1995)
- reduced (self-ventilating) tidal volume
- high airway pressure (from reduced volume)
- significant reduction in functional residual capacity
- pulmonary 'shunting' (V/Q below 0.8)

If high airway pressure persists, barotrauma and volotrauma cause progressive damage (see Chapter 4).

Proliferative/fibrotic stages

Early insults to lung tissue cause progression to diffuse problems. Damage to type I pneumocytes causes proliferation of type II cells (thick alveolar walls) and excessive collagen deposition, resulting in reduced lung compliance and increased alveolar dead space (Artigas *et al.* 1998). Other problems include

- emphysema-like lesions (Gattinoni *et al.* 1994)
- hyaline membrane formation
- capillary microembolism
- abnormal/inactive surfactant
- pulmonary hypertension (pulmonary artery pressures exceed 25 mmHg (White & Roberts 1991))
- cardiac output, initially high, falls as compensation fails (White & Roberts 1991)

Alveolar collapse predisposes patients to a sixfold increase in pulmonary infection (Sachdeva & Guntupalli 1997).

Treatment

Preventing further ventilator-induced injury and system support are the mainstays of treatment. Conventionally, treatment aimed to normalise blood gases, but the excessive peak airway pressures needed to achieve this accelerate alveolar damage (barotrauma, volotrauma). Current treatment has moved from short-term aims of normalising blood gases to longer-term aims of limiting damage and recruiting alveoli (Artigas *et al.* 1998) by

- limiting FiO_2 below 0.65
- optimising PEEP (10–15 cmH_20)
- limiting peak inflation pressure (maximum 30–40 cmH_2O end expiratory pressure)
- maximising mean inflation pressure (optimising gas exchange)

However, controversies persist, most evidence being from animal studies or anecdotal reports.

Fluid management necessitates balancing adequate perfusion without aggravating pulmonary oedema. Lung damage will prevent fluids given in the late stage of ARDS from reversing low-flow (oxygen debt) states (Shoemaker & Beez 1996).

Psychological support

As recovery is prolonged, patients with ARDS may remain on ICU for weeks, exposing patients and family to prolonged anxiety and stress that may exhaust their coping mechanisms. Nurses can offer valuable care and support (e.g. accommodation and facilities, enabling visiting whenever possible without causing sensory overload to patients or guilt to relatives, and being approachable and available).

Prolonged stays can enable close rapport between families and staff, but can become stressful for everyone; both bedside nurses and nurse managers need to recognise incipient distress. Families may seek hope where little exists, placing excessive trust/reliance/expectations on individual members of staff; as well as being a symptom of denial, this can be particularly stressful for staff.

Ventilation

Achieving 'normal' blood gases with reduced functional alveolar space necessitates forcing larger volumes of gas and/or higher concentrations of oxygen into remaining alveoli. Increased intra-alveolar pressures cause shearing damage ('volotrauma'), while higher concentrations of oxygen may become toxic. Hence, the focus has shifted from normalising blood gases to recruiting alveoli, using smaller tidal volumes and accepting abnormally high arterial carbon dioxide tensions (*permissive hypercapnia*): Thomsen *et al.* (1994) used 6 ml/kg, while MacNaughton and Evans (1992) recommend tidal volumes of 5 ml/kg to maintain airway pressures below 35 cmH_2O.

Permissive hypercapnia reduces mortality (Hickling *et al.* 1994), but may create life-threatening respiratory acidosis (Hickling 1996; Wilmoth & Carpenter 1996). Permissive hypercapnia should therefore be used cautiously or avoided with:

- raised intracranial pressure
- anoxic brain injury (e.g. following MI)
- severe ischaemic heart disease
- hypotension
- dysrhythmias

As hypercapnia is a respiratory stimulant, neuromuscular blockage may be needed (Bidani *et al.* 1994). Hypercapnia can be treated with IVOX (Keogh 1995).

Pressure limited/controlled ventilation limits peak inflation pressure, and so also limits further volotrauma (Hudson 1995). While preventing or limiting further damage remains the main priority, gas exchange can be optimised by manipulating other aspects of ventilation.

Alveolar recruitment is only likely to occur when PEEP exceeds 10 cmH_2O, so that levels of 10–15 are recommended (Artigas *et al.* 1998); DiRusso *et al.* (1995) argue that high levels of PEEP (above 15 cmH_2O) increase functional residual capacity and reduce intrapulmonary shunts, enabling reduction of FiO_2 to below 0.5, but Hickling (1996) suggests that once PEEP levels reach 16, inverse ratio ventilation should be attempted before further increasing PEEP. Preferences between increasing PEEP above 15 and extending inspiratory time (e.g. inverse ratio ventilation) remain controversial (Artigas *et al.* 1998).

High levels of PEEP may cause further oedema (especially pulmonary and cerebral), and so treatments should balance benefits against complications. Nurses detecting increases in pulmonary pressures (indicative of pulmonary oedema) should alert medical staff. Nursing patients with their head elevated reduces cerebral oedema formation.

Inverse ratio ventilation increases mean (but not peak) airway pressure (Mulnier & Evans 1995), and prolonged inspiratory phases promote alveolar recruitment, while shorter expiratory phases prevent alveolar collapse. But inverse ratio ventilation, which can cause air-trapping (auto-PEEP), is unphysiological and often uncomfortable, and so may require additional sedation (which may cause further haemodynamic compromise).

Lung rest may limit or reverse damage (Gattinoni *et al.* 1993), but evidence for benefits from treating ARDS with high frequency jet ventilation is limited (Artigas *et al.* 1998). Hypercapnia may be reduced by using intravenous oxygenators (IVOX) (Conrad *et al.* 1995) and extracorporeal carbon dioxide removal ($ECCO_2R$) (Morris *et al.* 1994) (see Chapter 29). Clinical use of these modes remains experimental rather than established.

Perfluorocarbon associated gas exchange (*liquid ventilation*, see Chapter 29) appears to have potential, and is likely to be evaluated rigorously in the near future.

Exogenous *surfactant*, effective with IRDS, has proved disappointing for ARDS, partly because volumes needed (about one litre) would cause drowning, and partly because exogenous surfactant only penetrates open alveoli, not the collapsed ones where it is needed (Mulnier & Evans 1995). However, Lewis and Veldhuizen (1996), while acknowledging that specific dose and intervals remain unknown and the prediction of which patients will benefit remains impossible, argue that exogenous surfactant has proved ineffective because it is given too late.

Positioning

In contrast to the often increasingly technological or pharmacological treatments, prone positioning and kinetic therapy have been used to treat ARDS. Lung damage occurs in dependent areas, so nursing patients prone for 4 to 8 hours (Brett & Evans 1997) may increase functional residual capacity, improve diaphragmatic motion and help removal of secretions (Mulnier & Evans 1995). Lateral positioning, potentially easier to achieve, also benefits gas exchange (Hinds & Watson 1996).

However, use of the prone position remains controversial (Thomas 1997). Studies consistently show improvements in oxygenation, reduction of shunting, reduced oxygen requirements and reduced mortality (Wong 1998), although available literature may be biased by reluctance to report unsuccessful cases (Ryan & Pelosi 1996). Chatte *et al.* (1997) found that most patients sustained improved PaO_2/FiO_2 ratios an hour after being nursed prone, while Gosheron *et al.* (1998) report (unspecified) 'remarkable' improvement, but Mulnier and Evans (1995) suggest that benefits do not last. Nursing prone may more usefully prevent potential problems rather than resolve existing ones, and so should be instigated early; too often, like other promising approaches, nursing prone is used once other approaches have failed (Gosheron *et al.* 1998). Prone positioning is less invasive than many therapies (e.g. ECMO) and so exposes patients to fewer risks (Chatte *et al.* 1997).

Recommended duration of prone positioning varies from 30 minutes to 12 hours; Vollman's (1997) 4–6 hours (drawn from literature review and substantial practice) is recommended until systematic evaluation provides more concrete guidelines. However, a major limitation on prone positioning is staff availability to turn patients. In the absence of suitable equipment (Thomas 1997), some units have experienced significant levels of staff injury from adopting prone positioning. Other nursing complications of prone positioning include access of intravenous lines, positioning of endotracheal and ventilator tubing and aggravation of cardiovascular instability (Thomas 1997).

Kinetic therapy can achieve short-term benefits (Hormann *et al.* 1994) but does not reduce incidence of ARDS (Wong 1998), perhaps because it is usually instigated to treat, rather than to prevent, problems.

Reducing pulmonary hypertension

Intra-alveolar damage increases pulmonary vascular resistance, causing pulmonary hypertension; but systemic hypotension from vasodilators (SNP, GTN, calcium channel blockers) outweigh pulmonary benefits (Brett & Evans 1997). Eicosanoid vasodilators (e.g. PGE_1 and PGI_2/prostacyclin) reduce

- platelet adhesion
- macrophage production
- T-lymphocyte function
- pulmonary hypertension

so reducing inflammatory response and pulmonary infiltration. Systemic vasodilation limits intravenous doses, but nebulised prostacyclin has little systemic effect, (half-life being 3–4 minutes (Brett & Evans 1997)). Coagulopathy, a frequent complication with ARDS, may be aggravated by prostacyclin. Doses of 7.5 nanograms (± 2.5 nanograms) may be as effective as nitric oxide (Walmrath *et al.* 1996), although Hudson's (1995) literature review suggests outcome is not improved.

Inhaled nitric oxide appears to have similar benefits (and problems) to nebulised prostacyclin. Prostacyclin and nitric oxide therapy are discussed in Chapter 28.

Inflammatory response

Sepsis is almost inevitable with ARDS (MacNaughton & Evans 1992). Viewing ARDS as the pulmonary manifestation of SIRS has led to attempts to counter circulating mediators. Steroids inhibit complement-induced leucocyte aggregation and reduce capillary permeability, and so may reduce lung injury (Meduri *et al.* 1998), but do not reduce incidence or mortality (Artigas *et al.* 1998). Antioxidants (e.g. glutathone) may prove useful (Brandstetter *et al.* 1997). In 1984 Gotloib *et al.* reported successful use of **ultrafiltration** for ARDS; the current interest in plasmapheresis is discussed in Chapter 35.

Lung transplant

Lung transplantation, a possible solution for end-stage respiratory failure, has yet to be adopted in the UK. Currently there is no consensus on the value or timing for transplantation with ARDS (Mulnier & Evans 1995); however, given the shortage of donor organs and the rapid progression of ARDS, lung transplantation will only be a viable option for a few (unpredictable) cases.

Fluid management

Fluid management in ARDS necessitates balancing problems from pulmonary oedema against perfusion needs, so that restricting fluid can reduce perfusion and mar right ventricular function (MacConachie 1991). Increased pulmonary permeability and pulmonary hypertension create excessive interstitial fluid (oedema); plasma albumin displaced into tissues creates an **osmotic** pull, accentuating tissue oedema and hypovolaemia. Fluid management therefore becomes a delicate balance of providing adequate total body hydration and adequate intravascular volume for perfusion without accentuating problems from oedema.

Myocardial dysfunction frequently occurs, compounding pulmonary (and systemic) hypovolaemia, so that central venous pressure (see Chapter 20) becomes an inaccurate guide to ventricular filling; left ventricular filling pressure is better indicated through pulmonary capillary wedge pressure measurement (PCWP), although infection risks from invasive monitoring should be remembered (see Chapter 15).

Traditional emphases on blood pressure (whether systemic or pulmonary) have limited value in complex pathologies such as ARDS. Since tissue perfusion is the aim of fluid management, delivery of oxygen (DO_2) is a more useful measurement, but usually necessitates invasive cardiac output studies. Factors reducing oxygen delivery to tissues (oxygen dissociation curve, see Chapter 18), such as alkalosis, should be avoided.

With PCWP, DO_2 and other cardiovascular parameters established, fluid management can be effectively approached. As intravascular volume is the likely main priority, colloids with long half-lives (see Chapter 33) increase colloid osmotic pressure, improving perfusion and potentially reducing oedema. Exogenous albumin has only transient benefits, increased membrane permeability allowing this to leak into tissue. Albumin levels will reverse as capillary permeability resolves with recovery. Early nutrition provides protein for endogenous albumin production, minimises muscle wasting and promotes immunity. Once commenced, nutrition should be adequate to meet metabolic needs (see Chapter 9).

Cardiac management

Cardiac management is a careful balance between attempting to meet systemic oxygen demand without causing excessive cardiac workloads. Inotropes may be used to increase cardiac output, with vasodilators to reduce afterload (so increasing perfusion).

Right ventricular workload will be increased by both pathology and treatments. PEEP above 20 cmH_2O can cause supraventricular tachycardias and ventricular dysrhythmias (DiRusso *et al.* 1995); although few advocate use of such high levels of PEEP with ARDS, DiRusso *et al.*'s (1995) suggestion of prophylactic digoxin may be beneficial.

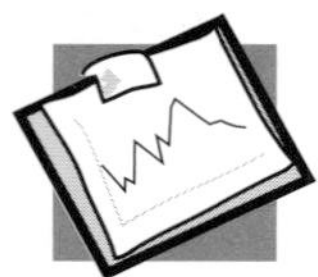

Implications for practice

- prolonged stay and poor prognosis place psychological stressors on relatives and staff; these stressors should be acknowledged; interventions should support everyone through an especially stressful time
- fluid management should optimise perfusion while avoiding fluid overload; colloids, especially those exerting high colloid osmotic pressure, are especially useful
- CVP is an inadequate guide for fluid management; invasive cardiac monitoring should balance benefits from information against risks from infection
- hypoalbuminaemia will occur; exogenous albumin gives only transient benefits, and may increase oedema
- early and continuing nutrition promotes early recovery
- ventilation is a delicate balance between optimising oxygenation and preventing further damage; nursing observations provide important information to guide medical management

- prone position remains controversial, and can neither be completely recommended nor rejected

Summary

ARDS, always secondary to another pathology, is the pulmonary manifestation of inflammatory responses. Like SIRS, it is largely a creation of the success of ICUs. For many years it has been responsible for many ICU admissions, and complicated the progress of many more. Mortality remains high, largely due to cardiovascular or other complications. Some novel medical treatments promise significant benefits, but the mainstay of treatment remains system support. Thus, patients with ARDS remain labour intensive for nursing staff; prolonged stays in ICU can place families, friends and nursing staff under much stress.

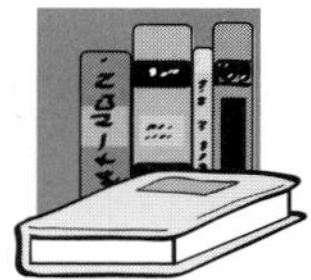

Further reading

Much has been written on ARDS, mainly in medical journals. Cutler (1996), Sachdeva & Guntupalli (1997) and Brandstetter *et al.* (1997) provide recent overviews, as will most current textbooks. Artigas *et al.* (1998) present a comprehensive (medical) conference perspective, identifying controversies and areas for future research. Recent nursing literature include Thomas (1997) and Gosheron *et al.* (1998).

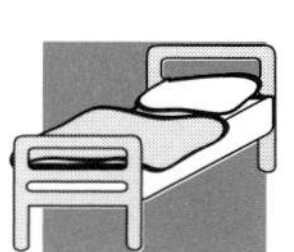

Clinical scenario

Ann O'Reilly, a 45-year-old mother of six children who weighs 104 kg, was admitted to hospital for elective ligation of fallopian tubes using keyhole surgery. Initially Mrs O' Reilly made a good recovery on the ward, but prior to discharge she presented with severe shortness of breath, fever and abdominal pains. Investigations revealed perforated bowel. Ann became septic, developed ARDS and was transferred to ICU for invasive ventilation and organ support.

On ICU pressure-controlled inverse ratio ventilation was commenced:

PEEP	10 cmH_2O
Pressure control	30 cmH_2O
FiO_2 of 0.8 (80 per cent inspired oxygen)	
Rate	14 per minute
Tidal volumes	600ml
I:E ratio of 2:1	

Arterial blood gases on these settings were:

pH	7.29
PaO_2	6.8 kPa
$PaCO_2$	8.4 kPa
HCO_3	16 mmol/l

Q.1 List the physiological processes, investigations and signs which led to Ann being diagnosed with ARDS.

Q.2 The interdisciplinary team decides to try prone positioning with Ann in an effort to improve her alveolar gas exchange. Analyse the rationale underpinning this approach, and the resources required to implement this in your own clinical area.

Q.3 Ann's gas exchange improves, allowing reduction in FiO_2 to 0.6 (60 per cent). Appraise potential adverse effects of prone positioning with Ann and propose nursing strategies to minimise or prevent occurrence (e.g. abdominal wound healing, pressure areas, breast, eye, mouth care, together with psychological effect on Ann and her family).

Chapter 28

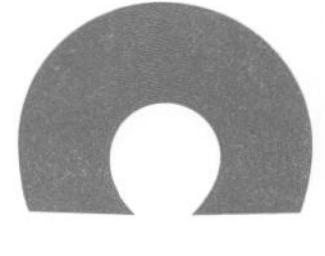
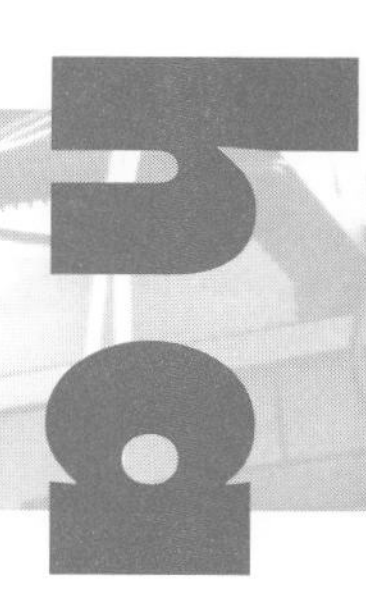

Nitric oxide

Contents

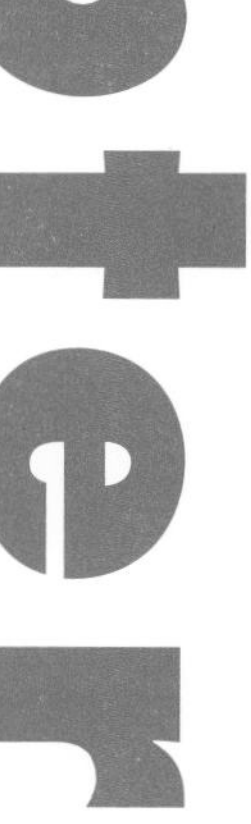

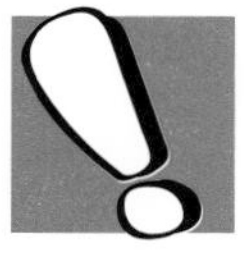

Fundamental knowledge

Alveoli: structure and pulmonary circulation

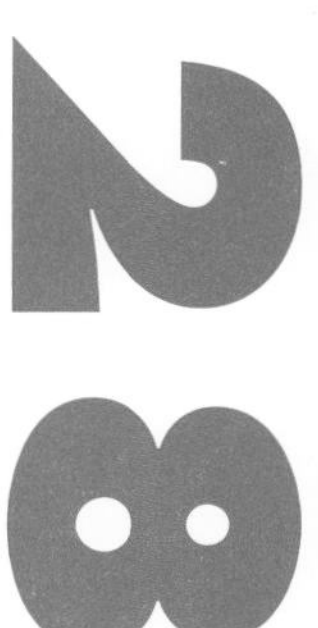

Introduction

Nitric oxide has diverse effects throughout much of the body, some beneficial some harmful. It is a potent vasodilator, possibly responsible for profound vasodilatation from septic shock (Groeneveld *et al.* 1996) and propofol (Quinn *et al.* 1995). It may cause AIDS-related dementia, Parkinson's disease (Quinn *et al.* 1995) and cerebral hypoxia/death following CVAs (Marieb 1995).

Inhaled nitric oxide (NO) has been used to treat many conditions; it may reduce sepsis-related pulmonary (Bloomfield *et al.* 1997), but is mainly used in ICU to treat ARDS. This chapter describes the chemistry of nitric oxide, which explains both its therapeutic benefits and problems. Nitric oxide therapy, doses and dangers are then explored. As nitric oxide is potentially toxic, nurses who are aware of potential problems can minimise risks to themselves and to others.

Nitrogen

Nitrogen can combine with oxygen in various forms; three of these are relevant here:

- nitrous oxide (N_2O) – an inhalational anaesthetic
- nitrogen dioxide (NO_2) – a poison
- nitric oxide (NO) – used therapeutically

Nitric oxide is a free radical (see Chapter 23), so inherently unstable, readily combining with another oxygen radical to form nitrogen dioxide. Nitrogen dioxide can be rapidly lethal.

Nitrous oxide has been clinically used for many years, but until recently nitric oxide and nitrogen dioxide (NO_2) were considered no more than toxic environmental pollutants (Grover 1993); nitrogen dioxide is used to measure air quality and pollution levels.

Greenbaum's 1967 animal experiments, following the fatal accidental exposure of two patients the previous year, confirmed concerns about nitric oxide. Exposing dogs to 5,000–20,000 parts per million (ppm) caused

- hypoxia from methaemoglobin
- right to left shunting from pulmonary oedema
- acidemia
- acid pneumonitis (from conversion of nitrous oxide into nitric oxide), reducing lung compliance

Greenbaum concluded that nitric oxide could rapidly be fatal (Frostell *et al.* 1991).

Endothelium derived relaxing factor (EDRF), an endogenous mediator discovered in 1980, was identified as nitric oxide in 1987.

Physiology

Hypoxia (from hypoperfusion or platelet aggregation) causes smooth muscle epithelium to release nitric oxide synthesase, which converts L-arginine into nitric oxide (Ganong 1995). Being a gas, nitric oxide diffuses rapidly across cell membranes, initiating a chemical cascade which dilates smooth muscle (see Figure 28.1). Nitric oxide is the medium used by endogenous vasodilatory hormones (e.g. acetylcholine, histamine, kinins) and exogenous nitrates (GTN, SNP) (Frostell *et al.* 1991; Gerlach & Falke 1995).

Similarly, nitric oxide easily diffuses into erythrocytes, binding readily with haem (nitric oxide has 1,500 times the affinity of carbon monoxide for haemoglobin (Frostell *et al.* 1991)). Binding inactivates nitric oxide, hence its very short half-life (under 1 second (Rykerson *et al.* 1995); 6–10 seconds (Holowaty 1995)) and selectivity of iNO to pulmonary vasculature (Frostell *et al.* 1991).

Negative feedback restores homeostasis: hypoperfused blood vessels release nitric oxide, causing vasodilation, and as perfusion increases, haemoglobin inactivates nitric oxide and stops endogenous production (Ganong 1995).

Although damage to erythrocyte membranes from entry of nitric oxide damage is probably insignificant (Frostell *et al.* 1991), haemoglobin should be monitored daily (Powronznyk & Latimer 1997).

Chemical reactions continue after therapeutic benefits end. Nitric oxide and haemoglobin (nitrosyl haemoglobin) is oxidised to methaemoglobin (Grover 1993), which impairs oxygen carriage (see Chapter 18).

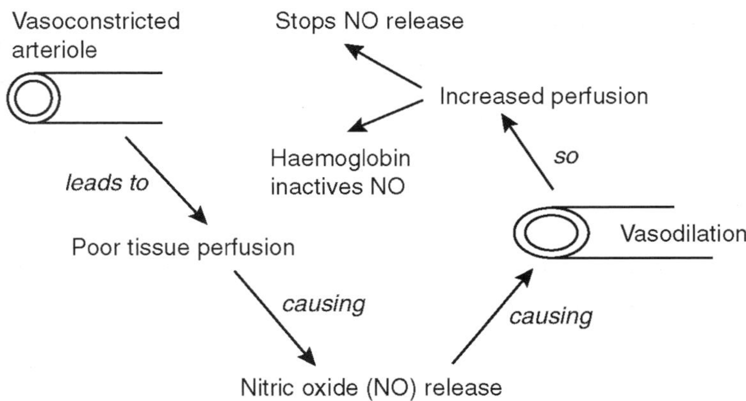

Figure 28.1 **The production of nitric oxide by endothelium**

Therapeutic use

Inhaled nitric oxide

- dilates pulmonary vasculature
- reduces pulmonary vascular resistance
- optimises gas exchange

but its effect varies. Gerlach and Falke (1995) report 20 per cent reductions in pulmonary vascular resistance, but their study combined nitric oxide with prostacyclin, so that the effect of nitric oxide alone is unclear.

Low levels of inhaled nitric oxide selectively vasodilate pulmonary capillaries in ventilated alveoli (Mulnier & Evans 1995), reducing pulmonary shunting, V/Q mismatch and improving arterial oxygenation (Abman *et al.* 1994). Young *et al.* (1994) measured mean improvements of 2.5–3 kPa in PaO_2.

Due to rapid inactivation, inhaled nitric oxide does not cause significant systemic vasodilation (Frostell *et al.* 1991, Holowaty 1995), and so will not compound hypotension. However, rapid inactivation also necessitates continuous delivery, including minimising any disconnection times.

Krafft *et al.*'s (1997) meta-analysis found average patient mortalities of 40 per cent when using nitric oxide; overall ARDS mortality of 50–80 per cent might suggest benefit from nitric oxide, but recent analyses question whether nitric oxide reduces mortality (Schewebel *et al.* 1997).

Compared with ECMO, nitric oxide is relatively cheap, requiring only minimal additions to familiar ventilator circuits (Grover 1993).

Levels

Therapeutic use of nitric oxide potentially exposes staff and others to toxic effects. Nitric oxide is quickly metabolised, and so long-term toxicity may be insignificant, but this has not yet been clarified (Mulnier & Evans 1995).

COSHH (Containment of Substances Hazardous to Health) regulations (Health & Safety Executive 1989) limit employee exposure to 25 ppm of nitric oxide and 3 ppm of nitrogen dioxide. The National Institute of Occupational Safety and Health is more cautious, recommending limits of 1 ppm nitrogen dioxide (Young *et al.* 1994).

Dose ranges vary greatly in literature. Animal studies have often used larger doses than those needed to treat ARDS, while doses needed to treat pulmonary hypertension in humans exceed those needed to treat ARDS. Recommended doses range from up to 100 ppm in Young *et al.*'s (1994) animal study to 0.1 to 18 ppm (Quinn *et al.* 1995). Lowson *et al.* (1996) found maximum haemodynamic and oxygenation responses at about 1 ppm. Many users agree with Abman *et al.*'s (1994) 3–10 ppm. Dellinger *et al.* (1998) suggest that arterial oxygenation is improved and pulmonary hypertension reduced with as little as 5 ppm, but that levels are safe up to 40 ppm.

As response is individual, dosages should be individually titrated, without exceeding permitted safety levels.

Literature gives a similarly wide range for toxicity. Frostell *et al.* (1991) found little evidence of toxicity below 100 ppm; Rossaint *et al.* (1993) extended this down to 50 ppm; doses used to treat ARDS appear to be safely below toxic levels and COSHH limits, although long-term effects remain unclear. Therapeutic doses appear small beside environmental nitric oxide and nitrous oxide pollution, heavy traffic, cigarette smoking (400–1,000 ppm (Frostell *et al.* 1991)) and indoor heating appliances, particularly gas-fired stoves (Greenough 1995).

Disconnection of closed circuits (e.g. endotracheal suction) exposes staff and others to possible danger. The short half-life may prevent this being problematic, but closed circuit suction should be used to protect others (and prevent loss of PEEP).

Possible problems

Nitrogen dioxide

Even small doses of nitrogen dioxide cause acute lung injury from pneumonitis and fulminant pulmonary oedema (Grover 1993). High concentrations of nitric oxide hasten nitrogen dioxide formation; Frostell *et al.* (1991) identified 50 per cent conversion from 10,000 ppm within 24 seconds (room temperature 20°C), compared with seven hours for 10 ppm. Dellinger *et al.* (1998) measured 1.5 ppm nitrogen dioxide from 80 ppm nitric oxide. Ventilator flow rates and I:E ratio do not affect conversion, but high oxygen concentrations (FiO_2 0.7–0.8) may (Miller *et al.* 1994). Nitrogen dioxide levels should be monitored if using more than 40 ppm nitric oxide (Dellinger *et al.* 1998).

Pulmonary complications

Inhaled nitric oxide enters functional alveoli, and so selectively vasodilates ventilated lungfields (Mulnier & Evans 1995), diverting blood from unventilated alveoli and thus delaying healing and recovery (Grover 1993). Nitric oxide also inhibits platelet-derived growth factor release, and so may inhibit smooth muscle proliferation and increase atherosclerosis (Foubert *et al.* 1993). It may also prolong coagulation (Greenough 1995); its brief half-life should limit systemic effects from inhaled nitric oxide, although pulmonary bleeding may occur with trauma (e.g. endotracheal suction).

The abrupt removal of nitric oxide can cause rebound pulmonary hypertension (Mulnier & Evans 1995; Rykerson *et al.* 1995), and so nitric oxide should be gradually weaned. The literature does not suggest rates for weaning, but pulmonary artery pressure monitoring can identify rebound hypertension.

Quinn *et al.* (1995) suggest prolonged exposure to as little as 2 ppm can decrease antioxidant defences and increase alveolar permeability. Although 'prolonged' is not clarified, both these effects may prolong critical illness.

Methaemoglobin

If nitric oxide binding to haem exceeds metabolism, methaemoglobin occurs (Greene & Klinger 1998), although therapeutic doses are usually sufficiently low to prevent this (Rykerson *et al.* 1995). Studies measuring methaemoglobin conversion found ranges of 1–3 per cent; Dellinger *et al.* (1998) measured 2.5 per cent conversion from 80 ppm nitric oxide. Most authors (e.g. Semple and Bellamy (1995), Mulnier and Evans (1995)) recommend measuring methaemoglobin levels to ensure they remain below 3 per cent, especially if the nitric oxide dose exceeds 40 ppm (Dellinger *et al.* 1998). Methaemoglobin makes pulse oximetry saturation unreliable (see Chapter 18).

Equipment

The short half-life necessitates quick access to spare cylinders. When changing cylinders, these should be flushed through before use to clear residual nitrogen dioxide (Greenough 1995).

As a possible toxic pollutant, environmental contamination by nitric oxide should be controlled. Scavenging systems may or may not be necessary (Mulnier & Evans 1995; Young & Dyar 1996) .

Nitrogen dioxide is far more toxic and should be monitored in both inhaled and exhaled gas (Grover 1993).

Professional issues

Nitric oxide is produced in the UK for medical use under special licence; the gas itself is not licensed for medical use (Young & Dyar 1996), and seems likely to remain unlicensed. This apparent contradiction means that manufacturers are not liable for any problems arising from its use (Young & Dyar 1996). Claims for compensation might therefore be made directly against nurses (or their employers).

Nitric oxide should therefore be considered as an experimental drug. Nurses using it must accept their professional accountability in accordance with the Code of Professional Conduct (UKCC 1992a), Scope of Professional Practice (UKCC 1992b), Standards for Administration of Medicines (UKCC 1992c) and local policies and guidelines.

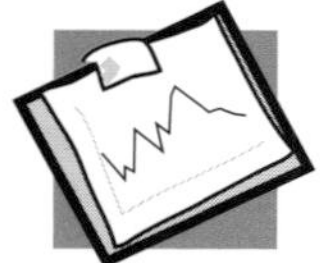

Implications for practice

- benefits from nitric oxide remain unproven
- nitric oxide can form nitrogen dioxide, a highly toxic environmental pollutant
- atmospheric levels should be controlled by measuring exhaled nitric oxide and nitrogen dioxide levels

- methaemoglobin levels are probably insignificant
- delivery should be continuous, disconnection from circuits being avoided whenever possible.
- closed circuit suction systems should be used for all patients receiving nitric oxide therapy
- staff and (where possible) patients and significant others should be informed about nitric oxide
- units using nitric oxide should consider the professional implications of its use, clarifying local protocols as appropriate

Summary

Nitric oxide is used to treat pulmonary hypertension and ARDS. Initial enthusiasm has now been tempered by studies debating its efficacy. Therapeutically, many aspects of nitric oxide and its use need further clarification, including benefits and long-term effects. Like many novel therapies, use has been largely confined to rescue attempts when more conventional therapies have failed; rather than attempting to repair damage, prevention of progression is a logical goal.

Nurses have a responsibility to maintain safe environments for patients, others and themselves, and may be responsible for monitoring environmental levels in ICU. They should understand therefore uses and dangers of nitric oxide.

Further reading

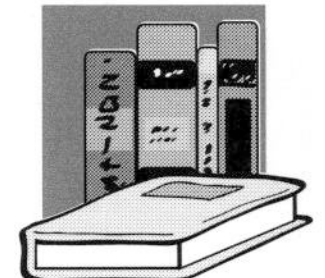

Many medical articles on nitric oxide have appeared; Greenough (1994) gives a useful overview, although rapid changes in knowledge base limit the use of material this old; Powronznyk & Latimer (1997) is a useful, more recent, overview, while Cuthbertson *et al.* (1997) give the most comprehensive guidelines to date for medical use of nitric oxide in the UK. Dellinger *et al.* (1998) is the most recent comprehensive trial to date. Rykerson *et al.* (1995) was one of the earliest comprehensive nursing perspectives; Camsooksai (1997) is a useful adjunct to this.

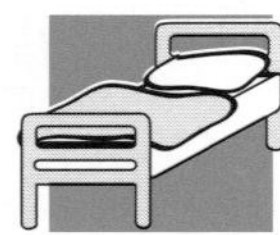

Clinical scenario

Ann O'Reilly, who is 45 years old and weighs 104 kg, is being treated on ICU for ARDS and sepsis. Despite inverse ratio ventilation, prone positioning and other therapies, Mrs O'Reilly's alveolar gas exchange remains poor. Her pulmonary vascular resistance (PVR) is double normal values and she has V/Q mismatch. The doctors decide to commence nitric oxide (NO) in order to reduce her PVR.

Q.1 List the equipment required to safely administer nitric oxide to Mrs O'Reilly via her ventilator. How are inhaled nitric oxide concentrations measured?

Q.2 How is the effectiveness of nitric oxide assessed with Mrs O'Reilly? Critically analyse the rationale for monitoring her methaemoglobin levels every 12 hours.

Q.3 After 24 hours Mrs O'Reilly's PVR is calculated to be 175 dyn/sec/cm^{-5}, her arterial oxygenation has improved and NO therapy withdrawn. Identify problems associated with withdrawal; examine local guidelines/protocols and the ICU nurse's role in this process.

Chapter 29

Alternative ventilatory modes

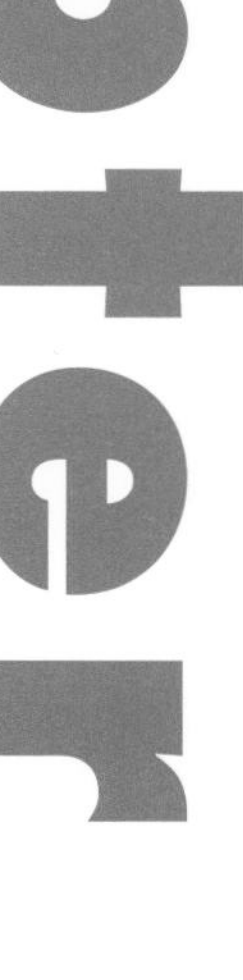

Contents

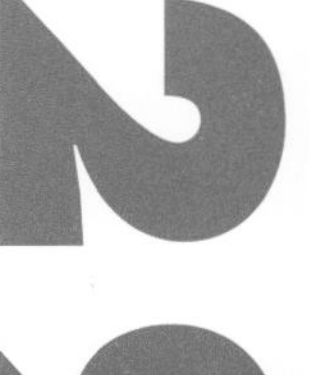

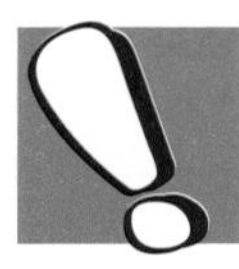

Fundamental knowledge

Alveolar physiology, gas exchange and pulmonary function
Surfactant production and physiology
V/Q mismatch

Introduction

Although conventional ventilators (see Chapter 4) remain the mainstay of ICU respiratory support, less familiar modes are available when conventional positive pressure ventilation proves unsuitable, although their use is often confined to specialist units. Modes discussed in this chapter are:

- extracorporeal membrane oxygenators (ECMO)
- extracorporeal carbon dioxide removal ($ECCO_2R$)
- intravenous oxygenators (IVOX)
- high frequency ventilation (HFV), especially oscillatory (HFOV) and jet (HFJV)
- liquid ventilation (perfluorocarbon – PFC)
- hyperbaric oxygenation

Alveolar recovery is optimised if

- inflated sufficiently to prevent further atelectasis
- movement is minimised
- overdistension (high peak inflation pressure) is avoided

Many modes discussed here achieve these aims, enabling improved alveolar recovery. The modes described may be useful for treating patients with ARDS, pneumothoraxes, poor lung compliance, contusion, fractured ribs flail chest and crush injuries.

These modes are often used as a last resort, when conventional techniques have already failed and prognosis is poor. Much literature on infrequently used, but not novel, modes is often either old or recycled, usually reflecting paediatric practice, so advantages and disadvantages identified do not always recognise changes in practice or applicability to adults.

When patients are critically ill, their conscious level is often severely impaired; where patients are conscious, the efficient carbon dioxide removal of most modes (carbon dioxide being more soluble than oxygen) reduces respiratory drive. Patients may find these modes more comfortable, and so require less sedation and analgesia (reducing complications from these drugs). However, hypocapnia may cause respiratory alkalosis (see Chapter 18).

ECMO

Extracorporeal membrane oxygenation (ECMO), initially developed as 'bypass' for open-heart surgery (see Chapter 30), can assist ventilation, usually supplementing conventional intermittent positive pressure ventilation. $ECCO_2R$ and IVOX (below) are variants of ECMO. There are two types of oxygenators; *bubble* oxygenators, simpler, cheaper and use less prime, but cause greater blood cell damage from turbulence; *membrane* oxygenators are therefore better for prolonged ICU use (Hug & Shanewise 1994).

ECMO can reverse neonatal 80 per cent mortality to 83 per cent survival (Bohn 1991), but survival with older children is only 50 per cent (Morton 1993) and most adult studies achieve only about 10 per cent survival (Mudaliar *et al.* 1991). However, some recent studies (e.g. Peek *et al.* 1997) found 60 per cent survival to hospital discharge (underlying mortality for ARDS and MODS approaches 100 per cent).

Like haemofiltration, ECMO pumps blood extracorporeally through a semipermeable membrane, usually at 70–120 ml/kg/min (Caron & Berlandi 1997). Circuits can be venoarterial (V–A) or venovenous (V–V); venoarterial circuits (usually from right jugular vein to right common carotid artery) are more likely to cause fatal emboli, and so are rarely used with adults (Greenough 1994), but venovenous circuits (usually right internal jugular vein to femoral vein) require adequate cardiac function.

Hollow fibres with silicone enable gas diffusion (Morton 1993), oxygenation being determined by membrane surface area and pump flow rate. Circuits require anticoagulation to prevent thrombus formation on synthetic tubing, although heparin-bonded tubing should not need additional heparin.

Low volume and rate IPPV is normally maintained during ECMO to prevent atelectasis.

The complications of ECMO include:

- *respiratory alkalosis*: supplementary carbon dioxide (e.g. carbogen – 5 per cent carbon dioxide, 95 per cent oxygen (Caron & Berlandi 1997)) may be needed (Morton 1993);
- *sepsis*: highly invasive cannulae enable microorganism migration; patients are usually severely immunocompromised;
- *haemorrhage*: from cannulation of major vessels;
- *coagulopathies/DIC*: circuits cause physical trauma to platelets (as with haemofiltration), compounding problems from anticoagulants and underlying pathologies; platelet and erythrocyte damage is reduced with transmembrane pressures below 300 mmHg (Caron & Berlandi 1997);
- *thrombi/emboli*: from stasis and coagulopathies;
- *cost*: from equipment, staff and extending life (or death) of very sick patients, usually consuming other costly treatments (Bohn 1991). Patients treated with ECMO incur double overall costs of other critically ill patients (Mudaliar *et al.* 1991).

ECCO$_2$R

Modified ECMO circuits using low blood flow (20–30 per cent of cardiac output) can be inserted intravenously (femoral vein, minimally invasive percutaneous saphenous vein) to remove carbon dioxide.

Supplementary oxygen will be needed, usually given as pressure-limited IPPV to reduce alveolar trauma (Gattinoni *et al.* 1986). Apnoeic intratracheal oxygen with PEEP can also be used (Mudaliar *et al.* 1991).

$ECCO_2R$ and ECMO have similar complications, although $ECCO_2R$ is less invasive.

IVOX

Intravenous oxygenators resemble miniature ECMO membranes placed percutaneously into the cardiovascular system (inferior vena cava (Young & Sykes 1994), right internal jugular vein (Conrad *et al.* 1995)). The heparin-coated membrane (Powell & Paes 1992) prevents thrombus formation.

Pure oxygen is passed through the fibres, potentially exposing tissues to toxic oxygen levels. Oxygen delivery may achieve 10–28 per cent of requirements (Young & Sykes 1994). Carbon dioxide removal is more efficient; Sim *et al.* (1996) suggest that IVOX should primarily be viewed as a carbon dioxide removing device.

IVOX shares most of the complications of ECMO; additional complications include:

- *internal placement* makes monitoring, adjustment and control more difficult than ECMO (Powell & Paes 1992);
- *time*: IVOX has been used for up to 29 days (Powell & Paes 1992), but users should remember their liability if exceeding manufacturers' recommended times;
- *haemorrhage*: from cannulation of major vessels;
- *thrombus formation*: Imai *et al.* (1994) measured average thrombus formation of 2 grams each day, accumulation being greatest in the first 96 hours. Thrombosis may also occur following removal;
- *oxygen toxicity*: although not reported in literature, prolonged exposure of endothelial cells to pure oxygen with IVOX presumably causes the same complications as pure oxygen from conventional IPPV (see Chapter 18).

High frequency ventilation (HFV)

High frequency ventilation includes various infrequently used modes, which have largely failed to establish a place in practice. High frequency jet ventilation (HFJV) is the one most frequently seen in ICU, although recent developments with high frequency oscillatory ventilation (HFOV) appear promising.

HFV delivers frequent (often above 100/min) but small (e.g. 1–3 ml/kg (ACCP 1993)) tidal volumes (usually smaller than dead space volume), providing efficient oxygenation with minimal chest movement and sheer damage to alveoli.

Carbon dioxide removal is normally achieved by manipulating inspiratory: expiratory time, pressure or volume. Hypocapnia can readily occur.

High frequency oscillatory ventilation (HFOV)

Traditional HFOV negative pressure cuirasses (e.g. Hayek oscillator) are rarely seen in ICU, but the introduction of a significantly different oscillatory ventilator appears promising for ICU use; this combines a mechanical diaphragm with a near-conventional ventilator to produce oscillatory tidal waves of gas (essentially superimposing 5–10 hertz oscillation onto CPAP) at up to 600 breaths each minute. Developed initially for paediatric use, adult versions are currently being tested.

Preliminary results with ARDS patients suggest this ventilator can deliver higher mean airway pressures (improved gas exchange) with lower peak pressure (less barotrauma) and reduced (potentially toxic) oxygen levels than conventional ventilators (Fort *et al.* 1997).

The complications of HFOV include:

- *prototype equipment*: mechanical breakdown currently limits adult use, although technological progress should resolve this problem;
- *novel therapy*: until current trials are completed, knowledge is largely limited to theory, anecdotes and preliminary reports;
- *peak intra-alveolar pressures*: these are higher than measurable peak airway pressure; excessive pressure may impair perfusion, so increasing mean airway pressure will achieve little (V/Q mismatch);
- *noise*: like CPAP, high frequency modes are usually noisy, provoking stress responses, inhibiting sleep, and contributing to sensory overload.

High frequency jet ventilation (HFJV)

HFJV (or 'jet'), the most widely used high frequency mode in ICU, uses tidal volumes of 1–5 ml/kg (Allison 1994) (with most adults, approximately the same volume as physiological dead space). Ultra-high frequency ventilation can deliver 600 breaths each minute (Gluck *et al.* 1993), but faster rates tend to cause gas trapping (thus raising peak pressures); peak airway pressure is minimised with rates of 60–100 (Sykes 1986). HFJV can be delivered through minitracheostomy (Allison 1994), thus preventing many complications of intubation.

Carbon dioxide clearance is efficient. Pulmonary secretions are mobilised, presumably due to constant chest wall 'quivering' resembling physiotherapy, so increasing alveolar surface area and gas exchange.

The complications of HFJV include:

- *safety*: most jet ventilators have few alarms, chest wall movement and air entry are barely perceptible, spirometry is impractical, and capnography inaccurate (Sykes 1986) so that nurses have to trust ventilators to deliver preset tidal volumes. Blood gas analysis and pulse oximetry are among the few remaining means of monitoring;

- *variable tidal/minute volumes*: these make effects of changes difficult to predict (Sykes 1986); Ackerman *et al.* (1985) recommend checking blood gases within a few minutes of changes, rather than waiting the standard 15–20 minutes;
- *gas trapping/shunting*: from minimal lung recoil (Kalia & Webster 1997);
- *mucosal injury*: if gas jets directly onto tracheal wall (Tan & Oh 1997a); this is especially likely to occur when ventilated through minitracheostomies;
- *peak intra-alveolar pressures*: as HFOV;
- *humidification*: large minute volumes cool and dry epithelium, causing sputum plugs (Molloy *et al.* 1992); over-humidification can cause fluid overload, but inadequate humidification may cause necrotising tracheobronchitis (ACCP 1993). Humidification of jet ventilation remains problematic, although pump-controlled instillation of fluid (Pierce 1995) and specialised humidifiers (e.g. high temperature vaporisers (ACCP 1993)) should enable adequate humidification. Nurses should actively assess humidification status, reporting and recording problems;
- *noise*: as HFOV.

Liquid ventilation

Perfluorocarbon (PFC) is an effective medium for gas carriage and exchange; currently few significant adverse effects or complications have been identified. After prolonged animal trials and more recent neonatal use, liquid ventilation is now being used in some adult ICUs to treat ARDS.

Perfluorocarbon can dissolve up to 50 ml of oxygen in every 100 ml (Greenough 1996) (plasma carries 3 ml per 100 ml); carbon dioxide, which is more soluble than oxygen, has a fourfold solubility in perfluorocarbon compared to water (Greenough 1996). Perfluorocarbon has very low surface tension (one-quarter that of water) so that lung compliance is increased (Greenough 1996). Animal studies have found that liquid ventilation (compared with conventional ventilation)

- reversed atelectasis (Leech *et al.* 1993; Tooley *et al.* 1996)
- improved macrophage response (Smith *et al.* 1995)
- produced fewer reactive oxygen radicals (Smith *et al.* 1995)
- improved shunt fraction (V/Q mismatch) from more even pulmonary capillary blood flow throughout the lungs
- reduced pulmonary oedema

Pneumoprotection protects pulmonary epithelium from inflammatory effectors of ARDS and SIRS (Kallas 1998).

Initial use was clumsy, relying on instillation and the removal of each tidal volume of oxygen-saturated perfluorocarbon through a liquid ventilator (Norris *et al.* 1994) (*total liquid ventilation*). This method has largely been superseded by *partial liquid ventilation*: instilling fluid daily (after endotracheal suction) over a couple of hours, until a meniscus is seen within the endotracheal tube (Kallas 1998). Partial liquid ventilation can be achieved using conventional ventilators, although perfluorocarbon lost through evaporation (Greenough 1996) should be replaced.

Whether ventilation is partial or complete, perfluorocarbon (heavier than water) should be trickled down to fill dependent alveoli, to prevent alveolar collapse (Dirkes *et al.* 1996). During instillation, patients should lie supine, and be ventilated with pure oxygen (Kallas 1998). Once instilled, the liquid maintains the patency of alveoli. Mucus, sputum and other lung fluids are lighter than perfluorocarbon, and so should float to the surface where they can be removed; failure to remove tenacious secretions can obstruct endotracheal tubes. Following suction, perfluorocarbon fluid level should be topped up and the volume instilled recorded. Secretions and fluid removed should be measured and recorded.

Complications of liquid ventilation include:

- *long-term effects unknown*: monkeys killed three years after one hour's treatment had analysable amounts of perfluorocarbon in lungs and fat tissue (Greenough 1996). Perfluorocarbon appears to be inert (Greenspan 1993), but animal studies do not always reflect human experience. Clinical usage may extend for many days, and so absorption (if problematic) may limit treatment (Greenough 1996). Despite extensive animal studies, human experience is relatively limited;
- *air trapping*: may cause pneumothoraces (Greenough 1996) or mucous plugs (Kallas 1998). Decreased tidal volume during instillation indicates possible air trapping, which should be confirmed through radiography with radio opaque dye;
- *increased intrathoracic pressure*: should logically occur through instilling intrathoracic fluid. Increased intrathoracic pressure should reduce cardiac output, but this does not seem to occur (Greenough 1996);
- *increased pulmonary vascular resistance* (Greenough 1996).

Hyperbaric oxygen

Ratios between gases in air remain constant; if temperature remains constant, water content (volume) of humidified air also remains constant. Thus changes in atmospheric pressure alter the volume of each gas that can be dissolved in plasma.

At normal sea-level atmospheric pressure (approximately one bar) only small volumes of oxygen are dissolved in plasma (3 ml oxygen per 100 ml blood); if haemoglobin carriage is prevented (e.g. carbon monoxide poisoning), tissues rely on plasma carriage.

Twenty-one per cent oxygen at 2.8 bar (= 18 metres depth of water) increases oxygen pressure from 21 kPa to 284 kPa, providing sufficient plasma carriage to meet normal metabolism (Pitkin *et al.* 1997).

Hyperbaric oxygen reduces half-life of carbon monoxide from 250 minutes in room air and 59 minutes with 100 per cent oxygen to 22 minutes with 100 per cent oxygen at 2.2 bar (Hinds & Watson 1996).

Hyperbaric chambers can be *single patient* or *rooms* which staff and equipment can enter. Hyperbaric pressure can be discontinued once haemoglobin oxygen carriage is available (at most, usually a few hours).

The complications of hyperbaric oxygen include:

- *evidence*: is largely limited to enthusiastic anecdotes rather than controlled trials;
- *high atmospheric pressures*: cause barotrauma to ears, sinuses and lungs, grand mal fits and changes in visual acuity (Oh 1997);
- *oxygen toxicity*: if prolonged (Oh 1997);
- *monitoring*: pulse oximetry has little value as oxygen carriage is not by haemoglobin (Pitkin *et al.* 1997);
- *access*: single-person chambers may prevent equipment (including ventilators) being used, while transfer of equipment (e.g. emergency equipment) between normal and hyperbaric pressures may be restricted or delayed. This may affect ventilation, inotropes and other infusions/mechanical support;
- *scarcity*: few units have hyperbaric chambers, necessitating long-distance transfer of hypoxic patients.

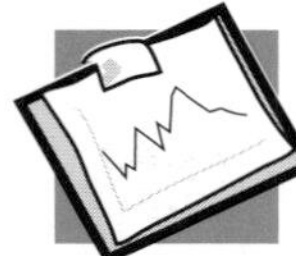

Implications for practice

- modes discussed in this chapter may be rarely seen; where used, staff should take every opportunity to become familiar with their use
- these modes are usually used with the sickest patients, so individual complications of each mode are compounded by complications of severe pathophysiologies; nursing care should be actively planned to optimise safety for each patient
- visitors and patients may be anxious about use of rarer modes, or frightened by particular aspects (e.g. liquid ventilation = 'drowning'), so should be reassured
- monitoring facilities are often limited with unconventional modes, and so nurses should optimise remaining facilities (e.g. pulse oximetry, blood gases), which may need to be measured more frequently
- particular problems of modes (e.g. humidification with HFJV) should be actively monitored
- highly invasive modes (e.g. ECMO) may cause haemorrhage; cannulae should (where possible) be easily visible
- sensory disruption (e.g. HFV noise) should be minimised

Summary

Modes discussed in this chapter are rarely used, but may offer significant benefits to some patients. ICUs not using these modes may transfer patients to units which do. This chapter provides an introduction to these modes for staff unfamiliar with them or new to units where they are used. More experienced users will wish to pursue supplementary material.

Whenever rarer modes or treatments are used the potential for unidentified complications is increased. Therefore the decision to use (or suggest) alternatives modes should be tempered by considerations of patient safety:

- How will the patient benefit?
- What are the known complications?
- What is the likely risk from unidentified complications (research base)?
- Do staff on the unit have the competence to use the mode safely?

Where unusual equipment is used, staff should take every reasonable opportunity to become familiar with it, but remember the focus of nursing should be the patient, not the machine.

Useful contact

Helpline for hyperbaric oxygen: 01705–822351, ext. 41769

Further reading

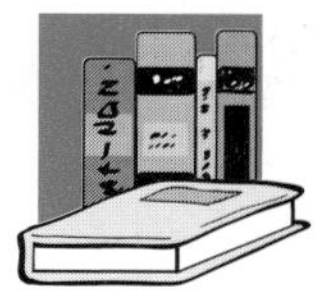

Most clinical literature on these modes is found in medical journals. Kallas (1998) provides a useful review of various modes. Peek *et al.* (1997) provide a recent review of ECMO. Allison (1994) offers a relatively recent overview of jet ventilation. Fort *et al.* (1997) offer a valuable preliminary report on HFOV. Greenough (1996) discusses liquid ventilation, while Smith *et al.* (1995) provide one of a number of more substantial studies.

Fewer nursing articles have appeared on these modes; Dirkes (1996) gives a reasonable summary of liquid ventilation, although discusses medical treatment rather than nursing care.

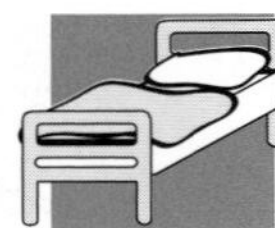

Clinical scenario

Gary Powers is a 22-year-old who, whilst working in construction, sustained a crush injury to his chest and head injury when a wall collapsed on top of him. Chest X-ray has revealed flail chest with multiple rib fractures, haemothoraxcis and lung contusions. He was invasively ventilated using high frequency jet ventilation (HFJV).

Q.1 List the ventilator settings usually recorded with HFJV and note other respiratory observations to be documented.

Q.2 Gary is unconscious with a closed head injury. Justify the use of HFJV with potentially increased intracranial pressures, explain the mechanism by which PCO_2 is reduced and suggest strategies to minimise environmental noise.

Q3 Analyse the effectiveness of humidification with HFJV and propose the most appropriate methods to ensure adequate humidification for Gary.

Chapter 30

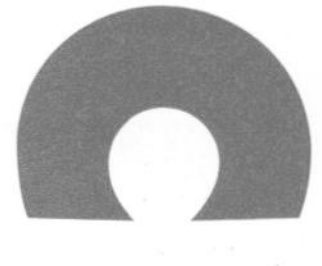

Cardiac surgery

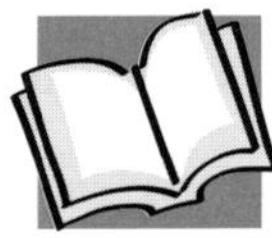

Contents

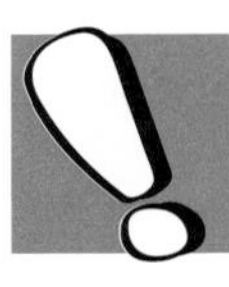

Fundamental knowledge

Cardiac anatomy: arteries and valves
Coronary artery disease

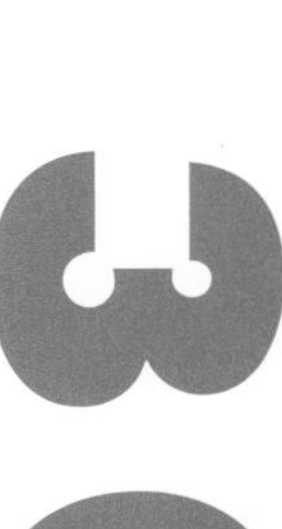

chapter 30

Introduction

Coronary artery and valve disease (see Chapter 24) remains a major cause UK mortality. When drug therapies cannot support cardiac failure, surgery is needed either to repair or replace damaged tissue. The NHS performed 33,000 open heart operations in 1993–4 (Bailey 1995), most admitted to ICUs. Hospitals not performing open heart surgery may still transfer patients to or receive patients from specialist centres. This chapter describes most open heart procedures, percutaneous ('closed') alternatives, means to support failing hearts (intra-aortic balloon pumps, ventricular assist devices), and transplant surgery. Much nursing care follows from problems and potential problems caused by surgical procedures; this chapter begins by briefly describing intraoperative procedures.

Aortic dissection and aortic root repair, although not discussed in this text, share many of the approaches and problems of open heart surgery.

'Bypass' can variously mean:

- blood pump oxygenators, or cardiopulmonary *bypass* (CPB; also called ECMO, see Chapter 29) which replaces cardiac and lung function during surgery;
- surgery which grafts vessels to *bypass* occlusion in coronary arteries.

In this chapter, 'bypass' refers to grafts; in practice, contexts often clarify intended meanings.

Perioperative

Open heart surgery usually uses median sternotomy incision. The heart is isolated and either arrested (with cardioplegia) or slowed (with β-blockers, usually to about 40 bpm). Sternotomy repair with permanent wire loops (usually five – visible on X-rays) leaves a distinctive permanent skin scar. Sternal wounds and chest drain tubing can cause considerable postoperative pain, making patients reluctant to breathe deeply (predisposing to chest infection).

CARDIOPULMONARY BYPASS This replaces heart (and lung) function, although not all surgery, or surgeons use CPB. Complications ascribed to CPB (some unconvincingly), include:

- neurological ('post-pump delirium')
- blood cell trauma (platelets, erythrocytes, leucocytes)
- clumping and consumption of clotting factors (especially reduced platelet counts)
- microemboli
- vasoactive mediators release
- protein denaturation

- fat emboli
- systemic immune response
- increased vascular permeability
- haemodilution (CPB circuits hold 1–2 litres)
- reduced haematocrit and colloid osmotic pressure (erythrocyte loss and damage)

Many problems (e.g. post-pump delirium) are blamed on nonpulsatile flow; pulsatile oxygenators may reduce systemic inflammatory responses (Driessen *et al.* 1995), but probably have few significant advantages (Chow *et al.* 1997).

The return of CPB circuit volume at close of surgery forces diuresis. Osmotic (e.g. mannitol) or loop (e.g. frusemide) diuretics may be given before leaving theatre to prevent fluid overload, but contribute to haemodynamic instability in ICU. Residual cardioplegia can cause hyperkalaemia.

Disconnection and reconnection of major vessels, together with surgery on heart tissue, exposes patients to possible air (micro)emboli, causing possible postoperative neurological and coronary dysfunction.

CARDIOPLEGIA A potassium-rich crystalloid used to arrest myocardium and so reduce metabolic oxygen demand, this can cause postoperative dysrhythmias. Traditionally, cold cardioplegia (4–10°C) was used to reduce metabolism, but hypothermia causes

- myocardial depression ('stunning')
- ventricular dysrhythmias
- increased blood viscosity
- reduced cerebral blood flow
- increased systemic and pulmonary vascular resistance
- cell dysfunction

and many other complications (Price & Donahue 1994; Barden & Hansen 1995). 'Warm' (normothermic) cardioplegia is more cardioprotective, and so increasingly used (Earp & Mallia 1997).

HYPOTHERMIA (CORE TEMPERATURE OF 28–32°C) This reduces metabolic oxygen demand and causes peripheral vasoconstriction (reducing venous capacity). To prevent hypervolaemia, 2 units of blood are usually removed for postoperative **autologous** transfusion. Postoperative rewarming causes vasodilation, necessitating fluid monitoring and replacement.

Postoperative complications

Common postoperative complications therefore include:

- pain

- neurological dysfunction
- multiple and various dysrhythmias
- hypothermia and hypervolaemia
- hypovolaemia on rewarming
- initial polyuria causing hypokalaemia
- haemodilution
- anxiety

Infection is a potential problem, but postoperative infection can usually be prevented through infection control and active care. Surgeons usually prescribe prophylactic antibiotics. Nurses should follow infection control guidelines and observe and report any signs of infection. Preventative care is identified in various sections below.

Valve surgery

Mitral valvotomy, a 'closed' or 'open' procedure, dilates encrusted mitral valves. Surgery does not require cardiac arrest. However, valvotomy merely replaces incompetent semiclosed valves with incompetent dilated ones; valve replacement has largely usurped valvotomy in First World countries.

Replacement valves

- tissue (human cadaver, **xenografts**: porcine, bovine, baboon)
- prosthetic (e.g. Bjork-Shirley®, Starr Edwards®)

Tissue valves avoid the need for long-term anticoagulation (Grotte & Rowlands 1992), but usually fail within 6–10 years (Hudak *et al.* 1998), and so are mainly given to older patients (Treasure 1995) whose life expectancy is limited. As tissue valve failure is usually slow, elective replacement is possible.

Prosthetic valves last longer (often for 10–12 years) but require lifelong anticoagulation to prevent embolisation. Failure is usually sudden (Grotte & Rowlands 1992), valve fracture causing incompetence. Most models have a distinctive click, which may be heard on auscultation.

Valve surgery causes greater cardiovascular and pulmonary dysfunction, especially dysrhythmias) than bypass grafts (Unsworth-White *et al.* 1995).

Percutaneous valvuloplasty, used less in the UK than in other First World countries (Lamerton & Albarran 1997), has similar success to mitral valve replacement without needing open-heart surgery (Lamerton & Albarren 1997). However, many postoperative risks remain, including:

- tamponade
- infarction
- emboli
- dysrhythmias (from oedema and manipulation)
- chest pain (Lamerton & Albarren 1997)

Coronary artery bypass grafts

Occluded coronary arteries can be bypassed by grafts to restore myocardial blood supply. Autoharvest avoids complications of rejection. Traditionally, grafts were saphenous vein or internal mammary artery (IMA, especially left – LIMA), but radial artery grafts (Shapira *et al.* 1997) are increasingly used. Other grafts include:

- pedicle (grafts remain attached to subclavian artery, distal ends being anastomosed beyond occluded coronary artery)
- cephalic vein from arm (if patient has varicose veins)
- homograft veins
- synthetic grafts (poor patency rates)
- porcine/bovine grafts (smaller in size and aneurysm more likely)
- gastoepiploic artery
- inferior epigastric arteries

Saphenous veins are easier to harvest, so reducing CPB time. One graft is needed for each occluded vessel; each additional graft increases CPB and complication risks.

IMA grafts have longer patency (and survival) rates than vein grafts (Ryan 1995); postoperative problems include:

- pain (parietal pleural incision, used for IMA harvest, disrupts richly innervated tissue);
- spasm (arterial muscle), causing angina-like pain and more bleeding from anastomoses (Ryan 1995).

Percutaneous coronary angioplasty (PTCA)

Compared with open heart surgery, percutaneous approaches enable quicker recovery and reduce short-term costs, although long-term benefits are more questionable (Hlatky *et al.* 1997), especially for elderly patients (De Gregorio *et al.* 1998).

Percutaneous coronary angioplasty dilates stenosed arteries through inflation of a balloon-tipped catheter. Endothelial damage from angioplasty may leave a flap of intima, which can cause sudden *occlusion* (Brady & Buller 1996). Implanting coronary stents widens the lumen, reducing severity of restenosis (Brady and Buller 1995).

Perioperative acute vessel closure requires urgent graft surgery, causing debate about whether on-site facilities are essential (Rowlands 1996b).

Minimally invasive cardiac surgery

Minimally invasive surgery exposes patients to fewer complications from wound healing and tissue repair; median sternotomy can be replaced by thoracotomy (Suen *et al.* 1997).

Transmyocardial laser revascularisation can supplement or replace bypass surgery or angioplasty, especially for patients with diffuse coronary artery disease or at high risk from conventional cardiac surgery (Trehan *et al.* 1998).

Complication rates are low (Morgan & Campanella 1998). Minimally invasive saphenous vein harvest significantly reduces postoperative pain (Horvath *et al.* 1998), but analgesia is still needed (Carlson 1997). Bleeding may occur, and so chest drains are inserted (Carlson 1997). Nasal cannulae can usually provide sufficient respiratory support (Carlson 1997).

Intra-aortic balloon pumps (IABP)

Intra-aortic balloon pumps can support a failing heart. Balloon inflation in the upper descending aorta (see Figure 30.1) is synchronised with diastole, displacing (usually) 40 ml of blood both upward (coronary and cerebral arteries, improving myocardial and cerebral perfusion) and downward (increasing systemic pressure, perfusion and preload, shown by augmented pressure on arterial blood pressure traces – see Figure 30.2).

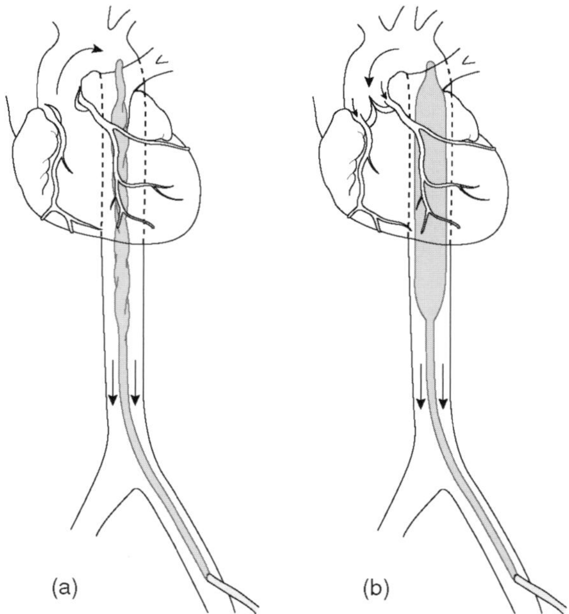

Figure 30.1 The catheter of an intra-aortic balloon pump (deflated and inflated)

Problems of IABP include complications of femoral artery cannulisation

- rapid haemorrhage
- difficulty observing the site
- infection

Balloon rupture (rare) or gas diffusion through the balloon exposes gas used to aortic blood, and so soluble gases (e.g. helium) are used. Gas cylinders maintain constant pressures to compensate for leaks. Alarms should sound before reserve gas in cylinders is exhausted, but nurses should still check cylinder volume and know how to replace them.

Ventricular assist devices (VAD)

VADs can be dual-chamber (see Figure 30.3), but single chamber left ventricular assist devices (LVADs) are usually used. Unlike intra-aortic balloon pumps, they replace, rather than support, a failing heart. This enables survival, but exposes severely immunocompromised patients to highly invasive equipment, infection and thromboembolism (Tsui & Large 1998).

Technological intervention (IABP, VAD) to support, but not cure, heart failure creates ethical dilemmas, and so balloon pumps are usually only used as a 'bridge' to transplantation, cardiac surgery, or postoperative recovery.

Tsui and Large (1998) describe cardiomyoplasty as the biological equivalent to artificial hearts, but long-term benefits and risks have not yet been clarified.

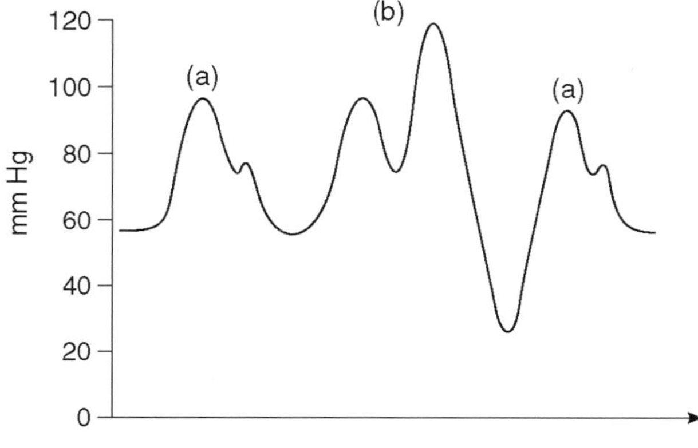

(a) Unassisted arterial pressure
(b) Augmented pressure with inflation increasing pressure after closure of the aortic valve creating a second pressure wave after the dicrotic notch

Figure 30.2 Arterial pressure trace showing augmented pressure from use of an intra-aortic balloon pump

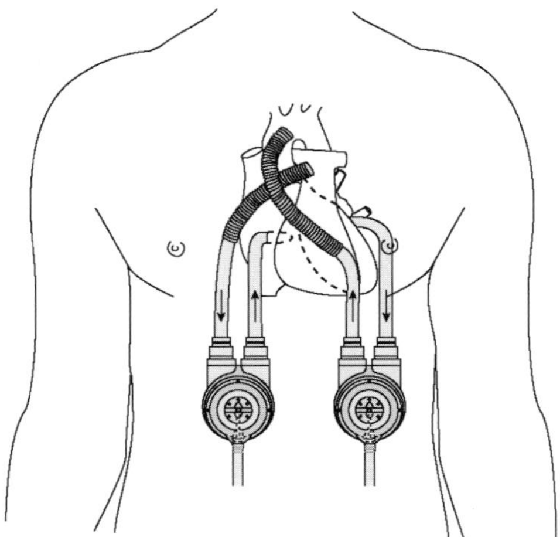

Figure 30.3 A ventricular assist device (VAD)

Transplants

Heart and heart/lung transplant can resolve endstage cardiac failure. Approximately 400 heart transplants are performed each year in the UK (MacLean Dunning 1997). Insufficient supply (approximately 6,000 waiting (MacLean & Dunning 1997)) and preoperative mortality (21–30 per cent on waiting lists (Tsui & Large 1998)), has encouraged interest in *xenograft* (including genetically engineered) and artificial alternatives, despite continuing problems with each alternative.

Postoperative nursing

In addition to the needs of any postoperative patient, cardiac surgery creates specialised needs.

Preparation

Any surgery is likely to be daunting for patients, but long-standing heart disease and traditional emotional connotations of the heart can heighten anxieties of patients undergoing cardiac surgery. Recovery is improved through preoperative information (Hayward 1975), and patients (and families) can find preoperative visits useful (Lynn-McHale *et al.* 1997).

Most patients undergoing cardiac surgery have only single organ failure and so recovery is usually rapid, patients usually being transferred to step-down units the following day. Seeing and helping patients progress rapidly can be very rewarding for nurses. Emphasis should therefore focus on normalisation, promoting homeostasis and encouraging patients to resume normal activities of living.

Ventilation

Traditionally, postoperative ventilation was routinely used until normothermia and homeostasis were restored. Fluid shifts, hypovolaemia, infusion of large volumes of intravenous fluids, and myocardial surgery (forming oedema and dysrhythmias from irritation) make cardiovascular status volatile in the immediate postoperative period. Artificial ventilation therefore ensures adequate ventilation and oxygenation while cardiovascular stability and pulmonary blood flow are restored. Extubation exposes patients to risks from atelectasis and hypoventilation, while pain or fear of pain cause reluctance to breathe.

Auscultation may detect possible atelectasis (a major risk given the area of surgery) or accumulation of secretions. *Suction* is necessary to remove secretions and secretions may accumulate without obvious sounds to indicate their presence but, like any other aspect of care, suction should not become routine; trauma from excessive endotracheal suction may delay recovery. Patients rarely need to be weaned from short-term ventilation.

Hypoventilation and *impaired cough* may be caused by

- pain
- fear
- impaired respiratory centre function

Pulmonary complications delay discharge for 25 per cent of patients following coronary artery bypass grafts (Johnson & McMahan 1997). With adequate analgesic cover, patients should be encouraged to breathe deeply and cough. Unstable sternal wounds may need support during coughing and deep breathing. Incentive spirometry is often useful.

Following cardiac surgery, patients are traditionally ventilated until stable; increasingly, centres encourage early extubation (often in theatre). Early extubation hastens recovery, patients needing less inotropic support, suffering less anxiety and developing fewer chest infections (Maxam Moore & Goedecke 1996; Jenkins 1997). Debate about early extubation arouses strong emotions, both sides having valid arguments, but it supports philosophies of normalisation.

Hypertension and hypotension

Initial hypertension from hypothermic vasoconstriction may damage anastomoses, causing bleeding. Medical staff usually indicate upper limits for systolic pressure, frequently 100–120 mmHg, prescribing vasodilators (e.g. glyceryl trinitrate – GTN, sodium nitroprusside – SNP). Persistent hypertension unresponsive to nitrates indicates neurological damage.

Hypotension is usually due to

- hypovolaemia on rewarming
- myocardial dysfunction.

Fluid is replaced to maintain CVP. Hypotension, despite adequate CVP, indicates myocardial dysfunction; inotropic support may be needed to maintain tissue perfusion.

Bleeding

Significant bleeding is usually from:

- anastomoses
- coagulopathies.

Any sutures can prove incompetent, but aortic (from CPB) and myocardial sutures are exposed to high pressure and heartbeat/pulse movements. Arterial spasm with IMA grafts usually cause more bleeding. Pericardial bleeding may cause rapid *tamponade*. Two or three drains are inserted in the following regions:

- pericardial
- mediastinal
- pleural (if pleura injured).

Low suction (-100 cmH_2O/-13 kPa) (Gordon *et al.* 1995)) assists drainage. Closed systems should be maintained, and clamps made available in case of disconnection.

On arrival, volumes in each drain should be marked. Drainage, usually recorded hourly, should gradually reduce, becoming more serious. Sudden cessation may indicate thrombus obstruction, with likely tamponade; if patency of drains cannot be re-established, this should be reported urgently as emergency thoracotomy may be needed. The value of milking drains is debated; they can restore patency, but large negative pressures may damage tissue (Gordon *et al.* 1995). Gordon *et al.* (1995) recommend drains should only be milked if a clot or other obstruction is visible. Dependent loops in chest drain tubing may inhibit drainage, so although evidence is lacking, they should be avoided (Gordon *et al.* 1995).

Coagulopathies are multifactorial (e.g. heparinsation using CPB), being monitored through clotting studies (e.g. **ACT** bedside measurements). Haemostasis may require

- platelets/FFP
- protamine sulphate (reverses heparin)
- vitamin K

- aprotinin (Trasylol®) (plasmin and kallikrein inactivator) (Rodrigus *et al.* 1996)
- tranexamic acid (Pinosky *et al.* 1997)

Fluid balance

Postoperatively, patients may have large negative fluid balances from

- fluid shifts (vasoactive mediators, low colloid osmotic pressure)
- forced diuresis.

Reversing hypothermia causes vasodilation, necessitating large volumes of fluid. Total body hydration is normally maintained with continuous low-volume crystalloid infusion (e.g. 5 per cent glucose), but tissue perfusion and cardiac return necessitate haemostasis so that most fluids replaced are colloidal (see Chapter 33).

Fluid charts may be divided between colloids (colloidal infusions against blood loss) and crystalloids (crystalloid infusion against urine output). Colloid replacement is given to maintain central venous pressure (e.g. above 10 mmHg); 'driving' central venous pressure hastens peripheral perfusion, and so rewarming. Blood is often transfused if haemoglobin falls below 10 g/dl (haematocrit below 33 per cent). Haemodilution with colloids usually necessitates blood supplements, and so patients should already have units crossmatched.

Temperature

Gradual rewarming should bring central temperature within 2°C of peripheral (pedal) temperature (avoid limbs from which saphenous veins are harvested). Use of artificial warming is controversial: it can cause burns, although recently marketed warming devices are generally safe and reliable; it hastens homeostasis and may prevent shivering (which increases metabolic rate, so increasing oxygen consumption and metabolic acidosis).

Hypermetabolism creates heat, so when rewarmed 'overshoot' pyrexia may occur.

Acid–base balance

Anaerobic metabolism from cold cardioplegia and hypoperfusion causes metabolic acidosis so that cardiovascular instability continues during rewarming. Acidosis can cause dysrhythmias. Although acidosis is closely monitored through blood gas analysis, it is not usually necessary to treat acidosis following cardiac surgery.

Dysrhythmias

Various dysrhythmias (often multifocal) often occur following cardiac (especially valve) surgery. Resolution is usually spontaneous and relatively quick. Causes include:

- chronic cardiomyopathy
- oedema (from surgery, disrupting conduction pathways)
- acidosis
- electrolyte imbalance
- hypoxia/ischaemia
- mechanical irritation (e.g. drain/pacing wire removal)
- hypothermia

Only symptomatic and problematic dysrhythmias normally need treatment (drugs, pacing or resuscitation).
Atrial fibrillation, the most common postoperative dysrhythmia (Ellis 1998), is relatively benign. *Bradycardia*, *blocks*, *junctional* and *tachydysrhymias* frequently occur; persistent blocks often require pacing, hence perioperative placement of epicardial wires. Epicardial wires are unipolar, a negative pole being created by inserting a subcutaneous needle. Pacing wires usually remain in place until dysrhythmias become unlikely (normally 5–10 days).

Myocardial infarction may necessitate emergency thoracotomy/sternotomy and internal massage/defibrillation (although limited infarction may cause little more than minor ECG changes and not require resuscitation). Staff should know, therefore, where thoracotomy packs are situated. Internal defibrillation avoids transthoracic bioimpedance, so uses lower voltage (e.g. 20–50 J).

Electrolyte imbalance

Other than potassium, imbalances rarely require treatment. Causes include:

- *fluid shifts* from vasoactive mediators
- *hyperkalaemia* from damaged cell membranes leakage
- *hypokalaemia* from forced diuresis; also cell recovery returning potassium to intracellular fluid
- *hormones* (e.g. aldosterone, ADH)

Hypokalaemia necessitates frequent potassium supplements, usually diluted in small volumes of maintenance crystalloid fluid to maintain plasma concentrations of 4.0–4.5. Hyperkalaemia may necessitate insulin and dextrose infusion (which can cause later rebound hyperkalaemia).

Renal function

Following initial polyuria, patients may become oliguric from

- reperfusion vasodilation
- increased circulating ADH (stress response).

Driving central venous pressure protects renal perfusion. Supplementary diuretics may be used, but some patients later require haemofiltration (see Chapter 35).

Urinary catheters can normally be removed the day after surgery.

Prolonged peri- and postoperative hypotension can precipitate acute tubular necrosis. Renal protection with dopamine is increasingly being replaced by dobutamine or dopexamine (see Chapter 32).

Pain control

Pain control is central to intensive care nursing; absence of pain is desirable for both humanitarian and physiological reasons (see Chapter 7); poor pain control may prolong recovery, circulating catecholamines impairing myocardial perfusion. Early postoperative pain usually needs opiate infusion, possibly supplemented by nonsteroidal anti-inflammatories.

Although Kuperberg and Grubbs (1997) found patients were satisfied with their analgesia, many studies (e.g. Valdix & Puntillo 1995; Cottle 1997) suggest postoperative pain control remains poor with nurses underestimating pain (Ferguson *et al.* 1997). Ferguson *et al.*'s (1997) finding that pain scores increased with time contrasts with (or may result from) reduced supply/strength of analgesia.

Pain is individual and so should be individually assessed rather than stereotyped by the operations performed. Since thoracic nociceptor innervation is relatively sparse, patients often experience relatively less pain from thoracic incisions than from saphenous incisions, although arterial graft spasm (e.g. IMA) can cause angina, and IMA harvest disrupts richly innervated tissue. Nitrates (e.g. GTN) dilate arteries, reducing spasm pain and tension on newly grafted vessels. Saphenous vein harvest necessitates a long incision, stimulating many nociceptors, thus causing considerable pain (Horvath *et al.* 1998).

Types of pain experienced following cardiac surgery include:

- bone pain (sharp/throbbing)
- visceral pain
- muscle pain (harvest site)
- cardiac/angina pain
- neurogenic pain
- psychogenic pain (anxiety)

Patterns may be:

- continuous
- sudden/spasm

Continuous analgesia may alleviate underlying/continuous pain (including anxiety-related pain), but nurses should observe for breakthrough (usually spasm) pain.

Sedation, a valuable adjunct to promote comfort, is usually limited to a few hours, and so rapidly cleared drugs (e.g. Propofol) are usually used. The hypotensive effects of Propofol can compound hypovolaemia from rewarming.

Neurological complications

Potentially fatal thrombi (and emboli) may be from

- cardiopulmonary bypass
- air emboli
- thrombotic vegetations (chronic preoperative atrial fibrillation).

Neurological deficits can cause

- impaired peripheral nerve function
- cerebral/cognitive deficits
- uncontrollable hypertension (injury to vital centres).

Neurological assessment is a priority, but cerebrovascular accidents may remain undetected until patients show deficits or fail to wake normally. Nurses suspecting abnormal neurological recovery should seek urgent assistance.

Psychological considerations

Psychological stressors of ICU (see Chapter 3) compound additional stressors through symbolic connotations which, despite anatomical knowledge, still surround the heart (people 'love with their heart', not with other vital organs). Postoperatively, mood is often labile, euphoria (induced by opiates and survival) being followed (day 2–4) by reactive depression.

Barris *et al.*'s (1995) small-scale study found that most patients experience transient neuropsychological dysfunction following graft surgery. Stress provokes tachycardia, hypertension and hyperglycaemia (see Chapter 3), all impairing recovery in patients least able to tolerate such insults. Providing information, achieving optimum pain control, relieving anxieties and minimising sensory imbalance are therefore important aspects of holistic nursing care.

Skin care

Wound breakdown or skin ulceration may occur from (Waterlow 1996; Lewicki *et al.* 1997):

- prolonged (often 2–4 hours) surgery
- hard operating tables
- profound hypothermia (with anaerobic metabolism).

Following transfer to ICUs, patients often remain unturned on canvasses for 2–4 hours (to allow surgical stabilisation). Significant pressure sores usually develop following transfer from ICU, but vigilance, active assessment of pressure areas when removing canvasses and early intervention can prevent many complications that delay discharge home.

On regaining consciousness, pain and anxiety often make patients reluctant to move. Good pain management and patient education can prevent many complications. Sternal instability can cause 'clicking' sounds; although not painful, external stabilisation with hands or a cushion helps deep breathing and coughing.

Wound dressings are usually removed within 24 hours, and then left exposed unless oozing. Debilitation and poor cardiac output may delay wound healing. Sternal wound dehiscence is rare (3 per cent), but can prove fatal (Kuo & Butchart 1995), especially following IMA grafts (which can reduce sternal blood supply by up to 90 per cent); complete sternal dehiscence necessitates surgical intervention.

Perfusion of graft sites (especially radial artery grafts; also arteriovenous shunts) should be protected, and so pressure (e.g. sphygmomanometer cuff, tourniquet) should be avoided.

Normalisation

Nurses can experience considerable satisfaction from assisting rapid postoperative recovery following cardiac surgery. Normalisation should be urged, and families and friends encouraged to visit, as they would on a surgical ward. The day following surgery, patients may enjoy breakfast before transfer.

Early mobilisation should be supported, musculoskeletal complications and pulmonary emboli being the main causes of delayed discharge (Johnson & McMahan 1997). Mobilisation may begin in ICU with active exercises.

Transplantation issues

The severing of the sympathetic and parasympathetic pathways causes loss of vagal tone, resulting in resting rates of about 100 beats/minute (Adam & Osborne 1997). Denervation also (usually) prevents angina, increasing risk of silent infarction (12 per cent of patients do experience pain (Tsui & Large 1998)).

A loss of sympathetic tone impairs cardiac response to increased metabolic demands, making atropine ineffective (Adam & Osborne 1997).

Surgery preserves recipients' right atrium, resulting in two P waves (one intrinsic, one graft) (Adam & Osborne 1997). Although not pathologically significant, the reasons for the presence of two P waves should be explained to patients, families and junior nurses.

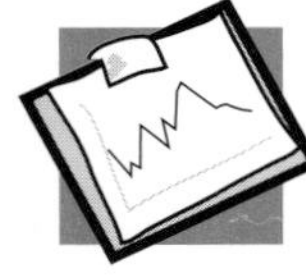

Implications for practice

- the care of patients following cardiac surgery has much in common with the care of other postoperative patients, but it requires continuing full individual assessment
- nursing care should focus on normalisation
- neurological events may prove fatal; report any indications of deterioration
- physical and psychological pain cause various complications; patients should receive adequate analgesia, its effect being monitored by frequent assessment
- preoperative visits and information can significantly reduce stress, but psychological care of both patients and their families remains a nursing priority
- relatively rapid recovery requires nurses to spend much time on the technical roles of assessing, observing and administering drugs, but the human elements of care should simultaneously be maintained

Summary

Most patients undergoing cardiac surgery are admitted to ICU following treatment for single system failure, and so usually recover rapidly. This can be both rewarding and time-consuming for nurses. Many possible postoperative complications result from the necessities of intraoperative procedures; increasing percutaneous surgery may significantly reduce numbers of open heart operations.

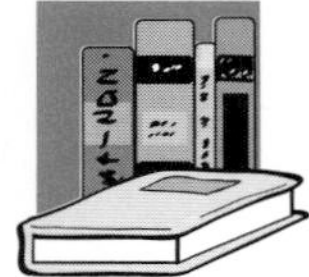

Further reading

Material on cardiac surgery often dates quickly, and so check ICU or hospital libraries which often stock current articles/journals; most texts and specialist journals include material on cardiac surgery. Gordon *et al.* (1995) provide a thorough literature review of chest drain management. Jenkins (1997) discusses nursing care following early extubation. Rowlands (1996b) describes percutaneous surgery. Dunning (1997) offers useful insights to artificial hearts.

Clinical scenario

Peter Da Silver is a 48-year-old man with a history of angina, hypertension and insulin dependent diabetes. He was admitted to ICU following a triple coronary artery bypass graft (CABG × 3) using saphenous vein and left IMA.

Q.1 Describe Mr Da Silver's preoperative preparation and explain relevance to ICU care (e.g. type of investigations, patient information, pre-admission visits, diabetes control, etc.).

Q.2 Examine the nursing priorities and identify potential complications for Mr Da Silver in the first 24 hours post-CABG surgery.

Q.3 Mr Da Silver develops dehiscence of his sternal wound and can feel his sternum moving on deep breaths and coughing. Review causative factors for this complication and propose a plan of care to stabilise sternum, promote healing and recovery (evaluate various treatment approaches, pharmacological/surgical interventions, equipment used to stabilise sternum, appropriate nutrition).

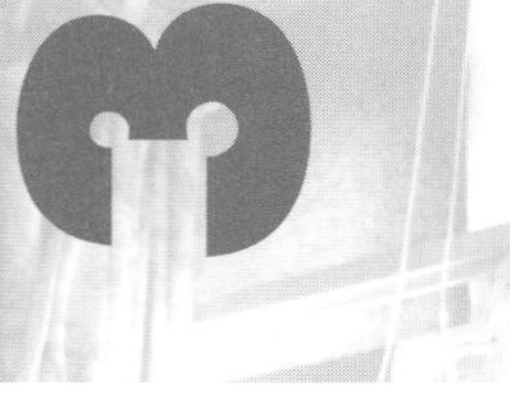
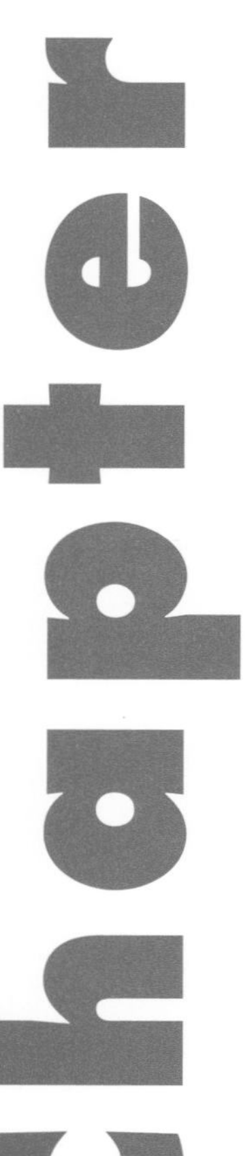

Chapter 31

Disseminated intravascular coagulation (DIC)

Contents

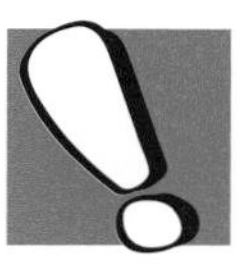

Fundamental knowledge

Normal intrinsic and extrinsic coagulation pathways

Introduction

Disseminated intravascular coagulation (DIC) causes one in every thousand USA hospital admissions, mortality exceeding 50 per cent (Thelan *et al.* 1990); ICU incidence and mortality is presumably higher. DIC is secondary to other pathologies, and has been called various other names (e.g. 'consumptive coagulopathy', 'defibrination syndrome').

DIC is uncontrolled systemic activation of coagulation, just as SIRS is uncontrolled systemic activation of inflammatory homeostatic responses. Haemostasis has four phases:

- smooth muscle contraction (vasoconstriction; myogenic reflex)
- formation of platelet plugs
- formation of fibrin clot (blood clotting/coagulation), followed by retraction of fibrin clots
- fibrinolysis.

Pathophysiology and treatments for this frequent complication of many other pathologies are described, together with three related syndromes:

- haemolytic uraemic syndrome (HUS)
- thrombotic thrombocytopenia purpura (TTP)
- heparin-induced thrombocytopaenia and thrombosis syndrome (HITTS)

Pathophysiology

DIC is a multifactorial syndrome caused by:

- bacteria (usually gram negative)
- viruses (especially varicella, hepatitis, CMV (Rutherford 1996))
- pregnancy (especially delivery/abortion – placenta and brain are especially rich in thromboplastin (Kelsey & Colvin 1997))
- crush injuries
- severe burns
- trauma
- hepatic failure (low-grade DIC) (Hambley 1995)

Whatever the initiating cause, pathological progression is similar.

Bacteria damage endothelium, exposing collagen and phospholipid, which activates factor XII (Rutherford 1996) (intrinsic clotting) and aggravates hypotension. Arterial hypotension triggers kallikrein and complements release. These highly vasoactive substances:

- further activate factor XII ('a' after a factor indicates activation: thus factor XII becomes factor XIIa)
- release kinin
- increase vascular permeability
- cause cell lysis

Cell lysis releases phospholipid, further activating factor XII. Proteolysis releases fibrin degradation products (FDPs), which aggravate microcirculatory obstruction and are potent anticoagulants. The hepatic reticulo-endothelial system, which normally clears FDPs, becomes overwhelmed by excessive degradation products or impaired liver function. Other circulating mediators of cellular injury, such as cytokines (e.g. IL-1, IL- 6, TNF) and antigen–antibody complexes, further complicate DIC, causing interstitial oedema and hypovolaemia.

The most effective diagnostic tests are **D-dimer** tests, platelet counts, antithrombin-3 levels and fibrin monomers (Jørgensen *et al.* 1992).

Progression

DIC causes four main complications:

- hypotension
- microvascular obstruction and necrosis
- haemolysis
- haemorrhage

Stagnation of capillary flow from prolonged hypotension and systemic arteriovenous shunting causes

- metabolic acidosis
- tissue and cell ischaemia
- intracapillary thrombosis

Procoagulant material from cellular injury enters the systemic circulation, activating widespread inappropriate clotting. Proteolysis stimulates further coagulation and fibrinolysis, causing disseminated generation of thrombin and plasmin. Excessive fibrin production and deposition consume clotting factors (hence 'consumptive coagulopathy') and cause inappropriate clotting.

Fibrin meshes

- obstruct blood flow (especially to arterioles, capillaries and venules) causing capillary ischaemia and tissue necrosis

- haemolyse the erythrocytes that do manage to penetrate the fibrin mesh
- trap platelets (hence low platelet counts).

Consumption of clotting factors leaves insufficient supply for homeostasis so that patients bleed readily (typically from invasive cannulae and trauma, such as endotracheal suction). DIC progresses rapidly, often occurring within a few hours of the initiating cause.

Signs

Early symptoms of DIC are typically nonspecific, such as

- mild cerebral dysfunction (e.g. confusion)
- dyspnoea
- mild hypoxia
- petechial bleeding (especially trunk)
- skin rashes
- purpura
- minor renal dysfunction
- spontaneous mucocutaneous bleeding

As DIC progresses, symptoms become more severe. DIC prolongs *clotting times*, with reduced counts of clotting factors (e.g. fibrinogen and platelets), with rising FDP levels. As coagulopathy progresses, patients bleed from multiple sites, clotting at bleeding sites taking progressively longer. Typically, ICU patients ooze blood from various cannulae sites; bleeding from arterial lines can become especially problematic due to pressure of arterial blood.

Skin symptoms are easily visible; subdermal haemorrhages cause purpura, the skin may appear cyanotic, mottled or cool, and in latter stages gangrene may develop.

Vascular fibrin deposits form throughout the cardiovascular system, progressive *organ failure* follows:

- lungs: especially ARDS, pulmonary emboli and pulmonary hypertension
- kidneys (intrarenal failure)
- liver failure
- cerebral: microthrombi may cause confusion or cerebrovascular accidents; unconsciousness may mask neurological symptoms

Highly vascular surface membranes are especially prone to haemorrhage. Bleeding may occur from traumatic endotracheal suction, further complicating respiratory function. The gastrointestinal tract is especially susceptible to haemorrhage, and so gastric drainage/aspirate and stools should be assessed for blood (including occult and melaena). If patients are not being fed enterally, stomach decompression (free nasogastric drainage) reduces stomach stretch and acid accumulation, thus helping to prevent haemorrhage.

Treatment

Treatments have varied over time and between units. Being secondary to another pathology, underlying causes should be treated, but symptom control is usually needed to ensure survival:

- control source of inflammation
- maintain tissue oxygenation
- minimise oxygen demand
- optimise nutrition
- support other organs

Consumption of clotting factors often necessitates exogenous infusions (fresh blood, fresh frozen plasma: FFP, fibrinogen, platelets) to reduce bleeding temporarily, but restoring endogenous haemostasis (including through nutrition) will resolve underlying problems. Vitamin K may also be given.

Platelet infusions should be handled carefully, as turbulence (e.g. shaking) damages platelets, and given quickly through dedicated administration sets. Used blood-giving sets should not be used for FFP and other clotting factors, as anticoagulant used with blood may adhere to plastic and neutralise FFP.

Enthusiasm for releasing endogenous clotting factors by giving anticoagulants has waned, although debate about the value of heparin for DIC continues. Early beliefs that heparin would release clotting factors from microthrombi for normal homeostasis proved unfounded. Heparin helps to prevent further thrombus formation, but it also delays systemic clotting; with misdiagnoses of DIC, heparin may cause life-threatening haemorrhage.

Critical illness halves plasma antithrombin III levels; replacement to normal concentrations has been advocated (Thelan *et al.* 1990), but results have generally been disappointing (Kelsey & Colvin 1997).

Like SIRS, the mainstay of treatment remains system support – buying time while underlying causes are resolved. Since hypovolaemia is a common complication, fluid replacement with whole blood and plasma substitutes is likely (see Chapter 33). Severe acidosis may need treatment. System failure will be supported by appropriate interventions (e.g. ventilation, inotropes, haemofiltration). A range of other symptoms may also occur requiring treatment (e.g. antibiotics and cytoprotective drugs to prevent gastric bleeding).

Related syndromes

Some syndromes, rarely encountered on general ICUs, are similar to DIC.

HAEMOLYTIC URAEMIC SYNDROME (HUS) This is DIC largely localised to the kidneys, fibrin deposits in renal microcirculation causing renal failure. Parker (1997) suggests that HUS is the paediatric counterpart to TTP, but other authors apply HUS to adults.

The pathology of HUS is unclear, but Kelsey and Colvin (1997) suggest that the abnormal interaction of platelets and vascular endothelium triggers microvascular coagulation. The deranged clotting figures of DIC are absent, and platelets transfusion can exacerbate the problem (Kelsey & Colvin 1997). Treatments include FFP, plasma exchange, steroids (Kelsey & Colvin 1997) and prostaglandin.

THROMBOTIC THROMBOCYTOPENIA PURPURA (TTP) This is a rare condition, traditionally considered a separate syndrome from HUS, but with similar symptoms, pathophysiology and treatments (Parker 1997), extending to systemic and central nervous system involvement. Symptoms typically include purpura, neurological deficits, multifocal neuropsychiatric disturbances and renal failure. TTP is usually treated by plasmapheresis and supportive therapies.

HEPARIN-INDUCED THROMBOCYTOPENIA AND THROMBOSIS SYNDROME (HITTS) This is a complication of heparin therapy. Heparin stimulates heparin-dependent anti-platelet antibodies, causing intravascular platelet aggregation, thrombocytopenia and arterial and venous stenosis (Cavanagh & Colvin 1997).

Like DIC, HITTS can become fulminant, causing major organ infarction (e.g. myocardial, cerebral) or other major vessel occlusion (Cavanagh & Colvin 1997). The treatment is to stop heparin (Cavanagh & Colvin 1997).

Nursing care

Although DIC is a medical problem, and treatments will be medically prescribed, quality nursing care can significantly reduce complications from trauma, sepsis and bleeding. Many nursing interventions may provoke haemorrhage:

- endotracheal suction
- turning
- cuff blood pressure measurement
- rectal temperature
- enemas

- rectal/vaginal examinations
- plasters and tape
- shaving
- mouthcare

Some interventions may be necessary, although alternative approaches should be considered. For example, wet shaves are likely to cause bleeding; electric shavers may be safely used (staff may need to ask families to bring electric razors in, as electric shavers are usually unavailable in hospitals for infection control reasons). Similarly, foam sticks are less traumatic than toothbrushes. Lubrication of skin and lips (e.g. with white petroleum jelly) helps to prevent cracking. Invasive cannulae and procedures should be minimised to reduce risks of haemorrhage.

The sight of blood can cause many people great distress, often out of all proportion to the amount of volume lost. The loss of 5 ml of blood is physiologically unimportant, but can cause a large enough stain on bedding to create distress, and possible fainting. Anxiety of both patients and relatives/visitors should be remembered. Visitors should be warned about the possible sight of blood, escorted to the bedside, and observed until staff are satisfied about their safety. Relatives experiencing stress may transmit their fears to patients; apart from humanitarian reasons for reducing stress, it may increases fibrinolytic activity (Thelan *et al.* 1990), so aggravating coagulopathy.

Implications for practice

- patients should be closely observed/monitored for complications in all body systems
- nurses should minimise interventions that will cause trauma/bleeding
- visitors should be warned of the possibility of seeing blood, and should be escorted and observed until safe

Summary

DIC is a complication caused by a variety of pathological processes. Early treatments with anticoagulants have been largely superseded by more conservative (temporary) approaches of replacing clotting factors and treating symptoms to buy time while the underlying pathology is treated.

Nursing care should focus on avoiding complications of trauma, while minimising anxiety to both patients and relatives.

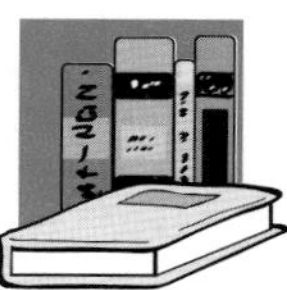

Further reading

Most intensive care textbooks contain sections on DIC. Of journal articles, Kesteven & Saunders (1993) and Rutherford (1996) give useful overviews.

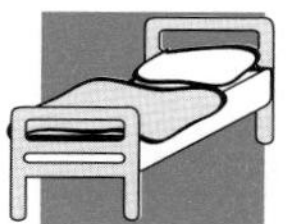

Clinical scenario

Kelly Jones, a healthy 18-year-old, ingested an unknown amount of MDMA (Ecstasy) at a local nightclub. On admission to ICU, Kelly was deeply unconscious, hyperthermic (40.1°C), tachycardic (140 beats per minute) with hypotension (80/40 mmHg). Treatments were commenced to correct her hyperthermia, hypotension and tachycardia; however, she later developed disseminated intravascular coagulation (DIC).

Kelly's haematological investigations included:

	Kelly's results	*Normal*
Prothrombin time	22 sec	1–15 sec
Partial thromboplastin time	60secs	39–48 sec
Thrombin time	15 sec	10–13 sec
Fibrinogen levels	0.1 g/100 ml	0.2–0.4 g/100 ml
Platelets	90×10^{-9}/l	150–400 $\times 10^{-9}$/l

Q.1 Identify which blood results are related to intrinsic activation and which are related to the extrinsic activation of Kelly's blood coagulation. With reference to physiology, explain why Kelly developed coagulation disorder from hyperthermia and hypermetabolic state.

Q.2 Cryoprecipitate, fresh frozen plasma and platelets are prescribed. Outline the rationale for this treatment and the nursing approaches which can maximise their therapeutic benefits (e.g. specify methods, routes and order of administration, storage, temperature, minimising bleeding points and/or further fibrinolysis, evaluating effectiveness).

Q.3 Kelly's prognosis is deemed poor and her family are informed. They begin to discuss the possibility of organ donation if she dies.

Reflect on how such a discussion should be managed, appraise the feasibility of organ donation (e.g. which tissues/organs can or cannot be used in the light of treatments, infusions of multiple blood products), ethical dilemmas, specialist services.

Chapter 32

Acute renal failure

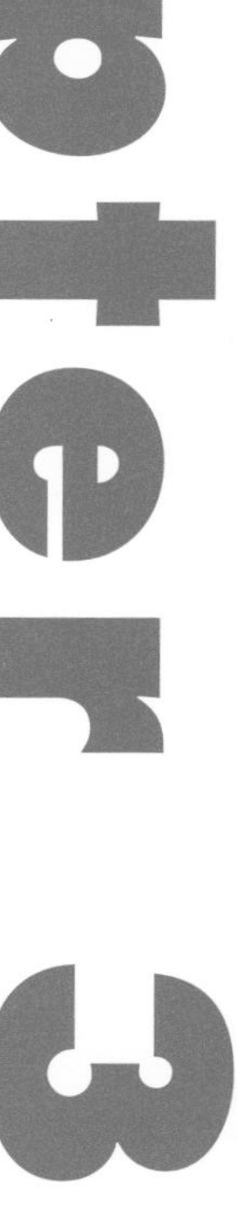
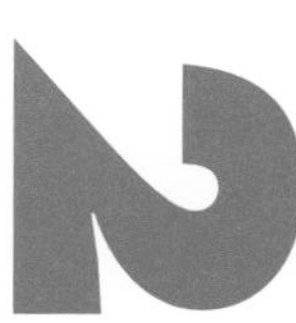

Contents

Fundamental knowledge

Renal anatomy and physiology

Introduction

Primary renal failure rarely occurs in ICUs, but renal hypoperfusion commonly complicates primary ICU pathologies, such as SIRS. Renal failure in ICU is therefore usually secondary and acute. When patients with pre-existing chronic renal failure are admitted, renal management usually continues previous care (e.g. peritoneal dialysis).

Distinctions between acute and chronic renal failure are arbitrary (often 100 days), but imply differences between potentially recoverable and incurable conditions. Acute renal failure is therefore potentially reversible; treatment aims to replace renal function while optimising recovery of renal tissue.

Acute renal failure can be classified as:

- prerenal
- intrarenal (intrinsic)
- postrenal

In this chapter, some treatments for renal failure are discussed, while haemofiltration is covered in Chapter 35. This chapter also describes some renal hormones (renin, atrial natriuretic factor and insulin-like growth factor) and rhabdomylolysis.

Renal failure is failure of the kidneys to perform normal metabolic functions (see Table 32.1). Oliguria (e.g. less than 0.5 ml/kg/min) is often a sign of renal failure, but functional failure can occur despite 'normal' or 'polyuric' urine volumes.

Table 32.1 The functions of the kidney

waste removal (urea and toxin metabolites)
maintenance of fluid balance
acid–base balance
electrolyte imbalance
renin production (hormone increasing blood pressure)
erythropoietin production (hormone stimulating erythrocyte production)
part of chain of vitamin D synthesis

Like most body systems, healthy kidneys have a large physiological reserve; adequate renal function can usually be maintained with urine outputs of about 450 ml/day. Renal failure indicates widespread (about three-quarters) non-function of nephrons. Endstage renal failure occurs when 90 per cent of nephrons fail, leaving a relatively narrow margin between recoverable and terminal failure.

Five per cent of hospital patients suffer acute renal failure (Appadu 1996), but the incidence in ICUs is higher; Sweny (1995) suggests that one-quarter of ICU patients require **dialysis**. As more patients survive primary pathologies, and the population becomes older, secondary renal failure is likely to increase.

Primary acute renal failure has a good outcome, but renal failure in ICUs is usually secondary to multiple organ failure, which carries a higher mortality. One-third of ICU patients with renal failure will die, but not usually from renal failure itself (Beale & Bihari 1992). Provided chronic failure is prevented, recovery of renal tissue (unlike other major organs) is usually complete.

Urea and creatinine

Most metabolites are excreted renally. Two easily measured metabolites (urea 60 kDa, creatinine 133 kDa) are useful markers of healthy renal function, but with critical illness become progressively unreliable (Stark 1998).

Blood nitrogen (see Chapter 9) is primarily transported as ammonia (NH_3). Nitrogen balance is restored by hepatic metabolism of ammonia to urea, which is excreted renally. Normal serum urea is 2.9–8.9 mmol/l; raised blood urea nitrogen (BUN) levels indicate failure of hepatic metabolism or renal excretion. Glomerular filtration of urea is influenced by many factors, such as tubular reabsorption of urea, metabolic rate, diet and drugs.

Creatinine, a waste product of muscle metabolism, varies with muscle mass; those with less muscle (children, older adults) usually produce less creatinine. In health, creatinine clearance reflects glomerular filtration rate, normal serum levels being 50–120 micromol/l. As creatinine clearance is highest in the afternoon (Sladen 1994), accurate measurement necessitates 24-hour urine collections.

Prerenal failure

Prerenal failure occurs where renal hypoperfusion causes failure of renal function. Critical illness (e.g. SIRS, cardiac failure) frequently causes profound and prolonged hypotension, in turn causing prerenal failure. Children are especially prone to hypovolaemia from diarrhoea and vomiting (Stewart & Barnett 1997). Prolonged ischaemia results in cellular damage and intrarenal failure. Cardiovascular complications will normally be apparent from routine ICU monitoring.

Since prerenal failure is caused by hypovolaemia rather than tubular damage, urinary sedimentation remains normal (Joynes 1996). As aldosterone increases renal reabsorption of sodium and water, urinary sodium can fall below 20 mmol/l (McHugh 1997), while urine **osmolality** rises (Joynes 1996).

In proportion to tissue weight, renal blood flow normally exceeds all other tissues except the carotid body (Ervine & Milroy 1997); however, renal tissue is especially susceptible to ischaemia. Damage to tubular epithelium from ischaemia causes cell dysfunction, allowing diffusion of filtered solute into interstitial tissue (Ervine & Milroy 1997). Intratubular accumulation of cellular debris further impairs tubular flow (Ervine & Milroy 1997), accelerating progression to intrarenal failure.

Intrarenal failure

Intrarenal failure is caused by:

- nephrotoxicity
- ischaemia
- inflammation

Intrarenal failure can be caused by acute glomerulonephritis and acute pyelonephritis, but intrarenal failure in ICUs is usually due to *acute tubular necrosis*.

Nephrotoxic drugs used in ICUs include amphotericin and gentamicin. Damage from nephrotoxicity is usually confined to epithelial layers; the epithelium readily regenerates, making recovery rapid (Carlson 1995).

Ischaemia or inflammation damages deeper tissue; if basement membrane damage occurs, regeneration is unlikely, leading to chronic renal failure (Carlson 1995).

Acute tubular necrosis used to be attributed to death of renal tubule cells, but pathology is more complex: while the problem is 'acute' and affects tubules, it is caused by ischaemia, rather than (necessarily) necrosis, of tubular cells. Hypoxia disrupts cell membranes (see Chapter 23) causing intracellular oedema and releasing vasoactive chemicals. Preglomerular vasoconstriction reduces glomerular perfusion, and so glomerular filtration. Widespread tubule intracellular oedema causes physical compression of lumens, obstructing flow of any filtrate produced.

Medullary damage from intrarenal failure reduces sodium reabsorption in the Loop of Henle, so that urinary sodium levels are high (above 40 mmol/litre (McHugh 1997)). Hypernatraemia in the *macula densa* activates the renin–angiotensin–aldosterone cascade, further reducing glomerular blood flow and filtration.

Intratubular sedimentation from cells rapidly obstructs flow, and the resulting retrograde pressure impedes filtration and can cause nephritis.

Tubular cells readily regenerate so that renal replacement therapy buys time until recovery. However, as with other body tissue, reperfusion injury (see Chapter 23) from calcium and oxygen radicals can reverse recovery.

Glomerulonephritis, inflammation of glomerular basement membrane, causes increased glomerular permeability. Large particles, such as erythrocytes and plasma proteins, may be filtered (Joynes 1996) or, with cellular debris, obstruct tubules, causing further back pressure (and damage) to glomeruli.

Postrenal failure

Postrenal failure, the main cause of renal failure in the community, rarely occurs in ICU. Caused by obstruction between the kidneys and meatus (such as bladder tumours, renal/bladder calculi or an enlarged prostate), the resulting back pressure reduces filtration (Carlson 1995) and can cause intrarenal damage. Postrenal failure is reversed by removing the obstruction.

Stages

The *oliguric* phase (urine production below 0.5 ml/kg/hr) of renal failure usually occurs within two days of precipitating events and usually lasts for 12 days, although it may persist for several weeks. Prognosis becomes bleaker with prolonged oliguria. As renal function fails, the volume of urine falls, while serum urea and creatinine levels rise.

Recovery begins with the *polyuric* (diuretic) phase. As damaged tubules begin to recover function and new (immature) tubule cells grow, filtration improves and obstruction to flow is removed. However, recovering and immature tubule cells function inefficiently. As selection tubular reabsorption of fluid and solutes is poor, large volumes of dilute urine are passed (up to 5 litres/day). Polyuric renal failure often persists for two weeks (Carlson 1995).

As tubular cells mature, *normal* function is recovered. Urea and creatinine levels fall, urine volumes return to normal, and electrolyte balance is restored. Full recovery can take 3–12 months (Carlson 1995).

Effects

Renal failure disrupts homeostasis, although some problems (e.g. vitamin D deficiency) are more likely to affect chronic than acute renal failure. The main complications to body systems which result from renal failure are:

Cardiovascular:

- pericarditis
- hyperkalaemia
- acidosis
- dysrhythmias
- anaemia
- hypertension (from renin)

Nervous system:

- confusion (from uraemia)
- twitching
- coma

Respiratory:

- acidosis
- pulmonary oedema
- hiccough
- compensatory tachypnoea

Gut:

- nausea
- diarrhoea
- vomiting

Metabolic:

- electrolyte disorders (see above)
- toxicity from active drug metabolites
- vitamin D deficiency

Passively and actively, peritubular reabsorption of sodium in exchange for potassium and/or hydrogen ions maintains homeostasis, and so renal failure usually causes electrolyte imbalance:

potassium: hyperkalaemia often occurs, although polyuria can cause hypokalaemia
sodium: hyponatraemia may occur, especially with polyuric failure
hydrogen: failure to excrete hydrogen ions causes metabolic acidosis

Hypocalcaemia, hypophosphataemia and hypomagnesaemia can also occur (Carlson 1995). Many of these electrolytes affect cardiac and other muscle cell conduction so that dysrhythmias and generalised muscle twitching/weakness may occur. Muscle weakness will limit the effectiveness of patient-initiated breaths and weaning.

Acid–base: normal renal function maintains acid–base balance by reabsorbing bicarbonate and excreting hydrogen atoms; urinary pH, normally about 5, can be as high as 8. Acidosis stimulates tachypnoea to compensate metabolic acidosis with respiratory alkalosis, but respiratory failure will limit effectiveness; excessive triggering (e.g. with SIMV or PSV) increases oxygen consumption, aggravating systemic hypoxia.

The main plasma protein creating colloid osmotic pressure, *albumin* weighs 66.5 kDa (Fleck & Smith 1998), and so is below renal threshold (68 kDa (Green 1976)); however, being an anion, it is repelled by negatively charged sialoproteins in glomerular capillaries (see Chapter 33), and so virtually no albumin is normally filtered.

With nephritis, albumin is filtered due to:

- loss of glomerular capillary negative charge
- increased glomerular bed permeability (inflammatory response).

Hypoalbuminaemia, common in ICUs, lowers colloid osmotic pressure so that intravascular fluid is lost into interstitial spaces ('third spacing'), resulting in hypovolaemia and oedema.

Afferent arteriole hypoperfusion causes juxtaglomerular cells to release renin. Renin initiates the *renin–angiotensin–aldosterone cascade*: angiotensin (a systemic vasoconstrictor) and aldosterone (increasing tubular reabsorption of sodium and water) increase systemic blood pressure and volume. Restoration of afferent arteriole perfusion pressure inhibits further renin release. This homeostatic mechanism therefore maintains renal perfusion pressure during hypovolaemia. But hypoperfusion from intrarenal problems (e.g. glomerulonephritis) still causes renin release, hence hypertension from chronic renal failure. Autoregulation fails when mean arteriole blood pressure falls below 70 mmHg (Carlson 1995); prolonged and profound hypotension frequently complicates critical illness. Similarly, prerenal failure from renal artery stenosis causes systemic hypertension which may compound cardiovascular complications.

Anaemia complicates renal failure due to:

- lack of erythropoietin (Schobersberger *et al.* 1998)
- platelet dysfunction (McHugh 1997)
- oxidative stress to erythrocytes from immunocompromise (Schobersberger *et al.* 1998)
- haemorrhage (e.g. from anticoagulants for haemofiltration).

Anaemia further compounds tissue (including renal) ischaemia.

Management

Too often prerenal failure remains undertreated, and so progresses to intrarenal failure; early intervention can prevent many complications. If renal failure is suspected, cardiovascular status should be optimised by providing adequate *fluids*. With relatively prolonged underlying pathologies (e.g. SIRS, MODS) inappropriate fluid shifts and hypoalbuminaemia will persist, so that fluids given to treat hypovolaemia should remain intravascularly. This necessitates using large-molecule fluids, such as hydroxethyl starches (unless patients are receiving renal replacement therapy, these can cause fluid overload, and so haemodynamic status should be closely monitored) rather than cheaper low molecular weight colloids (see Chapter 33). If cardiac failure is present, hypotension may require inotropic support.

Once blood volume and pressure are optimised, a *fluid challenge* helps to identify any failure of renal function. Although much debated, the choice between colloid and crystalloid for fluid challenges is probably less important than ensuring that glomerular beds receive sufficient volume to filter; fluid challenge should determine whether urine is produced, and so fluids well below renal threshold (crystalloid) are appropriate. However, fluids below capillary threshold will also be filtered into other body tissues, including alveoli. Pulmonary oedema can soon result from overload of low molecular weight fluids (such as crystalloid), so that fluid challenge volumes should be limited to sufficient to diagnose the problem.

If kidneys do not respond to fluid challenges, then medical management involves *drugs* (see below). Traditional *dietary* management aims to compensate for electrolyte imbalances and reduce glomerular workload (and so damage) by restricting protein (a 'renal' diet) (Uldall 1988), although this approach is now questioned.

When conservative measures fail, some form of *continuous renal replacement therapy* (see Chapter 35) is needed.

There are a number of possible new developments which may in time become established ways to manage renal failure, and these are discussed at the end of this chapter.

Diuretics

Frusemide blocks sodium reabsorption in the ascending loop of Henle; as reabsorption of water is passive, retention of sodium in filtrate increases urine volume. Increased intraluminal flow may prevent or remove tubular obstruction from debris (Adam & Osborne 1997). Frusemide is ototoxic and so should be given slowly; with high-doses this necessitates continuous infusion. Frusemide can cause hypokalaemia, so that with large doses ECG should be monitored and serum potassium levels checked.

Mannitol, an osmotic diuretic, also vasodilates renal blood vessels (Joynes 1996). Reducing interstitial fluid reduces tubular swelling, while increasing intraluminal flow clears obstructing debris (Joynes 1996). McHugh (1997) suggests that high-dose mannitol can reduce duration of dialysis, although this remains to be established. Mannitol is described further in Chapter 22.

Dopamine (DA_1) receptors (see Chapter 34) occur in the juxtaglomerular apparatus of afferent arterioles. Stimulation of dopamine receptors causes dilation, increasing glomerular blood flow, so increasing filtration volumes.

Dopamine does increase urine volume, but animal studies suggest that dopamine-mediated vasodilation only occurs with normal perfusion, urine volumes being increased by dopamine inhibition of sodium reabsorption in distal tubules (which contain more dopamine receptors than juxtaglomerular apparatus) rather than increasing glomerular filtration (Ervine & Milroy 1997).

Duke *et al.* (1994) found that creatinine clearance was not improved by dopamine, despite increased urine volumes, whereas dobutamine did improve creatinine clearance without significantly increasing urine volume. This confirmed Duke and Bersten's (1992) paper. Ervine and Milroy (1997) recommend dopexamine (at 2 mg/kg/min) to increase renal blood flow (this level exceeds recommended dose ranges).

Currently, there is growing evidence that dopamine treats staff and fluid balance charts rather than patients; it may have a place in removing fluid overload and preventing tubular obstruction, but dobutamine and other inotropes are increasingly replacing renal dopamine.

Renal rescue

A protocol from Charing Cross Hospital (London) aims to achieve normovolaemia, normotension and decreased ion pumping in the ascending loop of Henle by optimising fluid management (Palazzo & Bullingham 1994); this is effectively recognising and treating prerenal failure before it progresses. Early trials appear to reduce the need for dialysis. While management of multisystem-failure patients needs a holistic rather than a reductionist perspective, renal rescue protocols appear to be promising.

Renal rescue may also prevent progression necessitating ICU admission, and so is potentially valuable for critically ill patients outside ICUs.

Atrial natriuretic factor

Right atrial stretch causes release of the hormone atrial natriuretic factor (ANF, also 'atrial natriuretic peptide' – ANP; natriuresis = excretion of sodium in urine) so that distended atria resolve hypervolaemia through diuresis. Exogenous human atrial natriuretic peptide (extracted factor) can be given to improve creatinine clearance, reducing the need for dialysis and reducing mortality (Rahman *et al.* 1994).

Urodilatin (a renal peptide, similar to atrial natriuretic factor) improves diuresis without causing systemic hypotension (Cedidi *et al.* 1994).

Insulin-like growth factor

Animal studies show that this hormone (also called somatomedin C) stimulates anabolism, protein synthesis and renal perfusion. Being similar to insulin it may cause hypoglycaemia (Rennie 1996). Its therapeutic value for humans, if any, remains unproven.

Rhabdomyolysis

Awareness of rhabdomyolysis (muscle necrosis) is poor, but improving, yet it causes up to one-quarter of all cases of acute renal failure (Cunningham 1997). The causes of muscle damage include

- crush injuries
- thermal injury
- infection
- prolonged immobilization.

Myoglobin, the oxygen-carrying iron-containing pigment in skeletal muscle, is released; weighing 17 kDa, this is below renal threshold and so is filtered (colouring urine deep red or brown). Rapid renal clearance may prevent diagnosis from plasma levels. Precipitation (more likely with urinary pH below

5.6 (Sladen 1994)) in renal tubules or urinary catheters can obstruct flow, causing renal failure and further damage.

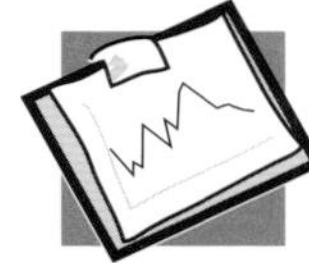

Implications for practice

- renal function should be measured by the ability of the kidneys to achieve and maintain homeostasis, not simply by the amount of urine produced
- the most useful biochemical markers of renal function are urea (blood urea and nitrogen – BUN) and creatinine
- factors outside the kidneys (e.g. metabolism) may affect glomerular filtration of urea, so blood urea alone is not a reliable marker
- the most common cause of renal failure in ICU patients is acute tubular necrosis caused by prerenal failure
- prerenal failure can often be prevented if patients receive adequate support to maintain perfusion
- renal failure prevents excretion of hydrogen ions from the body, so causes metabolic acidosis
- the many other metabolic functions of the kidney mean that renal failure causes complications for all other major systems
- diuretics may restore urine volumes; however, the value of many diuretics in renal failure is controversial

Summary

Acute renal failure frequently complicates other pathologies in ICU patients. While mortality from primary renal failure is encouragingly low, mortality from multisystem failure remains high.

Renal failure is failure of renal function, and so it causes fluid overload, electrolyte imbalances, acid–base imbalances and other metabolic complications; these further complicate underlying pathologies. Nursing care, therefore, should consider the holistic effects of renal failure. Haemofiltration, the main ICU renal replacement therapy, is discussed in Chapter 35.

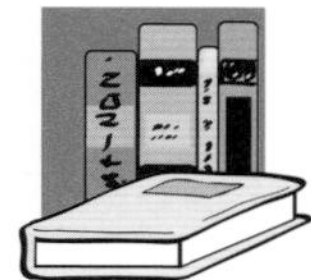

Further reading

Most applied physiology texts include overviews of renal failure, although recent changes in practice limit the value of older texts. Among journal articles, McHugh (1997) gives a useful general perspective; Stewart and Barnett's (1997) paediatric article is also useful. Cunningham (1997) describes rhabdomyolysis. Uldall's (1988) classic book on renal nursing is useful for basic principles, although its age necessitates cautious reading for changes in practice.

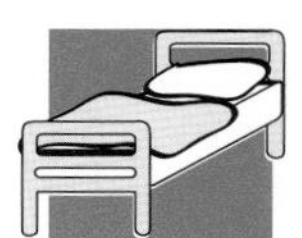

Clinical scenario

David Sinclair is a 58-year-old film critic who is known to suffer from hypertension, angina and gout. He has been taking large doses of ibuprofen, a nonsteroidal anti-inflammatory drug (NSAID) for joint pain, along with 150 mg of aspirin as part of his angina medication. Mr Sinclair collapsed at home and was found by neighbours after lying on the floor for approximately 18 hours. On admission to ICU he was unconscious with a swollen and bruised left leg. A urinary catheter was inserted and Mr Sinclair produced less than 15 ml/h of dark cloudy urine.

Blood investigations on admission:

Potassium	6.0 mmol/l
Sodium	134 mmol/l
Phosphate	2.6 mmol/ l
Bicarbonate	16 mmol/l
Lactate	2.3 mmol/l
Urea	18 mmol/l
Creatinine	310 μmol/l
Creatine kinase	45,000 IU/l
Vital signs:	
Temperature	36.8°C
Heart rate	78 beats/min
BP	130/70 mmHg
CVP	4 mmHg

Q.1 List Mr Sinclair's risk factors for developing acute renal failure (ARF) and for each factor explain the physiological processes resulting in ARF.

Q.2 Compare Mr Sinclair's results to normal values. Examine his abnormal values and risk factors and give a rationale for Mr Sinclair having pre-, intra- or post-renal failure.

Q.3 (a) Review the renal replacement therapy protocols used in your own ICU or clinical practice area.

(b) Analyse how best to restore Mr Sinclair's renal perfusion, renal functions and urine output (e.g. specify goals, types of fluid and electrolyte replacement: crystalloid/colloid, inotropes, diuretics, nutritional therapies, other drugs and therapies).

(c) Reflect on the evidence base available for each therapy (e.g. is there an evidence base for 'renal dose' dopamine?)

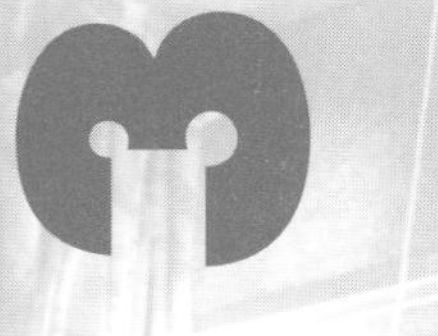
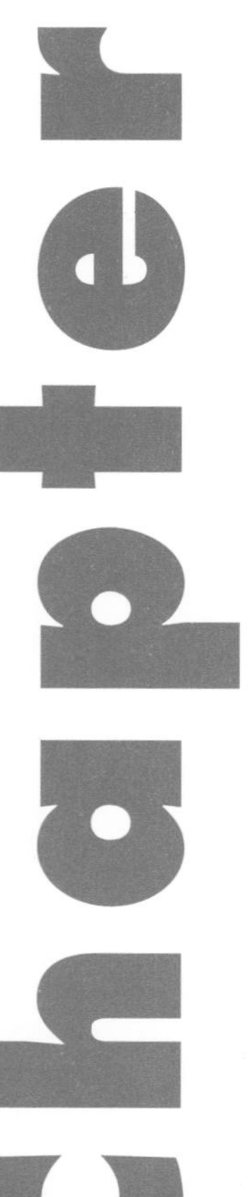

Chapter 33

Fluids

Contents

Fundamental knowledge

Blood groups (A, B, AB, O)

Introduction

Intravenous fluids require medical prescription, but ICU nurses begin and control infusions, and monitor fluid balance. As part of the multidisciplinary team, nurses should therefore understand how factors, such as likely extravasation, affect patients.

Fluid management of critically ill patients has aroused impassioned argument (e.g. colloid vs. crystalloid debate), but too often through oversimplistic approaches. Body fluid may be divided as:

- extracellular
- intracellular

Extracellular fluid is further divided into

- intravascular
- interstitial

Fluid balance is homeostasis of total body water. Although this chapter focuses on intravascular fluid resuscitation, these compartments are dynamic, not static, and problems with one compartment may compound other problems: critical illness is often complicated by both hypovolaemia and interstitial oedema. Therefore fluid management necessitates considering total body hydration and effects across all three compartments.

Fluid management should depend on patient needs:

- oxygen supply (haemoglobin, perfusion)
- blood volume
- other factors (electrolytes, clotting factors)

Schierhout and Roberts' (1998) meta-analysis concludes that colloids increase mortality, but this only reflects the debate that has persisted about the relative merits of colloids and crystalloids for fluid resuscitation.

Individual metabolism, capillary leakage, renal/hepatic failure and haemofiltration all affect *half-life*, and so ranges vary. Manufacturers' information often originates from animal and (usually) healthy volunteer studies, and information from clinical practice with critically ill patients can be sparse, especially with newer products. Thus, half-lives cited may not always reflect experience.

Half-lives cited vary both among literature and between people; figures often derive from measurements on healthy volunteers; increased capillary permeability and other complications of critical illness frequently alter (usually shortening) half-lives. Users should read manufacturers' information on data sheets; pharmacopoeias (e.g. BNF) also provide useful summaries about individual fluids.

Fluid balance

Total body water is approximately 600 ml/kg (Tonnesen 1994), although this varies with total body fat (fat repels water), which itself varies with

- gender (women have more fat than men)
- age (total body water reduces with age).

Infants have proportionally less fat (and so more body water) than adults, but reach near-adult levels by 2 years of age.

Fluid shifts between compartments are both passive (diffusion) and active (**hydrostatic** and **oncotic** pressure). Intravascular fluid regulates fluid gain and loss by

- absorbing ingested fluid
- osmoreceptor and baroreceptor regulation
- production of urine and other body fluids from plasma
- capillary oncotic pressure (normally 17 mmHg)

Intravascular volume is also the compartment normally measured/monitored (cardiovascular monitoring, blood chemistry).

Intravenous fluid therapy can:

- replace specific components (e.g. erythrocytes through blood transfusion)
- increase intravascular volume to improve tissue perfusion
- hydrate other fluid compartments

Oedema (excessive extravascular fluid) may occur from:

- leakage at site of vessel injury (e.g. puncture from cannulae)
- increased capillary permeability (e.g. SIRS)
- decreased removal of interstitial fluid (low plasma oncotic pressures)
- cell membrane damage and failure of sodium–potassium pump

The movement of solutes across capillary membranes varies according to:

- capillary pore size
- interstitial osmotic pressure
- capillary osmotic and hydrostatic pressures
- tissue resistance
- inflammatory response and vasoactive chemicals (e.g. interleukin-1)

In health, pore size varies between tissues, ranging from renal (largest pores) to the blood–brain barrier (smallest).

Inflammation enables antibodies and leucocytes (the largest blood cells) to migrate into infected tissue to destroy bacteria. Neutrophils, which enter first, secrete proinflammatory cytokines (e.g. interleukins, TNFα). Fluid exudation dilutes toxins, but causes oedema (which stimulates nociceptors, causing pain signals of tissue damage).

SIRS, ARDS and MODS are inappropriate system inflammatory responses, causing hypoperfusion from inappropriate fluid shifts: fluids are least likely to remain in the vascular spaces of patients needing them most. Fluid management of critically ill patients necessitates the careful evaluation of benefits against disadvantages of each, and this is the focus of this chapter. Nursing observations and records can identify the likely causes of oedema to guide appropriate fluid management: compounding extravasation only prolongs hypovolaemia and pulmonary complications.

Extravasation of fluids with high osmotic pressures (e.g. hydroxyethyl starches – HES) accentuates oedema, and so nursing monitoring of infusion volumes and sites is important to prevent additional complications.

Osmosis is the passage of fluid through semipermeable membranes (e.g. capillary walls) to form homeostasis (equilibrium of concentrations); **diffusion** is the opposing movement of solutes into fluid. **Colloid osmotic pressure** (COP) is the intravascular pressure exerted by large molecules (plasma proteins, mainly albumin) unable to cross capillary membranes that draws fluid (osmosis) into the bloodstream. Increased COP retains/attracts intravascular water, reduced COP allows more diffusion into tissues. Synthetic molecules (gelatins/starches) can also increase COP.

In health, COP is 3.7 kPa (28 mmHg) (Forbes 1997), but critical illness causes loss of larger molecules, reducing net pressure. Extravascular fluids create a counter osmotic pressure, aggravated by any extravasation/leak of low-weight 'colloids' from increased capillary permeability.

Fluid balance in critical illness is complex, and so *hypovolaemia* necessitates careful fluid management. Webb (1997) identifies three options for treating hypotension:

- crystalloids
- colloids
- inotropes

Using inotropes before correcting hypovolaemia ('dry drive') causes unpredictable maldistribution of blood flow, tachycardia and increased oxygen demand (Webb 1997).

Right ventricular stretching or displacement of the ventricular septum reduces left ventricular filling, which may limit fluid resuscitation (Robb 1997). Right atrial stretch causes release of atrial natriuretic factor (ANF – see Chapter 23), increasing diuresis and vasodilation.

Different fluids have various physiological functions and effects. A major factor in determining their effect is their molecular size (indicated by molecular weight, usually measured in **daltons (Da)** or **kilodaltons (kDa)**; where 'molecular weight' is cited, this is a slightly different measurement, but approximates to daltons). Like any 'normals', exact figures vary between authors; as vascular permeability varies with pathologies (see Chapter 25), precise molecular weights are less important than ranges within which molecules are measured.

Table 33.1 Summary of intravenous infusion fluids

Fluid	*Half-life(h)*	*kDa*	*COP (mmHg)*	*Benefits*	*Disadvantages*
blood	–	–	–	carries oxygen	possible viral contamination
albumin 4.5%	–	66.5	25	no evidence of viral infection; hypoallergenic	limited supply; exogenous albumin has only transient effect
albumin 20%	–	66.5	75–100	reduces oedema	as 4.5%
gelatins	2–3	30–40		cheap, stable during storage	short half-life (for colloids)
HES	10–14+	200–450	280–1088	prolonged effect; reduces oedema	expensive, prolonged clearance
oxygen carrying fluids	6–48			can carry oxygen	novel therapy with multiple problems; vary between products
crystalloids	<2			provide whole body hydration	aggravate oedema

Crystalloids

Crystalloid fluids are water with small molecule (below 10 kDa) solutes (e.g. 0.9% sodium chloride, 5% dextrose). Small molecules and water readily diffuse across cell membranes, providing intracellular hydration. Crystalloids provide total body hydration, but rapid extravasation (normal saline plasma half-life is 15 minutes (Tonnesen 1994)) makes them unsuitable for persistent hypovolaemia whether through external blood loss (e.g. surgery/haemorrhage) or internal fluid shifts and increased intravascular space (e.g. SIRS). Rapid infusion of large crystalloid volumes could cause pulmonary oedema (MacIntyre *et al.* 1985), although pump-controlled infusions and close monitoring should prevent this.

Five per cent glucose (in water) is often used to replace lost body water, but should be avoided with raised intracranial pressure as anaerobic metabolism of glucose produces lactic acid and water increasing oedema (North & Reilly 1994). Crystalloid fluid is unsuitable for the replacement of large volumes of intravascular fluid, and so is not discussed further here.

Perfusion

Tissue perfusion is needed to supply nutrients to cells and remove the waste products of metabolism. Tissue perfusion relies on pressure gradients across capillary walls. These gradients (see Figure 33.1) are the sum of

- resistance in tissues
- (mean) arterial blood pressure (MAP)
- colloid osmotic pressure.

At the arteriolar end, intracapillary pressure (average: 30–40 mmHg (Guyton & Hall 1997)) exceeds combined interstitial and COP, forcing fluid into tissues. As fluid extravases, intracapillary pressure falls while interstitial pressure rises; intracapillary pressure progressively falls, (average: 15 mmHg by venule end (Guyton & Hall 1997)), so interstitial and COP force most fluid to return into the capillary.

Capillary permeability varies greatly, ranging from the blood–brain barrier (least permeable) to renal glomerular beds (most permeable). Glomerular beds may filter positively charged substances up to 70 kDa (Adam & Osborne 1997), although clearance rate reduces as molecular size increases; the plasma half-life of crystalloids (low molecular weight) is brief, and the half-life of low molecular weight colloids (e.g. gelatine) is limited. Fluids with larger molecular structures remain intravascularly until metabolised into smaller molecules (which can be excreted). Thus the effects of intravascular fluids depend upon molecular size and metabolic rate.

Colloids

Colloids are fluids with large molecules (above 10 kDa according to Webb (1991)). They may be grouped as:

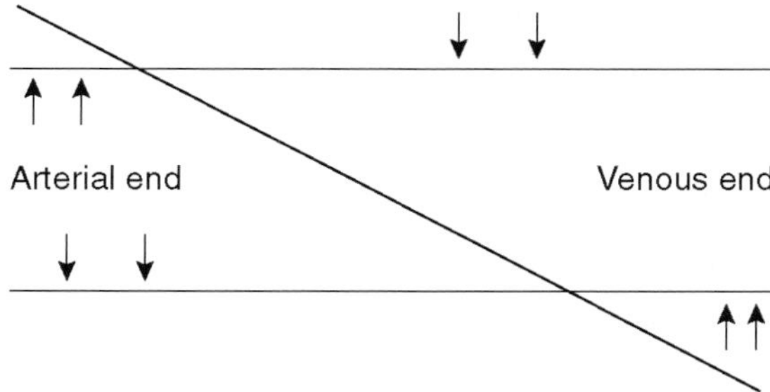

Figure 33.1 Perfusion gradients

Blood and blood products

- gelatins
- starches

Each group has advantages and disadvantages, and choice (and availability) depends upon the required effect and the benefit/burden balance. This chapter also describes

- oxygen-carrying artificial fluids

which have little effect on COP, and although not yet commonly used in clinical practice, may be increasingly used in the near future.

Blood

Blood for transfusion can be harvested from:

- donors
- recycling (usually perioperative) haemorrhage
- autotransfusion

Finite resources of blood, together with increasing concerns about infection from viruses (especially HBV and HIV) in donor blood, has caused reluctance to transfuse blood unless specific components (e.g. erythrocytes) are needed.

People can survive an 80 per cent loss of erythrocytes, but only a 30 per cent loss of blood volume (Williamson 1994), and so blood is normally only given when there is significant loss of erythrocytes (packed cell volumes below 33 per cent or Hb below 10).

Since donor blood is foreign protein, immunological reactions (both from cellular and plasma components) can occur; although these are usually limited to mild fever and slight hypotension, anaphylactic shock can occur. Reactions are normally minimised by crossmatching blood between recipient and donor, but emergency situations – where the risk from not giving blood exceeds the risk from the blood itself – may necessitate giving blood without crossmatching (Isbister 1997a).

Although whole blood is sometimes used, blood is more often separated into components. Packed cells, fresh frozen plasma, platelets and albumin are the most commonly encountered blood products, although there are a wide range of other products (including various other clotting factors) available to treat specific needs.

The increasing chemical instability of blood creates complications; expiry dates on each unit allow 40 days' shelf life, but as instability is progressive, nurses should be watchful for potential complications, especially as the units near their expiry dates.

As it is a living protein, blood is stored in a preservative. The most commonly used preservative is citrate, which is metabolised via Krebs' cycle. Citrate is acidic (Ali & Ferguson 1997); metabolism reduces plasma calcium (Isbister 1997a), potentially affecting muscle (including myocardial) contractility; thus large transfusions of blood may necessitate calcium supplements. A bag of approximately 500 ml whole blood contains 70 ml of preservative (Isbister 1997a), so that in addition to other complications, preservative causes mild haemodilution.

Cellular metabolism continues during storage (Ali & Ferguson 1997), and so storage time reflects increasing complications. Since the factor VII levels halve after one day, falling to 30 per cent after five days, and 6 per cent after 21 days (Hewlitt & Machin 1990), old blood provides fewer clotting factors. Problems are accentuated with whole blood as leucocytes create an adverse storage environment for most blood components (Isbister 1997a).

Adenosine triphosphate (ATP) is progressively depleted during storage (Isbister 1997a) causing oxidant damage to cell membranes, and allowing intracellular potassium to progressively diffuse into plasma (Isbister 1997a). Intracellular concentrations of potassium and sodium reverse plasma levels, causing progressive hyperkalaemia in stored blood. Potassium levels should therefore be checked when patients receive blood; however, with cell recovery following transfusion, potassium returns to intracellular fluid, causing potential rebound hypokalaemia within 24 hours (Isbister 1997a). Hypernatraemia can also occur from giving whole blood and fresh frozen plasma (FFP) (Isbister 1997a).

Up to one-third of cells may die during storage; metabolism of dead cells increases hepatic workload, potentially overwhelming hypofunctioning livers and causing jaundice. The age of blood transfused correlates with patient mortality (Purdy *et al.* 1997).

Blood is stored at 4°C to minimise metabolism; warming to 37°C consumes 1255 kJ (which is equal to one hour of muscular work, requiring 62 litres of oxygen) (Isbister 1997a); this extra workload may place significant strain on an already hypoxic patient. Blood and blood products should therefore be warmed at least to room temperature (20°C) before transfusion.

Blood stored at room temperatures (or other inappropriate temperatures) should not be used, but returned to the haematology department.

Filters can be used to remove components from blood. During the storage of blood, progressive microaggregate formation occurs; filters in standard blood-giving sets remove particles below 170 micrometers (Isbister 1997a). Concern about the effects of microaggregates stimulated the development of microaggregate filters; most commercial microaggregate filters remove particles of 40 micrometers (Ali & Ferguson 1997).

However, the effects of microaggregates are debatable (Isbister 1997a); filters slow transfusions and remove leucocytes (Ali & Ferguson 1997), and so the popularity of microaggregate filters has waned. Leucocyte filters may be beneficial to

- prevent febrile and other responses with immunocompromised patients (including those in renal failure)

- patients awaiting/recovering from organ transplantation (leucocytes potentially altering compatibility, complicating organ matching or increasing risk of rejection).

Albumin

Normal plasma (or serum) albumin levels are 42 ± 3.5 g/l (Fleck & Smith 1998), 12–15 g of the average total 500 g being synthesised by the liver each day (Friedman *et al.* 1996). As serum half-life is 20 days (Friedman *et al.* 1996), hypoalbuminaemia is a relatively late indicator of acute hepatic failure. Hypoalbuminaemia occurs in most ICU patients due to underlying liver failure. Albumin synthesis is inhibited by TNFα and interleukin 1 (Kulkarni & Webster 1996), prime mediators of cellular pathology (see Chapter 23). Hypoalbuminaemia is aggravated by a loss of albumin from the capillaries into tissues and dilution with intravenous infusions (Park & Evans 1997). However, restoring plasma albumin levels with exogenous albumin (Human Albumin Solution – HAS) is no more effective than using gelatins (Stockwell *et al.* 1992), although where loss of plasma proteins has occurred (e.g. burns), giving albumin is preferable to synthetic colloids.

Exogenous albumin is normally supplied in two strengths: 4.5 per cent (isotonic, 400 ml) and 20 per cent (hypertonic/salt-poor, 100 ml). The 4.5 per cent solution exerts COP of 20 mmHg (McDaniel & Prough 1996), whereas the 20 per cent solution exerts 75–100 mmHg. For colloid replacement, the 4.5 per cent solution is used. Standard bottles contain 17–19 g of albumin in 400 ml. Estimated molecular weight in solution is 66.5 kDa (Fleck & Smith 1998).

Albumin is heat-treated, and so there is no (known) risk of viral transmission, although albumin is not screened for all hepatitis viruses. It is stable, with a shelf life of five years at 2–8°C and one year at 25°C (Forbes 1997). However, benefits of exogenous albumin are transient; sustained recovery necessitates adequate nutrition for endogenous production of albumin.

Unlike most other colloids, albumin is negatively charged, which causes it to be repelled by similarly negatively-charged sialoproteins in glomerular capillaries, resulting in renal preservation of albumin. Thus, although albumin as a molecule is small enough (just) to be renally removed, glomerular filtrate albumin concentration is only 0.2 per cent of plasma concentration (Ganong 1995), and therefore protein is normally absent with urinalysis. In health, 80 per cent of exogenous albumin remains intravascularly, expanding the blood volume for about 24 hours (Forbes 1997); however, sepsis may limit this effect to little more than an hour.

Other benefits to albumin have been claimed: some anecdotal reports suggest it scavenges free radicals (so countering micropathophysiological mechanisms of critical illness).

Albumin supply is limited and costly (being derived from donated blood).

Cochrane Injuries Group Albumin Reviewers' (1998) meta-analysis suggested albumin infusion increased mortality; predictably, this initiated heated debate, with accusations of faulted methodology. Whatever the final outcome, further studies appear likely.

Other blood products

Most blood components are available individually for transfusion, but, except for albumin, these mainly carry potential for antigen–antibody reaction and virus infection and so are subject to similar crossmatching safeguards to blood transfusion, and are not given unless specifically indicated. Some of the most widely used blood products are fresh frozen plasma (FFP) and platelets, given to reverse haemorrhage. Solvent detergent (SD) plasma, which was given a UK licence in 1998, appears to be free of HIV and HBV, and may also have cytokines (which provoke SIRS) removed (Freeman 1998).

Gelatins

Gelatins (e.g. Haemaccel®, Gelofusin®), which are relatively inexpensive and stable plasma substitutes, are useful for resolving simple hypovolaemia, but have the lowest mean molecular weight of colloid fluids (30,000 (BNF 1998)); being below renal threshold, this limits their half-life to a few hours, and also their value for ICUs. Like most fluids, gelatins are iso-osmotic, only expanding blood by the volume infused. Both of these gelatins contain high concentrations of sodium (Haemaccel® 145 mmol/l, Gelofusin® 154 mmol/l (Gosling 1999)) and so may precipitate heart failure.

Haemaccel® is hypoallergenic, and so rapid infusion may (rarely) cause histamine release (Twigley & Hillman 1985; Hardy 1991).

Dextran

Dextran 40 and Dextran 70 (numbers referring to molecular weight), which are made from modified sugars, have largely fallen into disuse. They inhibit platelet aggregation and so are used to reduce perioperative risk of deep vein thromboses.

Hydroxyethyl starch (HES)

Starch has a complex chemical structure, giving solutions high molecular weights:

- Hespan® (molecular weight = 450,000 (BNF 1998))
- Pentaspan® (molecular weight = 250,000 (BNF 1998))
- eloHAES® (molecular weight = 200,000 (BNF 1998))
- HAES-steril® = 200 kDa (molecular weight = 200,000 (BNF 1998))

All starches are above renal threshold, so remain intravascularly until metabolised (half-lives of many being near to 24 hours). The colloid osmotic pressure (COP) of Hespan® is 30 mmHg and that of Pentastarch, the active component of HAES-steril® and Pentaspan® is 40 mmHg (McDaniel & Prough 1996). Prolonged plasma expansion (the main indication for their use) necessitates continued cardiovascular monitoring. Additionally, high COP attracts extravascular fluid, which further increases plasma volume and reduces interstitial oedema. This effect can be useful to treat ischaemia and injury from intracranial oedema (Schell *et al.* 1992).

Adverse effects of most starches include:

- anaphylactic reactions with Hespan® (Twigley & Hillman 1985)
- extravasation causing gross oedema from prolonged intravascular osmotic pressure
- coagulopathies
- hypervolaemia from overinfusion (most units limit to one litre per patient per day)
- circulatory overload in patients with impaired ventricular function

Expense (relative to other artificial colloids) also discourages use.

Oxygen-carrying fluids

Current plasma expanders increase blood volume without oxygen-carrying capacity resulting in dilutional anaemia; blood transfusion carries risks of viral infection, while supplies and shelf-life are limited. Oxygen-carrying fluids attempt to resolve both these problems.

There are two types of oxygen-carrying fluids:

- haemoglobin derivatives (modified human/other haemoglobin; neo-red cells)
- chemical (e.g. perfluorocarbon, see Chapter 29)

These fluids exert little colloidal osmotic pressure and so are not 'colloids'. Currently there are many problems and limitations to both groups (e.g. short duration of action, limited oxygen carriage). Limited licences have been granted in the USA, and some UK trials have been undertaken (Morris 1998); rapid improvements seem likely, and these fluids will probably be increasingly used for fluid replacement/resuscitation.

Implications for practice

- the prescription of fluids remains a medical decision, but nurses are professionally responsible and accountable for all fluids they administer (so should be aware of efficacy and adverse effects) and their choice of route (e.g. central or peripheral).

- crystalloid fluid is needed for cellular hydration
- despite varying assertions by some writers, debate continues between the value of colloids and crystalloids for intravascular volume expansion
- colloids have a higher molecular weight, and so remain for longer in the intravascular compartment and may reduce oedema formation (including pulmonary oedema)
- increasing COP draws extravascular fluid into the intravascular compartment
- microaggregate filters have no proven advantages
- massive blood transfusion creates various complications, including coagulopathies and hyperkalaemia
- blood should be warmed to room temperature before transfusion to reduce energy demand; blood should not be stored for prolonged periods at room temperature
- ICU nurses will frequently be exposed to blood and so should be vaccinated against hepatitis B
- hypoalbuminaemia reduces COP, thus reducing venous return; giving exogenous albumin causes only transitory increases of serum albumin levels; endogenous production, with adequate nutrition, is the most effective long-term treatment for hypoalbuminaemia
- cardiovascular function should be closely monitored continuously for as long as fluids exert an effect

Summary

Within the restrictions created by unit stock, as with any another therapy used, nurses should recognise the advantages and disadvantages of the fluids used. Crystalloid fluids are useful for cellular hydration, but for significant increase of intravascular volume colloids should be used.

Choice of colloids falls into three groups. Blood and blood products are usually essential if specific components are needed, but most carry potential risks of viral transmission. Blood transfusion also creates further complications. Gelatins are useful both for their relative cheapness and stability, but have the shortest half-life of all colloids and so are of limited use for critically ill patients. Starch solutions have the heaviest molecular weight of all colloids, and are clinically the most useful fluids for volume replacement, but expense and side effects limit their use. Oxygen-carrying solutions promise to be a useful development in the near future, but have not yet been licensed for UK use.

Further reading

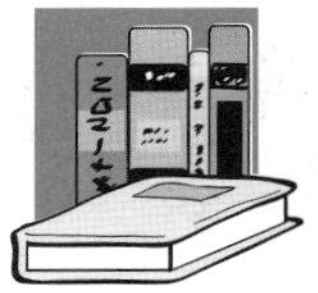

Most textbooks include chapters on colloids and/or fluid replacement; Webb's (1997) article also provides a useful overview. Separate articles, such as those cited above, can be found on each fluid, although vested interests (e.g. research sponsored by manufacturers) can limit objectivity.

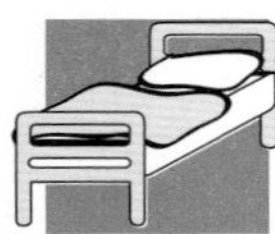

Clinical scenario

Rosemary Davies, a 34-year-old accountant with no previous medical history, was found unconscious and incontinent by her friends. She had been recovering from flu, and complaining of fever, thirst, tiredness and feeling confused.

Rosemary was admitted to ICU self-ventilating at 32 breaths/min:

Vital signs were:

HR	120 beats/min
BP	80/60 mmHg
CVP	0–1 mmHg

Core temperature 35.0°C (hypothermic)
Blood investigation revealed:

blood sugar	40 mmols/l
sodium	150 mmols/l
potassium	4.8 mmols/l
bicarbonate	19 mmol/l (with metabolic acidosis)

A diagnosis of Diabetic Hyperosmolar Hyperglycaemic Nonketotic coma (DHHNK) was made.

Q.1 Rosemary is extremely dehydrated. Identify signs associated with dehydration for each of the three fluid compartments. (e.g. unconsciousness is associated with which signs?; vital signs indicate?).

Q2 Select and give the rationale for the type of fluid replacement needed to correct Rosemary's hypovolaemia and hypotension (e.g. analyse choice of crystalloid, colloid).

Q3 Evaluate the use of 5% dextrose IV with Rosemary; consider its benefits to which fluid compartment, potential adverse effects and how these may be prevented or minimised.

Chapter 34

Inotropes

Contents

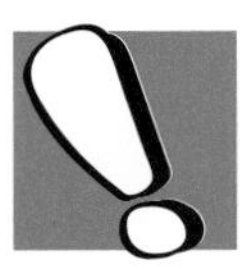

Fundamental knowledge

Renal anatomy: afferent arteriole, juxtaglomerular apparatus
Sympathetic nervous system
Negative feedback and parasympathetic effect
Renin–angiotensin–aldosterone mechanism

Introduction

'Inotrope' derives from the Greek word for 'fibre', and so inotropes alter the stretch of cardiac and other (smooth) muscle fibres. This effect is mediated through stimulation of the sympathetic nervous system, and can be affected positively (i.e. increased) or negatively (i.e. decreased).

Although some drugs and other chemicals are described as negative inotropes (e.g. digoxin, beta blockers, tumour necrosis factor), the word 'inotrope' is more commonly used without any prefix, referring to positive inotropes. This chapter discusses only positive inotropes. Positive inotropes, used to resolve hypotension from cardiac failure, are often assumed to primarily affect cardiac muscle fibres; while many do, some also affect muscle fibres (and so tone) in peripheral vasculature, thereby increasing systemic vascular resistance. Remembering that

blood pressure (BP) = cardiac output (CO) 3 systemic vascular resistance (SVR)

and

CO = heart rate (HR) × stroke volume (SV)

then

BP = HR × SV × SVR

Provided other factors remain constant, increasing heart rate, stroke volume or systemic vascular resistance necessarily increases blood pressure. Inotropes increase systemic blood pressure by increasing stroke volume (myocardial stretch) and/or systemic vascular resistance (vasoconstriction).

Chronotropes affect heart rate. Like inotropes, chronotropes can be positive (e.g. atropine) or negative (e.g. digoxin). The inclusion of digoxin in both groups illustrates how artificial the division between inotropes and chronotropes can be. Digoxin is primarily a chronotrope with inotropic effects; similarly, most positive inotropes cause tachycardia.

Positive inotropes may be divided into two main groups:

- adrenergic agonists
- phosphodiesterase inhibitors

Adrenergic agonists (adrenal stimulants), or 'catecholamines' (adrenaline, noradrenaline) are produced in the adrenal medulla and stimulate receptors in myocardium and vascular muscles. The enzyme phosphodiesterase is negatively inotropic, and so phosphodiesterase inhibitors (e.g. enoximone) increase cardiac output while relaxing vascular smooth muscle (inodilation).

Currently phosphodiesterase inhibitors are more frequently used in coronary care units than in ICUs.

Receptors

Cardiovascular receptors influence the sympathetic/parasympathetic control (feedback). For this chapter, receptors may be divided into three groups:

- alpha
- beta
- dopamine

Each group can be further subdivided.

Alpha receptors are primarily found in artery/arteriole smooth muscle; alpha stimulation (e.g. with noradrenaline) causes arteriolar vasoconstriction, thus increasing systemic vascular resistance. Visceral vasculature is especially susceptible to alpha stimulation, potentially causing major adverse effects:

- heart (dysrhythmias, ischaemia, infarction)
- liver (accentuating immunocompromise and coagulopathies)
- kidneys (renal failure)
- gut (translocation of gut bacteria)
- skin (peripheral blanching or cyanosis; extreme ischaemia may precipitate gangrene, necessitating amputation of digits)

Restoring central perfusion may necessitate such extreme adverse effects, but careful monitoring and observation may enable prevention of some of these. Observations include visual observation of peripheral blanching and cyanosis, and peripheral temperature (feeling hands and feet for warmth; monitoring with temperature probes). Monitoring will usually include cardiac output studies to measure systemic vascular resistance, and titrating alpha stimulants to prescribed parameters. Alpha stimulants inhibit insulin release (Moss & Craigo 1994), predisposing to hyperglycaemia.

Beta (β) receptors are found primarily in the heart and lungs. This chapter identifies β_1 and β_2; other beta receptors also exist. Beta$_1$ receptors are almost solely found in the myocardium: in the SA node, AV node and ventricular myocardial muscle. Beta$_1$ stimulation increases cell membrane permeability, thus increasing spontaneous muscle depolarisation. The effects of β_1 stimulation include (Moss & Craigo 1994):

- increased contractility
- improved atrioventricular conduction
- quicker relaxation of myocardium
- increased stroke volume
- increased heart rate (with potential dysrhythmias)
- therefore net increased cardiac output

- increased release of insulin, renin and antidiuretic hormone (Moss & Craigo 1994)
- transient hyperkalaemia: as potassium moves out from hepatic cells
- followed by prolonged hypokalaemia as potassium moves into blood and muscle cells

Beta$_2$ receptors are found mainly in bronchial smooth muscle, but a significant minority are also found in myocardium (15 per cent of ventricle and 30–40 per cent of atrial beta receptors (Moss & Craigo 1994)). Beta$_2$ stimulation is especially chronotropic, increasing myocardial workload and predisposing to dysrhythmias (hence tachycardic/dysrhymthmic effects of bronchodilators such as salbutamol). Beta$_2$ receptors are also found in other smooth muscle, such as blood vessels and skeletal muscle, vasodilating arterioles and reducing systemic vascular resistance (afterload).

Dopamine (DA_1) receptors are found in various organs. Insufficient brain stem production causes neurotransmission failure in Parkinson's disease, but dopamine cannot permeate mature blood–brain barriers (van den Berghe & de Zehger 1996), and so intravenous dopamine does not affect cerebral receptors. Gut and renal dopamine receptors have been the main targets of dopamine therapy.

Renal juxtaglomerular apparatus contains dopamine receptors; stimulation dilates afferent arterioles, increasing blood flow to the Bowman's capsule, so increasing urine output. Provided sufficient drug is given to stimulate dopamine receptors, stimulation continues regardless of dose. Gut receptors similarly increase splanchnic perfusion, but attempts to reduce the translocation of gut bacteria with low-dose dopamine have proved disappointing (Azar *et al.* 1996).

Prolonged beta stimulation causes 'down regulation' – progressive destruction of beta receptors, requiring progressively larger doses of inotropes to achieve the same effect. Destruction starts within minutes of exposure to stimulants, reaching clinically detectable levels by 72 hours (Sherry & Barham 1997). Beta receptors regrow once beta stimulation is removed (Sherry & Barham 1997).

Monitoring

Ideally all drugs would be titrated to a patient's weight; in practice, most drugs have a wide enough therapeutic range to enable 'standard doses', making both production and prescription safer and simpler. Most inotropes have very short half-lives (a few minutes); overdoses can cause massive, life-threatening hypertension, necessitating close monitoring and careful titration. While short half-lives make accumulation unlikely, flushing or failure of delivery (pump failure; change of syringe) can make blood pressure labile.

Monitoring inotropes necessitates both careful monitoring of cardiovascular effects and careful recording of amounts delivered. Short half-lives of inotropes and gross hypertensive effects necessitate continuous (or very frequent – every minute) blood pressure measurement. Most inotropes are dysrhythmic, and so ECGs should be continuously monitored. Other cardiovascular monitoring, such as cardiac output studies, will probably be required. Peripheral vasoconstriction, especially from alpha stimulants, necessitates frequent monitoring of peripheral oxygen saturation (SpO_2).

Traditionally inotropes are measured in micrograms per kilogram per minute (see below), or variants (e.g. micrograms per minute):

dosage (mcg/kg/min) = drug (mcg) ÷ dilutant (ml) × infusion rate (ml/min) ÷ patient's weight (kg) [1]

Thus if 500 mg dobutamine diluted in 250 ml, runs at 9 ml/hr, for a patient weighing 75 kg:

dosage (mg/kg/hr) = 500 mg ÷ 250 ml × 9 ml/hr ÷ 75 kg
∴ mcg/kg/min = 500 × 1,000 ÷ 250 × 9/60 ÷ 75
= 2,000 × 3/20 ÷ 75
= 2,000 × 1/20 ÷ 25
= 100 ÷ 25
= 4 mcg/kg/min [2]

Some units have replaced these potentially cumbersome calculations with simpler measurements (e.g. recording milligrams, as with most other drugs), titrating amounts given to the desired effects (e.g. systolic blood pressure). As normotension is the desired end of inotrope therapy, the value of investing nursing time in complex calculations is questionable, especially with calculations based on estimated weights, necessitating recalculation when one guess is replaced by another.

Adrenaline (adrenalin, epinephrine)

The adrenal medulla produces two hormones, both called 'catecholamines'. Adrenaline, the main adrenal medullary hormone, stimulates alpha, β_1 and β_2 receptors, triggering the 'fight or flight' stress response via the sympathetic nervous system:

- vasoconstriction (alpha receptors)
- increased cardiac output (β_1,β_2)

Acting on both alpha and beta receptors, adrenaline effectively increases all factors contributing to blood pressure; it has therefore become the major inotrope used during cardiac arrests, where immediate short-term restoration of systemic blood pressure and circulation is essential. Since prolonged critical illness is more complex, it necessitates careful balancing of factors. The place of adrenaline is therefore limited in intensive care.

Its bronchodilatory qualities (β_2) make nebulised adrenaline useful during asthma crises, especially with children.

Adrenaline causes gross tachycardia; with critical illness, increased myocardial oxygen consumption in already hypoxic patients may provoke angina or infarction. Adrenaline can also cause ventricular dysrhythmias.

Alpha effects include peripheral shutdown, including reductions in glomerular filtration rates; the short half-life of bolus adrenaline does not make this problematic during resuscitation, but continued infusion during critical illness may aggravate impending renal failure.

Adrenaline depresses insulin secretion, while blocking peripheral insulin receptors; with depressed insulin secretion and increased glycogenolysis, this causes stress-induced diabetes (whether adrenaline is endogenous or exogenous). Normoglycaemia may be restored once intravenous adrenaline is removed, although depleted intracellular glucose supply may prolong cellular recovery.

Almost uniquely among drugs, adrenaline is marketed in the virtually obsolete form of ratios. Ampoules normally contain 1:1,000 (or 1 in 1,000) and 1:10,000 (or 1 in 10,000). The ratio represents grams per ml, so that 1:1,000 = 1 gram per 1,000 ml = 1,000 mg per 1,000 ml = 1 mg per ml; similarly, 1:10,000 = 1 mg per 10 ml; 1:1,000 is usually marketed in 1 ml ampoules and 1:10,000 in 10 ml ampoules (so that both contain 1 mg per ampoule). While 1:10,000 may be used neat for an infusion, 1:1,000 should be diluted before administration.

Noradrenaline

Noradrenaline, a natural catecholamine, primarily stimulates alpha receptors, causing intense arteriolar vasoconstriction. With conditions such as SIRS which cause gross vasodilation (and so hypotension), noradrenaline effectively increases systemic blood pressure. However, as identified above, alpha stimulation can cause severe ischaemia, and so nurses should observe for pale/mottled skin and cold digits. Ideally, doses will be titrated to systemic vascular resistance measurements from cardiac output studies; however, where this necessitates invasive monitoring, infection and other risks from monitoring will be weighed against benefits from measurement.

Vasoconstriction increases cardiac afterload, in turn increasing left ventricular work; noradrenaline is usually given to restore a normal systemic vascular resistance (see Chapter 20), but excessive doses can be counterproductive. As hypotension is often multifactorial, problems with cardiac output should be resolved independently where possible, and not compensated for by excessive vasoconstriction.

Stimulation of alpha receptors in the kidneys and gut may cause or aggravate renal failure and translocation of gut bacteria. Extravasation of noradrenaline can cause necrosis and peripheral gangrene, and so should be given centrally.

Isoprenaline

Isoprenaline, a synthetic catecholamine, directly stimulates β_1 and β_2 receptors, enhancing atrioventricular node conduction. Previously a standard inotrope and chronotrope, isoprenaline has been replaced by more sophisticated drugs and is now rarely used (except for heart block unresponsive to atropine). As it is more chronotropic than inotropic, it increases myocardial oxygen consumption and is very dysrhythmic.

Dobutamine

Dobutamine, a synthetic analogue of dopamine, is currently the most widely used β_1 positive inotrope, although Tighe *et al.* (1998) argue that it causes significant alpha stimulation, aggravating hepatic damage. It also has slight β_2 effects, but is less chronotropic and dysrhythmic than most β_1 inotropes, and, despite common practice, does not need to be given centrally. Dobutamine achieves greater blood flow and oxygen transport to tissues than inotropic dopamine, probably due to the fact that it causes some vasodilation (Shoemaker *et al.* 1989).

Dopexamine (hydrochloride)

Dopexamine, a synthetic dopamine derivative, primarily causes arterial vasodilation (β_2 agonist) (Millar 1997); it also has weak β_1 and dopaminergic effects (Millar 1997), promoting diuresis (Gray *et al.* 1991), but causes tachycardia and dysrhythmias (BNF 1998). Tighe *et al.* (1998) recommend using dopexamine rather than dobutamine during sepsis. It can be given peripherally, but being an irritant it should be given through a large vein (MacConnachie 1996). Its half-life is 5–10 minutes (MacConnachie 1996). Expense and licence restrictions have limited its use, but its main current use is before and during cardiac surgery and to treat splanchnic ischaemia (Evans 1998).

Dopamine

Dopamine, an endogenous catecholamine and noradrenaline precursor, targets dopamine receptors in various parts of the body, including juxtaglomerular apparatus of afferent arterioles. It can also stimulate alpha and beta receptors, although levels at which these occur are disputed.

Traditionally, low-dose (renal) dopamine is given during renal failure, larger (inotropic) doses also stimulate β_1 receptors and high doses additionally stimulate alpha receptors. Its uses for cardiac support have largely been replaced by dobutamine, and in recent years doubt has been cast increasingly on its renal benefits.

Dopamine has a half-life of two minutes (DBL 1991). Since it is highly acidic, it is inactivated by alkaline solutions and alkalosis. As an alpha stimulant, it causes peripheral vasoconstriction and so should be given through a central line.

Low ('renal') dose dopamine supposedly targets only dopamine receptors in the kidneys. Dopamine also inhibits the sodium–potassium pump, reversing the fluid retention that predisposes to oedema (Evans 1998). DBL's data sheet (1991) gives renal range as 1–5 mcg/kg/min, but even 'low doses' cause significant inotropic effects (Juste *et al.* 1998). 'Renal' doses are tenfold those of endogenous secretion (van den Berghe & de Zehger 1996). Most literature is more conservative with the ranges given, many units aiming for about 2.5 mcg/kg/min (where units estimate patients' weights, this usually provides a safe margin to avoid inotropic effects).

Once standard practice on most ICUs, the benefits to patients of renal dopamine have been questioned (see Chapter 32). Some units have therefore its abandoned use in favour of other 'renal' drugs (e.g. Duke *et al.* (1994) found dobutamine gave better creatinine clearance than dopamine). Other units continue the use of renal dopamine, arguing that it 'buys time' by maintaining urine output until normal renal function recovers.

Van den Berghe and de Zehger (1996) suggest that (renal) dopamine may reduce prolactin and growth hormone secretion, potentially aggravating immunocompromise.

Inotropic dopamine has similar effects to dobutamine, but is more dysrhythmic. Inotropic range is given by DBL (1991) as 5–20 mcg/kg/min, but practice (and most authors) suggests inotropic effects at lower doses; Fitzgerald (1992) gives the cardiac range as 1–5 mcg/kg/min, but Graver's (1992) 4–8 mcg/kg/min is more realistic. In practice, inotropic dopamine is unlikely to be used unless an inotrope is urgently needed with a patient already receiving renal dopamine, but nurses should be aware of the unwanted inotropic effects of renal dopamine. Being more chronotropic than dobutamine (often causing heart rates around 140 bpm), myocardial oxygen consumption in increased and left ventricular filling time is reduced (so reducing stroke volume).

Dopamine and β_1 receptor stimulation continue with increasing doses, but *high dose* dopamine also stimulates alpha receptors. As more specific alpha stimulation can be achieved with noradrenaline, high dose dopamine is an undesirable overdose. The range for high dose dopamine begins where cardiac doses end. Alpha stimulation causes greater renal vasoconstriction than the vasodilation from dopamine receptor stimulation, and so high dose dopamine reduces urine output.

Phosphodiesterase inhibitors (PDIs)

Phosphodiesterase is a coronary artery enzyme which removes guanosine monophosphate, the enzyme that removes nitric oxide (see Chapter 28). Synthetic phosphodiesterase inhibitors (e.g. Amrinone/Inocor®, Milrinone/Primacor®, Enoximone, Bipyridine, Imidazole) therefore prolong vasodilatory effects of nitric oxide, causing

- inodilation
- positive inotropy.

Thus, increasing both cardiac output and diastolic relaxation, without down-regulation.

Cyclic adenosine monophosphate (cAMP) assists the slow calcium channels of muscles, increasing action potential, and in turn increasing myocardial conductivity. Phosphodiesterase inactivates cAMP (negative inotropic effect), so that inhibiting phosphodiesterase (i.e. inhibiting the inhibitor) has a positive inotropic effect, without increasing myocardial oxygen consumption. Unlike β_1 stimulants, down-regulation does not occur (Powell & Whitwam 1990).

PDIs affect action potentials of all muscles, causing relaxation of vascular smooth muscle (Broughton & Filcek 1990) and reducing cardiac afterload. As PDIs affect action potential, electrolyte imbalances, especially hypokalaemia, should be resolved before administration.

Prolonged use during severe heart failure has shown increased mortality (Myburgh & Runciman 1997), although this is unlikely to be an issue for ICU management. Phosphodiesterase inhibitors have far longer half-lives than adrenergic agonists, and so may be given by bolus. They should be given through a central line (Graver 1992).

Significant proportions (often around one-half) of PDIs are protein bound, giving them longer half-lives than inotropes (e.g. Enoximone half-life is 3–6 hours (Powell & Whitwam 1990)). Protein binding, and so effectiveness of PDIs, is impaired with hypoalbuminaemia (most ICU patients). Prolonged half-life can also cause plasma accumulation, so that PDIs should either be given intermittently or titrated.

Adverse effects of PDIs include

- thrombocytopaenia (especially from high dose amrinone)
- gastrointestinal disturbances
- hepatic dysfunction/failure
- dysrhythmias
- hypotension

Implications for practice

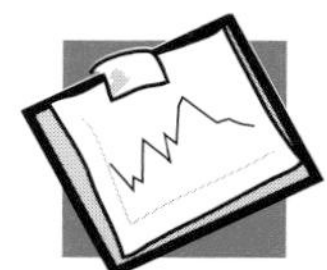

- inotropes (alpha and β_1 stimulants) should be given by continuous controlled infusion
- infusion pumps should maintain a constant flow rate
- syringes should be horizontal (to prevent precipitation)
- ideally inotropes should be diluted in 5% dextrose (to prevent oxidation)
- although some (not all) inotropes may be given peripherally, with hypoperfusion (e.g. SIRS) central administration is usually safer, and is generally used in ICU

- within prescribed limits, inotrope doses should be titrated to achieve desired effects, while minimising adverse effects
- observations of patients receiving alpha stimulants should include: continuous or very frequent blood pressure monitoring; peripheral temperature (all four limbs); peripheral colour; systemic vascular resistance (via cardiac output studies)
- most inotropes (but not phosphodiesterase inhibitors) have half-lives of only a very few minutes; blood pressure monitoring should ideally be continuous; if intermittent, intervals should not exceed half-lives of drugs
- many patients become highly dependent on inotropes, becoming hypotensive when infusions are changed; a 'spare' syringe ('double pumping') can reduce changeover time of infusions, so minimising hypotensive effects
- indications for renal dopamine now appear questionable; while further research is needed, units should review its value in the light of existing studies which generally favour dobutamine
- traditional practices of measuring inotropes by body weight and calculations, rather than monitored effect, should be reconsidered, especially where units lack facilities to accurately weigh patients on a regular basis
- the potent effects of most inotropes necessitate careful weaning (usually slow) with continuous monitoring
- the place of phosphodiesterase inhibitors in ICU is currently limited, largely to cardiac surgery, but may increase in the future
- use of alpha stimulants necessitates monitoring for peripheral ischaemia; ideally this should be through cardiac output studies measuring systemic vascular resistance, but visual and tactile observation of patients' peripheries is a useful adjunct to care
- most inotropes are given in 5% dextrose, as they oxidise in saline; but manufacturers' data sheets should be checked before preparation

Summary

Drugs inhibiting myocardial contraction are labelled 'negative inotropes'; drugs increasing muscle contraction should be called 'positive inotropes', but practice usually limits the label 'inotropes' to positive inotropes.

Central blood pressure can be increased by increasing heart rate (chronotrope), increasing stroke volume (β_1 stimulation or phosphodiesterase inhibition) or increasing systemic vascular resistance (alpha stimulation). Beta$_1$ stimulation, the traditional mainstay on inotrope practice, creates problems of down-regulation, necessitating progressively higher doses.

This chapter has also discussed renal dopamine since it is classified as an 'inotrope'; however, there is little indication for the use of inotropic dopamine. For β_1 stimulation, most units rely on dobutamine or adrenaline. Alpha stimulation (from adrenaline or noradrenaline) can usefully raise central blood pressure by increasing systemic vascular resistance, but complications from peripheral (and gut) ischaemia should be considered.

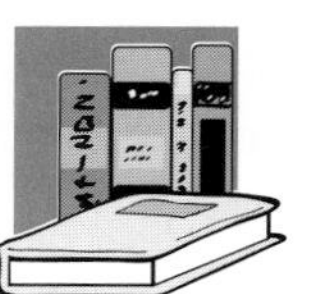

Further reading

Nurses wishing to read more about specific drugs should follow up references cited in relevant sections of the text. A nursing overview is given by Graver (1992), but most literature is inevitably medical or pharmacological. Of medical texts, Hinds & Watson (1996) offers comprehensive application of drugs; Evans (1998) is a valuable recent addition to the nursing literature. Many articles discuss individual inotropes, or the specific effects of individual drugs.

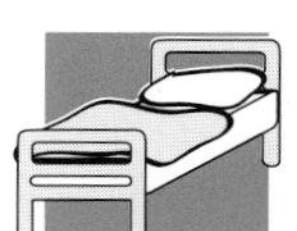

Clinical scenario

Rita Goodwin, who is 56 years old, has been admitted with severe chest pain and her ECG shows sinus rhythm and an anterior wall MI. Mrs Goodwin has no previous cardiac history; she is 165 m (5 ft 6 in) tall and weighs 63 kg (139 lb) with BSA of 1.7 m^2. She is self-ventilating and conscious.

Her vital signs include:

BP 85/60 mmHg (MAP 68–70 mmHg)
HR 125 beats/min
CVP 11 mmHg

(*See page 218 for calculation of Mrs Goodwin's SVR and other haemodynamic monitoring results.*)

Mrs Goodwin is commenced on an intravenous infusion of Dobutamine. Infusions of GTN and milrinone were also considered.

Q.1 Describe the therapeutic action of GTN, dobutamine and milnirone. Explain their action on specific receptor sites and intended effects.

Q.2 Identify the haemodynamic parameters which should be assessed and recorded when evaluating effectiveness (and monitoring for adverse effects) of Mrs Goodwin's inotropes.

Q.3 Evaluate nursing strategies which can promote and enhance the effectiveness of these inotropes. Consider resources, methods of administration (e.g. IV equipment, dilution, double pumping, etc.), titration, other medications (e.g. analgesics, oxygen), patient position, psychosocial, behavioural and other interventions in order to stabilise Mrs Goodwin's endogenous catecholamine release.

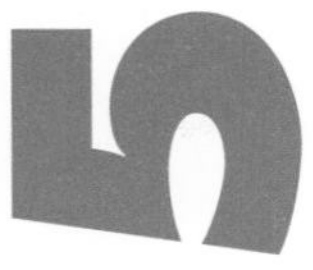
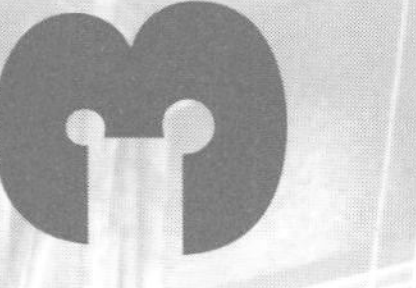

Chapter 35

Haemofiltration

Contents

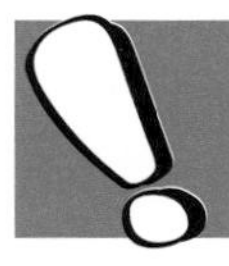

Fundamental knowledge

Normal renal anatomy and physiology
Acute renal failure (see Chapter 32)

Introduction

Haemofiltration is the major continuous renal replacement therapy (CRRT) used in ICU, and so it is important that nurses should understand the principles of haemofiltration and have a working knowledge of whichever system their unit uses. Manufacturers' recommendations differ between systems, and so readers should adapt the material in this chapter to the systems used. Peritoneal dialysis and haemodialysis are briefly described, but nurses regularly using these therapies should resource specific texts on them. Plasmapheresis uses similar circuits to haemofiltration (usually used intermittently rather than continuously), and so most principles of haemofiltration apply to plasmapheresis.

Haemofiltration considerably increases nursing workload; while caring for patients receiving haemofiltration can be rewarding, nurses should understand the potential complications.

The terminology used to describe modes often varies between units (and in literature); 'haemodialysis' and 'haemofiltration' are interchanged and variously interpreted (Table 35.1 lists the commonly used terms). Material referring to 'haemofiltration' in this chapter also applies to variants (diafiltration, plasmapheresis) unless stated otherwise.

Renal replacement therapies mimic normal renal function by placing semipermeable membranes between the patient's blood and a collection

Table 35.1	**Commonly used terms for continuous renal replacement therapies (CRRT)**
CAPD	chronic ambulatory peritoneal dialysis
CAVH	continuous arteriovenous haemofiltration (= ultrafiltration, see below); rarely now used in ICU
CAVHD	continuous arteriovenous haemodialysis
CAVHDF	continuous arteriovenous haemodiafiltration
CRRT	continuous renal replacement therapy (blanket term used to describe any mode)
CVVH	continuous venovenous haemofiltration
CVVHD	continuous venovenous haemodialysis
CVVHDF	continuous venovenous haemodiafiltration
dialysis	movement of particles from a highly concentrated to a lower concentration solution, using a semipermeable membrane
haemodialysis	renal replacement therapy primarily using extracorporeal dialysis
haemofiltration	renal replacement therapy primarily using extracorporeal convection of solutes
haemodiafiltration	haemofiltration adding a countercurrent, thus adding principles of dialysis to haemofiltration
plasmapheresis	haemofiltration, usually with smaller filter pores (sometimes called 'continuous plasma adsorption')
SCUF	slow continuous ultrafiltration removal of ultrafiltrate, usually using a small-pore filter, so minimising solute removal (used only for removing/reducing fluid overload)
ultrafiltrate	solution removed through a small-pore semipermeable membrane

conduit. *Filtration* is the passage of fluid through this filter; *dialysis* is a similar movement of solutes. In the human kidney, both occur passively at the glomerular bed and actively as filtrate passes through renal tubules. While technically separate functions, in practice filtration necessarily contains solutes, while *osmotic pressure* of solutes on either side of the filter inevitably influences filtration.

Dialysis

PERITONEAL DIALYSIS The earliest modern CRRT, this uses the highly vascular and permeable peritoneal membrane. Peritoneal blood and dialysis fluid (infused through an abdominal catheter) achieves equilibrium of most solutes. Using fluids with large (glucose) molecules, excess body fluid is drawn by osmosis into dialysate, then removed by negative pressure (usually gravity).

Chronic ambulatory peritoneal dialysis (CAPD) may be encountered when patients with pre-existing chronic renal failure are admitted. Peritoneal dialysis has many limitations, including:

- limited dialysate volumes (abdominal distension causes pain, lung splinting and impairs major organ perfusion)
- solute removal is limited by filtrate-to-plasma concentrations (toxin levels are reduced, not eliminated)
- loss of albumin and other large molecules (the peritoneum is highly permeable)
- peritonitis
- contraindications (e.g. abdominal surgery)

HAEMODIALYSIS This overcomes many limitations of peritoneal dialysis by pumping large volumes of blood rapidly through an extracorporeal circuit, so that the countercurrent dialysate flow enables the rapid removal of fluid and electrolytes by exposing high blood levels to 'clean' fluid. Haemodialysis (and haemodiafiltration) combines diffusion, ultrafiltration and convection; toxin removal is so efficient that a few (3–5) hours treatment once or twice each week enables people with chronic renal failure to live fairly normal lives. Haemodialysis is the most widely used renal replacement therapy, but is usually only seen in ICUs if hospitals have renal units attached; renal nurses normally perform the dialysis.

However complications of haemofiltration include

- cardiovascular instability
- disequilibrium syndrome
- immunological deficiency
- limited water and solute removal

These complications can be especially problematic with critical illness.

CARDIOVAACULAR INSTABILITY Haemodialysis rapidly removes large volumes from plasma, creating potential *hypovolaemia* and *hypotension*, while priming fluid and blood loss from intermittent treatments may cause dilutional *anaemia* ('flushing back' circuits inevitably remaining incomplete). Hypotensive episodes are twice as likely with haemodialysis as with haemofiltration (Henderson 1987).

DISEQUILIBRIUM SYNDROME This is traditionally attributed to the rapid removal of urea and uraemic toxins, creating an osmotic gradient between cerebral spinal fluid (CSF) and blood, although the exact cause of disequilibrium remains unclear (Mercer 1996); complement activation by non-biocompatible filters may have contributed to disequilibrium in the past. However caused, disequilibrium syndrome rarely occurs, but when it does it can be distressing for both patients and others; neurological effects include confusion, aggression, nausea/vomiting, muscle twitching, lethargy, blurred vision and possible coning. Critical illness and sedation can mask many of these symptoms, but not the discomfort problems for patients.

IMMUNOLOGICAL DEFICIENCY Unlike human kidneys, artificial filters are non-selective, with no tubular reabsorption, so that immunological deficiency may result from the removal of complements and other small-weight components of both non-specific and specific immunity. Highly invasive equipment provides access for pathogens.

WATER AND SOLUTE REMOVAL This is limited to intravascular fluid, but most body fluids (and solutes) are extravascular (see Chapter 33); oedema further increases extravascular volume. Removing intravascular fluid encourages replacement by extravascular fluid, but limited transfer occurs during the few hours of haemodialysis, whereas continuous treatments (e.g. haemofiltration) enable greater indirect removal of extravascular fluid/solutes. Patients with primary or chronic renal failure are usually hypertensive, and so tolerate rapid reduction of plasma volume better than the typically hypotensive ICU patient.

Haemofiltration

Haemofiltration resolves many of the problems of haemodialysis. It mimics human glomerular filtration, as plasma is forced under pressure through a semipermeable membrane (*ultrafiltration*), and solutes are drawn across the membrane by *convection*. Unlike the human kidney, haemofiltration (and haemodialysis) cannot selectively reabsorb. Ultrafiltrate volumes are large (although smaller than healthy human ultrafiltrate), so that large infusions are needed to mimic reabsorption.

Early haemofilters, adapting principles of haemodialysis, consisted of a filter placed between arterial and venous cannulae: continuous arteriovenous haemofiltration (CAVH). Driving pressure was therefore the differential between a patient's arterial and venous blood pressures. Anticoagulation was added to prevent thrombus formation in extracorporeal circuits; replacement fluid was given to mimic tubular reabsorption.

CAVH is simple and, unlike haemodialysis, able to be performed by ICU nursing staff. But as flow relies on patients' blood pressure, solute removal by CAVH is relatively inefficient and circuits frequently occlude (clot) due to hypotension. Slow Continuous Ultrafiltration (SCUF), a variant of CAVH, remains useful in renal units for relieving fluid overload, but CAVH/SCUF is relatively inefficient at removing solutes, and has largely been replaced in ICU.

Adding a driving ('arterial' or afferent) pump to CAVH circuits provided adequate driving pressure to maintain patency. Mechanical pumps replaced the need to cannulate arteries; continuous venovenous haemofiltration (CVVH) requires only two central venous cannulae (usually combined in one double-lumen catheter). CVVH rapidly became the standard ICU renal replacement therapy. Descriptions of 'arterial' and 'venous' circuits persisted, even though CVVH circuits contain no arterial blood (so are unsuitable for arterial blood gas analysis). Manufacturers are rationalising terminology by renaming 'arterial' circuits 'afferent' and 'venous' circuits 'efferent'; this follows human renal physiology, and is logical, and so although not (as yet) universal, it is used here.

Compared with haemodialysis, haemofiltration:

- enables filtration despite hypotension
- improves cardiovascular stability
- enables more gentle removal of solutes (less disequilibrium)
- removes significantly larger fluid volumes

High-speed haemofiltration for short periods may achieve better clearance than haemodialysis, but circuits are relatively costly and time-consuming to prime, and the use of intermittent filtration is almost exclusively confined to hospitals with on-site renal units (Amoroso *et al.* 1992).

Haemodiafiltration

Ultrafiltrate countercurrent was not used with early haemofilters, so solute clearance remained poor once ultrafiltrate concentrations in filters approached plasma levels. To improve solute clearance, countercurrent ('dialysate') was added to haemofiltration to create haemo*dia*filtration (CAVHDF/CVVHDF, sometimes called continuous haemodialysis – CAVHD/CVVHD). Most units now add countercurrent to haemofiltration, calling it simply 'haemofiltration' (literature describing haemofiltration may not always clarify whether it refers to systems with or without countercurrents).

Theoretically, countercurrent clearance is proportional to countercurrent volume, but exchanges above 2–3 litres per hour do not significantly increase clearance (Miller *et al.* 1990); most units use 1–2 litres each hour.

Factors affecting filtration

Whatever CRRT is used, filtration (like human kidneys) relies on *blood flow* through filters and *pressure gradients* across the semipermeable membrane. Transmembrane pressure gradients are affected by:

- driving pressure
- resistance
- *oncotic*/osmotic pressure
- negative pressure

BLOOD FLOW This is primarily created by *driving pressure*. In human kidneys and CAVH driving pressure is afferent arteriole blood pressure; CVVH driving pressure is afferent pump speed. Inadequate flow (e.g. occlusion with changes of the patient's position) causes arterial/afferent pressure alarms; readjusting the patient's position usually restores blood flow.

Blood flow through filters is also affected by blood *viscosity* (see Chapter 18). Prediluting blood (before the filter) reduces viscosity, increasing filtrate volume, urea clearance and filter life (reducing need for anticoagulation) (Kaplan 1985a); but anecdotal reports suggest predilution both hastens coagulation and reduces filter life, perhaps due to activation of clotting factors; further research is needed both to identify mechanisms and to guide practice.

RESISTANCE Dialysate flow rate with haemodiafiltration creates counter-pressure resistance to afferent pump speed. Usually exchanges are 1–2 litres every hour (16.6–33.3 ml/min), creating a relatively low resistance against afferent flows of 150 ml/min.

ONCOTIC AND OSMOTIC PRESSURE These are created by plasma proteins and other large molecules. Predilution reduces oncotic pressure in filters. Some dialysate fluids (e.g. hypertonic glucose) increase osmotic pull.

NEGATIVE PRESSURE This is suction pressure drawing plasma across filter membranes. Free-flow ultrafiltrate relies on gravity (height difference between the filter and collection bag) to create negative pressure, but most systems now control ultrafiltrate with volumetric pumps, so that the ultrafiltrate pump speed determines negative pressure.

Filter membranes

Cuprophane or cellulose, used for early filters (Kwan 1997), activate the immune complement system, releasing highly vasoactive substances (e.g. interleukin 1, TNFα) (Kwan 1997). These cause:

- hypotensive crises
- neutropenia

- thrombocytopenia
- hypoxia (neutrophil sequestration in pulmonary circulation).

Modern filters use *biocompatible* materials; as these are more porous, they can remove larger molecules (cardiodepressant and vasoactive mediators), hence the potential of plasmapheresis to treat SIRS.

Hollow fibres are usually used. Often containing more than 20,000 fine capillary tubes, they have large surface areas (often 2 m^2 (Ervine & Milroy 1997)), a small volume and, being cylindrical, they are also sturdy. Small capillary tube diameter (65 micrometres (Ervine & Milroy 1997)) usually necessitates anticoagulation to prevent thrombosis and obstruction. Ervine and Milroy (1997) suggest hollow fibre threshold is usually about 30 kDa, but various pore-size filters are available: most of the filters now used can double this threshold. Fibres are glued with polyurethane, making them less biocompatible than flat plate filters (Molnar & Shearer 1998).

Flat plate filters contain a series of plates. Although overall surface area is smaller than with hollow fibres, flat plates can clear small molecules more efficiently (Hinds & Watson 1996) and are less prone to clotting, and so require less anticoagulation. As they are less sturdy, they are more easily damaged (e.g. by clamping).

High **transmembrane pressure** (TMP) can rupture ('blow', 'burst kidney') the filter, necessitating immediate cessation of filtration. Most systems now measure transmembrane pressure directly, although some older systems may still rely on indirect indications (e.g. falling venous pressure and ultrafiltrate volumes). The maximum transmembrane pressure is stated on filters. Transmembrane pressure is created by various factors, but rising pressure usually suggests significantly decreased filtration surface area from thrombus formation (efferent filters protect patients from emboli).

Recommended *priming* volumes normally exceed total circuit volume. While priming removes air emboli, its main purpose is the removal of glycerol and ethylene oxide used to protect filters during storage and transportation. These chemicals can cause convulsions, paralysis, renal failure and haemolysis (Martindale 1996), so that priming volumes should follow manufacturers' recommendations and not be abandoned once circuits are filled with fluid. Similarly, circuits left standing unused should be reprimed before use.

As with human nephrons, *solute clearance* is limited by ultrafiltrate concentrations, ending once equilibrium is reached. Pore sizes of human nephrons and artificial filters are normally large enough to clear anything potentially in blood apart from blood cells. Solutes are often referred to as either small or middle (above 500 Da = 0.5 kDa) sized.

Human nephrons normally clear molecules up to 69 kDa (McClelland 1993a). Early filters allowed solutes of 30 kDa to pass – many are now more porous – but actual clearance varies with:

- molecular size
- ultrafiltrate concentration
- protein binding.

Weight reflects molecular complexity. Electrolytes weigh very few daltons (urea 60 Da; creatinine 133 Da; glucose 180 Da); drugs are heavier, but weigh less than **inulin** (5,200 Da; NB not insulin).

The use of lactate-based dialysate fluids can accentuate problems with *acidosis*; bicarbonate filtration (Hilton *et al.* 1998) can resolve this problem.

Problems

Haemofiltration, the main CRRT in ICU, is impractical for prolonged use with mobile patients. Most ICU patients are already *immobile*, and so ICUs are one of the few areas where continuous haemofiltration becomes practical.

Haemofiltration *increases nursing workload.* Patients who are being haemofiltered are often ventilated, unconscious, monitored and receiving many drugs (often including large dose inotropes); their dependent state necessitates fundamental aspects of care (comfort, hygiene, pressure care), while family and friends of critically ill patients are often anxious, needing more time spent with them. Care may have to be prioritised to maintain safety; such workloads illustrate the dangers of assuming that one-to-one nurse–patient ratios are always safe.

Large filtrate and replacement volumes, together with many other inputs and outputs, can make calculations complex, increasing risks of *fluid balance calculation error*. Hammond *et al.* (1991) found errors in one-quarter of all fluid balance charts; while many of these errors may have been slight, filtration exchanges can exceed a litre, so that cumulative miscalculations, or forgetting a single running total, can equate to total blood volume.

The risk of fluid balance error can be reduced by rationalising fluid balance charts. Insensible loss in health is about 500 ml each day, rising to a litre or more with critical illness: fluid balance charts are necessarily inaccurate by 500–1,000 ml. Measuring decimal points of millilitres achieves little beyond pedantry and possible carelessness with larger figures (centilitres and litres); fluid balance charts and calculations are safer if rationalised.

Calculators can assist complex calculations, but major errors can occur by accidentally catching keys, and so larger figures (e.g. centilitres) should be checked to see whether they are appropriate, and periodically (e.g. 4–6 hourly) calculations should be rechecked.

Extracorporeal circuits are (usually) continuously *anticoagulated* to prevent thrombus (and embolus) formation. Although efferent filters should remove emboli before reaching patients, adsorption of blood proteins onto foreign surfaces (e.g. extracorporeal circuits) occurs within milliseconds of exposure, triggering platelet adhesion, rapidly occluding narrow pores of filter membranes, thus reducing their efficiency. Thrombus formation is increased by slow blood flow. The signs of thrombus formation include:

- dark blood in circuits
- kicking of lines
- high transmembrane pressure
- reduced filtration (if not pump-controlled).

Anticoagulation may be unnecessary with prolonged clotting times or when afferent flow exceeds 300 ml/min (McClelland 1993a). Heparin prime reduces initial platelet aggregation, enabling a lower dose of subsequent anticoagulants. Anticoagulants are below filter threshold, but some inevitably reach patients, aggravating coagulopathies; reversal agents (e.g. protamine) can be added after the filter.

Heparin remains the most widely used anticoagulant, but *prostacyclin* (epoprostenol; prostaglandin I_2 – PGI_2) is also used with or instead of heparin. Prostacyclin inhibits platelet aggregation, but it is also a powerful endogenous vasodilator, and so it can cause hypotension (BNF 1998). Kirby and Davenport (1996) suggest that up to 40 per cent of prostacyclin is removed by filtration (i.e. over one-half remains).

Storing reconstituted vials in refrigerators may (or may not) be chemically safe, but nurses (and condoning managers) who are contravening manufacturers' data sheet instructions to discard reconstituted prostacyclin after 12 hours should consider their legal liability.

Prostacyclin is more expensive than heparin, and so tends to be used if coagulopathies from heparin become problematic.

Despite the extensive monitoring of respiratory and cardiovascular systems on ICUs, many units rely on haematology departments and daily blood samples to monitor the effects of haemofiltration on clotting. On-unit facilities to monitor clotting (e.g. activated clotting time – ACT) can enable speedier identification and treatment of problems. Clotting should be 1.5–2 times normal baseline (normal PTT = 40 seconds; normal ACT = 80–100 seconds) during haemofiltration.

Freeflowing *ultrafiltrate volumes* vary with the above factors, particularly functional filtration surface. New filters function effectively; initial volumes using free drainage usually exceed one litre every hour. Pump speeds should not be reduced to reduce filtrate volume, as this rapidly causes thrombus damage to filters. Excessive filtrate should be countered with additional fluid replacement (possibly necessitating a second volumetric pump). Large volume infusions should be pumped directly into filtration circuits to avoid overloading peripheral veins.

Afferent pump speeds of 150 ml/min are a minimum, not maximum. Circuits can safely run at 250–300 ml/min, which may prolong filter life and/or reduce anticoagulation requirements. Renal units often run circuits faster; however such aggressive treatment is normally unnecessary with continuous filtration, and may not be tolerated by critically ill patients, and so ICU nurses are wise to be more cautious.

Volumes below 300 ml per hour in circuits without countercurrent dialysate (haemofiltration) or below 180 ml per hour with diafiltration provide ineffective solute clearance, consuming nursing time without benefit to patients, and so should be discontinued. Outflow volumetric pumps prevent ultrafiltrate volumes falling, but as functional filtration area decreases, transmembrane pressure will increase.

Recommended *afferent pump speed* varies between systems (readers should check the manufacturers' recommendations and local protocols), but should be commenced slowly (e.g. 100 ml/min) in case hypotensive crises occur from the rapid removal of blood volume. If stable, speeds should usually be increased to a minimum 150 ml/min within 10 minutes.

Concern about *drug clearance* by haemofiltration is justified, but factors are complex, requiring advice from unit pharmacists. Some factors are described here to illustrate how problematic this issue is.

All drugs (except some colloidal fluids) used in clinical practice are smaller than filter pore size, and so potentially may be filtered. Studies of drug clearance may refer to peritoneal dialysis, haemodialysis, haemofiltration or haemodiafiltration. Even within a single technique, different filter pore sizes influence clearance. Clearance may also differ between animal or healthy human volunteers and critically ill patients.

Kaplan (1998) identifies four main factors affecting drug clearance:

- molecular weight (5–10 kDa readily cleared by haemofiltration)
- degree of protein binding
- drugs' volume of distribution (water solubility/lipid affinity)
- drugs' endogenous clearance (hepatic)

Drugs are usually only active if unbound, so that binding is normally weak, with volatile shifts between bound and unbound drug molecules. Protein binding alone is affected by

- acidity (pH) of blood
- molar drug concentrations
- bilirubin levels
- uraemic inhibitors
- presence of heparin
- numbers of free fatty acids
- other (displacing) drugs

Predilution increases transfer (and so clearance) of protein-bound urea (and other molecules) into plasma (Kaplan 1998).

Large ultrafiltrate volumes are often smaller than human glomerular filtrate so that drug clearance by filters may be no higher than the Bowman's capsule. But selective reabsorption in the human kidney may restore plasma concentrations. Drug prescriptions may therefore need increasing or decreasing during haemofiltration. Where drugs are titrated to therapeutic effects such as measured laboratory levels (e.g. vancomycin) or clinical parameters (e.g. blood pressure with inotropes), dosages can safely be adjusted within prescribed limits to achieve specified aims. With other drugs, advice from unit pharmacists is valuable.

Many colloids in clinical use are below filter pore size; volume replacement should either use cheaper crystalloids or large molecule colloids (e.g. hydroxyethyl starch – see Chapter 33).

Most manufacturers recommend *changing circuits* every 72 hours. Anecdotal reports suggest filters and circuits can function considerably longer, but circuits are highly invasive and so major sources for infection; nurses contravening (and managers condoning) the manufacturer's instructions may be legally liable for harm.

Plasmapheresis

Plasmapheresis ('extracorporeal purification') resembles haemofiltration, usually with smaller filter pores. Intermittent treatments, usually spread over several days, enables removal of

- drugs (e.g. overdoses)
- mediators (e.g. of ARDS, SIRS and MODS)
- fluid, electrolyte and acid–base imbalance (Kaplan & Epstein 1997)

Cytokines weigh under 80 Da (Marshall 1995) and so can be readily filtered provided they remain unbound. Interleukin 1 (IL-1) and tumour necrosis factor (TNF) are absorbed onto filter membranes, while interleukin 6 (IL-6) and platelet activating factor are lost in ultrafiltrate (Kirby & Davenport 1996). At present, it is unclear whether removing mediators improves patient outcome (Kirby & Davenport 1996), but Ronco *et al.*'s (1995) laboratory study found removal of platelet activating factor by CAVH effective, suggesting potential benefit for treating SIRS and MODS.

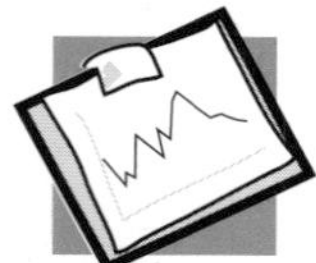

Implications for practice

- nurses who have not used haemofiltration equipment should take every opportunity to learn how to manage it before caring for patients being haemofiltered
- principles of haemofiltration are similar to the human nephron so that, although machines can appear daunting, circuits can be followed through by comparing them with nephron function
- when checking circuits, start from the beginning of the afferent line and work through the circuit until the end of the efferent line
- check the circuit and equipment at the start of each shift and whenever necessary
- nursing workload usually increases significantly when haemofiltration is commenced, necessitating careful prioritisation of nursing care

- large fluid balance errors can quickly accumulate; fluid balance should be kept as simple as possible, avoiding volumes under 1 ml; recheck calculations and running totals
- alarms normally halt circuits; identify and resolve problems urgently, restarting the system before coagulation blocks the filter
- involve unit pharmacists to identify how therapeutic drugs are affected by filtration
- hypotension can occur quickly, especially when commencing filtration so that haemodynamic status should be closely monitored
- unless instructed otherwise, start afferent pumps at 100 ml/min; once stable (after 10 minutes) increase pump speed to at least 150 ml/min

Summary

Renal replacement in most ICUs is provided by haemofiltration (and variants), although hospitals with renal units may use haemodialysis; there is also growing interest in plasmapheresis to treat pathologies such as SIRS/MODS.

Haemofiltration has proved to be a valuable medical adjunct to intensive care. While technology has made circuits and machines safer, haemofiltration is highly invasive, exposing patients to various complications and dangers. Renal failure in ICU patients is usually secondary, and caring for patients receiving haemofiltration can create high nursing workloads. Care should be prioritised to ensure a safe environment. Nurses unfamiliar with using haemofiltration are encouraged to find out how to use it in practice before having to care on their own for patients receiving haemofiltration.

Further reading

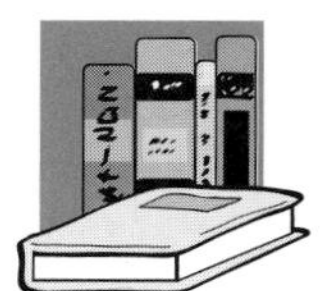

Despite widespread use in ICUs, few ICU textbooks discuss haemofiltration in sufficient depth. Some useful articles have appeared in specialist journals; Kirby and Davenport (1996) offer a useful recent overview; despite their age, articles by Miller *et al.* (1990) and McClelland (1993a) are worth reading.

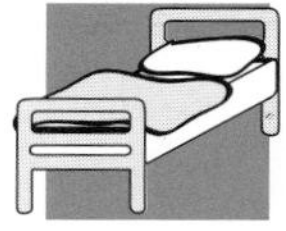

Clinical scenario

David Sinclair is 58 years old. He developed rhabdomyolysis and acute renal failure from compression injury as a result of collapsing, lying on the floor for over 18 hours and ingesting nephrotoxic medication. He is known to suffer from hypertension, angina and gout. He was commenced on continuous venovenous haemofiltration (CVVHF).

Q.1 List the range and approaches of continuous haemofiltration and haemodiafiltration available in your practice area. Identify and explain any differences in equipment and patient application between haemofiltration and haemodiafiltration (e.g. in condition of patients, nursing skills, knowledge, pump devices, filters, catheters, access, dialysate and intravenous fluid replacement solutions, adverse effects, etc.).

Q.2 Mr Sinclair has been taking aspirin and ibuprofen (NSAID's) prior to ICU admission.

(a) Analyse how these drugs may affect Mr Sinclair's coagulation while on CVVHF.
(b) Note from which cannulation site (venous/arterial) or area of CVVHF circuit blood is best sampled to assess Mr Sinclair's clotting. How frequently should his clotting be assessed? Describe and explain the observational assessment of Mr Sinclair's coagulation status.
(c) Review the choice of anticoagulation therapies and select the most appropriate approach for Mr Sinclair (e.g. administration route, dose and titration of heparin, prostacyclin, low molecular weight heparin, no anticoagulant, use and cost of biocompatable filters, other therapies, etc.).

Q.3 Appraise the role of the ICU nurse in maintaining effectiveness and patency of CVVHF until Mr Sinclair's kidneys are sufficiently recovered to be able to dispense with the CVVHF by:

(a) explaining the nurse's role in monitoring, trouble shooting and maintaining patency of filter and patient safety with circuit (e.g. blood flows, leaks, air, fluid and electrolyte management, patient position);
(b) justifying other nursing approaches aimed at promoting renal recovery (e.g. drugs, nutrition, psychological support, infection control, weaning CVVHF, etc.).

Chapter 36

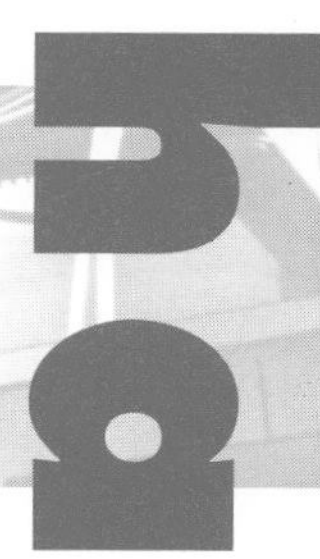

Gastrointestinal bleeds

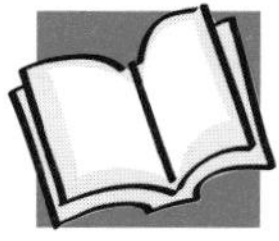

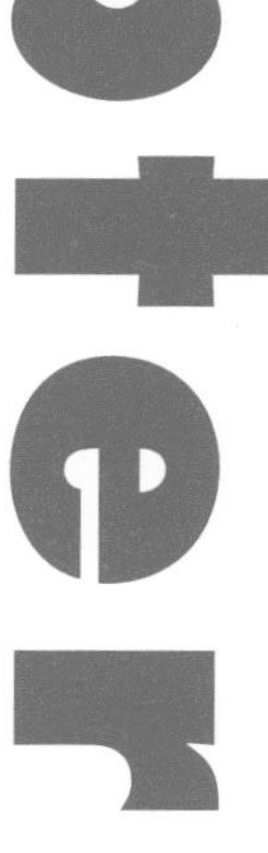

Contents

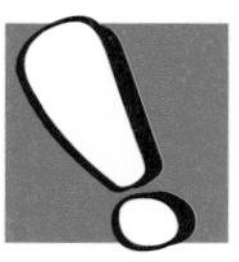

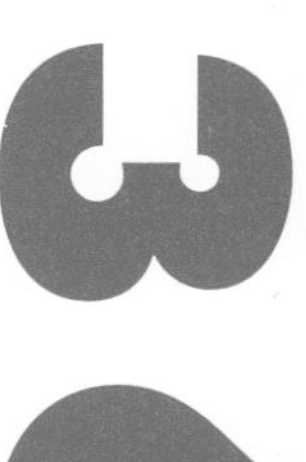

Fundamental knowledge

Gastrointestinal anatomy

Introduction

The importance of gastrointestinal failure to critical care pathophysiology has been increasingly recognised; major gastrointestinal bleeding poses more obvious threats to survival. The gastrointestinal (GI) tract is highly vascular; although bleeding can be a primary pathology, coagulopathies and haemorrhage complicate other disease processes.

Acute upper GI bleeds are usually larger, more rapid and more likely to cause or complicate ICU admission than lower GI bleeds; first bleeds usually indicate liver failure, often from alcoholic liver disease, which has a high incidence of re-bleeding. Most clotting factors are produced by the liver, and so hepatic dysfunction disrupts haemostasis. Oesophageal varices can haemorrhage so rapidly and profusely that one-half of patients die from their first bleed (Schoenfield & Butler 1998). Lower GI bleeds are less immediately life-threatening, but are briefly mentioned at the end of this chapter.

Variceal bleeding

The portal vein carries blood (and nutrients) from the stomach to the liver; portal hypertension can be caused by portal vein thrombosis or (more often) cirrhosis (McCaffrey 1991). Alcoholic liver disease, the main cause of cirrhosis (Quinn 1995), is often complicated by malnourishment and gastric ulceration. Collateral veins (e.g. oesophageal varices) are a compensatory mechanism, returning splanchnic bed blood to the inferior vena cava (Quinn 1995); like other collateral vessels, varices have weak walls and are tortuous (McCaffrey 1991), and so rupture easily.

Portal vein pressure is normally 5–10 mmHg. Pressures exceeding 15 mmHg can cause rupture (Lisicka 1997); obstruction may create pressures exceeding 30 mmHg (McCaffrey 1991). Rupture of varices can cause massive haemorrhage, with 30–50 per cent mortality (Sung *et al.* 1993). Urgent treatment should:

- stop the haemorrhage
- provide fluid resuscitation
- replace clotting factors

Haemorrhage is usually stopped by:

- balloon tamponade
- sclerosis
- stents

Medical treatments

Direct pressure to bleeding points is possible using **balloon tamponade** (Sengstaken, Sengstaken-Blakemore, Minnesota tubes; see Figure 36.1). Tubes usually have four ports:

- oesophageal balloon (to stop bleeding)
- oesophageal aspiration port (omitted on 3-port tubes)
- gastric balloon (to anchor tubes)
- gastric aspiration port

Balloon tamponade controls 85–92 per cent of bleeds, but re-bleeds are common (Boyer & Henderson 1996), so that balloon tamponade is often only a temporary (emergency) treatment.

Tubes are large and relatively difficult to introduce, especially during major haemorrhaging. Despite oesophageal aspiration channels, patients will usually be intubated to prevent aspiration; decreased consciousness and other complications usually necessitate ventilation.

Unlike digital pressure on radial arteries, balloon pressure on oesophageal varices creates various problems:

- surrounding tissue cannot be seen, and so ischaemia from arterial/capillary occlusion may remain undetected until damage occurs

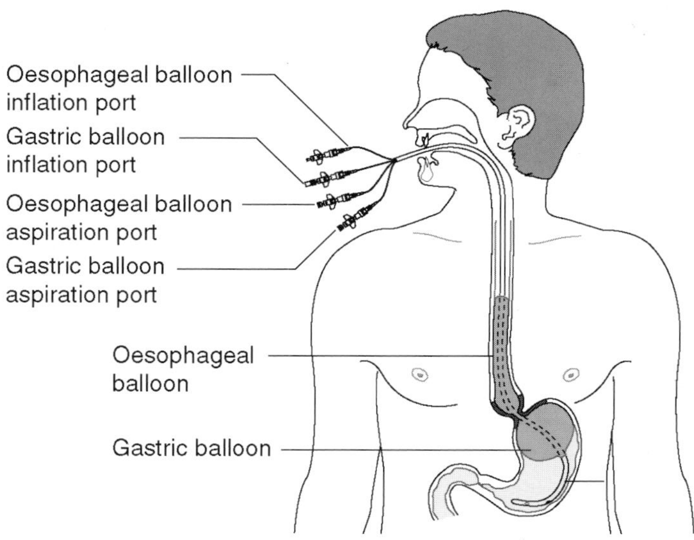

Figure 36.1 **A Sengstaken tube**

- staff usually soon tire of digital pressure, but balloon tamponade does not provide staff with sensory feedback
- efficacy is seen only by presence or absence of frank bleeding; extent of subcutaneous bleeding (bruising) remains unseen

Oesophageal pressure should be sufficient to control haemorrhage, but not to cause rupture, ischaemia or necrosis.

Oesophageal balloons can hold up to 60 ml of air. Recommended pressures vary from 25–40 mmHg (McCaffrey 1991) to 50–60 mmHg (Sung 1997) (see section on capillary occlusion pressure in Chapter 5). Pressure can be measured by connecting a sphygmomanometer or continuous monitoring system to the oesophageal inflation port. McCaffery (1991) recommends measuring oesophageal pressure half-hourly, but higher priorities may prevent this aspect of care, and with lack of consensus on optimal pressure, frequent measurement has dubious benefits.

Using external traction (weights) to further compress oesophageal varices with the gastric balloon (Hudak *et al.* 1998) is controversial. Gastric varices, already compressed by the gastric balloon, should prevent flow to higher varices. Many centres avoid using traction, but, if used, lifting weights should be avoided as tube movement may dislodge clots.

Since deflation can traumatise friable healing tissue, some centres avoid inflating oesophageal balloons, relying on occlusion of flow from inflation of gastric balloons to stop the haemorrhage. Gradual deflation may limit trauma, but again the effects cannot be seen.

Complications from prolonged pressure (e.g. oedema, oesphagitis, perforation, ulcers) limit balloon use to 24 hours (Hudak *et al.* 1998); McCaffery (1991) recommends balloon deflation to prevent complications, but, given the friable nature of varices, this practice seems difficult to support.

VASOPRESSIN This antidiuretic hormone and its derivatives (desmopressin, terlipressin) cause splanchnic arterial vasoconstriction, thus reducing portal hypertension. They can temporarily control haemorrhage for 28–70 per cent of patients, although up to one-third may re-bleed during treatment (Boyer & Henderson 1996); like tamponade, vasopressin can buy time for more definitive treatments.

Vasopressin causes systemic vasoconstriction, and extravasation may cause necrosis, and so it should be given into central veins (Boyer & Henderson 1996). Vasoconstriction can provoke angina, necessitating ICU admission for monitoring; angina can be alleviated by (sublingual) nitrates (Boyer & Henderson 1996).

SCLEROTHERAPY (endoscopic injection of alcohol into varices) This usually involves progressive obliteration through a series of treatments (usually over 1–4 weeks) so that patients may be transferred from ICU before treatment is completed. Sclerosis stops most bleeds, although re-bleeds are common (Dobb 1997).

BANDING Endoscopic ligatation with bands ('*banding*') is more effective than sclerotherapy (Stiegmann *et al.* 1992; Gimson *et al.* 1993).

BETA-BLOCKERS These also cause splanchnic vasoconstriction, thus reducing portal pressure in about 60 per cent of patients with cirrhosis, making β-blockers as effective as sclerosing agents (Boyer & Henderson 1996).

The hormone *somatostatin* inhibits gastrin secretion, reducing gastric acid secretion. Schoenfield and Butler (1998) claim that the longer-acting synthetic analogue *octreotide* is as effective as endoscopy, but anecdotal reports suggest it is ineffective.

TRANSJUGULAR INTRAHEPATIC PORTOSYSTEMIC SHUNT (TIPS) An angioplasty-type catheter, inserted under radiography, can create a fistula between the portal and hepatic veins (Schoenfield & Butler 1998); patency is maintained using expandable metal stents (usually 8–12 mm diameter) (Boyer & Henderson 1996).

Early complications (Boyer & Henderson 1996, Roessle *et al.* 1994) include:

- capsular hepatic rupture
- arteriovenous fistula
- venous biliary fistula
- stent migration
- hepatic encephalopathy
- raised blood ammonia from portocaval shunting
- dysrhythmias

Encephalopathy can usually be limited with protein restriction and lactulose, so is rarely problematic (Lisicka 1997).

GASTRIC IRRIGATION to remove blood may also prolong or restart haemorrhage. Cold water may also cause vagal stimulation, increasing gastric motility and irritation to ulcers.

SURGICAL oesophageal transection or implantation of portocaval shunts effectively controls bleeding, but without improvement in long-term survival (Sung 1997), and so tends to be tried when one or more of the above measures has failed.

Peptic ulcers

Most upper GI bleeds are from peptic ulcers – 10 per cent of the UK population develop peptic ulcers (Cotterill 1996). Treatment may be preventative (protecting against gastric acidity), supportive (replacing blood volume and clotting factors), medical (treating bacteria – see below) or surgical.

Gastric mucus maintains wide pH differences between gastric acid (or alkaline bile) and epithelium. Mucosal failure may be caused by

- excess acid production (from gastromas)
- lack of neutralising factors (absence of enteral nutrition)
- bile reflux
- irritant drugs (e.g. aspirin and non-steroidal anti-inflammatories).

The bacterium *Helicobacter pylori* is particularly associated with peptic ulceration.

About one-half of the population harbour this gram negative bacterium, with colonisation often starting in childhood (MacConnachie 1997a). As it is found in water, enteric transmission seems likely (Cotterill 1996), and it is particularly prevalent when sanitation is poor.

Most people colonised by *Helicobacter pylori* remain asymptomatic (Cotterill 1996), but most people with ulcers are infected by it (MacConnachie 1997a), and it appears to cause gastritis, ulcers and gastromas (Cotterill 1996). According to MacConnachie (1997a) it provokes:

- local inflammatory responses (disrupting mucosal barriers)
- systemic immune response

and inhibits endogenous somatostatin release (so increasing acid production).

Since *Helicobacter pylori* requires an alkaline environment, in stomach acid it produces urease to convert urea to ammonia (the alkaline environment it needs) and carbon dioxide (Cotterill 1996).

Helicobacter pylori is destroyed by combination drug therapy (e.g. omperazole, metronidazole and another antibiotic) (MacConnachie 1997a). Once eliminated, UK recurrence rates are low, but they can reach 40 per cent in developing countries (Cotterill 1996), probably due to re-infection through poor sanitation.

Helicobacter pylori can be detected by carbon dioxide production on ingesting urea isotopes (carbon 13 or 14), but, being costly, tests are not often performed (Cotterill 1996).

Complications

Severe haemorrhage rapidly causes *hypovolaemic shock*, hypoperfusion predisposing to SIRS and MODS. Urgent fluid resuscitation is usually required, especially with colloids, clotting factors and blood transfusions. Massive blood transfusions further disrupt homeostasis, predisposing to DIC and electrolyte imbalance (necessitating close haemodynamic and electrolyte monitoring).

Gastrointestinal tract bacteria digest blood, releasing *ammonia*. Normally cleared hepatically, liver failure causes toxic circulating levels. Ammonia is neurotoxic, causing rapid *encephalopathy* and confusion. Lactulose inhibits ammonia absorption (Quinn 1995).

Prevention

Enteral feeding helps to protect against gastric ulceration; however, enteral feeding should include rest periods to enable gastric pH to fall (see Chapter 9). H_2-blockers (cimetidine, ranitidine), once used to reduce gastric acid secretion, do not reduce incidence of bleeding (Sung 1997).

Sucralfate, an aluminium salt, stimulates mucosal blood flow and mucus secretion, together with local prostaglandin production (Sung 1997), thus increasing endogenous defences. Sucralfate does not reduce gastric acidity so that gram negative colonisation is inhibited; it can also cause constipation, and aluminium toxicity can provoke renal failure (Sung 1997).

Lower GI bleeds

Bleeds below the duodenum are rarely life-threatening; most stop spontaneously and seldom require ICU admission. However, many ICU patients have coagulopathies, and so may bleed from the highly vascular lower GI tract.

Stools should be observed for frank blood; occult bleeding can be confirmed by testing. Observations should be recorded and reported; samples may be required for testing. Bleeding may be fresh (red; usually lower GI bleeds) or old (black, tarry; usually upper GI bleeds).

Most bleeds are small, but if large bleeds do not resolve spontaneously, early surgery (e.g. hemicolectomy) may be needed.

Implications for practice

- emergency situations necessitate prioritising of care ('patients before paperwork')
- large bleeds need urgent fluid resuscitation and close haemodynamic monitoring; computerised memory and appropriate alarm limits can be particularly valuable
- with balloon tamponade, oesophageal aspiration is usually continuous; periodic gastric aspiration should be performed to assess blood loss and prevent digestion of blood metabolites (the source of ammonia)
- elevating the patient's head reduces portal blood flow
- burst stomach balloons usually rise (especially if traction is used), potentially causing airway obstruction
- keep scissors handy (if tubes need removing quickly, tapes/ties should be cut)
- blood is hazardous, potentially carrying viruses such as hepatitis B and HIV; maintain a safe environment for yourself, other staff and visitors
- seeing blood can make patients and families especially anxious; psychological support and care can help them cope and warn them about the possibility of seeing/smelling blood; if possible, remove soiled linen

- escort visitors to the bedside, encouraging them to sit down (so they do not harm themselves on equipment if they faint)
- mouthcare helps to remove the vile taste of blood

Summary

Helicobacter pylori is increasingly recognised as a major cause of peptic ulceration. Liver failure (often due to alcoholism) often leads to oesophageal varices, but, however caused, upper gastrointestinal bleeding can be rapid and fatal, requiring ICU admission and intensive treatment. ICU nurses necessarily have an important role in assisting doctors to control and monitor bleeds, but they also have an important role in maintaining a safe environment for themselves and others, and in meeting the psychological needs of patients and visitors.

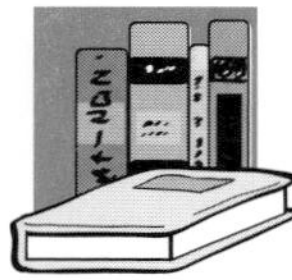

Further reading

In general, chapters in ICU books (e.g. Quinn (1995), Sung (1997) give practical overviews of GI bleeding. McCaffrey (1991) gives a simplistic description of Sengstaken tubes, useful for those unfamiliar with using them. Schoenfield and Butler (1998) provide a useful review of oesophageal bleeding. *Helicobacter pylori* is described by Cotterill (1996).

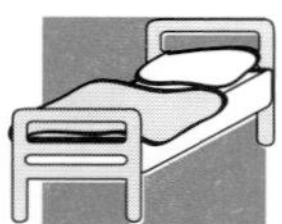

Clinical scenario

Kevin Brown is a 45-year-old mobile phone salesman. He smokes an average of 20 cigarettes each day and usually drinks several pints of beer after work during the week, with more at the weekends. Kevin has recently experienced epigastric pain for which he has taken oral antacids. A colleague accompanied Kevin to the Accident & Emergency Department (A & E) after he had vomited 'dark fluid' and collapsed in a business meeting. In A & E he had further haematemesis, estimated volume of 3 litres, and was quickly admitted to ICU in hypovolaemic shock from suspected peptic/duodenal ulcers or bleeding oesophageal varices.

Q.1 List the nursing priorities when preparing for and admitting Kevin Brown with an emergency GI bleed. Include resources needed such as equipment, drugs, investigations and specialists.

An emergency endoscopy is performed which confirms bleeding oesophageal varices. Kevin then has endoscopic banding ligation to obliterate the ruptured and bleeding vessels. His hypovolaemia is resolved and Kevin becomes more haemodynamically stable.

Q.2 Analyse nursing interventions following endoscopic variceal ligation which monitor and minimise potential complications (e.g. if elastic bands are found in Kevin's mouth, melaena, metabolic effects of blood in lower GI tract).

Q.3 This was Kevin's first hospital admission. His initial experience of haematemesis and speed of emergency interventions have made him highly anxious.

(a) Review probable causes of his ruptured varices and the risk of reoccurrence. Specify the liver function investigations he may undergo.

(b) Design a plan of care for Kevin that focuses on reducing his anxiety and the risk of re-bleeding in ICU and later in transfer to ward and discharge from hospital care.

Advice should include the reason for and practical strategies on:

- Avoiding vigorous coughing and sneezing
- Recognition of early signs and symptoms of re-bleeding
- Relaxation techniques
- Drug action affected by his condition and hepatic impairment, e.g. benzodiazepines, aspirin, paracetamol, some antibiotics, alcohol, cigarettes/nicotine.
- Lifestyle changes
- Use of specialist nurses, referral groups.

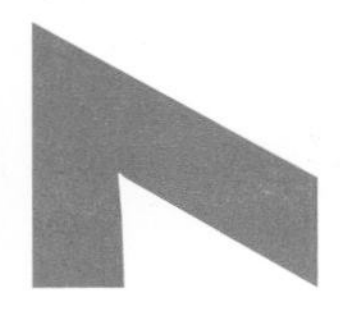
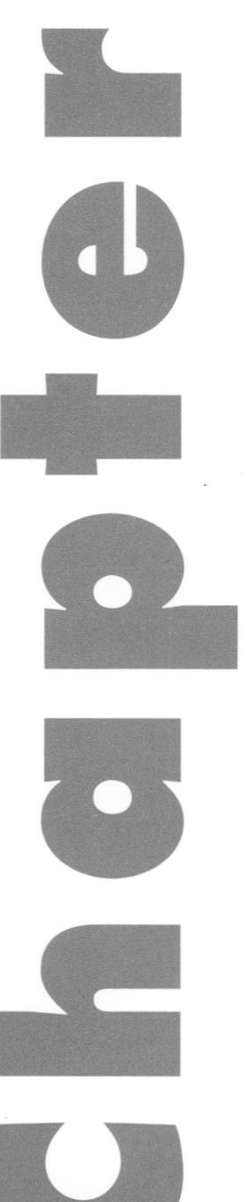

Chapter 37

Pancreatitis

Contents

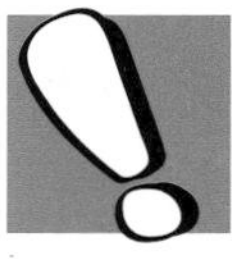

Fundamental knowledge

Pancreatic anatomy and physiology
Endocrine and exocrine functions
Sphincter of Oddi

Introduction

Pancreatitis is a relatively common disease affecting people of all ages, normally caused by

- alcoholism (usually in men under 40)
- biliary reflux (usually in older women)

Most district general hospitals treat between 50 and 100 cases each year (Mitchell & MacFie 1991); pancreatitis is usually mild and self-limiting, and so not needing ICU admission, but severe cases often progress rapidly (sometimes within one week (Johnson 1998)) to multisystem dysfunction requiring ICU support. Mortality from severe pancreatitis remains high with most deaths resulting from complications (SIRS, MODS); medical and nursing management, therefore, focuses on system support to minimise or limit complications. This chapter describes the possible effects of severe pancreatitis.

The pancreas normally secretes 1,500 ml of digestive juices each day as secretion is a reflex vagal response to acidic chyme in the duodenum. Pancreatic juice, which enters the duodenum at the sphincter of Oddi, is strongly alkaline (pH about 8.0) and contains phospholipidase A, a powerful protein-digesting enzyme. Phospholipidase A, released as an inactive proenzyme to prevent autodigestion, is normally activated in the duodenum by trypsin; activation in the pancreas or outside the gastrointestinal tract (via fistulae) causes autodigestion and fat necrosis.

Obstruction of the ampulla of Vater (e.g. gallstones) causes reflux of pancreatic enzymes (Venables 1991); acid chyme, which remains unneutralised, continues to stimulate further pancreatic juice production. Congestion eventually ruptures the pancreatic ductules, releasing pancreatic juice directly into the gland.

Pancreatic damage releases a cascade of vasoactive mediators, including

- kinins
- interleukins
- platelet activating factor
- free oxygen radicals (Gunning 1997).

Gross vasodilation causes hypotension and ischaemia and further release of mediators from ischaemic endothelium, often progressing to multisystem dysfunction. Gut ischaemia facilitates translocation of bacteria, and so prophylactic antibiotics are usually prescribed (Johnson 1998).

Serum amylase levels usually increase up to tenfold (Reece-Smith 1997) within 6 hours, but may return to normal within 48 hours (Santamaria 1997). Chronic underlying pancreatic disease (from alcoholism) may prevent a rise in serum amylase (Johnson 1998) so that normal levels can not preclude diagnosis.

Pathology

The terminology for types of severe pancreatitis varies. Acute pancreatitis can progress to fulminant stages, most texts identifying these as *acute oedematous* or *toxic pancreatitis*, and *necrotizing* or *fulminant pancreatitis*.

ACUTE OEDEMATOUS/TOXIC PANCREATITIS This lasts a few days, the pancreas being congested and swollen. Tissue damage causes release of vasoactive mediators (see above), triggering massive extravasation of plasma, hypovolaemic shock and gross oedema.

NECROTIZING PANCREATITIS Acute oedematous pancreatitis can progress to necrotizing pancreatitis. Disruption of vessels in and around the pancreas causes systemic release of enzymes and toxic chemicals, resulting in inflammation, haemorrhage and fat necrosis. Translocated gut bacteria suppurate in necrotic tissue, leading to SIRS and MODS. The problems may not be apparent until patients relapse some weeks following apparent recovery from acute pancreatitis.

CHRONIC RELAPSING PANCREATITIS This is a rare complication occurring when pancreatic function remains insufficient after four weeks (necessarily a retrospective classification). ICU admission is seldom needed.

PANCREATIC ABSCESSES These can occur after two or more weeks (Reece-Smith 1997), with high (60 per cent) mortality (Venables 1991); once confirmed by *CT scan*, open surgical drainage is necessary (Reece-Smith 1997).

PANCREATIC PSEUDOCYSTS These are inflammatory exudate, often collecting as fluid within the lesser sac around the pancreas (Venables 1991); pseudocysts occur in up to one-half of patients suffering acute pancreatitis (Reece-Smith 1997) during the fulminant stages. Most pseudocysts resolve spontaneously (Venables 1991), but until resolution, surrounding tissues can be compressed and fistulae into surrounding tissue can develop, causing haemorrhage (especially hepatic or splenic) or infection (especially with bowel fistulae).

Pseudocysts unresolved after six weeks should be drained percutaneously, under endoscopy, or removed surgically (Venables 1991).

Symptoms

Oedema and distension of the pancreatic capsule, biliary tree obstruction or chemical peritoneal burning (phospholipidase A) cause severe acute *abdominal pain* (Krumberger 1995), requiring opiate analgesia.

Use of morphine is controversial; theoretically, morphine constricts the sphincter of Oddi, accentuating pain, but Krumberger (1995) suggests morphine has minimal effects on the sphincter of Oddi. Pethidine may avoid this problem (Reece-Smith 1997; Johnson 1998), although Santamaria (1997) suggests both drugs cause constriction, but that pancreatic secretions through the sphincter will be minimal so that differences are largely theoretical. Mitchell and MacFie (1991) similarly support the use of either pethidine or morphine. Hence, as reasonable alternatives exist, using morphine appears unnecessary.

Thoracic epidural analgesia may also be useful (Johnson 1998), provided that clotting is not impaired. Epidural blockade can cause further vasodilation (Johnson 1998), and so blood volume should be monitored and replaced as appropriate.

Increased capillary permeability from vasoactive mediators causes massive and rapid intra-abdominal *fluid shifts*, hypovolaemia and gross oedema. Patients may need up to 10 litres of intravascular fluid replacement in the first day (Mitchell & MacFie 1991); Hypovolaemia is intravascular rather than total body fluid so that most fluid replacement will be with colloids (Johnson 1998) and should be closely monitored (CVP and probably PCWP).

Hypermetabolism is the main cause of *pyrexia*, although infection can also occur. Temperature should be monitored; if problematic (e.g. excessive oxygen consumption), antipyretics may be needed (see Chapter 8).

Possible *skin discoloration* includes Turner's sign (bluish-purple discoloration of flanks, from retroperitoneal haemorrhage); this occurs in about 1 per cent of cases, indicating probable mortality (Gunning 1997).

Pancreatitis causes *electrolyte imbalances*:

- *hyperglycaemia* (from impaired insulin secretion, increased glucagon release, circulating antagonists such as catecholamines, and glucose in parenteral feeds); blood sugars should be closely monitored; sliding scales of insulin may be prescribed
- *hypocalcaemia* is usually caused by hypoproteinaemia (Santamaria 1997)
- *hypomagnesaemia* is common, especially with alcohol-related pancreatitis (Santamaria 1997)

Multisystem complications

Pancreatitis compromises most major systems.

Gross ascites causes physical splinting of both lung bases, precipitating *respiratory failure*, the main cause of deaths (Krumberger 1995). Atelectasis and pleural effusions may occur, especially in the left lung (Gunning 1997). Surfactant damage from phospholipidase A can lead to ARDS.

Cardiovascular instability is caused by

- continuing massive fluid shifts
- myocardial depressant factor (pancreatic hormone released in response to pancreatic ischaemia)
- pericardial effusions
- electrolyte imbalances.

Cardiac output studies will probably be needed to monitor haemodynamic status. Dysrhythmias, especially ST segment, often occur.

Autodigestion of arteries near the pancreas (especially splenic arteries) by pancreatic juices can cause aneurysms (Chalmers 1991). Damage to the splenic vein can cause portal venous thrombosis (Chalmers 1991).

Raised fibrinogen and factor VIII levels provoke hypercoagulopathy (Krumberger 1995), predisposing to DIC.

The cardiovascular system should be closely monitored, with supports to maintain homeostasis.

Direct damage to the *gastrointestinal system* can cause

- peptic ulceration
- gastritis
- bowel infarction
- paralytic ileus
- translocation of gut bacteria.

Hypermetabolism increases energy expenditure, necessitating additional nutritional support. If possible, feeding should be enteral (Johnson 1998), but paralytic ileus and/or duodenal damage may prevent enteral feeding, although jejunal feeds (which unlike gastric feeds do not stimulate pancreatic secretions (Santamaria 1997)) may be possible; parenteral nutrition may be necessary, but will expose patients to potential infection, hyperglycaemia and other complications.

Severe systemic hypotension often causes *acute tubular necrosis*; in these circumstances, haemofiltration will be needed.

Medical treatments

Gallstones should be removed with early endoscopic retrograde cholangiopancreatography (ERCP) (Neoptolemos 1992; Johnson 1998). Surgical removal is also possible, but has a worse prognosis than ERCP (Neoptolemos 1992). Fat necrosis and slough may need surgical removal (Reece-Smith 1997).

Dialysis does not remove vasoactive mediators effectively (Gunning 1997), but *plasmapheresis* appears promising.

Antiproteases to reduce or neutralise pancreatic enzyme release (e.g. aprotinin, gabexate mesylate) should theoretically improve outcome (Gunning 1997). Most studies have proved disappointing (Johnson 1998), with the result that antiprotease treatment has largely been abandoned.

Leucocyte by-products cause most damage, and so possible treatments (needing further evaluation) include (Neoptolemos 1992):

- antioxidants
- tumour necrosis factor antagonists

- leukotriene antagonists
- plasminogen activation factor antagonists

Lexipafant appears promising, but antioxidant therapy remains untested (Johnson 1998) and trials of antibodies for tumour necrosis factor-alpha have proved detrimental, so that this treatment is not now recommended.

Implications for practice

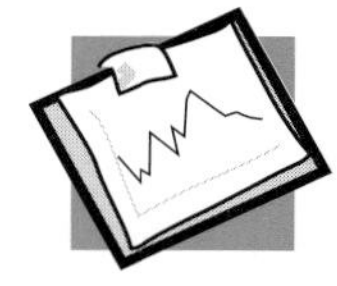

- pain is severe; analgesia (usually opiate) should be provided and its effectiveness assessed
- morphine may aggravate pain (contracting the sphincter of Oddi), and so pethidine or other non-morphine opiates are recommended
- large fluid shifts can rapidly cause oedema (including pulmonary) and hypovolaemia; arterial blood pressure and fluid balance charts give little indication of intravascular volume; haemodynamic monitoring should include CVP, ECGs, electrolyte balance, and possibly PCWP with cardiac output studies
- hyperglycaemia may occur; blood sugars should be monitored regularly, and insulin infusions may be needed
- nurses should ensure nutrition is optimised; if possible use enteral routes; consider jejunostomy

Summary

Pancreatitis can cause rapid and severe complications in most other major systems. Severe pancreatitis, seen in ICUs, continues to cause high mortality. The current treatment is largely support systems, with pain control being a particularly important nursing role.

Further reading

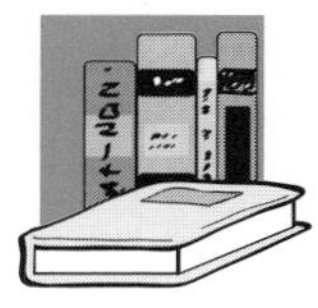

Pathophysiology is well described by Reece-Smith (1997), although Johnson's (1998) article draws on more recent material. Textbook chapters (e.g. Krumberger (1995), Gunning (1997), Santamaria (1997)) usually provide useful overviews.

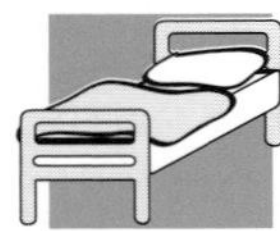

Clinical scenario

Gita Kumar is 56 years old and was admitted to ICU with severe respiratory distress and considerable abdominal pain. She is 1.52 m (5 feet) tall and weighs 70 kg (154 lb/11 stone). Prior to this Gita was attending a large family wedding where she experienced worsening of left-sided epigastric pain. She had experienced this pain intermittently over two days. The pain radiated towards her back and was accompanied by nausea and vomiting.

On admission her abdomen was distended, ultrasound scan revealed gallstones. Other abnormal results from admission assessment included:

Vital signs		*Blood serum*	
Temperature	38.9°C	Glucose	15 mmol/l
Respiration	35 per min	WBC	16×10^{-9}/l
SpO_2	85%	Amylase	1,265 IU/l
Heart rate	125 bpm	Alkaline phosphate	350 IU/l
3-lead ECG	sinus rhythm, ST elevation	Potassium	3.1 mmol/l
		Calcium	0.8 mmol/l
BP	90/45 mmHg	Magnesium	1.2 mmol/l
MAP	60 mmHg		

Q.1 Review the anatomy and endocrine functions of the pancreas. Explain Gita's abnormal results using physiological processes (i.e. why has her temperature and respiratory rate increased, why does she have low potassium with presenting symptoms and diagnosis?).

Q.2 A nasogastric (NG) tube is sited.

(a) Debate the rationale for siting a NG tube with Gita, noting both benefits and potential complications (e.g. decompressing abdomen for improved diaphragmatic movement versus risk of nosocomial respiratory infection).

(b) Discuss appropriate nutritional interventions for Gita. Consider the type, route and amount of nutritional support suitable for her increased metabolic demands, impaired digestion and carbohydrate metabolism, control of blood sugars.

Q.3 Gita recovers from this acute episode of pancreatitis. Appraise the ICU nurse's role in health promotion. What advice and information can you give to Gita to enhance her short-term recovery and longer-term health?

Consider: infection risks, metabolic disturbances from pancreatic insult, advice on diet/medications/activities, etc., changes to lifestyle, body image, social and family role.

Chapter 38

Neurological pathologies

Guillain Barré syndrome, critical illness neuropathy, autonomic dysreflexia

Contents

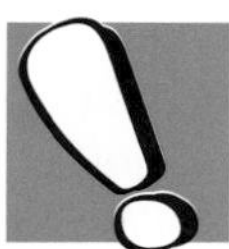

Fundamental knowledge

Nerve anatomy and conduction: myelin, nodes of Ranvier
Sympathetic/parasympathetic function and negative feedback mechanisms for homeostasis
Autonomic nervous system

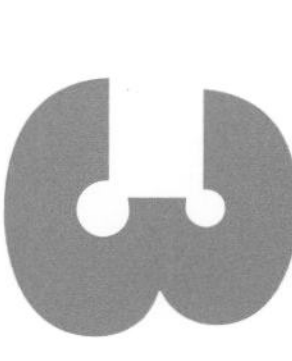

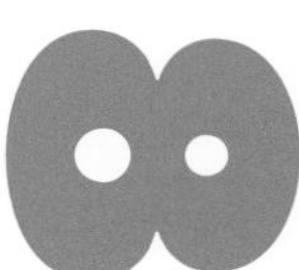

Introduction

This chapter discusses three conditions seen with varying frequency on ICUs:

- Guillain Barré syndrome
- critical illness neuropathy
- autonomic dysreflexia

All three conditions cause nerve dysfunction, so that normal homeostatic balance between sympathetic and parasympathetic controls (through feedback mechanisms) is disrupted. Impaired voluntary nervous function may be frustrating for patients, but autonomic nervous system dysfunction may prove life-threatening. The problems are similar in all three conditions: muscle weakness (including respiratory), underlying hypotension and bradycardia with potentially excessive inappropriate episodes of hypertension and tachycardia.

Nursing patients with these conditions can be labour intensive and stressful; they need care and support with many activities of living, while minimising complications significantly improves recovery and survival. Nursing care is therefore especially valuable for such patients.

Head injury, the major neurological cause of general ICU admission, is included in Chapter 22, while meningitis is discussed in Chapter 13.

Management of all three conditions centres on

- attempts to remove underlying causes
- prevention of complications
- system support.

While there is some research evidence, practice varies between units; some approaches described below are anecdotal rather than evidence-based.

Guillain Barré syndrome (GBS)

This syndrome describes acute inflammatory demyelinating polyneuropathies of peripheral nerves. One of the most prevalent neurological disorders (Waldock 1995), GBS occurs in 1.7 per 100,000 population per year (Fulgham & Wijdicks 1997). While the literature is consistent on incidence, it is inconsistent about possible gender, age, racial and seasonal prevalence.

Although the precise mechanism remains unclear, GBS is probably caused by either

- viral infection or
- autoimmune response.

GBS usually occurs following minor viral infections (Desforges 1992), especially respiratory or gastrointestinal, often from cytomegalovirus (CMV)

(Hund *et al.* 1993). GBS can also occur following vaccination, especially tetanus, influenza or measles (Waldock 1995). Immunosuppression (e.g. lymphomas, HIV, Hodgkin's disease) can also trigger GBS (Waldock 1995).

Immune system dysfunction results in T-lymphocyte migration to peripheral nerves causing inflammation oedema (Ross 1993) and myelin destruction (Desforges 1992), creating lesions (especially in spinal nerves and near dorsal root ganglia) (Waldock 1995) and the progressive destruction of the nodes of Ranvier. This, in turn, causes ascending motor and sensory paralysis, resulting in diffuse muscle weakness.

Medical attempts to treat the underlying causes of GBS remain controversial. Prolonged artificial ventilation is often needed, and many units favour early tracheostomy. Steroids, once used widely, are not recommended in Desforges' (1992) literature review. Circulating mediators may be removed through plasma exchange (Fulgham & Wijdicks 1997), plasmapheresis (Hund *et al.* 1993) and intravenous gamma globulin (Desforges 1992) – although this may cause meningitis and acute renal failure (Fulgham & Wijdicks 1997).

If basement membrane remains intact, recovery begins once Schwann cells' mitosis remyelinates damaged nerves (usually 2–4 weeks (Skowronski 1997)). Within six months, 85 per cent of patients recover completely, although a minority suffer residual disability, especially older patients (Waldock 1995), presumably because GBS compounds neuronal loss from ageing. Overall mortality from GBS is 5 per cent (Winer 1994), but ICU mortality is higher (25 per cent (Skowronski 1997)). Death is usually caused by respiratory or cardiac arrest (McMahon-Parkes & Cornock 1997), so that the prevention of complications improves survival.

Muscle weakness and autonomic dysfunction can cause:

- *pain* from nerve dysfunction, exacerbated by touch (Coakley 1997) and anxiety, which is usually worse in the evening (Mirski *et al.* 1995). Analgesia (often opiates) is needed. Patients should be positioned comfortably; TENS, massage and other interventions may alleviate pain.
- *respiratory failure*, the usual cause of ICU admission (Fulgham & Wijdicks 1997). Many GBS patients need ventilatory support, although intubation is avoided if possible by CPAP/noninvasive positive pressure ventilation and intensive physiotherapy.
- *hypersalivation* and loss of gag reflex from autonomic dysfunction necessitate oral suction to prevent aspiration.
- *hypotension* from extensive peripheral vasodilation (poor sympathetic tone).
- ***hypertensive*** episodes caused by failure of normal negative feedback opposition to sympathetic stimuli. Prophylactic beta blockers can control hypertension (Hinds & Watson 1996), although Fulgham and Wijdicks (1997) recommend caution with vasoactive drugs.
- *dysrhythmias* (sinus tachycardia, bradycardia, asystole) frequently occur (Hund *et al.* 1993). As hypoxia can cause bradycardias (Hough 1996),

patients should be given 100 per cent oxygen before suction; during suction, ECG should be monitored closely (Fulgham & Wijdicks 1997). Routine atropine (Hinds & Watson 1996) or sequential pacing may prevent bradycardias.

- *profuse sweating*; frequent washes and changes of clothing help to improve comfort.
- *thrombosis* from venous stasis (immobility) and hypoperfusion. Two per cent of deaths are caused by pulmonary emboli (Coakley 1997); cerebral and myocardial infarction may also occur. Thrombosis risk can be reduced by

  - frequent changes of position
  - prophylactic subcutaneous heparin (Winer 1994)
  - thromboembolytic stockings (Winer 1994)
  - early and aggressive rehabilitation, including active and passive exercises

- *limb weakness*, ascending from distal to proximal muscles, affecting hands, feet or both. Passive exercises may prevent contractures (Winer 1994) and promote venous return.
- *bilateral facial muscle weakness* occurs in one-third of GBS patients (Desforges 1992), causing dribbling of saliva and opthalmoplegia.
- *incontinence* from bladder muscle weakness.
- *immunocompromise* (stress response, hepatic dysfunction), and so infection control and the prevention of opportunistic infection are especially important.
- *catabolism* (McMahon-Parkes & Cornock 1997), thus early nutrition should be given. Paralytic ileus may necessitate parenteral nutrition, but if possible enteral feeding should be used (McMahon-Parkes & Cornock 1997); paralytic ileus may be bypassed through jejunostomy.
- *psychological problems* occur from experiencing progressive weakness for some weeks.

Mentally fit (often young) adults, forced to rely on others to perform fundamental and intimate acts of daily living, develop stressors that compound the environmental stressors of ICUs (see Chapter 3) and fears about prognosis (many GBS sufferers have extensive knowledge about their disease); this can cause hallucinations and acute depressive disorders.

Depression reduces the motivation that is needed with protracted debility. Antidepressants are often useful, but should not become a substitute for active human nursing (e.g. making environments as 'normal' as possible). Psychological support should be extended to family and friends.

Patients with critical illness neuropathy, autonomic dysreflexia and other prolonged disease processes may suffer similar psychological problems.

Critical illness neuropathy ('acute axonal neuropathy')

Critical illness neuropathy, acute axonal neuropathy (Hund *et al.* 1996), occurs in one-half of the patients who are ventilated for over a week, and the incidence increases with the severity of multiorgan failure (Leijten *et al.* 1996); muscle flaccidity delays weaning and causes myocardial fibrillation (Hund *et al.* 1996). Many causes have been speculated, but none clearly established.

Currently there are no specific treatments for critical illness neuropathy; recovery usually occurs between 1–6 months following resolution of sepsis and MODS, often necessitating prolonged rehabilitation (Hinds & Watson 1996).

Autonomic dysreflexia ('hyperreflexia')

The autonomic nervous system controls homeostasis (including vasodilation/constriction and heart rate). Spinal injury severs normal inhibitory pathways, so that parasympathetic compensation occurs only above lesions, with exaggerated sympathetic responses below.

Most patients with spinal injuries above T6 develop autonomic dysreflexia at least 4 weeks, and often 6 months, following injury; it can occur with injuries above T10 (Keely 1998). Although this is usually after transfer to spinal injuries units, ICU nurses may encounter it, especially with patients who have old spinal cord injury (Keely 1998); nurses should therefore be aware of its existence to enable them to provide appropriate information for patients and their families, especially as the incidence of spinal cord injuries is increasing (Witrz *et al.* 1996). Until the injury resolves (usually after a few years), labile blood pressure and pulse may cause cerebral bleeds, damage and death.

Problems include

- *hypotension* from extensive peripheral vasodilation (poor sympathetic tone) (Naftchi & Richardson 1997).
- *paroxysmal hypertensive crises* (up to 250/150 mmHg) (Naftchi & Richardson 1997) from the failure of negative feedback opposition to sympathetic stimuli. Hypertension causes various symptoms: blurred vision, pounding headaches, nasal congestion, nausea, pupil dilatation and profuse sweating and flushing above, with pallor below, the lesion.
- *bradycardia vasodilation* from baroreceptor-mediated vagal responses.
- *infarction* (of any vital organs) from excessive hypertension.

Three-quarters of the crises are provoked by bladder distension (sometimes as little as 200 ml), bowel distension accounting for most (19 per cent) of the remainder (Finocchiaro & Herzfeld 1990). Other sympathetic stimulants include:

- cutaneous (pressure sores, ingrowing toenails, tight/restrictive clothing, seams/creases in clothing and splints)
- skeletal (spasm – especially limb contractures, passive movement/exercises)
- visceral (internal distension: usually bladder or faecal; also gastric ulcers, uterine contractures during labour)
- miscellaneous (bone fractures, vaginal dilation, ejaculation)

Since the patient is unable either to feel stimuli or move, spinal reflexes occur without normal protective responses (e.g. changing position).

Treating such crises requires urgent intervention – immediately elevating the bedhead (Hickey 1997b) and removing possible causes (e.g. straightening creased sheets). Blocked urinary catheters are usually replaced: 30 ml bladder washouts should be attempted, but, if unsuccessful, catheters should be immediately replaced (Hickey 1997b). Constipation may require manual evacuation under topical anaesthetic cover – for example, lignocaine (Hickey 1997b). Blood pressure should be recorded very frequently (continuously or every 5 minutes (Hickey 1997b)). Antihypertensive (e.g. hydralazine) may be used – once sympathetic stimuli for hypertension are resolved, circulating drugs and bradycardia may trigger excessive rebound hypotension (Finocchiaro & Herzfeld 1990).

Thermoregulation is impaired and labile due to

- inappropriate cutaneous vasodilation (hypothermia)
- inability to shiver (hypothermia)
- impaired sweating predisposes (hyperthermia) (Moss & Craigo 1994).

When autonomic dysreflexia occurs during rehabilitation from spinal injury, patient and carer education becomes progressively important. Quadriplegia creates continuing dependency (on carers) for the fundamental aspects of living, including movement; pressure area care regimes are carefully staged to build up skin tolerance until patients can remain in one position for prolonged periods (possibly all night) without developing sores or dysreflexic crises.

Carers should be increasingly involved in all aspects of care which they will have to perform following discharge (e.g. changing urinary catheters, performing manual evacuations). While later stages of rehabilitation are unlikely to be reached before transfer to spinal injury units, ICU nurses may initiate rehabilitation, and should therefore supply appropriate information to patients and carers, as well as being able to recognise and treat complications of autonomic dysreflexia.

Implications for practice

- prolonged admission makes nursing care an especially important factor in recovery for these patients

- holistic assessment enables many complications to be avoided
- depression and sensory imbalance can easily occur; psychological care should be optimised
- neurological deficits impair normal homeostatic mechanisms, and so nurses should avoid interventions or lack of interventions that may provoke crises
- providing information to patients and families can help them cope and develop any skills they may need following discharge

Summary

This chapter has described three neurological conditions that may be encountered with varying frequency on general ICUs. For nurses with specialist neurological training, these conditions can create very real challenges, which – more than in many pathological conditions – are largely resolved by nursing rather than medical interventions.

Useful contact

The Guillain Barré helpline: 0800 374803

Further reading

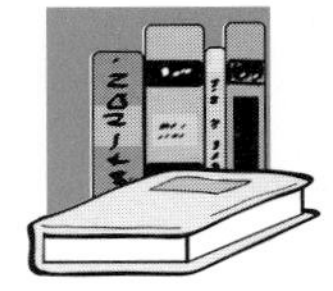

Useful medical articles on Guillain Barré syndrome include Desforges (1992) and Fulgham & Wijdicks (1997) literature reviews, Hund *et al.*'s (1993) overview of treatments, and Winer's (1994) focus on ICUs. McMahon-Parkes & Cornock (1997) give nursing perspectives.

Literature on critical illness neuropathy and autonomic dysreflexia is limited. Hund *et al.* (1996) describe seven patients with critical illness neuropathy; Bolton (1996) describes the syndrome and its variants. Finocchiaro and Herzfeld (1990) provide almost the only easily accessible nursing article on autonomic dysreflexia; Keely (1998) gives a useful critical care update.

Reading reports of patients' experiences is useful. Some have been published in nursing and medical journals, but can be difficult to obtain. Bauby (1997) vividly describes paraplegia following a CVA.

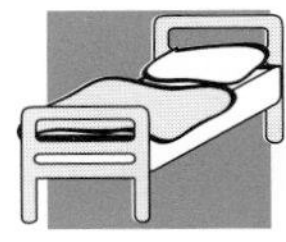

Clinical scenario

Duncan Munro, 46 years old, presented with tachypneoa (over 40 breaths/min), tachycardia (110 beats/min), hypertension (170/110 mmHg), difficulty swallowing, general fatigue with numbness in both legs and feet. During the previous three weeks, he had been travelling abroad on business and recovering from an upper respiratory tract infection. Guillain Barré syndrome (GBS) is suspected and Duncan has been admitted to ICU for ventilatory support. Noninvasive positive pressure ventilation (NPPV) via a full-face mask was commenced with inspiratory pressure of 12 cmH_2O and expiratory pressure of 4 cmH_2O.

Q.1 In order to confirm the diagnosis, respiratory function tests (lung volumes, FEV_1 and FVC), a lumbar puncture (for CSF) and electromyography were performed. Discuss how Duncan is prepared for these investigations by the ICU nurse (e.g. patient explanation, equipment needed, physical preparation whilst on NPPV etc.).

Duncan's respiratory and motor function deteriorated, a tracheotomy was performed and invasive positive pressure ventilation initiated.

Q.2 Analyse the main GBS complications (physical and psychological) experienced by Duncan during his ICU stay and with his treatment of plasmapherisis. Propose specific nursing interventions to minimise these.

Q.3 Identify and reflect on a range of approaches which may support and strengthen the immune response in Duncan and promote an early recovery, for example, immunonutrition, sleep, administration of intravenousimmunoglobulin, psychological support, mobilisation, pain management.

Chapter 39

Hepatic failure

Contents

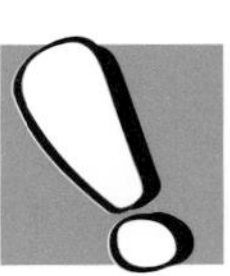

Fundamental knowledge

Hepatic anatomy and physiology
(Main) hepatic functions: nutrition, immunity, coagulation
Kupffer cell function

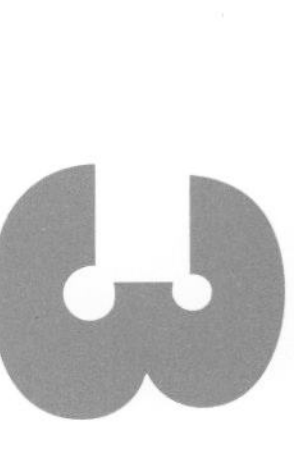
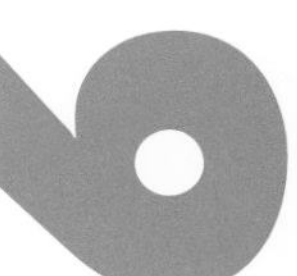

Introduction

Most ICU patients suffer liver dysfunction, usually due to hypoperfusion. The liver has more functions, and a wider range of functions, than any other major organ, so that hepatic failure causes many problems. This chapter describes its pathophysiology, major complications and treatments. While failure in ICU is usually acute, patients with existing chronic failure may be admitted (e.g. oesophageal varices or following liver transplantation). Liver function tests indicate the degree of liver failure; if severe, referral to specialist centres may be necessary.

The term *fulminant* hepatic failure (liver disease together with encephalopathy occurring within 8 weeks of onset) is still used, but it is increasingly being replaced by

- *hyperacute* (0–7 days)
- *acute* (8–28 days)
- *subacute* (29 days–12 weeks).

This chapter follows the terminology of the sources cited.

Acute hepatic failure may be caused by

- drugs
- chemicals
- viruses.

Although scientifically questionable (drugs are chemicals), this apparently arbitrary division is clinically useful. Symptoms of acute failure are similar from all causes, but are included here in the section on paracetamol.

The main cause of liver failure in the UK (unlike most other countries) is paracetamol overdose (Langley & Pain 1994; Stanley *et al.* 1995). Many other therapeutic drugs (such as chlorpromazine) can also provoke failure (Hawker 1997a).

The main chemical cause of liver failure in this country is alcohol. Occasionally (but only rarely), liver failure can be caused by industrial solvents, such as carbon tetrachloride (CCl_4, which is widely used, especially in the dry cleaning business) or by mushroom poisoning – usually *Amanita phalloides* ('death cap') (Sussman 1996).

Hepatic failure may be caused by hepatitis and many other viruses (e.g. herpes simplex, varicella, CMV, Epstein–Barr (Hawker 1997a)). Outside the UK, the cause of liver failure is usually viral (Karnik & Freeman 1998).

Hepatocyte recovery is good following acute hepatic failure, and so treatment is largely a matter of system support to minimise complications (especially cerebral oedema and cardiac failure) and allow hepatocyte recovery. Progression to chronic failure usually causes

- hyperdynamic circulation

- portal hypertension
- oesophageal varices and bleeding.

Survivors of these complications usually progress to end-stage failure, necessitating transplantation (see Chapter 44). Most of the complications identified here occur with acute failure, but some complications of chronic failure are also specifically identified.

Paracetamol

Severe hepatocellular necrosis can be caused by as little as 10–15 grams of paracetamol (BNF 1998). Paracetamol poisoning causes over one hundred deaths each year in the UK (O'Grady *et al.* 1991); the increasing incidence, possibly due to its easy access through supermarkets and other retail outlets (Leighton 1995; Budden & Vink 1996) resulted, in 1998, to the limitation of its sale in the UK to 32 tablets (maximum) in pharmacy packs and 16 tablets (maximum) elsewhere.

Hepatic metabolism of paracetamol (= *acetaminophen* in USA) forms the potentially toxic metabolite N-acetyl-p-bezoquinone imime (NAPQI) (Lockhart-Wood 1996); toxicity causes hepatocyte necrosis. Plasma paracetamol levels exceeding 250 mg/litre after 4 hours or 50 mg/litre at 12 hours usually result in hepatic damage (Weekes 1997), although severe symptoms may be delayed for 2–3 days, appearing only after significant, possibly fatal, damage. Hepatocellular necrosis peaks at 72–96 hours (BNF 1998), leading to the late complications of liver failure:

- metabolic acidosis – pH 7.3 (Leighton 1995)
- hepatorenal syndrome
- intracranial hypertension
- coagulopathies (*prothrombin time* exceeds 100 seconds) (Leighton 1995)

If conscious, patients experience abdominal pain (Hawker 1997a). Acetylcysteine (Parvolex®) and methionine can prevent hepatic failure within 10 to 12 hours of paracetamol overdose; it may still be hepatoprotective up to 24 hours (BNF 1998). Plasmapheresis can remove circulating toxins.

Hepatitis viruses

Long-standing classifications of hepatitis viruses between A and B (HAV, HBV), with subsequent identification of non-A-non-B, have led to recent classification of more specific viruses. In the UK, hepatitis B, sometimes complicated by hepatitis D, is the only significant viral cause of hepatic failure.

HEPATITIS A This infection is common, but rarely causes acute liver failure. Human transmission is only through faeces (not blood or other body fluids), infection being endemic where sanitation is poor (Pratt 1995). Hepatitis A can also be transmitted from shellfish (Halliday *et al.* 1991). HAV can cause fulminant hepatic failure (Pratt 1995).

HEPATITIS B This is a major cause of liver failure, although most infections do not cause acute failure (Sussman 1996). Transmission can be

- parenteral (most body fluids)
- sexual
- (possibly) through insect bites (Pratt 1995).

Chronic carriers rarely develop infection (Raeside 1996), but can spread infection (Pratt 1995).

Like HIV, HBV replicates through reverse transcription so that it is similarly prone to mutation (Shields & Neuberger 1997). Viral incubation takes three months (Murray *et al.* 1994); all staff working in ICUs should therefore be prophylactically vaccinated.

HEPATITIS C Identified in 1989, this is parenterally and (rarely) sexually transmitted. 300,000–600,000 people have been infected in the UK (Dolan & Hughes 1997); HCV causes progressive chronic failure. Mortality rates are 1–2 per cent (Booth 1997). Hepatitis C usually recurs following transplantation, but most patients remain asymptomatic.

HEPATITIS D (OR 'DELTA') Uniquely among hepatitis viruses, this has defective RNA and so can only replicate in the presence of hepatitis B (Pratt 1995); therefore all patients with hepatitis D must be infected by hepatitis B (although hepatitis B infection does not necessarily lead to hepatitis D). Hepatitis D complicates hepatitis B infection, making fulminant hepatic failure more likely. In Europe and North America, hepatitis D is primarily transmitted through drug injection; elsewhere infection is usually sexual (Pratt 1995). Lamivudine and interferon are the most effective drugs against hepatitis D.

HEPATITIS E This was originally named 'E' for 'enteric' (Shields & Neuberger 1997). Infection is endemic in many Third World countries (Karnik & Freeman 1998), but rare in the UK. HEV usually causes mild and self-limiting disease (Pratt 1995).

HEPATITIS F This is a poorly defined virus whose existence is still in doubt (Shields & Neuberger 1997).

HEPATITIS G This may have caused a few cases of severe hepatitis, but there are only scattered reports. Infection usually occurs with HBV and HCV.

GB VIRUS This group was identified from a 1967 serum sample called 'GB' (Shields & Neuberger 1997). To date, three related viruses have been identified: GB-A, GB-B and GB-C (Shields & Neuberger 1997).

Complications

Liver dysfunction affects most other major systems of the body. The effects are cumulative, often provoking multisystem dysfunction. The description below is reductionist, and specific management of other systems is covered in other chapters.

Fulminant Hepatic Failure by definition includes *encephalopathy*. While not necessarily included in other classifications, toxins increase blood–brain barrier permeability (Lockhart-Wood 1996), facilitating entry into the CSF of:

- gamma aminobutyric acid (GABA)
- electrolytes
- plasma proteins

Leaked plasma proteins further increase CSF osmotic pressure, escalating oedema formation (Lockhart-Wood 1996). Cerebral oedema provokes intracranial hypertension, impairing cerebral perfusion pressure (see Chapter 22). Nurses should therefore assess and monitor neurological function.

GABA, an inhibitory neurotransmitter (see Chapter 6) produced by gut bacteria, is normally cleared hepatically (Lockhart-Wood 1996); increasing plasma concentrations and increased blood–brain barrier permeability cause high CSF concentrations and impaired consciousness (Lockhart-Wood 1996). Prolonged effects from exogenous sedation may delay recovery and make assessment difficult; debate continues on whether to avoid sedating patients with hepatic failure. Whichever medical practice is followed, nurses should actively assess the level of sedation and effects of drugs.

Despite intracranial hypertension, fitting may remain subclinical (e.g. detectable by cerebral function analysing monitoring, see Chapter 22). Normal sleeping patterns may be reversed, with patients remaining awake overnight. Increased muscle tone may cause decerebrate postures (Hawker 1997a).

Treatment should optimise cerebral perfusion pressure by reducing intracranial pressure while maintaining mean arterial pressure (see Chapter 22). Persistent intracranial hypertension (above 25 mmHg) may be reversed with mannitol.

The liver synthesises all coagulation factors except Factor VII and von Willebrand's Factor (vWF), so that hepatic failure provokes *coagulopathies*.

Chronic failure compounds dyscrasias from

- splenatomegaly (from portal hypertension), which reduces platelet counts
- depressed bone marrow function (from alcoholism or paracetamol) which reduces erythropoiesis.

Gastrointestinal and respiratory (although not cerebral) *bleeds* frequently occur (Hawker 1997a). ICU nurses should therefore minimise trauma and observe for bleeding on endotracheal suction or from nasogastric tubes. Oozing around cannulae or healing of sites after removal may also cause problems. Cannulae, especially arterial, should remain visible whenever possible. Replacement factors, such as vitamin K (Cowley & Webster 1993) or blood components, may be prescribed.

The liver contributes significantly to immunity through production of complements (see Chapter 23) and Kupffer cells – specialised reticuloendothelial cells in the liver which destroy any bacteria translocating from the gut. Liver dysfunction therefore causes *immunocompromise*; infection frequently occurs. Asepsis, high standards of infection control and continuing vigilance can minimise risks to patients; early detection of infection enables early treatment.

Blood from the liver soon reaches pulmonary vessels so that surviving gut bacteria readily cause *pulmonary* infection; increased capillary permeability enables pulmonary oedema formation, and possible shunting. Endotracheal suction is needed to reduce sputum retention. As suction raises intracranial pressure, patients should be preoxygenated and duration and number of passes should be minimised (see Chapter 22). Suction may also cause trauma, so that catheters withdrawn should be observed for blood (type, amount) as well as sputum (type, colour, amount).

Hepatopulmonary syndrome occurs in up to 30 per cent of patients with endstage failure (Isaac & Manji 1997). Pathology is unclear; there is no specific treatment and resolution can be spontaneous, but mortality remains high. Hepatopulmonary syndrome is an indication for liver transplantation (Isaac & Manji 1997.).

Cardiovascular compromise is caused by

- hypovolaemia
- vasodilation
- increased capillary permeability
- reduced cardiac return.

As prolonged hypotension predisposes to multiorgan dysfunction, nurses should closely assess and monitor cardiovascular function. Inotropes will probably be needed, although may have little effect if sympathetic pathways are damaged.

Stress responses (see Chapter 3) increase blood and intracranial pressure, and so patients should be nursed in quiet environments with minimal sensory stimulation.

Renal failure frequently occurs following paracetamol overdose as NAPQI is nephrotoxic (Lockhart-Wood 1996). Hypotension can also cause acute tubular necrosis.

With chronic failure, *hepatorenal syndrome* (hepatic nephropathy) may develop. There is no detectable histological change to renal tissue, and kidneys resume normal function following hepatic transplantation (Hinds & Watson 1996); without transplantation, mortality exceeds 90 per cent (Hinds & Watson 1996). Unlike acute tubular necrosis, relatively normal sodium reabsorption and urine concentration is maintained during hepatorenal syndrome.

The liver has more than 500 metabolic functions, and so hepatic failure causes complex disorders. *Electrolyte* disorders from hepatic hypofunction are often compounded by renal and capillary epithelial changes. Reduced free water clearance can dilute electrolyte concentrations, causing *hyponatraemia* and *hypokalaemia* (Sussman 1996). Prolonged malnourishment (especially with alcoholism), vomiting and nasogastric drainage may compound hypokalaemia, while dehydration (e.g. mannitol infusion) may cause *hypernatraemia* (Sussman 1996). Paracetamol toxicity can cause hypophosphataemia (Sussman 1996). Electrolyte imbalances have varied systemic effects, including dysrhythmias from hypokalaemia and oedema formation from hyponatraemia.

Metabolic *acidosis* may occur from

- hypoperfusion (anaerobic metabolism)
- renal impairment
- gastric acid loss (vomiting, aspiration) (Adam & Osborne 1997)

Impaired *toxin* metabolism and clearance increases sensitivity to, and effects of, many drugs and metabolites.

With chronic failure, hepatocellular necrosis prevents glycogenolysis, which causes potential *hypoglycaemia* (Lockhart-Wood 1996), necessitating frequent blood sugar monitoring and probably glucose supplements.

Artificial livers

The development of artificial livers has been slow and problematic, but shortage of donor livers prompted experiments with xenoperfusion. Cadaver and baboon livers have achieved extracorporeal support for up to 75 days (Conlin 1995), although immunologic intolerance makes xenoperfusion impractical (Sussman 1996). Temporary support is possible from hepatocytes grafted onto semipermeable hollow-fibre devices (visually similar to those used for haemofiltration), which provide support until transplantation (Fristoe *et al.* 1993), although support is (so far) limited to 168 hours (Riordan & Williams 1997). At present, devices are cumbersome, expensive and not used clinically in the UK; however, technology will doubtless improve their function – perhaps to permanently implantable devices.

Implications for practice

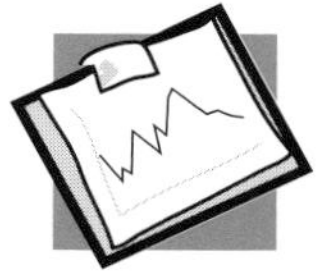

- most ICU patients suffer hepatic dysfunction, usually due to hypoperfusion; nurses should actively assess liver function (e.g. clotting, consciousness), documenting their observations

- impaired consciousness increases forgetfulness; patients may need information to be repeated frequently
- whenever possible, exposure of invasive sites enables continuous observation
- if clotting is prolonged, reassess the traumatic aspects of nursing care (e.g. shaving, mouthcare – see Chapter 31)
- seeing blood can distress families and friends, and so they should be warned about possible bleeding; soiled sheets and dressings should be replaced if possible
- blood loss should be assessed (e.g. marking limits of ooze on dressings)
- hepatic dysfunction impairs immunity, so that infection control is essential to maintain a safe environment
- endotracheal suction is necessary, but causes trauma, and so should be individually assessed
- suicide attempts (paracetamol overdose) and (alcoholism) may cause guilt and/or anger among families and friends. Nurses should encourage families to express their needs and emotions, but it may be necessary to involve counselling or other services. Listening is often more useful (cathartic) than replying to guilt and anger.

Summary

The liver can be the forgotten vital organ in ICU; other than transplantation centres, few units specialise in hepatic failure, but it frequently adds complications to most pathologies seen in ICUs. Liver function affects many other organs and systems, and so the care of patients with liver dysfunction requires a range of knowledge and skills. Intracranial hypertension, a major complication of hepatic failure, is discussed further in Chapter 22. Extracorporeal liver devices are currently only experimental; for the present, ICU nurses should actively assess liver function and minimise potential complications.

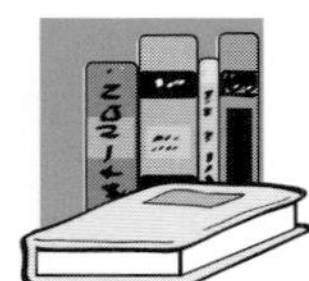

Further reading

Hawker is a leading authority on hepatic failure; her chapter (1997a) is an accessible and useful source. Cowley and Webster's (1993) literature review is also useful. Lockhart-Wood (1996) is one of the few articles from ICU journals to focus on nursing care. Langley and Pain (1994) discuss some of the options for medical treatment, while Stanley *et al.* (1995) give a useful surgical perspective. Artnal and Wilkinson (1998) give a case study of fulminant failure from paracetamol.

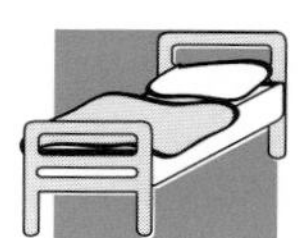

Clinical scenario

Fabio Galvani is a 26-year-old male who has recently completed a six-month backpacking trip to southeast Asia. Since his return he has been feeling increasingly unwell with nausea, vomiting, fever with influenza-like symptoms. He was admitted to hospital for investigations after behaving in a confused and agitated manner. While in hospital, Fabio lost consciousness and was transferred to ICU for invasive ventilation and organ support. Doctors made a diagnosis of fulminating hepatic failure and grade 3 hepatic encephalopathy. Blood investigations revealed the presence of hepatitis B surface antigen (HB_sAg) and 'e' antigens (HB_eAg).

Q.1 Explain how hepatitis B infection resulted in Fabio's fulminating hepatic failure. Review your understanding of hepatitis B virus:

- Likely route (portal of entry) and mode of transmission
- Incubation period
- Survival outside host cells (how long virus can live outside body)
- Infectious risk to friends, family and health care workers.
- Significance of HB_sAg, HB_eAg and HB_cAg (core antigen)
- The effects on Fabio's liver and other body systems, particularly cerebral function.

Q.2 Analyse the infection control procedures applicable to Fabio while he is nursed in ICU (e.g. should 'protective isolation' be implemented or 'universal precautions', labelling and disposal of laboratory specimens, equipment, body fluids).

Q.3 Reflect on the contribution that ICU nurses can make to enhance Fabio's recovery from hepatic encephalopathy. Specify proactive nursing strategies, which can minimise potential complications (prioritising care, type of psychological support, nutrition, health promotion, use of specialists).

Chapter 40

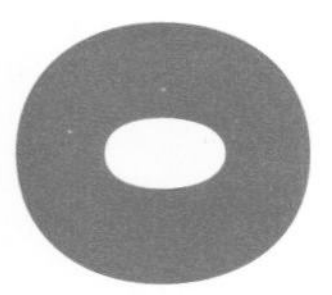

Immunity

Contents

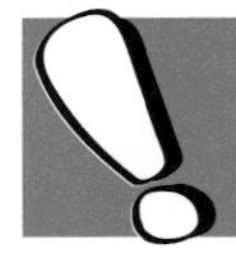

Fundamental knowledge

Universal precautions

Introduction

Immunity enables us to resist many potential pathogens; most ICU patients are immunodeficient. This chapter describes normal immunity, illustrating dysfunction through the human immunosuppressive virus (HIV) and acquired immune deficiency syndrome (AIDS). Many mediators of immunity (e.g. complement) have been described in Chapter 23.

Immunity

Classifications of immunity derive from historical schools of immunology, which increasingly recognised that different modes of immunity existed concurrently. Immunity may be

- nonspecific (innate)
- specific (adaptive) (Johnson 1994).

Nonspecific immunity is any defence mechanism not targeting specific micro-organisms. Much human nonspecific immunity is present at birth. Specific immunity is necessarily acquired through exposure to various organisms or antibody vaccination.

Immunity may also be classified as cell mediated and humoral. Cell-mediated immunity causes T-lymphocytes to respond to (nonspecific) protein by producing various lymphokines; humoral immunity is mediated by antibodies (B-lymphocytes) in the blood, and is antigen-specific.

Nonspecific immunity

Many body systems include defence mechanisms against foreign material, all potentially compromised by critical illness and treatments (e.g. intubation, steroids). Examples of nonspecific immunity include:

- stickiness of mucous membrane and cilia (trapping airway particles smaller than 2 μm)
- body 'flushes' (tears, saliva), many including antibacterial lysozyme
- sebrum (from sebaceous glands) preventing bacterial colonisation of skin
- acidity/alkalinity of gastrointestinal tract
- pyrexia (see Chapter 8)
- inflammatory response: increases and activates phagocyte and complement concentrations
- interferon: inhibits viral replication and enhances action of killer cells (Johnson 1994)
- lactoferrin: binds iron (needed by microbes for growth)

Nonspecific chemical defences inhibit bacteria and viruses, but place stress on the body: inflammation can become pathological (SIRS, see Chapter 25), while graft-versus-host disease threatens viability of transplanted tissue (foreign protein), necessitating immunosuppressant drugs.

Specific immunity

Specific immunity is achieved through two types of lymphocytes: T and B. Antigen recognition by T-lymphocytes usually precedes B-lymphocyte production.

T-lymphocytes

T-lymphocyte precursors originate in bone marrow, migrating to and maturing in the thymus gland (Abbas *et al.* 1994). Older people (most ICU patients) have decreased immunity due to:

- progressive auto-antibody accumulation (Wilson 1997)
- decreased maturation of T-lymphocytes (Kilner & Janes 1997).

Antigen recognition by T-lymphocytes causes enlargement and differentiation into (Johnson 1994):

- *killer cells* (cytolytic) attach to invading cells, then secrete
  - lymphotoxins (kill invading cells)
  - lymphokines (attract lymphocytes and macrophages)
  - interferon (inhibits viral replication, enhances action of killer cells)
- *helper cells* assist B-lymphocytes increase antibody production (Johnson 1994). Most helper T-lymphocytes contain surface protein $CD4^{+}$ (Abbas *et al.* 1994), a major mediator of AIDS (CD = cluster designation).
- *memory cells* enable future antigen recognition by T-lymphocytes.

B-lymphocytes

B-lymphocytes, produced in the bone marrow, respond to foreign antigens by becoming antibody producing cells (Abbas *et al.* 1994) which release immunoglobulin. These are antibodies in cell membranes (Young-McCaughan & Jennings 1998). Three (IgA, IgG, IgM) primarily neutralise toxins and viral activity, promoting bacterial lysis and phagocytosis.

IgA Relatively unimportant for systemic humoral immunity, this is found mainly in mucus membranes (Abbas *et al.* 1994): mucus, saliva, tears, sweat and breast milk.

IgD Only trace amounts are found in serum (Bassion 1996).

IgE This attaches to cell membranes of basophils and mast cells, triggering histamine (Young-McCaughan & Jennings 1998). Normal serum contains only trace amounts (Bassion 1996).

IgG A major cause of allergic reactions (Abbas *et al.* 1994), this is secreted during secondary immune responses (Young-McCaughan & Jennings 1998). Readily entering tissue spaces, IgG coats micro-organisms prior to phagocytosis (Hudak *et al.* 1998).

IgM This is the first immunoglobulin secreted during primary immune response to antigens (Young-McCaughan & Jennings 1998).

Immunodeficiency

Failure of the immune system is usually secondary to either autoimmune pathologies (e.g. HIV, leukaemia, hepatic failure) or drug-induced (e.g. steroids, cyclosporin A, chemotherapy). The immune system can also be overwhelmed by infection or complex surgery/invasive treatment, exposing patients to opportunistic infections (e.g. MRSA) that may colonise, but not infect, healthier people (e.g. staff).

During healthy maturation T-lymphocytes are exposed to self-antigens, developing tolerance so that surviving T-lymphocytes tolerate the body's own tissue (Abbas *et al.* 1994). Failure of this selection process causes autoimmunity.

Steroids

Despite variable use over many decades to treat various conditions, steroid therapy remains controversial, tending to treat symptoms (inflammation) rather than causes. Symptom treatment may be justified when 'cures' prove evasive.

Graft-versus-host disease (GvHD)

This reaction occurs when immune cells react against transplanted tissue; severe cases may cause organ failure or death. GvHD causes fibrosis, necrosis and necrosis in skin, liver and gut epithelium (Abbas *et al.* 1994). The incidence increases with older donors, older recipients or those with human leucocyte antigen (HLA) mismatch.

Symptoms include:

- skin rashes (typically: face, palms, soles, ears)
- jaundice
- diarrhoea

Treatments include corticosteroids and chemotherapy (e.g. cyclosporin, methotrexate, thalidomide (Isbister 1997b)), often with system support.

HIV

Two HIV viruses have been identified: HIV-1 and HIV-2. HIV-1, prevalent in the West, is primarily described here. HIV-2, predominant in Africa, is structurally different from HIV-1, but causes similar symptoms (Abbas *et al.* 1994).

Autoimmune dysfunction syndrome (AIDS) only occurs with symptoms from opportunistic infection; HIV+ people who remain symptom-free are colonised, but not infected. Thus, while HIV can lead to AIDS, it is not the same as AIDS. Three-quarters of all HIV carriers will probably develop full AIDS within 10 years (Weller & Williams 1995), although a few early carriers remain AIDS-free.

While HIV is rightly seen as a major threat to modern healthcare, hepatitis B causes more disease and death than HIV.

History

First reported in 1981 (Pratt 1995), this virus quickly created levels of fear and stigma unknown since syphilis epidemics. Hysteria was heightened by it being a sexually transmitted disease and its early association with homosexuals and, to a lesser extent, intravenous drug users – a stereotype ignoring global statistics: 71 per cent is transmitted heterosexually (Pratt 1995).

In the West, infection among 'high risk' groups has declined, but it has grown amongst heterosexual non-drug users, (1994 UK figures showed over one-quarter of new cases were from heterosexual contact (Francome & Marks 1996)).

The UK incidence varies: over 70 per cent occurs in central London, especially the North Thames region (Pratt 1998). In 1994, 1 in 400 women in London were HIV+ (in some areas, 1 in 200) (Evans 1997). By March 1998, of the 31,000 cases of HIV+ diagnosed in the UK, over 5,000 were women and over 700 were children (Pratt 1998). Even these figures may be underestimates; the Thames region 1993 figures found only 15 per cent of seropositive newborns had mothers diagnosed as HIV+ (Evans 1997).

Seeing HIV as a 'gay plague', or a disease of homosexuals and drug abusers, not only propagates homophobia, but ignores histological trends, thereby exposing many to unnecessary risk. Initiatives intended to protect others can reinforce stigmatisation (e.g. disposable paper toilet seats); sexually transmitted viruses are very fragile, and unable to survive long outside the human body. Universal precautions minimise infection risks to healthcare workers from all infections, without stigmatising specific groups. Nurses can valuably promote health education for patients, their friends and families, and healthcare colleagues.

The virus

The human immunosuppressive virus primarily infects CD4$^+$ molecules, found mainly on T-lymphocyte helper cells (Abbas *et al.* 1994). Once inside host cells, HIV transmits genetic information as a single RNA strand. Using the enzyme reverse transcriptase, it then replicates RNA into a DNA copy (hence 'retrovirus'). This clumsy arrangement is complicated by inaccuracies of enzyme replication, causing frequent mutations (Abbas *et al.* 1994).

The virus may avoid detection because

- seroconversion can take 8–24 weeks to detect (Pratt 1995)
- HIV-2 may evade tests relying on antibody detection (Abbas *et al.* 1994)
- HIV-1 subtype O (a West African subgroup) may remain undetected by either HIV-1 or HIV-2 tests (Loussert-Ajaka *et al.* 1994).

Thus, HIV-negative results do not necessarily confirm absence of the virus.

Low CD4 and T-lymphocyte counts may indicate HIV infection (Smith *et al.* 1993). In 1993 the USA's Centre for Disease Control extended definitions of AIDS to include all severely immunocompromised patients (CD4$^+$ counts below 200×10^6 per litre), but this definition is not accepted in either the UK or Europe (Weller & Williams 1995), causing possible discrepancies with future statistical comparisons.

Problems

Autoimmune dysfunction exposes patients to opportunistic infections:

- respiratory
- gastrointestinal
- central nervous system

The anxieties and stigma that surround HIV and AIDS often increase the psychological needs of patients and their families and friends.

RESPIRATORY FAILURE This causes high mortality (Weller & Williams 1995); untreated, over 80 per cent will develop *Pneumocystis carinii* pneumonia (PCP) (Miller & Roberts 1991). The protozoa *Pneumocystis carinii* forms cysts in the alveoli and interstitial lung tissue; these cysts inhibit perfusion and disrupt surfactant production, probably progressing to ARDS (Ong 1993). Tuberculosis (TB) infection increasingly complicates AIDS (Brudney & Dobkin 1991; Snider & Dooley 1993), and the problem is aggravated by the development of resistant strains (Neville *et al.* 1994).

Whether artificial ventilation is justified for PCP remains debatable; survival rates have fallen to between 10 and 25 per cent, reviving doubts about appropriateness of admission and artificial ventilation (Cowan *et al.* 1997). CPAP may support respiratory failure without the trauma of intubation, although even this raises dilemmas of whether life or the process of death is being prolonged. Further studies may clarify when and where aggressive treatment is more appropriate than palliative care.

GASTROINTESTINAL DYSFUNCTION This includes malnourishment and increased motility. Many patients are malnourished (with weight loss) from prolonged illness on admission. Breathlessness often causes reluctance to eat or drink. Malnourishment further impairs immunity and healing. Increased motility from both disease and drugs causes diarrhoea, vomiting and nausea. Nutrition should therefore be a priority; gut malfunction may necessitate parenteral nutrition (Macallan 1994). Vitamin supplements may be needed as deficiency from malnutrition is likely. Drugs to prevent nausea and diarrhoea help to restore comfort and dignity; mouthcare provides comfort and helps to prevent opportunist infection.

CENTRAL NERVOUS SYSTEM Damage in this respect and encephalitis are usually seen at post-mortem. Many patients suffer both cognitive and behavioural changes, such as memory loss, apathy and poor concentration. Dementia occurs in up to two-thirds of people with AIDS (Abbas *et al.* 1994). Cognitive changes can be especially distressful for families and friends.

Psychological stressors include

- stigma surrounding HIV/AIDS
- anxieties about dying

Psychological distress needs human care and interaction, spending time with people and allowing them to express their needs. Isolation, whether in side rooms or by hanging signs over beds, merely reinforces stigmatisation (hence the value of universal precautions); however, using side rooms to provide privacy can be valuable for patients and their families and friends. Some healthcare workers still refuse to go near HIV+ patients; such behaviour is professionally unacceptable for nurses (UKCC 1996).

Drug treatments

Frequent viral mutations frustrate the development of ideal anti-HIV drugs, but combination therapy delays the development of resistance (French 1997). Some of the more successful drugs include:

CO-TRIMOXAZOLE This is the standard treatment for PCP (Vilar & Wilkins 1998).

ZIDOVUDINE (AZIDOTHYMIDINE, AZT) This inhibits reverse transcriptase, and so prevents further viral replication. It crosses the blood–brain barrier, reducing incidence of AIDS-related dementia (Slade & Churchill 1997). Its side effects include bone marrow depression and anaemia.

PENTAMADINE (Intravenous, nebulised) This can be used instead of co-trimoxazole (BNF 1998), but has more toxic effects, including hypo-/hyperglycaemia, dysrhythmias and renal failure (Vilar & Wilkins 1998).

Other reverse transcriptase inhibitors include *didanosine* (ddI), *lamivudine* (3TC), *stavudine* (d4T) and *zalcitabine* (ddC).

Protease inhibitors include *indinavir*, *ritonavir* and *saquinavir*.

Ethical and health issues

HIV and AIDS have raised more ethical dilemmas and issues than any other disease in recent years. HIV tests, even when negative, may threaten insurance and mortgage policies and employment prospects. Technically, any non-consensual touch is (legally) assault. The testing of blood for HIV without consent brought the leading bodies of nursing (UKCC) and medicine (BMA) into rare open conflict: UK nurses must not be involved in anonymous HIV testing (UKCC 1996).

Relatives may only discover the diagnosis of HIV/AIDS from death certificates; they may have been unaware, and perhaps disapproved, of the deceased's lifestyle. This can cause additional distress following bereavement, but a nurse's duty of confidentiality to patients is absolute (apart from specific legal requirements), and extends beyond the death of patients.

Dilemmas raised through clinical practice can usefully be discussed among unit teams and thus contribute to the professional growth of all involved. Goffman (1963) and Sontag (1989) raise provocative insights. Support agencies are identified below.

HIV and AIDS are not included in the Public Health (Control of Diseases) Act, 1984 (Dimond 1995), probably due to the historical accident of this act being drafted before AIDS became a significant problem in the UK. HIV and AIDS are therefore not notifiable diseases. However, the AIDS Control Act (1987) places obligations on health authorities to report the number of people with AIDS, and a statutory instrument of 1988 extended requirements regarding AIDS to HIV (Dimond 1995).

Universal precautions should apply to all body fluids from any patient. Although complacency should be avoided, risk from occupational exposure is small – under 1 per cent of healthcare workers exposed to HIV through work have seroconverted (Jeffries 1991; Pratt 1995). Of 176 significant UK healthcare workers' exposure to HIV between 1985 and 1992, only four have definitely been infected (Pratt 1995).

Implications for practice

- many ICU pathologies and treatments impair immunity, and so high standards of infection control are needed to protect patients from opportunistic infections
- observe for signs of GvHD with any patient receiving any human tissue/cells
- problems of HIV/AIDS are compounded by widespread stigma; nurses should promote positive attitudes, and consider the implications of all their actions
- HIV+ patients and their families may need additional psychological support; involving specialist agencies may be beneficial
- unit discussions (ethical forums, case review) can stimulate useful debate for professional development

Summary

Most patients in ICU are immunocompromised. Treatments and interventions increase infection risks, but proactive infection control can reduce risks from nosocomial infection.

HIV and AIDS have created medical and ethical challenges to healthcare. The unique role of nurses in ICU teams enable them to challenge and resolve stigmas and negative attitudes in order to meet the psychological and physiological needs of their patients.

Useful contacts

National AIDS helpline: 0800 567123
Terrence Higgins Trust: 0207 2421010
AIDS Healthline: 01392 59191
Body Positive: 0207 8332971
Frontliners: 0207 8310330
Red Admiral (bereavement counselling): the telephone number is available from the Terrence Higgins Trust

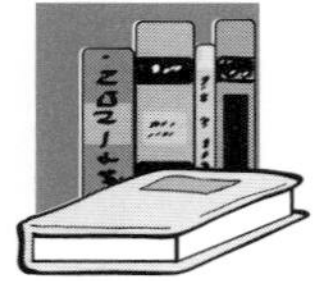

Further reading

Immunology is discussed in most physiology and microbiology texts; Abbas *et al.* (1994) provides a clear text on immunology, while Johnson (1994) is one of the few ICU-specific articles.

Pratt (1995) is an excellent text on HIV and nursing, although has little specifically related to ICU. Cowan *et al.* (1997) give a comprehensive recent overview of issues, while Evans (1997) offers a useful paediatric perspective.

Ethical dilemmas raise issues from wider contexts; Goffman's (1963) classic work on stigma (written before HIV was identified) and Sontag's

(1989) outstanding investigative journalism offer valuable sociological insights, raising many ethical issues. Extreme reactions to the stigma of a fictional killer virus are effectively illustrated in the film *Outbreak* (Warner Brothers 1995). Many experiential accounts exist; Gunn (1992) is a leading contemporary poet who has chronicled the death of friends from AIDS.

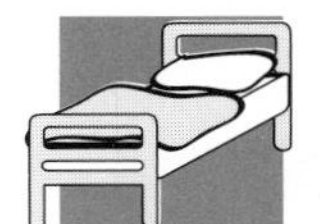

Clinical scenario

Paul Edwards is 24 years old and was admitted to intensive care for invasive ventilation following a respiratory arrest. Microbiology results confirm pulmonary tuberculosis and HIV. It is not known if he was aware of his HIV status prior to this investigation. The infection control nurse has been asked to approach Paul's girlfriend and flatmates for screening.

Q.1 Explain the differences in immune response between HIV positive and HIV negative people on exposure to tubercle bacilli. (Why is an HIV positive person more likely to develop pulmonary TB?)

Q.2 Discuss the nursing interventions that support Paul's immune system; include the value and limitations of these interventions (e.g. protective isolation, drug therapies of antibiotics and antiviral, nutrition, psychological support, therapeutic relationships).

Q.3 Should the infection control nurse approach Paul's girlfriend and flatmates for screening? Reflect on your legal, ethical and professional responsibilities towards Paul. (Consider the Public Health Act (1984), patient confidentiality, duty of care to public, disclosure of information to patient.)

Chapter 41

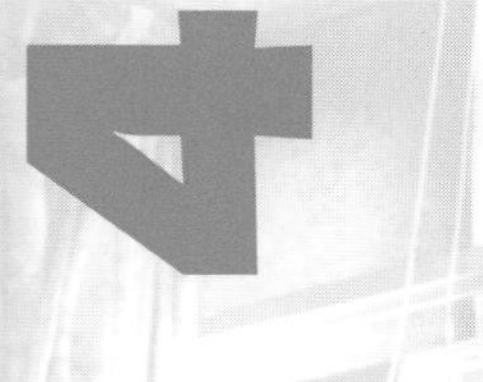

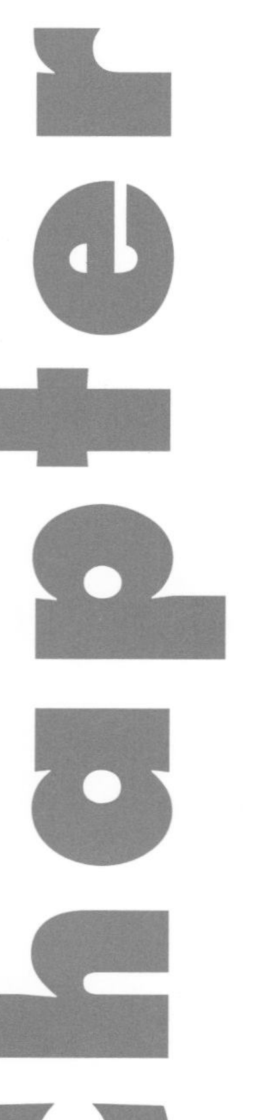

Ecstasy overdoses

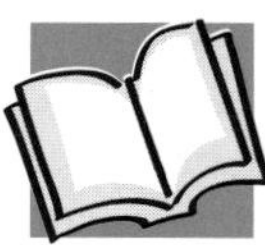

Contents

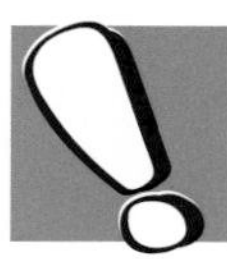

Fundamental knowledge

Neurotransmission synapse

Introduction

Patients may be admitted to ICUs following a range of both deliberate and accidental overdoses. This chapter describes one popular recreational (illegal) drug, MDMA (**Ecstasy**). (Paracetamol overdose is described in Chapter 39) Many wider issues of nursing care discussed in this chapter can be applied to overdose of other drugs, although readers should check applicability before transferring specific treatments.

Although Leah Betts' death in 1995 from one uncontaminated tablet of Ecstasy (Towers 1997) captured popular media attention, this death was not isolated; nurses working in acute care increasingly admit patients who have taken overdoses.

Illegal drugs and popular subculture trends change rapidly, and trends may have already changed by the time studies appear. There is a paucity of material available on these drugs, and unfortunately this means that even relatively recent material is potentially out of date by the time it is published. This chapter therefore relies on a relatively few key (and reliable) texts. Trends in drug use often have significant geographical, cultural and social variations, limiting generalisability of studies. Media influence on public perceptions can also be misleading. Although drug abuse can occur at any age, drugs such as Ecstasy tend to be taken by adolescents and young adults; at the risk of stereotyping, this chapter refers to this group.

With illegal drugs, users and friends are often understandably reluctant to seek medical help until dehydration and collapse occur (Cook 1995). When help is sought, friends may be reluctant to share information with hospital staff, fearing anything revealed may be passed on to the police (Jones and Owens 1996). Overdoses from drugs which rarely cause immediate life-threatening problems (e.g. cannabis) are seldom admitted to hospital (Jones and Owens 1996), and so are not discussed here.

The realisation that drugs are not as safe as patients and their friends previously thought may make them receptive to health education, and ICU nurses can provide useful information and contacts. However, users often have greater knowledge about street drugs than nurses, and they may also have different values and beliefs, so that adopting a moralistic or righteous attitude may cause alienation. Abusers may continue to take drugs, but health education can raise awareness of the dangers and suggest safer ways to take drugs so that users can make their own informed decisions.

MDMA (3–4 methylenedioxymethamphetamine) is an amphetamine derivative (MacConnachie 1997b) that remains unlicensed in the UK (O'Conner 1994). It has many street names, Ecstasy ('E' for short) being the most familiar. It is listed as a class A drug under the 1971 Misuse of Drugs Act (Wake 1995), so may only be legally possessed if authorised by the Home Office (Dimond 1995).

Ecstasy stimulates feelings of *euphoria* and *benevolence* (Wake 1995), breaking down social inhibitions and heightening *emotional attachment* to others (Cook 1995), hence the names 'Ecstasy' and 'love drug' (ironically, it impairs libido (Cook 1995)). Ecstasy contains amphetamine, causing hypermetabolism, providing *energy* which enables users to dance continuously for (literally) hours (Cook 1995). The attractions of Ecstasy may be seen in raves; the miseries are more often seen in ICUs.

Abuse

The 'pleasure centre' in the hypothalamus is activated by neurotransmitters (e.g. dopamine). Exogenous drugs that induce euphoria trap endogenous dopamine in the synapses of the pleasure centre. Constant stimulation of the pleasure centre causes a 'high' (Marieb 1995); but exogenous drugs also inhibit production of endogenous dopamine so that, once trapped, dopamine is metabolised and, if the central nervous system cannot meet demand, a 'low' follows. Exogenous drugs can restore the 'high', and so victims take further doses; progressive damage to endogenous neurotransmitters cause addiction, with addicts taking ever larger doses (Jones & Owens 1996) to prevent the 'lows'.

The purity of illegally produced drugs (e.g. Ecstasy) often varies greatly (Wolff *et al.* 1995); as Ecstasy is complicated and expensive to produce, active drugs are often adulterated with other substances (Cook 1995): the purity of street specimens varies between 50 and 100 per cent (O'Conner 1994), usual street doses being between 30 and 150 mg. Different tablets often have dissimilar strengths, so that even users with previous experience of the drugs cannot be sure how each dose will affect them. Hence, an accidental overdose can easily occur, and individual metabolism and tolerance can further influence the effect.

Ecstasy is often taken at 'raves', where users dance for hours in hot, humid, poorly ventilated conditions (Jones & Owens 1996). Ten or more tablets are usually taken at once, often together with other drugs (Cook 1995) and alcohol, so that variable doses of 50–200 mg/tablet can be multiplied tenfold. Ecstasy is usually taken orally, although rectal use, enabling quicker absorption, is also popular (Cook 1995). Oral tablets begin working within one hour, usually lasting for up to six hours, but excessive doses may continue working for more than 24 hours (MacConnachie 1997b). Toxicity can develop quickly and unexpectedly (MacConnachie 1997b), and misunderstandings by users may compound problems (e.g. alcohol accentuates dehydration, therefore drinking water can prevent dehydration – but excessive water can cause water intoxification).

Illegal drugs are often transported in body cavities ('body packing') (Jones & Owens 1996), especially the rectum. The rectum is highly vascular, so that if bags break, drugs are efficiently absorbed; drug traffickers may be admitted with accidental overdoses. Understandably, they may be reluctant to admit that they have a continuing rectal drug infusion, while attempts to remove bags may cause further internal spillage (Jones & Owens 1996). If drugs have not yet been absorbed, an activated charcoal slurry washout may limit absorption within two hours of ingestion (MacConnachie 1997b).

Widespread misuse of Ecstasy is a recent phenomenon; in 1990, four deaths were recorded in the USA, but none in this country; by 1991, seven UK deaths were attributed to Ecstasy (Wake 1995), but mortality may exceed official figures; Cook (1995) speculates that Ecstasy may have caused 50 deaths in the UK. Death usually occurs 2–60 hours after admission (O'Conner 1994).

Tober (1994) estimated that 20,000–30,000 doses of Ecstasy were taken each weekend in the UK; Cook (1995) raised this figure to 750,000. Ecstasy is now among the most widely used illicit drugs in this country (McGuire *et al.* 1994): Tober's (1994) survey of 186 university students found that over one-half had tried the drug, and 10 per cent took it at least every fortnight. Although trends change quickly in popular culture, these worrying statistics suggest that Ecstasy overdoses will continue to cause significant numbers of ICU admissions.

Reticular activating system suppression (see Chapter 3) overloads the cerebral cortex with impulses, causing psychedelic mood changes (Cook 1995), enhanced perception (Wake 1995) and potential psychiatric complications. Animal studies show long-term destruction of serotoninergic axons and terminals from as little as 20 mg; re-innervation is possible, but often abnormal (Green & Goodwin 1996).

Mortality figures often bear little relation to the amounts of Ecstasy taken (Jones and Owens 1996): single-tablet fatalities (serum MDMA levels of 0.424 mg/l) contrast with 42-tablet survival (serum MDMA 7.72 mg/l) (Wake 1995).

Metabolic problems

Ecstasy increases both aerobic and anaerobic metabolism; early complications from sympathomimetic action are largely cerebrovascular, but later effects include hyperpyrexia and muscle rigidity (MacConnachie 1997b). Most Ecstasy-related deaths are caused by fulminant hyperthermia, with temperature increasing by up to 2°C every hour (Wake 1995) (starting from systemic absorption of the drug, not admission to hospital) until death occurs at, on average, 41.6°C (O'Conner 1994). Dantrolene infusions to reverse hyperpyrexia and muscle relaxants (e.g. atracurium) to stop heat production (Wake 1995) are therefore priority treatments.

Increased metabolism causes hypercapnia and lactic acidosis which, if profound, lead to a syndrome of cell damage, increased capillary membrane permeability, increased oxygen consumption and electrolyte imbalance (calcium, potassium, creatinine, phosphokinase and myoglobin release from muscle cells (Wake 1995)). Hyperventilation (double/triple minute volumes) compensates both for metabolic acidosis and increased tissue oxygen delivery (Wake 1995). Profound metabolic acidosis may require reversal with sodium bicarbonate (Wake 1995; MacConnachie 1997b) (see Chapter 19).

Hyperkalaemia and hypercalcaemia cause dysrhythmias, and so ECGs should be continuously monitored. Hyperkalaemia may be reduced by intravenous insulin and dextrose (Wake 1995), which facilitates potassium transfer to intracellular fluid (rebound hyperkalaemia may occur later). Serum potassium monitoring should therefore continue after returning to 'normal'. Increased intracellular calcium also causes erratic, uncontrolled, but constant, muscle contractions (fuelling further hypermetabolism and hyperpyrexia) and muscle rigidity, lockjaw and teeth grinding. Hepatic hypoperfusion often causes dysfunction and hypoglycaemia. Water intoxification can cause severe hyponatraemia (118–110 mmol/l), necessitating hypertonic saline infusions. Blood sugars should be closely monitored and glucose supplements given as prescribed.

Cardiovascular problems

Sympathetic stimulation causes

- dysrhythmias/tachycardia (especially ventricular: VEs, VT, VF)
- vasoconstriction (including coronary and cerebral arterial spasm)
- hypertension
- peripheral tissue hypoxia

and possible myocardial infection – problems not usually associated with younger people. Vascular damage from intravenous drug abuse ('mainlining') and heavy smoking (Jones & Owens 1996) may make cannulation difficult.

Cardiovascular assessment should include vital signs (ECG, ABP, CVP and possible cardiac output studies).

Beta stimulation can be reversed by β-blockers (e.g. labetolol, esmolol) (MacConnachie 1997b) and stabilise tachycardias, but this will not ease α-mediated vasoconstriction (Jones & Owens 1996). Hypertension may necessitate systemic vasodilators (e.g. SNP, GTN, nifedipine) (Jones & Owens 1996; MacConnachie 1997b). Myocardial infarction is treated with thrombolysis (Jones & Owens 1996) (see Chapter 24). Adrenaline should be avoided, as it exacerbates adrenergic storm (Jones & Owens 1996).

DIC may, on rare occasions, occur through thromboplastin-C release and increased vascular permeability (Wake 1995; Cook 1995).

Renal problems

Hypermetabolism causes muscle breakdown (rhabdomyolysis); myoglobin deposits obstruct renal tubules, causing acute renal failure (Wake 1995) and myoglobinuria (orange-brown urine) (Jones & Owens 1996). Renal failure accentuates hyperkalaemia.

Neurological/psychological problems

Labile blood pressure and cerebral oedema (e.g. from hyponatraemia) can cause

- confusion
- grand mal fits (Jones & Owens 1996)
- intracerebral bleeds/CVAs
- SIADH (see Chapter 22)

Medullary depression may cause bradypnoea (Jones & Owens 1996).

Psychological complications include depression, anxiety and memory disturbance (McCann *et al.* 1998). Habitual use damages serotonin and dopaminergic neurones (Day 1996), causing permanent cognitive impairment (Parrott *et al.* 1998) and possible Parkinsonian traits. Survivors often experience frequent and persistent panic attacks ('bad trips'), believing death to be imminent (McGuire *et al.* 1994; Cook 1995; Lehane & Rees 1996).

Treatment for cerebral oedema is discussed in Chapter 22. Cerebral perfusion and oxygenation should be optimised, together with antiepileptics (usually benzodiazepines, although these can exacerbate cardiac instability) (Jones & Owens 1996).

Anxiety states may necessitate tranquillisers (e.g. diazepam), but major tranquillisers (e.g. chlorpromazine) should be avoided as they lower seizure threshold, aggravate hypotension and provoke dysrhythmias (MacConnachie 1997b).

Implications for practice

- overdoses can affect all major body systems; vital signs should be closely monitored
- peak effect often occurs 7.5 hours after ingestion, although wide variations occur, partly depending on dose, individual tolerance and metabolism
- friends and victims are often reluctant to share information with staff, and often experience guilt and fears
- victims are often young, giving friends (and nurses) an uncomfortable reminder of their own mortality
- nurses should maintain their duty of confidentiality (unless specifically exempted by statute law)
- ICU nurses may be able to offer health information about drugs or support groups

Summary

Ecstasy is one of a number of street drugs that may cause ICU admission. Unlike licensed drugs (e.g. morphine), its production is illegal; impurities and differing doses compound problems caused by the active drug. In addition to multisystem physiological problems (not usually occurring in younger people), users (and friends) often experience anxiety or guilt. Care is needed, therefore, to integrate urgent multisystem physiological support with skilful psychological care. Caring for such patients is challenging and can cause distress, but holistic nursing care can contribute significantly to every aspect of recovery.

Useful contacts

Families Anonymous: 0207 498–4680
Drugline Ltd, Drug Advisory Bureau: 0208 692–4975
Turning Point, Grove Park, Camberwell, London: 0207 274–4883

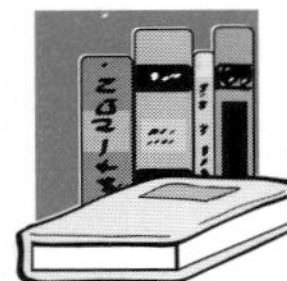

Further reading

Useful specialist nursing articles include Jones & Owens (1996), Wake (1995) and Cunningham (1997)). For other fields, Cook (1995) is brief, but gives information for health promotion, while Tober (1994) is an excellent piece of research.

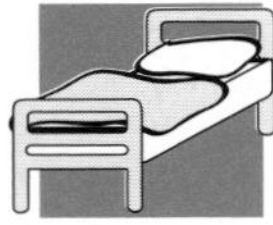

Clinical scenario

Kelly Jones is a healthy 18-year-old who had ingested an unknown amount of MDMA (3,4 methylenedioxymethamphetamine, or Ecstasy) at a local night-club at 11 p.m. She collapsed at about 1 a.m. and was taken to hospital. On admission to ICU, Kelly had become deeply unconscious, hyperthermic (40.1°C), tachycardic (140 beats per minute) with hypotension (80/40 mmHg). Blood investigations revealed metabolic acidosis and hypoglycaemia.

Q.1 (a) List the five main endogenous neurotransmitters and identify which is excessively released in response to Ecstasy.
(b) Review the physiological processes occurring from ingestion of Ecstasy to unconsciousness. Explain why Kelly became euphoric, hypermetabolic, hyperthermic, tachycardic, hypotensive, acidotic and low blood sugar, etc.

Q.2 Kelly is prescribed dantrolene and one litre fluid challenge in an attempt to reduce her hyperthermia. Analyse the effects of these treatments on other vital signs (blood pressure, central venous pressure, heart rate, ECG, temperature, arterial blood gases, etc.) and discuss other nursing strategies which may be used to monitor and minimise associated complications such as DIC, acute renal failure, SIADH, intracerebral haemorrhage.

Q.3 Kelly recovers from this life-threatening episode but is left with renal and hepatic dysfunction, depression and paranoid ideation. Evaluate advice and support offered to patients such as Kelly in your clinical practice area. Review the availability of specialist referrals, resources, discharge clinics, support groups.

Chapter 42

Obstetric emergencies in ICU

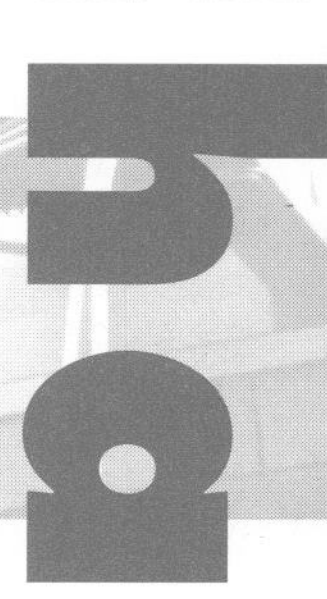

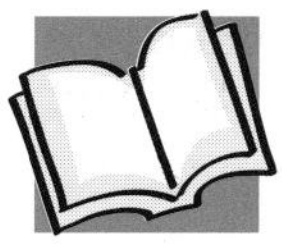

Contents

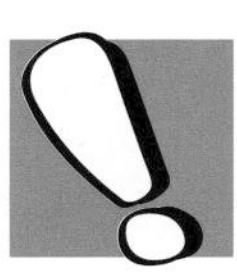

Fundamental knowledge

Normal pregnancy

Introduction

This chapter describes obstetric complications that necessitate ICU admission. Most deliveries are 'normal': for every thousand deliveries between 1 and 9 mothers need ICU admission (Kilpatrick & Matthay 1992), so that ICU admission is rarely needed (although incidence varies between units), but obstetric patients can be among the sickest patients in ICU. Since there is limited literature on obstetric emergencies in ICU texts and journals and few ICU staff are qualified as midwives, this can provoke special anxieties among staff (especially as most nurses are female, of a similar age, and possibly planning or raising families of their own).

The Department of Health's triennial report *Confidential Enquiries into Maternal Deaths in the United Kingdom* (DoH 1996b) provides valuable information on obstetric mortality. This 1996 report, which covers 1991–3 shows maternal mortality to be 9.8 per 100,000 pregnancies, a total of 320 deaths of which 104 deaths were in ICUs (40 per cent of all maternal mortalities); bed shortages had also caused refusal of further obstetric admissions (DoH 1996b). The numbers of obstetric admissions to ICUs are likely to rise, due to

- improved survival from simpler pathologies
- increased risks from social changes (e.g. older primigravidae, more multiple births from fertility treatments)

The 1996 Confidential Enquiry introduced a specific section on ICU nursing.

Most crises result from the physiological changes of pregnancy; since antenatal emergencies usually necessitate early delivery or termination of pregnancy, they are rarely admitted to ICUs. Antenatal ICU admissions are more likely to occur for non-obstetric conditions (e.g. road traffic accident); specific obstetric care (if any) depends on fetal age and condition, so nurses should seek advice from their midwifery colleagues. Antenatal care should optimise conditions for both mother and fetus. Fetal mortality may occur in addition to, or independently of, maternal mortality. However, most ICU obstetric admissions are postnatal (Bird 1997).

Postnatal admission is usually necessitated by complications such as respiratory or cardiovascular failure. Thus, while pregnancy and delivery may trigger crises, medical and nursing care centres on complications, medical treatments supporting failing systems (e.g. ventilation) and the human care familiar to ICU staff. Although ICU nurses do not need midwifery expertise to care for these admissions, an understanding of obstetric pathophysiology is useful. Midwives visit between 10 and 28 days following delivery, and so should be actively involved in the multidisciplinary teams. Midwifery expertise may provide both psychological reassurance and practical care (e.g. expressing breast milk, assessing and monitoring uterine contraction).

Normal pregnancy

Normal physiological changes during pregnancy favour fetal growth but place stress on the mother's body, altering 'normal' biochemical/haematological values from non-pregnant levels.

In the first **trimester** (weeks 1–12) the *cardiovascular* system becomes hyperdynamic:

- blood volume increases by up to one-half
- stroke volume and heart rate increase
- thus, cardiac output increases about 40 per cent (McNabb 1997) and
- systemic vascular resistance increases.

If cardiac reserve is limited, increased cardiac work may precipitate cardiac failure.

Fetal growth displaces the mother's heart upward, causing left axis deviation on ECGs. Patients should not be nursed supine as aortocaval compression may compromise circulation to both mother and fetus (Bird 1997).

Reduced colloid osmotic pressure (dilution), hypertension and vasoconstriction encourage *oedema* formation, including

- pulmonary oedema (impairing gas exchange)
- airway oedema (obstructing airways)
- cerebral oedema (causing intracranial hypertension).

Erythropoietin levels rise during trimesters 2 and 3, but erythrocyte count increases by only one-quarter, creating (dilutional) *anaemia*; reduced blood viscosity improves capillary flow, and so (highly vascular) placental perfusion but, with increased systemic vascular resistance from *prostacyclin*, reduces the mother's peripheral perfusion; auscultation for diastolic blood pressure may be difficult and expose mothers with pregnancy-induced hypertension to the risk of undetected strokes. Hypertension is discussed below.

Fetal haemoglobin (HbF) contains more 2,3 DPG (see Chapter 18) than adult haemoglobin (HbA), increasing HbF affinity for oxygen (with improved perfusion, this compensates the fetus for normal anaemia of pregnancy).

Pregnancy causes a *procoagulant* state with:

- doubling of prepregnant fibrin levels (400–600 mg/l)
- increased factors IV, VII, VIII, X
- decreased factors XI, XIII
- thrombocytopaenia

Onset of labour accelerates cardiovascular changes. In first stage labour, pain and anxiety increase circulating catecholamines, increasing cardiac output by nearly one-half. Second stage labour (contractions and delivery) creates a valsalva effect, reducing both venous return and cardiac output. Third stage labour (delivery of placenta) causes a 500-ml autotransfusion from uterine contraction. Stroke volume increases but systemic vascular resistance decreases.

Between 1991 and 1993, cardiac complications caused 41 UK maternal deaths (DoH 1996b). Maternal hearts are usually robust enough to cope with demands of pregnancy, but the number of maternal deaths from congenital defects is increasing (DoH 1996b), a trend likely to continue as the advances made in neonatal surgery 20–30 years ago allow more survivors to reach childbearing age.

Increased maternal oxygen demand (up by one-third during pregnancy, and a further 60 per cent during labour) increases the *respiratory* and cardiovascular workload. Minute volume increases by about one-half, mainly from larger tidal volumes, increasing PaO_2 and decreasing $PaCO_2$ (respiratory alkalosis). However, functional residual capacity, and thus respiratory reserve, is reduced by one-fifth from the upward displacement of the diaphragm (4–7 cm (Zerbe 1995)) by fetal growth, while pulmonary oedema impairs gas exchange (especially oxygen).

Nasal and airway mucosa become more vascular and oedematous, increasing the risk of epistaxis (Zerbe 1995), and necessitating smaller endotracheal tubes (especially with nasal intubation) while increasing airway resistance and pressures.

The incidence of acute respiratory distress syndrome (ARDS, see Chapter 27) is increasing, causing 44 UK obstetric deaths between 1988 and 1990 (DoH 1994b); in the 1996 report ARDS deaths are dispersed among other headings.

Neurological changes are not normally seen, but cerebral oedema and hypoxia can cause fitting from eclampsia (see below).

Gastrointestinal motility is reduced, contributing to nausea/vomiting, malnutrition and potential acid aspiration ('Mendelsohn's syndrome'). Hypertension can cause *liver* dysfunction, resulting in potential hypoglycaemia, immunocompromise, jaundice, coagulopathies, encephalopathy and other neurological complications. However, gestational hyperglycaemia occurs more often as catecholamines and other hormones increase insulin resistance. Maternal hyperglycaemia may facilitate fetal supply, but maternal blood sugar levels should be monitored regularly as insulin supplements may be needed.

Glomerular filtration increases by one-half (McNabb 1997), and so drug clearance may be increased. Increased urine output and antenatal bladder compression from the fetus cause urgency.

The depression of cell-mediated and humoral *immunity* during the third trimester prevents fetal rejection, but increases viral infections (especially varicella/chicken pox and colds).

Pregnancy-induced hypertension

Hypertension caused 20 UK maternal deaths between 1991 and 1993 (a 26 per cent reduction from the 1988–90 period); eleven of these were from eclampsia (DoH 1996b).

Pre-eclampsia (hypertension and proteinuria, with or without oedema) frequently occurs; full eclampsia only occurs about once in every 2,000 UK deliveries, but 38 per cent of these cases were not diagnosed pre-eclamptic (Douglas & Redman 1994).

Systemic release of thromboplastin in severe pre-eclampsia (probably from damaged placental tissue) causes intense arteriolar vasoconstriction and DIC (Bewley 1997), compounding hypertension and coagulopathies.

Eclampsia is grand-mal type fitting (Fraser & Saunders 1990). Over one-half of eclamptic deaths occur following only one or two fits, and so convulsions should be controlled (Bewley 1997). Delivery is essential to resolve eclampsia, so that Caesarian section or termination of pregnancy are usually necessary (Fraser & Saunders 1990). Eclamptic fits can also occur up to ten days following delivery (Abbott 1997), and so monitoring should be continued.

Acute fatty liver is a rare variant of pre-eclampsia; gross microvascular fatty infiltration occurs, without hepatic necrosis or inflammation. Normal hepatic function resumes postnatally (Kaplan 1985b), so that early delivery resolves the problem (Sussman 1996).

Hypertension should be controlled; antenatally, placental perfusion must be maintained. Hydralazine is often used, but it crosses the placenta (Hanson 1990) and animal studies have identified toxicity (BNF 1998). Eclampsia should be controlled with intravenous/intramuscular magnesium (Eclampsia Trial Collaborative Group, 1995; DoH, 1996b); doses vary, but most texts recommend plasma levels of 2–4 mmol/l (Idama & Lindow 1998). Toxicity (>5 mmol/l) can cause the loss of tendon reflexes (Idama & Lindow 1998) and respiratory paralysis in both mother and newborn (Adam & Osborne 1997), so that 1 g calcium gluconate should be immediately available (Idama & Lindow 1998). Magnesium also reduces the incidence of pulmonary emboli (Coetzee *et al.* 1998).

Analgesia should be given both for humanitarian reasons and to reduce sympathetic stimulation (stress response), which contributes to hypertension.

Plasmapheresis (see Chapter 35) can remove mediators, preventing pre-eclampsia from progressing to eclampsia or other complications (e.g. HELLP syndrome, see below).

Thromboembolism

The largest single cause of maternal mortality remains 'obstinately static', causing 35 UK deaths between 1991 and 1993 (DoH 1996b). Oral anticoagulants (e.g. warfarin) cross the placenta and may cause placental/fetal haemorrhage, and so should not be given antenatally (especially during the final weeks of pregnancy) (BNF 1998). For high-risk pregnancy, the CLASP collaborative group (1994) recommend low dose aspirin for high-risk pre-eclampsia, although some recent studies (e.g. Caritas *et al.* (1998)) have found low-dose aspirin non-beneficial.

Amniotic fluid embolus

This rare condition occurs most frequently in older women with higher **parity**; it progresses rapidly and is usually diagnosed at post-mortem (Nelson-Piercy & Hanson 1997). Maternal mortality remains virtually static at 80 per cent (10 UK deaths 1991–3) (DoH 1996b). For the first time, over one-half of those with amniotic emboli survived to reach ICUs during the period 1991–3 (DoH 1996b).

Amniotic fluid (derived from plasma) includes vasoactive mediators (e.g. prostaglandins, leukotrienes and thromboplastins). Animal studies with clear amniotic fluid are rarely symptomatic (Gin & Ngan Kee 1997), but uterine/cervical rupture (e.g. induction of labour) causes mixing with fetal debris/meconium (Adam & Osborne 1997).

Amniotic fluid emboli cause severe respiratory complications (oedema, hypertension, arrest) and DIC (Lindsay 1997). Pulmonary artery catheterisation can detect complications and enable the reduction of mortality (Vanmaele *et al.* 1990).

Haemorrhage

The Department of Health (1996b) recorded 15 UK deaths between 1991 and 1993 from haemorrhage, 8 being postpartum.

Bleeding from normal third-stage labour is reduced by arterial constriction and the development of a fibrin mesh over the placental site; placental circulation, about 600 ml/minute at term (Lindsay 1997), is autotransfused by uterine contraction. Incomplete contraction, therefore, causes a major haemorrhage. Bleeding can also occur from genital tract lacerations and coagulopathies (DIC is a common complication of pregnancy).

Postpartum haemorrhage volume is easily underestimated (e.g. from loss on sheets) (Lindsay 1997). Specific management of primary postpartum haemorrhage (e.g. oxytocin) is usually supervised by obstetricians or midwives before transfer to an ICU for fluid resuscitation and monitoring.

HELLP syndrome:

Haemolysis
Elevated Liver enzymes and
Low Platelets

This syndrome causes severe hypertension, coagulopathies and grossly disordered liver function, although the classification and criteria for HELLP are inconsistent (Geary 1997). Up to 8 per cent of severe pre-eclampsias progress to HELLP (Sibai 1994) and maternal mortality can reach 25 per cent (Geary 1997); HELLP is often the main obstetric emergency requiring ICU admission.

Platelet activation causes thrombi in small blood vessels, while narrowed lumens trigger erythrocyte haemolysis, further reducing haemoglobin levels (aggravating hypoxia) and raising serum bilirubin levels (Turner 1997).

Early symptoms are often vague and non-specific (e.g. epigastric pain, nausea and vomiting; hypertension and proteinuria may not even be present (Sibai 1994)), so that HELLP may become life-threatening before it is diagnosed.

Treatments include:

- urgent delivery of fetus (induction, Caesarian section) (Sibai 1994)
- antithrombotic agents (heparin, prostacyclin, fresh frozen plasma)
- plasmapheresis (removes circulating mediators) (Sibai 1994; Turner 1997)
- system support (e.g. ventilation)

Brain-death incubation

Technology can support body systems following brain death, enabling fetal growth despite maternal death (Diehl *et al.* 1994). Although rare events, the admission of brain-dead mothers creates stress for families and places nurses in a similar (but more prolonged) situation to that of caring for organ donors (see Chapter 43).

Drugs and pregnancy

Additional considerations when giving drugs during pregnancy include:

- will they cross the placenta?
- are they expressed in breast milk (if breastfeeding)?
- the fetal/newborn clearance of toxic metabolites

Being professionally accountable for each drug given, nurses should withhold drugs and seek advice (e.g. BNF, hospital pharmacy) if unsure of likely effects. Pharmacists should be actively involved in multidisciplinary teams.

Implications for practice

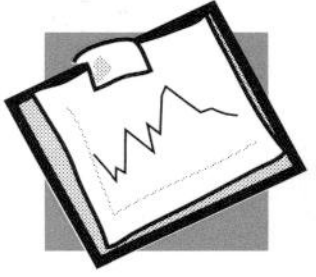

- ICU admission will usually be to provide respiratory and/or cardiovascular support, and so care should follow from problems necessitating admission
- do not nurse pregnant patients supine; aortocaval compression occludes circulation

- pregnancy causes immunocompromise, so minimise risk factors
- psychological stressors (especially with miscarriage/abortion) may cause feelings of guilt (mother, partner, children), and so plan care holistically to include the psychological needs of all concerned
- involve midwives

antenatally:

- the mother's body should provide an optimal environment for fetal development

postnatally:

- obstetric examinations should include vaginal examination (amount and type of discharge) and uterine contraction
- mothers wishing, but currently unable, to breastfeed should be offered opportunities to express breast milk (breast pump); this also relieves breast pain
- photographs may be wanted; hospitals usually have facilities for instant photographs

miscarriage/abortion:

- fathers and other family should be given an opportunity to view the body
- bereavement counselling and care may be needed
- photographs may become treasured mementoes of lost children; parents may not think to ask for photographs at the time

Summary

Pregnancy is a normal physiological function, and most pregnancies occur without serious complications. However, life-threatening complications can and do occur, necessitating ICU admission, usually for cardiovascular or respiratory failure. Antenatal admissions should consider fetal health; however, most admissions are postnatal and, as the precipitating cause (fetus/placenta) has been delivered, system support may be all that is required until homeostasis is restored, although some problems may require more aggressive treatments.

Interventions used will be familiar to most ICU nurses, but terminology and pathophysiology may differ. This chapter has described the main causes of ICU obstetric admissions.

Useful contacts

Miscarriage Association, c/o Clayton Hospital, Northgate, Wakefield, WF1 3JF: 01924 200799

Stillbirth and Neonatal Death Society (SANDS): 28 Portland Place, London, W1N 4DE

Further reading

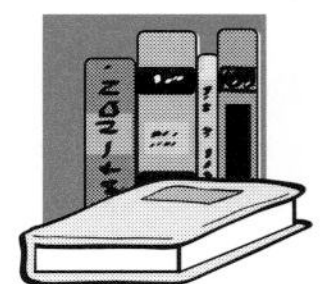

Most ICU textbooks include an overview of obstetric emergencies; articles in ICU journals tend to describe one pathology, but Bird (1997) gives a comprehensive overview of the main causes of obstetric admissions and provides a useful review. Hanson (1990) provides a useful description of drug management, despite its age. Sweet (1997) is a classic midwifery text.

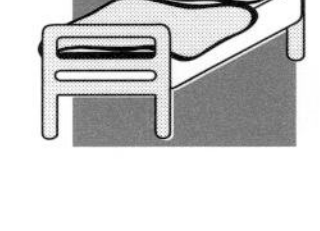

Clinical scenario

Elizabeth Franklin, a multiparous 37-year-old, presented in labour at 35 weeks gestation. She was hypertensive with BP of 180/115 mmHg with large proteinuria. Following an emergency caesarean delivery, Elizabeth had an eclamptic convulsion and was admitted to ICU. Elizabeth was ventilated and intravenous infusions of hydralazene, magnesium, phenytoin were commenced.

Q.1 Review emergency protocols and cardiopulmonary resuscitation guidelines used with obstetric patients in your clinical area. What modifications or adaptations to normal procedures are made for pregnant or postpartum patients and why?

Q.2 Explain the purpose (pharmodynamics) of hydralazine, magnesium and phenytoin infusions in Elizabeth's treatment. Consider how you would check their effectiveness and monitor for potential adverse effects or signs of toxicity.

Q.3 Analyse the role and responsibilities of the midwife for Elizabeth while she is ventilated and a patient on ICU. Specify the nature of collaborative care which can be provided (e.g. assessment of vaginal discharge, uterus, breasts, equipment and tips on expressing breast milk etc).

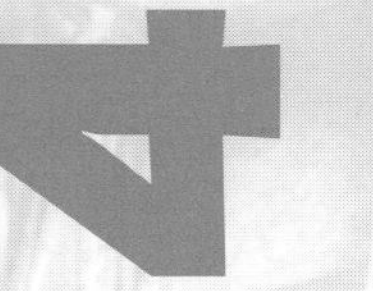
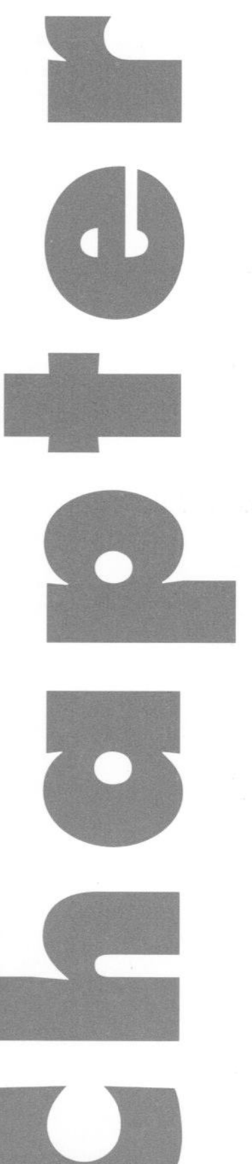

Chapter 43

Transplants

Contents

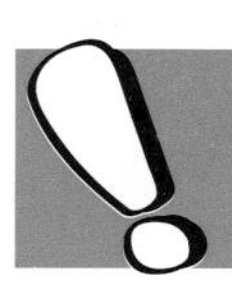

Fundamental knowledge

Brainstem and cranial nerve function

Introduction

Since the introduction of the immunosuppressant cyclosporin A and the University of Wisconsin preservation solution, transplantation has become a viable treatment for endstage failure of all major body systems (except the brain), and increasing numbers of other pathologies are treated by donor grafts (e.g. skin, bone marrow). Some ICUs receive patients following transplantation; all care for potential donors. Yet increasing donor shortage is causing increased waiting time which, with endstage failure, often means increased mortality.

Kidneys were the first organs to be successfully transplanted. Approximately 12,000 people in the UK receive renal replacement therapy for endstage renal failure (ESRF) (Williams *et al.* 1997); renal grafts offer the only possible cure. Most people on UK transplant waiting lists are waiting for renal grafts (5,000 out of 6,000), and about 1,500 renal transplants are performed each year.

Few centres currently perform lung transplantation; although the quality of life is improved (MacNaughton *et al.* 1998), persistent surfactant impairment limits graft function (Hohlfeld *et al.* 1998). Cadaver lungs are usually split, enabling two patients to receive transplants from one donor (Dark 1997).

Further discussion on specific organs can be found in Chapter 30 and Chapter 44.

Brainstem death

Historically, death was synonymous with cessation of breathing and/or heartbeat. The development of technologies to replace breathing (ventilators) and heartbeat (pacing) coincided with the transfer of organ donation from science fiction to science fact, necessitating a revision of the concepts of death.

The brainstem, extending between the cerebrum and spinal cord and consisting of the pons, medulla oblongata and midbrain, contains the vital centres (respiratory, cardiac and other), so that if the brainstem is dead, higher consciousness and control cannot be regained. Brainstem death, first described in 1959, is established in the UK through the Code of Practice (DoH 1998b), although UK legislation is limited to two main acts (see p.465), clarifying contentious issues.

Brainstem death is typically caused by

- intracerebral bleed/infarction
- head trauma
- cerebral hypoxia
- cerebral tumour
- drug overdose
- intracranial infection

Diagnosing brainstem death is not required for every death (it is used for 10 per cent of ICU deaths (Frid *et al.* 1998)), but provides protection for vulnerable patients and diagnosing doctors where

- there is any reasonable doubt about whether the patient is dead
- organs/tissues may be harvested for transplantation.

Any medical conditions that could prevent brainstem function must be excluded (see Table 43.1) before testing for brain death. The reflexes and responses of each cranial nerve are then tested (individually or in combination; see Table 43.2). If higher centre responses are absent, brainstem death may be diagnosed; any response from higher centres (however abnormal or limited) prohibits brainstem death diagnosis. Reflex responses from below the brainstem (e.g. spinal cord reflexes, which can occur with electrical stimulation to corpses) are insignificant, but may make relatives or other witnesses anxious if misinterpreted as signs of life. The legal time of death is the first test, although death is not pronounced until confirmed by the second test (DoH 1998b).

Table 43.1 Code of Practice for Brainstem Death diagnosis: preconditions

There should be no doubt that the patient's condition is due to irremediable brain damage of known aetiology
The patient is deeply unconscious
There should be no evidence that this state is due to depressant drugs
Primary hypothermia as a cause of unconsciousness must be excluded
Potentially reversible circulatory, metabolic and endocrine disturbances must be excluded as a cause of the continuation of unconsciousness
The patient is being maintained on a ventilator because spontaneous respiration has been inadequate or has ceased altogether

***Source*: DoH 1998b**

Table 43.2 Brainstem death tests

Brainstem death tests should establish the absence of:
pupil reaction
corneal reflex
vestibulo-ocular reflex
motor response
gag reflex
cough reflex
respiratory effort

Two sets of identical tests (each following all the criteria in the Code) should be carried out by two doctors, both of whom have been qualified for more than five years, and at least one of whom is a consultant; in practice, the patient's consultant is usually involved with the tests. Neither doctor making the test should be a member of the transplant team. Timing between the two sets of tests is often relatively brief, partly to facilitate the presence of the same team and partly to reduce anxiety for families waiting for confirmation of death, but it should be long enough to ensure that the second set of tests is meaningful.

The *Human Tissues Act* (1961) established that after death the body becomes the property of the next of kin, and so they must not object to the donation (Morgan 1995). The *Human Organ Transplants Act* (1989) legislated against making or receiving payment for organs so that unrelated living people cannot become donors during their lifetime (living related donors are discussed below).

Nursing care

Caring for donors and their families can be psychologically stressful. Unlike other terminal care, where (hopefully) peaceful death is followed by the last offices, the diagnosis of brainstem death is followed by the process of optimising organ function for harvest. While logical, this conflicts with normal nursing values where actions should be to the benefit of the patients being cared for. Once death has been diagnosed, and following harvest of the organ(s), the body is then normally transferred to the mortuary; the last offices ('letting go') are performed elsewhere. During this dehumanising experience, nurses are usually supporting the donor's family; less than one-half of Watkinson's (1995) sample of nurses found caring for donors to be a rewarding experience.

In such potentially undignified situations, nurses should optimise their patient's dignity, both before and after the diagnosis of death. Privacy can be helped by drawing curtains around patients' beds or transferring them into siderooms. Relatives facing bereavement should be allowed to grieve; they may also gain comfort from knowing their loved one's organs will help others to live. Relatives' responses vary; transplant coordinators are experienced at comforting relatives and may prove a valuable resource, although some relatives prefer to speak to staff with whom they have already established a strong rapport and trust.

Donors

At the end of December 1998, there were 6,502 people in the UK waiting for a solid organ transplant (UKTSSA 1999); growth in the waiting list continues to exceed organ availability. Donation criteria attempt to optimise the supply of viable transplantable organs/tissue without endangering recipients. What is viable varies with specific organs or tissue, but in many respects medical progress has enabled progressive relaxation of donation criteria. There are very few exclusions for surface tissue (e.g. corneas), but the criteria for vital organs usually exclude donors with malignancies or other transferable life-threatening conditions. Normally, transplant coordinators can clarify whether potential donors meet the required criteria.

Medical ethics requires that any treatment must be for the patient's benefit: intubation and ventilation cannot be initiated in a living person solely to preserve organs for harvest (DoH 1998b). Donor pools are therefore largely limited to patients who are already being artificially ventilated (i.e. ICU patients); unfortunately, multiorgan dysfunction, often the cause of death on ICUs, leaves few viable organs for harvest.

Road safety measures (e.g. seat belts, crash helmets) have reduced the numbers of fatal injuries, and UK road deaths are lower than in most developed countries. While reduced mortality is commendable, this has reduced organ availability for transplant. Austria, which operates a system of presumed consent, has the highest transplant rate in Europe (27.2 per cent per million population); the statistics for road deaths in Austria in 1995 were 15 per 100,000 population, compared to 6 per 100,000 population in the UK (Caldwell *et al.* 1998).

In the UK, available donor organs are matched and allocated through the United Kingdom Transplant Support Service Authority (UKTSSA). Organs are used for the benefit of UK patients, but where this is not possible, rather than waste a precious resource, they are offered to other European organ sharing organisations.

Inevitably, regional variations exist, sometimes from pragmatic considerations (e.g. services available), sometimes from the local criteria of transplant teams. Occasionally, controversial values cause national debate (e.g. should persistent alcoholics receive livers, or smokers be given hearts), but the increasing development of multidisciplinary teams, including recipient transplant coordinators (often from nursing backgrounds), is encouraging greater objectivity and fairness.

Ethical issues

Transplantation has always maintained a high public profile, ensuring widespread discussion of ethical issues. Organ donation relies on public goodwill, and so healthcare staff should encourage public awareness. Nurses experienced in caring for donors tend to display more positive attitudes towards donation (Duke *et al.* 1998), thus continuing educational development is needed (Watkinson 1995).

Organ donation can literally be life-saving; the *moral duty* to facilitate transplantation creates dilemmas between whether the onus should fall on society or on individuals. Some nations, such as France, Belgium, Austria, Sweden and Norway, operate systems of presumed consent, whereby people have to actively opt-out if they do not wish to donate. The UK, like most countries, however, has an opt-in system in which organs are freely donated without coercion, and seen as a gift.

Publicity has a significant influence on donor supply: positive publicity (e.g. transplant games) encourages donation, while any negative publicity can increase refusal rates. Although three-quarters of the UK population appear to favour donation, only one-quarter carry donor cards (Gibson 1996). Studies from other countries show similar statistics (Gibson 1996). The NHS Organ Donor Register, which is administered by UKTSSA on behalf of the Department of Health, enables people to record their willingness to be organ donors; however, most people remain unregistered (Wright & Cohen 1997).

Relatives may object to donation for various reasons (see Table 43.3), but according to a DoH report (1995), only one-fifth of relatives' refusals 'resulted from knowing that patients did not wish to donate organs' (cited Clacy 1998). Rather than asking relatives for their consent to organ donation, it would probably be preferable if they were asked to indicate their lack of objection (DoH 1998b); this change of approach could possibly reduce the incidence of relatives posthumously over-ruling a patient's wishes, and might also reduce the feelings of guilt often experienced by relatives and ease the dilemma in which they find themselves.

Table 43.3 Common reasons for next-of-kin refusing consent for organ donation

Relatives did not want surgery to the body (24 per cent)
Patient had previously said they did not wish to donate (21 per cent)
Relatives felt patient had suffered enough (21 per cent)
Relatives divided over decision (19 per cent)
Relatives not sure whether patient would have agreed to donation (18 per cent)
Relatives feared patient's body would be disfigured (15 per cent)

***Source*: DOH 1995 report, cited Clacy 1998.**

Except for Rastafarians, none of the major religions opposes organ donation (Randhawa 1997), although some ministers (e.g. some Jewish rabbis (Levine 1997)) may discourage donation, believing that the body should remain unmutilated.

Distressed relatives, facing inevitable bereavement, may not think to ask about organ donation, but may subsequently find not having been approached more stressful than being asked (Pelletier 1992). Staff should therefore offer the opportunity of donation to relatives. They should be approached openly, without coercion; the best time for doing this will be individual to each case, but the approach will probably benefit from teamwork, possibly involving the transplant coordinators. It should be remembered, however, that if subsequent tests exclude the possibility of donation, relatives may then feel rejected, although, if criteria do prove problematic, the donation of tissue (e.g. corneas) may still be possible, which may provide some compensatory comfort. Donor HIV testing is required, and if results are unexpectedly positive, nurses must maintain patient confidentiality.

It is normal for transplant coordinators to thank the donor families by letter, describing beneficiaries, without directly identifying them (for mutual safety). The letters are sent out at an early stage in case the recipients suffer rejection of the organs.

Macro-economically, transplant surgery can be highly cost-effective by replacing the cost of years of chronic treatment (e.g. renal dialysis). The units that provide donors receive financial remuneration through the transplant services, but some hidden costs can be difficult to quantify, and the demand for ICU beds may discourage the facilitation of donations (Wright & Cohen 1997), or cause refusal of other admissions.

Spain has the highest donor procurement in Europe (Talbot 1998). The Spanish transplant coordination services (established in 1989) employ a coordinator in every hospital (Talbot 1998), which enables closer supervision of potential donors and provides more support for staff. The greater availability of ICU beds there (50 per 1,000 hospital beds) removes many of the pressures experienced in the UK. Thus, investment in the transplantation services may increase the supply of donor organs (although like Austria, Spanish road deaths in 1995 were 15 per 100,000 population (Caldwell *et al.* 1998)), but of course such investments have to be paid for, usually through taxes.

Live donors

The limitation of cadaver organs has encouraged the use of live donors; this is especially true for renal transplants, but it is also the case for liver, lung and pancreas transplants.

Between 1991 and 1995, the numbers of unrelated living donor transplants in the USA tripled (Suzuki *et al.* 1997). However, in the UK, under the 1989 Human Tissue Transplants Act, live donor transplants must be genetically related and not receive financial payment. This means that considerably fewer transplant operations are therefore performed in the UK.

Exeter experiment

In Exeter, medical ethical approval was given to resuscitate patients who suffered massive strokes, then intubate, ventilate and transfer them to ICU, where they were allowed to die; following diagnosis of brainstem death, organs could be harvested (Feest *et al.* 1990). However, this experiment was ended by a Department of Health letter which stated that proxy consent was only valid when procedures were in a patient's interest (Dunstan 1997). The British Transplantation Society protocols were subsequently amended in 1995, limiting elective ventilation for harvest to terminal conditions following spontaneous intracranial haemorrhage, preferably after cessation of spontaneous breathing (Dunstan 1997).

Asystolic donors

Patients who do not survive cardiopulmonary resuscitation provide another source of potential donors. As warm ischaemia adversely affects the function of harvested organs, external compression pumps (mechanical cardiac compression) can perfuse organs until harvested, with oxygen provided through an endotracheal catheter or ventilation and metabolism reduced through induced hypothermia (Kootstra *et al.* 1997). Kootstra and colleagues report function (usually delayed) in 60 per cent of asystolic (non-heart-beating) donor kidneys.

However, since asystolic donors will not have been diagnosed brainstem dead, some hospitals delay touching cadavers for a stated time (Kootstra *et al.* (1997) adopted a no-touch rule of 10 minutes) to avoid the problems raised by the Exeter experiment.

Xenografts

Genetic engineering has made xenografting (animal tissue) a realistic option. Cloning could resolve the problems of supply, but macro-ethical concerns surrounding animal rights and genetic engineering were illustrated by 'Dolly' (the cloned sheep), and legislation on xenografting is currently being considered (Fulbrook & Wilkinson 1997). The possibility of widespread xenografting in the near future means that nurses need to clarify their own values on these issues.

Implications for practice

- organ donation offers families the opportunity to salvage something positive from bereavement
- donor families should be asked whether they have any objection (rather than whether they consent) to organ/tissue harvest
- ICU nurses should assist relatives to make informed decisions about organ donation
- organ donation in the UK remains a gift; coercion (or apparent coercion) should be avoided
- the timing and method for approaching families has to be appropriate for each individual case, but teamwork can support both staff and bereaved relatives
- regional transplant coordinators can offer useful support and information at all stages of donor harvesting
- any medical conditions that may affect brainstem function must be excluded before brainstem death tests
- both sets of brainstem death tests must show absence of all higher responses on both occasions

- spinal reflexes may occur despite the absence of brainstem function; staff and relatives should be warned about these – they are not a sign of life
- time of death is determined by the first set of tests, but is only confirmed after the second set of tests
- harvest and transplantation of organs raise many ethical issues; staff should clarify their thoughts and feelings on these issues; unit discussion forums can provide useful opportunities for the sharing and developing of ideas

Summary

The transplantation of organs and tissues can offer possible cures and improved quality of life to people with endstage and life-threatening pathologies, but a continuing shortage of donors often causes long waiting lists with many patients dying before suitable organs are found. Since most organs for transplant are harvested from patients already in ICUs, ICU nurses should promote (without coercion) awareness about transplantation. The (usually) close rapport with families enables nurses to offer valuable support during crises and discussion.

Nurses are normally present during brainstem death testing, and so should be aware of the Code of Practice (DoH 1998b) and its requirements.

Useful contact

UK Transplant Support Service Authority (UKTSSA), Fox Den Road, Stoke Gifford, Bristol BS34 8RR: tel. 0117 975–7575.

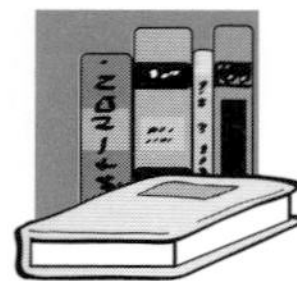

Further reading

Every ICU should have a copy of the current Code of Practice (DoH 1998b) (also available from transplant coordinators). The British Medical Bulletin, Vol. 53, issue 4 (1997) is devoted to the subject of transplants; Dunstan's article on ethics is especially valuable. Articles by transplant coordinators, such as Gibson (1996) and Morgan (1995), offer useful insights. Johnson (1992) outlines nursing care of donors and their families, while Randhawa (1997) provides a wider nursing review. Ethical dilemmas raised by non-therapeutic ventilation are discussed by Shaw (1996).

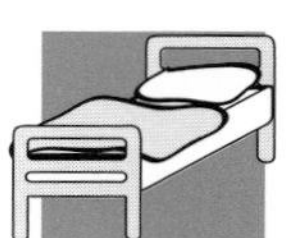

Clinical scenario

Kelly Jones is a healthy 18-year-old who ingested an unknown amount of Ecstasy (MDMA: 3,4 methylenedioxymethamphetamine) at a night-club. Kelly's progress was complicated by the development of DIC (Disseminated Intravascular Coagulation). While her condition was at its most critical her parents brought up the topic of organ donation (see scenarios for Chapters 31 and 41).

Q.1 Who, legally, can give permission (or consent) for organ donation on Kelly's behalf?

Q.2 Kelly has DIC and acute renal failure. Outline the range of tissues and organs that can be used for transplantation from Kelly.

Q.3 Kelly's parents request that if she dies, her ovum (eggs) are harvested and stored for future use by her siblings. Reflect on the legal and ethical aspects of this request. How do you think such a request would be dealt with in your own clinical practice area?

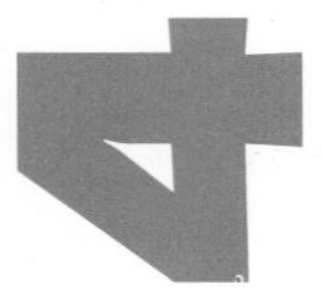
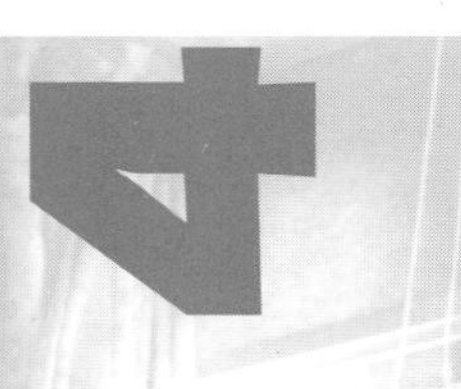
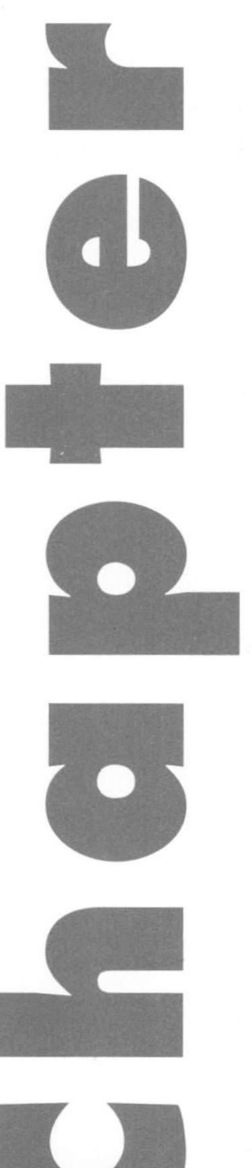

Chapter 44

Hepatic transplants

Contents

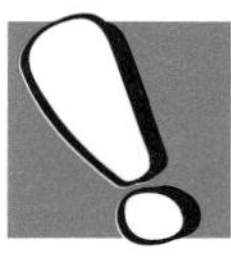

Fundamental knowledge

Effects of liver failure (see Chapter 39)
Immunity and effects of immunosuppression (see Chapter 40)

Introduction

Specialist ICUs may receive patients following transplant surgery. This chapter outlines early care following hepatic transplantation; while much care is similar to that of patients following any post-transplant care, hepatic surgery has been selected as it is performed at fewer centres than cardiac or renal transplantation. This chapter provides an insight for nurses unfamiliar with or new to post-transplant care.

Most early hepatic transplants attempted to cure liver cancer, but the cancer usually recurred within two years (Klintmalm 1998). In recent years, a number of developments – namely, cyclosporin A, venovenous bypass and the University of Wisconsin preservation solution – have combined to make hepatic transplantation viable treatment for endstage failure. After France, the UK performs the highest number of liver transplants in Europe; three-quarters of these are performed on adults (Malago *et al.* 1997). Although most patients develop complications, there is a one-year survival rate of 70–80 per cent (Reich *et al.* 1998).

The liver is the largest organ in the body; it is also highly vascular. Ideally, grafts should be of a similar size (within 10 per cent) to that of the recipient's premorbid one, but, as with other graft organs, the demand exceeds supply. Splitting livers between two or more recipients (Coinaud, a French surgeon, has divided a single liver into eight segments) can provide additional grafts (Malago *et al.* 1997)). Despite recent advances in genetic engineering, *xenografting* remains experimental with hepatic complement production causing complications.

Perioperatively, circulation is hyperdynamic, and major haemorrhage can occur peri- and postoperatively. Twenty units of blood are normally cross-matched, and clotting times should be closely monitored. In addition to an arterial line for monitoring, patients have a second (unheparinised) line for sampling; both lines remain in place postoperatively.

Priorities on arrival in ICU are normally

- ventilation
- restoring haemostasis
- rewarming

Extubation may occur between 1 and 4 hours postoperatively, allowing transfer to High Dependency Units; the Denver centre has pioneered immediate postoperative extubation. The removal of positive pressure ventilation improves venous return and splanchnic perfusion, and removes one source of infection (ventilator-associated pneumonia).

Complications

Rejection is classified as follows:

- Hyperacute rejection occurs within minutes of anastomosis, with pre-existing mediators provoking thrombotic occlusion of graft vasculature and irreversible ischaemia
- Acute rejection occurs with necrosis of individual cells
- Chronic rejection is caused by fibrosis and loss of normal organ structure

Although hyperacute rejection is rare, the failure of grafts necessitates retransplantation.

Most patients experience acute rejection; immunosuppression therapy usually enables graft survival, but predisposes patients to infection, especially from bacteria. High-dose steroids may also be used (Park *et al.* 1996).

Vascular occlusion (hepatic artery, portal vein) rapidly leads to hepatic necrosis, necessitating urgent retransplantation.

Biliary leaks commonly occur, especially following retransplantation (although the incidence varies between centres).

Many patients have pre-existing *pulmonary* shunting ('hepatopulmonary syndrome'); postoperative pleural effusions (especially right-sided) and atelectasis are common (Hawker 1997b). Chronic liver failure can cause pulmonary hypertension, and may prevent transplantation unless a heart–lung transplantation can also be performed.

Late complications are often similar to early complications, usually occurring after transfer from ICU. Chronic rejection necessitates retransplantation. Other late complications include

- vascular (especially arterial) occlusion
- biliary strictures
- infection
- recurrence of preoperative hepatitis B (or C) or tumours.

Immunosuppression

Cyclosporin has enabled liver (and other) transplants to become viable treatments. The current practice with immunosuppressant agents varies, but triple therapy (e.g. prednisolone, azathioprine, cyclosporin) reduces adverse effects from each drug. Cyclosporin is nephrotoxic and can cause hypertension.

Tacrolimus (FK 506; Prograf®), a fungal metabolite, is increasingly replacing cyclosporin. Tacrolimus inhibits the expression of interleukin-2 in T-lymphocytes and inhibits T-lymphocyte growth and proliferation (Tsui & Large 1998). Tacrolimus is a hundred times more active than cyclosporin (Heaton 1997), and oral doses are commenced the day following surgery. As Tacrolimus is protein-bound, displacement by other protein-binding drugs (e.g. warfarin) can cause toxicity; it is also nephrotoxic (Mihatsch *et al.* 1998) and neurotoxic (BNF 1998).

Immunosuppression by **monoclonal antibodies** (ATG, OKT3) has been abandoned due to lymphoedema from T-lymphocyte and leucocyte destruction.

Immunosuppression exposes patients to greater risk of infection, and so prophylactic antibiotics are given, often for 48 hours, and aciclovir is given to prevent herpes simplex.

Postoperative nursing

The reception of patients into ICUs following liver transplantation requires skilful management of surgical complications; patients will need

- *a safe environment*; the layout of equipment should be planned to ensure access (e.g. cardiac output monitors and ventilators are probably best placed on different sides of the bed)
- *infusions* for drugs; ensure sufficient syringe drivers are available
- *two nurses* (usually) on arrival; identify which staff will coordinate and which will support care.

Perioperative communication with the theatre can identify what equipment and drugs will be needed; the postoperative handover should identify specific complications and requirements (e.g. extubation plan).

Hypotension (from hypovolaemia and low systemic vascular resistance) necessitates haemodynamic monitoring. Inferior vena cava pressure should reflect central venous pressure, but it rises with haemorrhage or graft failure. Hypotension, intra-abdominal bleeding and sepsis can cause renal failure.

Dysrhythmias are often caused by vasoactive and toxic mediators from reperfusion injury. Increased vagal tone and toxins also make bradycardia likely (Park *et al.* 1996). Cardiovascular instability is usually limited to the first quarter of an hour, but can persist longer, so that close cardiovascular monitoring should be continued.

Hypotension will be potentiated by haemorrhage. As the liver produces most clotting factors, **coagulopathies** (e.g. DIC, thrombocytopenia) are likely from both presurgical chronic liver failure and massive blood transfusion (Park *et al.* 1996).

Although postoperative intra-abdominal haemorrhage is rare, it can be extensive, both from surgical causes and coagulopathies. Blood loss should be assessed through measuring drainage volume and content, and two nurses may be required for infusion of replacement blood. Drainage should be serous, with haemoglobin below 3 g/dl; if levels are above 5 g/dl or volumes above 200 ml/h, medical staff should be alerted. Bedside monitoring of clotting times (e.g. ACT) is essential.

Haemoglobin levels are usually maintained at between 8 and 10 g/dl to reduce viscosity and so improve perfusion.

Various *electrolyte* and *acid–base imbalances* can occur. If biochemistry does not stabilise over the first postoperative day, graft failure should be suspected.

Potassium absorption by the graft liver, together with *autologous* blood transfusion, make *hypokalaemia* likely (Park *et al.* 1996); this will cause further cardiac instability, and so should be closely monitored and supplements given. Autologous blood can also cause **hypernatraemia** (autologous blood suspends cells in saline) (Park *et al.* 1996). **Hypercalcaemia,** causing further cardiac instability, often occurs, but usually stabilises quickly (Park *et al.* 1996).

Hyperglycaemia can be caused by stress, steroids (ibid.) and parenteral nutrition. Blood glucose will need to be checked frequently, and so nurses should ensure that glucose monitors are nearby when preparing bed areas. The prescribed sliding scales of insulin should be followed.

Metabolic acidosis is caused by prolonged ischaemia.

Hypothermia from prolonged abdominal exposure during surgery is likely. Patients may be warmed with space blankets. Vasodilation accentuates hypotension.

Pain is surprisingly unproblematic, and patients often need relatively small doses of analgesic. However pain management should neither be forgotten nor trivialised.

Infection control is especially important (see Chapter 15), as immunosuppressant drugs and multiple invasive lines make patients particularly susceptible to infection.

Implications for practice

- immediate postoperative care requires careful planning of roles (e.g. identify staff who will help to provide infusion fluids) and equipment (ensure layout is safe and patients easily accessible)
- clarify from theatre staff what special infusions and equipment will be needed
- early hepatic hypofunction can be expected; this will affect all major systems; monitor homeostasis (vital signs, blood gases, electrolytes, blood sugar)

- postoperative infection usually occurs; minimising risk factors (e.g. early extubation) and controlling infection can reduce complication

Summary

Liver transplantation has enabled the survival of many patients who previously would have died. However, it is one of the most complex organs to transplant, and probably creates more complications than any other type of transplant surgery. Hence, postoperative nursing requires skill and expertise to avoid and minimise risks to each patient.

Further reading

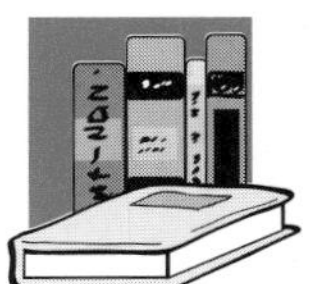

Hawker (1997b) is a comprehensive chapter covering issues of transplantation, while Heaton (1997) gives a paediatric perspective.

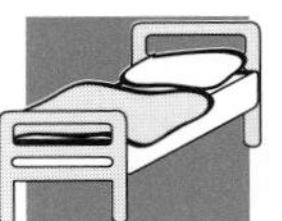

Clinical scenario

Catherine White is a 53-year-old with a diagnosis of chronic hepatic failure from primary biliary cirrhosis (PBC). She has a degree of portal hypertension from PBC and an increasing serum bilirubin above 200 µmol/l (normal range 5–17 µmol/l). Catherine was placed on the elective waiting list and had the appropriate preparation for a liver transplant. A compatible liver became available and she underwent a successful transplantation of donor liver.

Postoperatively, she is cared for in ICU. She has a large abdominal wound closed with skin staples and two wound drains (positioned right and left of the wound) to collect acetic fluid.

Q.1 An early complication of liver transplantation is haemorrhage.

(a) Describe nursing assessment for major haemorrhage with Catherine (e.g. monitored and non-monitored values, blood tests and normal values relevant to PBC, liver transplantation and associated coagulopathies.).

(b) List the priorities of care for treating such a major haemorrhage (e.g. type of volume replacement, route and rate of administration, potential complications from large blood transfusions, etc.).

Q.2 (a) Critically examine Catherine's post-operative pain management.

(b) Identify location, type and intensity of potential pain in liver transplantation.

(c) Analyse appropriate analgesics (specify drugs and format of administration), include non-pharmacological nursing interventions focused on minimising any perceived pain.

Q.3 To prevent graft rejection, Catherine is prescribed immunosuppression drugs. She has some understanding of this therapy from her pre-operative preparation, but asks for more information.

(a) Evaluate the advice the ICU nurse can give to Catherine on her drug therapy, including adverse effects and how these may be assessed.

(b) Propose other health promotion strategies which Catherine can implement to:

- Enhance acceptance of the donor liver (including psychological acceptance).
- Minimise tissue rejection and
- Strengthen her immune system against opportunist infections.

Part IV

Developing practice

Nursing exists in the context of society, healthcare and other professions. This section explores aspects of professional practice and career development: the first chapter considers what professional practice means in an ICU context; the second chapter looks at how nurses cope (or fail to cope), and how staff can help support their colleagues. Chapter 47 offers an introduction to complementary therapies, which in recent years have generated considerable interest in many areas of nursing practice. The next chapter suggests ways readers can develop practice on their own units; the penultimate chapter offers advice on managing their units, and the final chapter revisits the fundamental question of whether ICUs can be justified.

Chapter 45

Professionalism

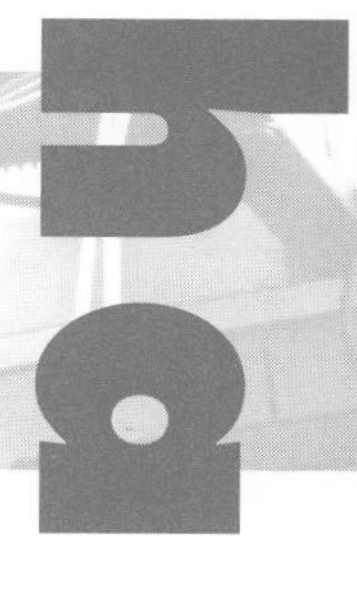

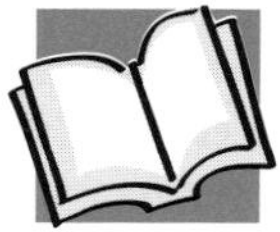

Contents

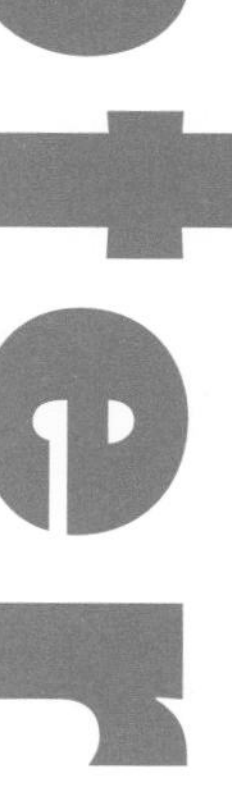

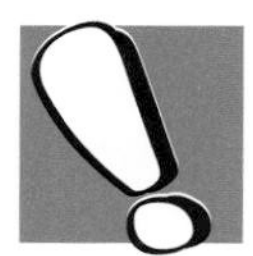

Fundamental knowledge

UKCC publications:

The Code of Professional Conduct for the Nurse, Midwife and Health Visitor
The Scope of Professional Practice
Guidelines for Professional Practice
Standards for the Administration of Medicines

Local hospital and unit policies, procedures and guidelines

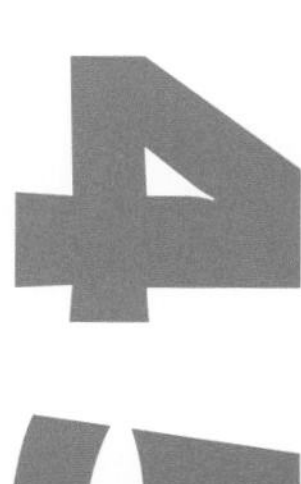

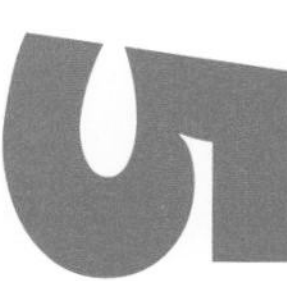

Introduction

As nursing has emerged from the shadows of medicine to claim its own professional autonomy, nurses have increasingly had to consider the problems, as well as benefits, of individual accountability. UKCC publications have both stimulated and reflected changes in professional practice. This chapter explores issues of what professional practice means, the accountability of nurses, and professional standards, in particular *The Scope of Professional Practice* (UKCC 1992b – hereafter referred to as 'SCOPE') and the civil law of negligence – issues affecting all registered nurses. This chapter uses general nursing texts; every nurse is accountable for their own practice (UKCC 1996), but ICU nursing often heightens problems due to the

- increased technology
- critical condition of patients
- differing roles of ICU nurses (see Chapter 1).

Enthusiasm to develop skills and knowledge has been rewarded by the positive inter-professional relationships of ICU staff. Nurses are often trusted to perform specialised tasks, but the enthusiasm to develop skills should be tempered by considerations of safety; professionalism includes accepting

- autonomy
- accountability
- responsibility.

Traditionally, nursing roles have been defined by other professions; SCOPE seeks to realign working boundaries in the best interests of patients. Ideally mistakes should never happen, but humans are fallible and mistakes will occur. Experience is needed to develop skills. Practice, and SCOPE, attempt to facilitate professional development while maintaining patient safety by emphasising the individual accountability of each nurse for their practice.

The references to civil and criminal law in this chapter cite texts such as Dimond (1995), to which most nurses (through libraries) should have access. At the time of writing (1999), the UKCC and national boards seem likely to be replaced; the UKCC is also considering revising *Standards for the Administration of Medicines* (UKCC 1992c); whatever changes occur in structure and documentation, the central principles of individual professional accountability are likely to remain.

Accountability

UKCC documents frequently refer to 'accountability', especially the *Code of Professional Conduct for the Nurse, Midwife and Health Visitor* (UKCC 1992a – hereafter referred to as 'CODE') and SCOPE (UKCC 1992b). The UKCC has consistently promoted nurse autonomy, but privileges of professional autonomy necessarily entail individual accountability for practice, as shown through evidence-based bedside nursing care.

Dimond (1995) identifies four arenas of professional accountability:

- criminal law
- civil law
- employer's contract
- professional body (UKCC)

adding that accountability between arenas may conflict.

For civil actions of *negligence* to succeed, three conditions must be met:

- a duty of care must exist
- that duty of care must have been breached
- resulting harm must have been reasonably foreseeable.

Civil cases failing to establish any one condition on the 'balance of probabilities' cannot make a conviction. The word 'negligence' used in different contexts, such as industrial tribunals or the UKCC's Professional Conduct Committee, need not carry these same conditions.

A *duty of care* clearly exists to patients allocated to nurses' care; there is, however, no legal requirement to be a 'good Samaritan' (Dimond 1995), so that legal duty of care to passers-by (e.g. in the street) is at best questionable (from legal perspectives). A breach of that care will usually be the basis of any case. Thus, any case reaching court almost certainly fulfils the first two criteria.

The third condition is the one least likely to be established. There are two parts to this third condition:

- breach of care must directly cause harm
- harm suffered must have been reasonably foreseeable.

If the *harm* may reasonably have been caused by other factors (judged by the balance of probabilities), links to breach of duty of care cannot be clearly established. For instance, the administering of large overdoses of penicillin is reprehensible, but *Kay* v. *Ayrshire and Arran Health Board* (1987) failed to establish that a child's deafness (harm) was caused by a penicillin overdose rather than meningitis (Dimond 1995), and the case was dismissed. Even where harm can be linked to breach of care, it may not be *reasonably foreseeable*: all drugs and treatments have adverse effects, and nurses should be aware of the common effects of whatever they give and the recorded allergies of patients, but they cannot reasonably know, or be held accountable for, every possible effect.

Nurses are primarily accountable to their patients (Pyne 1992), a view endorsed by the UKCC, most notably in Clause 1 of CODE (UKCC 1992a):

> A registered nurse … must:
>
> (1) act always in such a manner as to promote and safeguard the interests and wellbeing of patients and clients.

However, employers pay salaries; nurses failing to satisfy their employers' requirements may find themselves unemployed. Pragmatically, resisting the instructions of employers, managers or senior staff can prove difficult.

While all four of Dimond's arenas can apply to nurses, conflicts with criminal law are rare. Few laws specifically mention nurses or nursing, and so legal accountability and the rights of nurses are usually the same as for any other citizen. Any individual suffering harm from another may sue that person through civil law; negligence and assault with battery are the charges most frequently brought against healthcare staff. Negligence is briefly outlined later; assault is covered in Chapter 16; nursing accountability through civil law is comprehensively covered in Dimond (1995).

Employment contracts and expectations vary; breach of contract can lead to litigation, or more often dismissal. Although this chapter focuses on professional accountability (through the UKCC), readers should remember their concurrent accountability to other arenas.

- What are the limits of accountability?
- How can conflicts of accountability be reconciled?

Limits of accountability

Individual accountability and professional autonomy may seem desirable ideals, but quality healthcare also relies on multidisciplinary teamwork. Responsibility is inevitably partly shared between disciplines and members of the same discipline. The delegation of particular tasks varies between units, and may vary within each unit, depending on whoever is best able to perform that particular task at that time – endotracheal suction may be performed by anaesthetists intubating patients, and later by physiotherapists and nurses.

Each mentally competent adult remains legally accountable for their actions. Civil law precedent (*Nettleship* v. *Weston* 1971) establishes learner/student accountability, despite their inexperience or lack of knowledge (Dimond 1995). Learners and junior staff may be individually sued if they cause harm (hence the importance of professional indemnity). Both CODE and SCOPE emphasise that nurses must ensure their knowledge is current and adequate for practice (monitored through periodic re-registration). Evidence-based practice helps to identify aspects that are appropriate and those based on myth and ritual. Each nurse must individually decide whether (and, if so, how) they should perform tasks; following guidelines, although normally reliable, is no defence from individual professional accountability (Tingle 1997b).

Conflicts of accountability

Few tasks are ascribed by law to particular professions; even the traditional medical role of prescription is being eroded by nurses prescribing (as yet, not including ICU nurses). SCOPE (UKCC 1992b) removes traditional and rigid role demarcations, but some employers, responding to dangers created by this freedom, specify roles (e.g. whether nurses should change ventilator settings) and issue guidelines/protocols/standards for practice.

In civil law, the standards of care expected from qualified nurses are those of the ordinary skilled nurse ('Bolam test' (Brazier 1992)). Various UKCC documents establish these standards; many include 'standard' in their titles. Failure to meet professional standards may also cause removal from the professional register.

SCOPE was published when traditional professional boundaries were changing, partly in response to reduction in junior doctors' hours (Dowling *et al.* 1996). ICU nurses should cooperate with other members of multidisciplinary teams (UKCC 1992a), while maintaining their professional autonomy. If each person is accountable for their own actions, then patients' best interests are served by professional collaboration rather than power conflicts.

Attempts to restructure nursing has caused a proliferation of terms, such as advanced practice; terminology and appropriate educational development for practice have generated much debate but little consensus, and the UKCC has yet to clarify what advanced practice means (Fulbrook 1996b). Whatever terminology, educational structures and requirements are established, continuous professional development will remain integral to individual professional accountability.

Accountability in practice

DISPOSABLE EQUIPMENT Much equipment used in ICUs is disposable. Disposable equipment should not be reused (Medical Devices Agency 1995). Single-use items should be clearly identified by manufacturers (de Jong 1996); if disposable equipment is recycled, manufacturers' liability may be transferred to the recycler (e.g. individual nurses). Small savings through recycling disposable equipment may incur greater costs from healthcare litigation. Nurses should therefore follow manufacturers' instructions.

COMPLAINTS These are a familiar aspect of contemporary healthcare. They have unfortunately encouraged defensive nursing, but do highlight deficiencies in services provided, afford a conduit for public accountability, and may diffuse concerns that would otherwise end in litigation. Most complaints result from failures of communication; ironically, it is those least ill who often complain the most, so encouraging diversion of time away from those with the greatest need. Nurses have a professional duty to prioritise care (acts and omissions) so that actions can be justified.

LITIGATION UK healthcare litigation increased from £50m. in 1991 to £250m. in 1996 (Marian 1997); Tingle (1997b) suggests that healthcare litigation will increase by one-quarter each year for the next five years, diverting substantial funds from patient care to pay compensation. Minimising risks of litigation is effectively substantial income generation.

Personal costs of litigation can also be substantial: cases may take years to reach court; protracted (employer, UKCC) investigations until, and eventual stress from, the hearing, with possible loss of registration and/or loss of employment can cause significant financial, personal and professional hardship to nurses involved.

The scope of professional practice (UKCC 1992b)

Despite being much quoted, SCOPE is arguably the least understood and least practised of all major UKCC publications. Traditionally, preregistration training was assumed to prepare nurses for possible lifelong practice. Such stasis in nursing became increasingly inappropriate to modern, dynamic society: 'certification has tended to freeze and narrow the profession, has tied it to the past, has discouraged innovation' (Rogers 1980: 247).

The 1977 circular establishing 'extended roles' (DoH 1977; now withdrawn), enabled doctors to delegate tasks to nurses provided

- delegation was recognised by employers
- appropriate training was given
- competence was assessed and certified.

Few tasks are unique to specific professions (Wainwright 1994), especially in ICU. The 1977 criteria eventually proved cumbersome and restrictive, hindering the progress of intensive care and the delivery of patient care; nurses became increasingly competent to perform tasks which they were not allowed to carry out because they did not have appropriate pieces of paper (e.g. cardiac output studies). Often those allowed to perform these tasks (junior doctors) did not have the knowledge to do so, and learned under verbal instruction from nurses who did know how the task should be done, but were not allowed to do it. Such restrictive practices might leave cardiac output studies unmeasured (and so inotropes unaltered) between the doctor's last round at night and first round in the morning (possibly an eight-hour gap).

SCOPE reversed traditional approaches to the role of the nurse. Until 1992 nurses were expected to perform up to, but not beyond, their level of (formal) training. SCOPE recognised that nurses could develop roles to include aspects of care for which they did not necessarily hold certificates (e.g. changing ventilator settings). Rather than specify what each individual nurse could do through certification, SCOPE enables nurses to do what they are competent and confident to do; this places responsibility firmly on each nurse for their own actions.

SCOPE also stressed the centrality of holistic care, a welcome reversal of 1977 emphasis on tasks. SCOPE warned that nurses 'must ensure that any enlargement or adjustment of the scope of personal professional practice must be achieved without compromising or fragmenting existing aspects of professional practice and care' (UKCC 1992b). What aspects of care should be prioritised will differ between patients; SCOPE avoids giving examples of care, but performing 'glamorous' tasks at the expense of fundamental care contradicts the ethos of SCOPE.

SCOPE and the third edition of CODE appeared in the same month (June 1992). The interdependence of each is clarified within SCOPE, and by similarities of principles for practice with clauses of CODE. Both emphasise that each nurse must maintain their own knowledge, skill and competence, acknowledging any limitations. With CODE's first edition in 1983 nursing emerged as a profession; with SCOPE the profession reached maturity.

Implications for practice

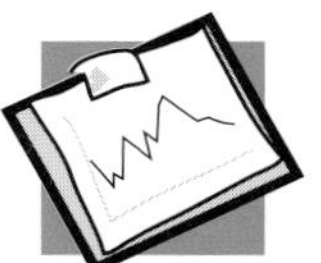

- each nurse remains individually accountable for their actions
- nursing care should be prioritised by patients' best interests
- all nurses have a responsibility to ensure that individually they have adequate and current knowledge for their practice
- each nurse should refuse any task they do not feel they can safely perform
- SCOPE provides the opportunity for nurses and nursing to respond nuickly to changing needs
- Nurses should be familiar with local policies/procedures/guidelines/standards

Summary

The demands of society and the pace of change are both likely to continue to increase. Nursing's professionalism, exemplified by SCOPE, enables nurses to meet changing needs. ICU nurses often respond positively to challenging and changing work, but enthusiasm should be tempered by considerations of safe practice, and how far care meets the holistic needs of each patient. The human and financial costs of professional malpractice can be high for each nurse, employer and patient.

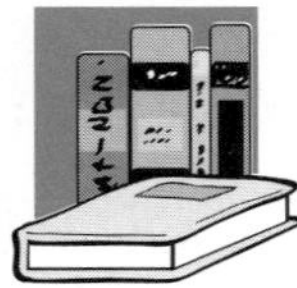

Further reading

Dimond (1995) remains the key text on the legal aspects of nursing, although Brazier's (1992) book on medicine and the law is also useful. Nurses should possess and read the core UKCC documents, such as CODE (UKCC 1992a) and SCOPE (UKCC 1992b). Most articles on SCOPE have been disappointing, although Land *et al.* (1996) offer a clear overview. Hunt and Wainwright's (1994) book is valuable reading. Much has been written on professionalism; Pyne's (1992) book offers valuable perspectives from an influential member of the UKCC. The RCN's (1994) standards for critical care provide a useful guide to support accountable, evidence-based practice, while de Jong (1996) provides a salutary warning against the false economies of recycling disposable equipment.

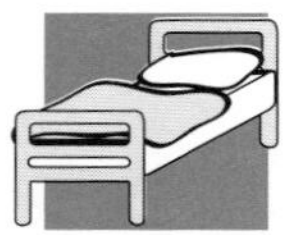

Clinical scenario

Q.1 Clarify your own understanding of accountability and responsibility within the ICU. Identify to whom you are accountable and the main areas of accountability in your practice.

Q.2 You are asked to administer a new trial drug yet to be licensed in the UK. The patient suffers associated adverse effects and dies. Who is accountable for the patient's death? Examine the extent of nurse accountability in this situation (re *The Scope of Professional Practice*, a nurse's knowledge of drug administration, awareness of adverse effects, appropriateness of drug, etc.).

Q.3 Reflect on the re-use of equipment designed to be 'single use only' or disposable in your ICU practice. How often are intravenous administration sets for blood transfusions used with more than one unit of blood and/or non-blood products (e.g. 5% dextrose)? Justify this practice with reference to physiology, patient safety, manufacturer's information, hospital or unit policy, established practices in your area.

Chapter 46

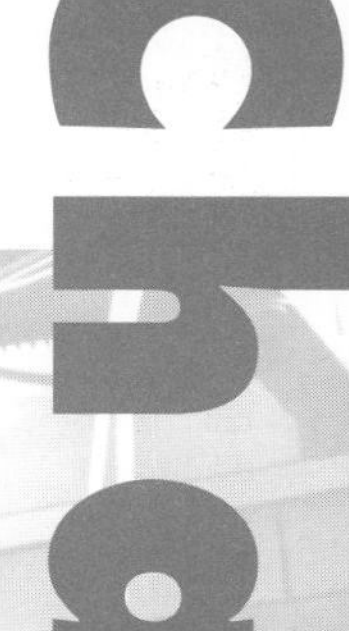

Stress management

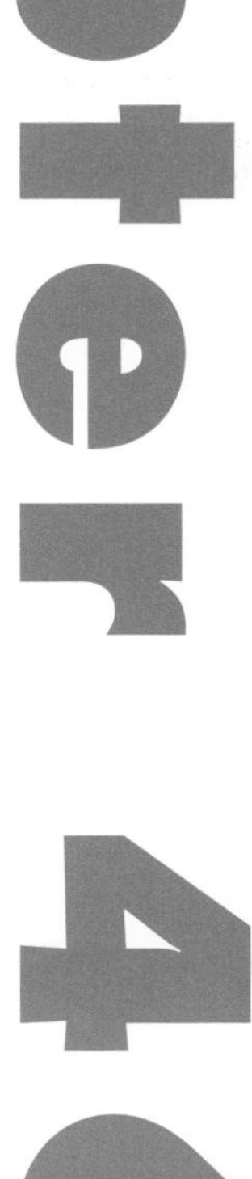

Contents

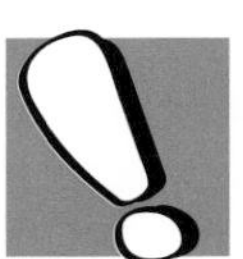

Fundamental knowledge

'Fight or flight' response – see Chapter 3

Introduction

Stress is a widely used word, but concepts of stress are often poorly defined. Physiological and psychological effects of stress on patients were discussed in Chapter 3. Stressors in ICU may affect patients, relatives and other staff; this chapter explores ways for nurses to recognise and cope with their own and colleagues' stress. Stress management, at all levels, is therefore fundamental to both good nursing and good health.

Although a popular topic, much literature on stress remains anecdotal, cathartic or dubious. Human responses to stress change little between generations, and so the literature dates less quickly than with most topics in this book; however, contexts of practice do change so that older literature should be placed within the context of changes in nursing practice. ICU nursing is often described as stressful, but as stress is a subjective response to stimuli, whether ICU nursing is more or less stressful than other fields is ultimately unquantifiable.

This chapter opens with a stark reminder of some of the extreme responses to stress, before describing and applying stress theory to help ICU nurses manage their own stress and support their colleagues.

Stress: a problem

Nurses experiencing distress work less efficiently, and are less able to support others; unresolved distress usually escalates. The Office of Population Census Surveys for 1979–1990 identified an average yearly suicide rate of 29 female nurses every year; this rate increased to 50 per year between 1990 and 1992 (Seymour 1995b). The highest level of female suicides in the UK is among nurses (Farrington 1997); even though nurses form the largest single group of working women, these statistics raise worrying questions, especially as suicide rates are higher among general nurses than among mental health nurses (Farrington 1997). While not all suicides necessarily result from work-related pressures, nurses need to look after themselves as well as others, and need staff support systems.

What is stress?

Stress is both a psychological and physical phenomenon. Physiological ('fight or flight') responses (e.g. hypertension, tachycardia, tachypnoea, hyperglycaemia) are identified in Chapter 3.

Psychological aspects of stress are less precise as stress is an individual subjective response, so that while stressors may be common, what one person finds stressful another person may enjoy (e.g. 'white knuckle rides').

'Stress' is popularly used to describe negative experiences, but it can be enjoyable and rewarding: the 'stress' of ICU nursing may make it more attractive to nurses than working in, say, out-patients. Selye (1976) identified two types of stress: 'eustress' and 'distress'. Eustress (*eu* = good) is stress that stimulates people to function more efficiently and enjoy life; 'distress' is a familiar concept. Eustress is not a problem and so is not pursued here.

Time out 1

- Identify what you find 'eustressful' and 'distressful' about ICU nursing.
- Share these ideas with a colleague, identifying differences between your responses to similar stressors.

Is ICU nursing stressful?

Because responses to stressors are individual, what is eustressful and distressful will vary between people; excessive exposure to *eu*-stimuli can become distressful. Most stressors for ICU nurses arise from patient care issues (Sawatzky 1996), so that although ICU nurses may find caring for critically ill patients rewarding (eustressful), the human cost of caring and empathy is high for ICU nurses (Rushton 1992), with overexposure and overwork potentially causing emotional exhaustion (Stechmiller & Yarandi 1993). Not surprisingly, the literature is variable about whether ICU is more stressful than other areas of nursing (Coombs 1991; Lloyd-Jones 1994), inevitably reflecting both the ethos and management of units where studies are undertaken, and the individual responses of different groups of staff.

Foxall *et al.* (1990) found that ICU nursing created similar levels of stress to hospice and medical nursing, but that stressors were different. Various researches have identified different stressors among ICU nurses.

Stechmiller and Yarandi (1993) identified six variables affecting stress levels for critical care nurses:

- (their own) family demands
- (their own) health difficulties
- supervision
- pay
- job security
- situational stress

Sawatzky (1996) found major (situational) stressors for ICU nurses were:

- unnecessary prolongation of patients' life
- perception that (medical or nursing) colleagues are incompetent
- inadequate knowledge/unfamiliar situations

while Lally and Pearce (1996) identified:

- death of patients
- perceived unnecessary prolongation of life
- inability to meet patients' needs
- overwhelming workload
- inadequate staffing

Stress is individual, and so varies between individual people and individual units.

Feeling powerless is a major stressor (Seligman 1975); ICU nurses may feel powerless because of

- patients
- relatives
- managers (Boeing & Mongera 1989)

Adonat and Killingworth (1994) found that organisation and management caused most ICU burn-out; Curry's (1995) small study found that ICU nurses felt inadequately prepared to cope with relatives' stress. Feeling inadequate is a stressor which is likely to increase inefficiency. If relatives perceive nurse-stress, their loss of confidence may accentuate their own stress levels (although Ramos's (1992) American study of general nurses suggested emotional involvement with patients provided potential support).

Exposure to, and feelings of inadequacy with, technology can be a major stressor for ICU nurses (although not identified widely in literature). Developing technical skills can obscure the human focus central to nursing (see Chapter 1); however nurses choose to develop their knowledge, they should ensure that they maintain and develop the interpersonal/human skills they already possess.

Time out 2

- What made you choose to work in ICU?
- Look at your own list from Time out 1; compare the eustress and distress lists to your experience of other areas of nursing.
- How do you hope to develop professionally over the next three months?

Stimulus-based model

Following the behaviourist philosophy (see Chapter 2), stressful stimuli would cause a response of stress. Therefore, reducing environmental stressors should reduce stress (Lloyd-Jones 1994). However, this approach fails to recognise the individuality of people and their stress responses (Lloyd-Jones 1994.).

Response-based model

This model focuses on internal responses: fear (stimulus) causes catecholamine-induced hypertension (response). Selye's *General Adaptive Syndrome* (1976) has three stages:

- alarm reaction
- resistance
- exhaustion.

Remembering simple but familiar stressful situations (e.g. cardiac arrest) can usefully illustrate these stages:

- *alarm reaction* is the initial transitory response to stressors, before mobilisation of compensatory mechanisms; individuals may experience 'freezing' or 'paralysis', functioning inefficiently
- *resistance* mobilises compensatory coping mechanisms, so that pituitary gland ACTH release initiates catecholamine release, which heightens awareness and ability for 'fight or flight'
- *exhaustion* follows when prolonged exposure to stressors overwhelms resistance; the length of time before reaching exhaustion varies between individuals and stressors.

The benefits from eustress are therefore limited by both time and intensity.

Transactional model

This theory largely combines the previous two: stress results from dynamic interaction between both stressors and individuals. Neuman's (1995) model of nursing develops this theory, suggesting that each person has variable lines of resistance to stressors. Stress is a mismatch between perceived demand and perceived ability to cope.

Therefore stress response has three aspects:

- source of stress
- mediators of stress
- manifestations of stress (Lloyd-Jones 1994).

Coping mechanisms

Exposure to stress initiates various coping mechanisms (responses). The fight and flight response is a simple physiological response, but there are more complex cognitive responses. When something causes distress we can try and change either the stressor or ourselves. These coping mechanisms may be positive or negative/palliative, so that attempts to escape reality (changing ourselves) with drugs (e.g. alcohol) seldom resolve the initial (external) problems. However, taking antidepressants (again, changing ourselves) can be a positive coping mechanism, the problem (depression) being internal.

Palliative coping mechanisms include:

- denial
- smoking
- excessive drinking
- excessive overeating.

Significantly, many of these are physically harmful. Similar palliative coping mechanisms encourage ICU nurses to control and limit communication with their patients (Leathart 1994). However, when stressors cannot be altered (e.g. bereavement), attempts to change oneself (without self-harm) can become positive.

Positive coping mechanisms attempt to change stressors, which may require finding out further information about them, just as preoperative information can reduce postoperative pain (Hayward 1975). Positive coping mechanisms include:

- catharsis (e.g. discussions with colleagues during breaks)
- emotional discharge (crying, exercises, meditation, massage, guided fantasy).

Permitting and enabling people to express and release their stress may be more beneficial than trying to offer advice (cf. Rogerian counselling, see Rogers 1951, 1967).

Recognising stress

Recognising distress in others is often relatively easy, but recognising signs of stress in ourselves can be harder. The stressors may be common to all, but their responses (types of stress) differ from person to person; in order to recognise stress, therefore, we must recognise how each stressor affects each person by trying to understand experiences from their viewpoint (i.e. empathy).

Unrecognised distress can progress, causing multiple problems, such as staff conflict, absenteeism, low morale, inefficient/poor work and (eventually) burn-out (Stechmiller & Yarandi 1993). Problems usually prove increasingly difficult to resolve, possibly causing potentially valuable staff to leave the unit and even, perhaps, nursing.

Tyler and Ellison's (1994) recommendation that nurses should attend stress management study days could be extended to other self-awareness courses, such as time management. Enabling staff to recognise their own (and others') stress can help to limit crises.

Burn-out, ultimate failure of coping mechanisms, causes:

- decreased energy
- decreased self-esteem
- output exceeding input
- a sense of hopelessness and helplessness
- the inability to perceive alternative ways of functioning
- cynicism
- negativism
- feelings of self-depletion

(Farrington 1997)

When burn-out is reached, work becomes hard, unrewarding and of poor quality. Burn-out is a form of mental ill-health, potentially ending in suicide (see the opening of this chapter).

Positive/negative thinking

Blaming others (e.g. management) for our stress is easy, but over simplistic. Everyone should recognise their own areas for development. Being stressed is not a personal failure; recognising and acknowledging our own stress helps us to resolve it.

Stress and response to stress are complex effects, which are often not helped by over-simplistic behavioural explanations. As most ICU staff leave because of career development and grading (Gibson 1994), staff resignations do not necessarily indicate distressful working environments.

Humanistic stress management seeks to identify the motivation underlying apparent behaviour. This necessitates discussion, but to be effective neither person should feel threatened by the other. Anyone seeking to help distressed colleagues should adopt Rogers' (1967) 'unconditional positive regard', respecting the person for whom they are and what they are. Recognising the rights of both yourself and others is fundamental to assertiveness: everyone has the (moral) right to disagree with others and openly state disagreement, but not to deny others the right to their own opinion. By respecting others it becomes easier both to respect oneself (self-esteem) and be respected by others; self-esteem and the esteem of others form the penultimate level of Maslow's hierarchy of needs (Maslow 1987 [1954]). Positive thinking about ourselves helps us to believe that we can (and should) change harmful stressors rather than change (harm) ourselves.

Type A and type B personalities

Much of the early literature on stress identifies two types of personalities: type A and type B.

Type A describes active, competitive, potentially aggressive people, highly stressed but also seeking out stress (Rentoul *et al.* 1995). Type B is placid, with the opposite characteristics. Traditional links between the type A personality and coronary disease have been questioned by more recent studies, and Case *et al.* (1985) found no link between type A behaviour and the mortality or progression of cardiac disease. However, these over-simplistic stereotypes, more appropriate to behaviourist approaches than humanist, are still being used.

Time management

Lack of time is often a major stressor: managing our time effectively reduces stress, especially when under pressure. Work, pleasure (recreation) and rest (restoration/sleep) should be balanced; watching television is a positive pastime if enjoyed (recreation), but a negative one if the viewer simply cannot be bothered to do something else. Many nurses are good at giving, but weaker at receiving. Effective time management enables nurses to work well while enjoying a full social life.

Time out 3

Think back over the past week; note down how you have spent your time, for example:

What are my overall feelings about the past week?
How much time did I spend on things I enjoy?
How much of my time has been taken up on things I do not enjoy?
How much time have I wasted, and in what ways?
Are there things which I had hoped to achieve which did not get done?
What can I learn from this for next week?

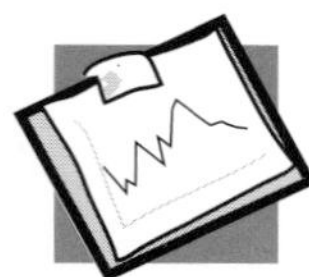

Implications for practice

- stress in an individual reaction to stressors (stimuli)
- externalisation (blaming others) is oversimplistic; recognising our areas for development (while acknowledging our strengths) enables us to grow as individuals
- stress can be beneficial (eustress), but exposure to intense or prolonged stimuli is likely to cause distress
- nurses are best able to promote the health of others if they are healthy themselves
- nurses often receive insufficient support to cope with their stressful jobs
- insufficient support is a major stressor for many ICU nurses
- recognising signs of stress, whether in ourselves, colleagues, patients or their families, is necessary to proactively resolve distress

- support can be improved through structures such as clinical supervision and regular constructive feedback
- active teamwork, rather than relying on top-down managerial direction, can support staff at all levels
- assertion skills and non-judgemental acceptance enable those helping others to resolve their own stress
- the knowledge needed for confident, safe ICU practice is greater than in many areas of nursing, and needs support and development through orientation and continuing staff development programmes
- optimising time management reduces stressors

Summary

The debate about how stressful ICU nursing is likely to continue, but constructive stress management necessitates a more analytical approach. The absence of all stress is not desirable, but achieving eustress without distress can be difficult. Stress is a complex individual reaction to stressors, with both physiological and psychological manifestations. When stressors exceed individual coping abilities, whether through prolonged exposure to, or intensity of, stressors, distressed begins; unresolved distress may progress to burn-out. Therefore, recognising the signs of stress in ourselves and others is a necessary foundation for managing distress. Coping mechanisms may be negative (attempting to alter oneself, which is usually harmful) or positive (attempting to alter stressors).

Further reading

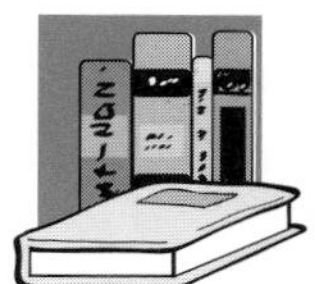

Lloyd-Jones (1994) offers a comprehensive review of stress, applied to ICU nursing. Farrington (1997) provides constructive ways to recognise and manage stress from a wider nursing perspective. Selye's classic work on stress is simply presented in his 1976 book. Of the many popular books on assertion, Harris (1970) provides a simple self-help text while Dickson (1982) is especially thought provoking.

Clinical scenario

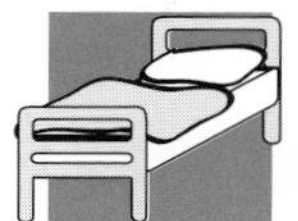

Q.1 From your personal experience as a nurse on ICU:

(a) List causes of your own work-related stress.
(b) Rank these in order of greatest to least stressful, e.g. interpersonal conflicts (specify with whom, doctors, colleagues, family, etc.), communication, emergency situations, death and

dying, workload, shift patterns, study, uncertainty/unfamiliar situation, decision making, lack of experience and skill, job satisfaction/dissatisfaction.

Q.2 Identify which patients you find most stressful to nurse on ICU and analyse why they cause you stress.

Q.3 Evaluate how you would identify and manage signs of stress or burn-out in yourself and others. Specify:

(a) behaviours (adaptive/maladaptive), emotions (positive/negative) and thoughts
(b) verbal comments
(c) typical coping mechanisms (effective/ineffective, beneficial/harmful).

Chapter 47

Complementary therapies

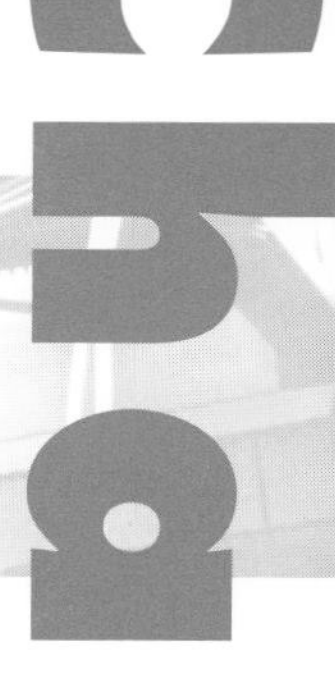

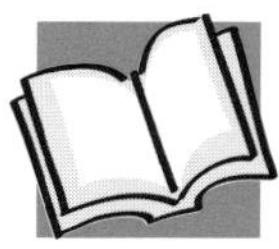

Contents

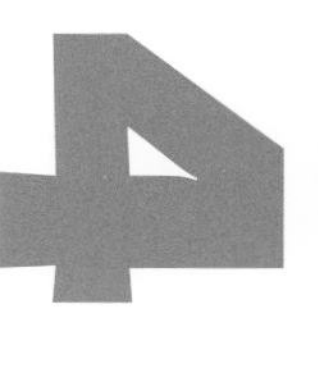

Introduction

The recent growth of interest in complementary therapies is reflected in their increasing use in nursing and healthcare. The literature varies between introductory and anecdotal texts to substantive studies. This chapter is intended to raise awareness about complementary therapies, their underlying beliefs, and specialist application to ICU nursing. Like any other beliefs, these may (and should) be questioned.

In 1993 the British Medical Association estimated that there were 180 different types of complementary therapy practised in the UK (Byrne 1995); a small sample of these are included here. The placebo effect is also discussed, before concluding with practical application and professional perspectives.

Although discussed under separate headings, the use of various complementary therapies may be mixed, just as orthodox medicine may use combination therapy; thus essential oils may be used for massage, with benefits potentially being gained from both the massage and the oil itself. While research studies need to specify causal relationships, for clinical practice the end results to patients is (from utilitarian perspectives) more important than precisely how results are achieved.

Concepts and terminology

The term 'complementary therapy' is increasingly replacing 'alternative therapy'. 'Complementary' suggests additional to standard medical treatments, whereas 'alternative' implies a conflict, necessitating a choice between them. Both supporters and opponents of complementary therapies have used 'alternative', usually to try and devalue the other approach. This text follows Rankin-Box (1988) in using the term 'complementary' rather than 'alternative'.

Many complementary therapies are derived from traditional Chinese medicine, and conflicts can occur from the differing cultural contexts and translation. Yin and Yang, which are popularly and often over-simplistically assimilated into Western culture, involve balances between the various kinds of energy necessary for health (Downey 1995) – this carries similar connotations to orthodox medicine's concept of 'homeostasis'.

In Chinese medicine, Ki (Qi or Chi), the universal energy which links people to their environment, is dispersed through twelve main channels (meridians) that connect the internal organs to the skin (Downey 1995). Manipulation of the skin (e.g. acupuncture) therefore affects organs along the same meridian.

Orthodox medicine

Many complementary therapies are very old; reflexology is depicted in pyramids of *c.* 2300 BC (Griffiths 1995). Since knowledge of the therapies has been mainly transmitted through oral traditions and folklore, the lack of regulation led some practices into disrepute, while the Cartesian focus on atoms largely replaced European folklore medicine with an 'orthodox' (and increasingly regulated) medical profession. Orthodox medicine has adopted some of the tried and tested remedies, such as foxglove (digitalis – digoxin) for dropsy (oedema) and willow bark (aspirin) for analgesia, so that, refined and analysed, 'orthodox medicine' has preserved elements of herbal medicine.

Orthodox medicine's pursuit of diagnosing anatomically specific problems led to targeting specific problems with specific drugs (e.g. antibiotics target specific bacteria). Complementary therapies focus attention on the whole person, and recognise the complex interactions contributing to disease (literally, dis-ease). Such holistic and humanist perspectives make complementary therapies attractive to many nurses; the absence of regulation (compared with orthodox medicine) enables nurses to initiate complementary therapies. The resurgence of interest in complementary therapies therefore parallels the growth of the nursing profession's autonomy and advocacy of therapeutic nursing.

Until recently, the knowledge bases of most complementary therapies was largely limited to anecdotes and unsupported assertions. However, the recent growth in demand for, and availability of, complementary therapists has encouraged some substantive studies, although research bases vary widely between therapies (Stevensen 1997), and ICU studies are complicated by the physiological crises with which most patients are admitted (Dunn *et al.* 1995).

Complementary therapies are often sought when orthodox medicine fails to resolve chronic problems, although some people seek interventions purely for pleasure (e.g. massage). Any complementary therapies used in ICUs must co-exist with orthodox medicine, but providing pleasure (rather than 'cure') is a legitimate nursing end.

Therapeutic touch

This intervention, conceptualised into nursing by Krieger (1975), develops the traditional laying-on of hands, and is included here mainly because its name can create confusion. Neither the laying-on of hands nor Krieger's Therapeutic Touch involve skin-to-skin contact. Building on Martha Rogers' philosophy that humans are made up of energy, and that humans and their environments are continuously, simultaneously and mutually exchanging energy with each other (Sayre-Adams 1994), Therapeutic Touch attempts to touch the energy or force field of the person.

Any intervention that increases qualitative staff–patient interaction is potentially beneficial. Cox and Hayes (1998) report using Therapeutic Touch in ICUs, although Rossa *et al.*'s (1998) study of 21 experienced Therapeutic Touch practitioners who were blindfolded found that they were unable to identify peoples' force fields. Whatever merits Therapeutic Touch may or may not have, its name is unfortunate. Qualitative touch (skin-to-skin contact) is much underused by nurses, and can significantly reduce sensory imbalance (see Chapter 3): touch can be therapeutic. Labelling Krieger's intervention 'Therapeutic Touch' may imply that other nursing touch is not therapeutic – an erroneous presumption. Therefore, when discussing therapeutic touch nurses should clarify whether they mean it in Krieger's sense or in the broader humane sense. This text uses the broader meaning.

Massage

Massage, which has been defined by Feltham as a 'systematic form of touch using certain manipulations of soft tissue of the body to promote comfort and healing' (1991: 27), is one of the most widely practised complementary therapies in nursing, with a reasonable body of research (some significant studies being undertaken in ICUs).

Nursing without touch is a contradiction, but where ordinary touch becomes massage is unclear: washing patients arguably fulfils Feltham's definition. Where guidelines and professional practice limit the use of massage, nurses should defend the value of touch (especially qualitative).

Nineteenth century attempts to regulate masseurs (many with nursing backgrounds) within medicine eventually led to the Chartered Society of Physiotherapists, so that dilemmas of professional boundaries with massage are not new.

Dunn *et al.* (1995) compared the use of simple massage (15–30 minutes) with aromatherapy massage (1 per cent lavender oil – relaxing, hypotoxic, hypoallergenic) against rest periods. Although physiological differences were insignificant, patients receiving aromatherapy described feeling better and less anxious. Hill (1993) justifiably questions how critically ill these patients were (over three-quarters could report effects), but such benefits on less critically ill patients are presumably transferable to those more sick. If nursing itself is therapeutic (person-to-person interaction, 'presence') then Dunn's use of a number of nurses to measure the effects of specific interventions (e.g. massage) introduces variables of personalities between different nurses.

Stevensen (1992) used twenty-minute foot massage on patients following cardiac surgery, both with and without neroli oil (relaxant). Other than relaxing respiratory rates, no physiological benefits were observed, but, when interviewed five days later, patients who had received the neroli oil massage reported psychological benefits. Ai *et al.* (1997) similarly report better psychological recovery following cardiac surgery when complementary therapies were used.

These studies suggest that massage may give psychological benefits to ICU patients, although some may result from sexual misinterpretations of female nurses performing massage on male patients (Hill 1993). Likely (but unproven) physiological benefits include improved lymphatic drainage, returning plasma proteins to the circulation. However, even this most widely used complementary therapy has not yet become established practice in ICU nursing.

Reflexology

Although there are ancient precedents, modern Western reflexology derives from the work of William Fitzgerald, a nineteenth-century doctor who accidentally found that the use of pressure could replace anaesthesia during minor operations (Griffiths 1995). Fitzgerald believed that organ malfunction resulted in tiny crystalline deposits of calcium and uric acid on the nerve endings of the feet, and that breaking down these deposits with massage would heal the organ (Griffiths 1995). Fitzgerald identified ten energy zones of life-force running longitudinally through the body (not too dissimilar to the twelve meridians of Ki), reflecting the organs in specific parts of the feet (and hands). Reflexologists can therefore treat any part of the body using specialised foot massage that breaks down the crystalline deposits. If reflexology's assumptions are correct, it is possible that nurses manipulating feet and hands (e.g. bed baths, passive exercises) could inadvertently cause undesired effects.

Griffiths (1995) warns that reflexology initiates a 'healing crisis' which can last up to 24 hours, although this is less likely to occur with the gentler Western approaches than the more vigorous approaches used in the East. The absence of any reported complications suggests this may not be an actual problem, but it leaves a (currently) unanswered question.

Anecdotal reports of the sedation grip (a form of acupressure) helping hospital patients to sleep suggests that this could be applied in ICUs in order to support (not replace) chemical sedation, and so merits further study.

Shiatsu

Although derived from the Japanese for 'finger pressure', Shiatsu practice has gained wider connotations; it usually treats the whole meridian system (of vital energy/life force) in order to harmonise Ki (Stevensen 1995). Like other variants of massage, shiatsu is best left to those with specialist knowledge. However, one popular application, sea bands, which has been used to reduce postoperative nausea (Phillips & Gill 1993), has possible application to ICU.

Aromatherapy

Aromatherapy implies the use of essential oils with direct chemical effects, not just burning something which emits pleasant smells (although boundaries between pleasure and therapy can become blurred when evaluating psychological benefit): burning neroli (see Massage above) can reduce anxiety. As active chemicals, essential oils can be considered to be drugs, albeit not restricted by regulations governing traditional medicines.

Because of the nature of this therapy, the effects of aromatherapy may affect anyone (staff, other patients) in the immediate environment, so although relaxation may help some patients, it could be harmful to others, while possibly reducing staff efficiency. Aromatherapy sessions in ICUs should therefore normally be limited to patients in single cubicles.

Placebo effect

Throughout history significant minorities of people have benefited from inactive medicines (placebos); Hippocrates was familiar with the problems of patients who had been given unhelpful (and often harmful) treatments. Complex interactions between human physiology and psychology can make it difficult to ascribe a particular effect to a particular cause. When evaluating any treatment (complementary or orthodox), placebo, rather than active components, can benefit 35–52 per cent of patients (French 1989). Double-blind trials are designed to identify the extent of placebo effects, thus measuring whether any significant further benefit is gained from active ingredients. However, the value of quantitative research methodology for qualitative interventions is questionable.

With their focus on the health of the whole person, rather than dysfunction of single organs, complementary therapist–client time typically exceeds the amount of time doctors can afford to spend with the majority of their patients. Thus, the benefits claimed for complementary therapies may result from prolonged human interaction rather than from active treatment. Similarly, the twenty-minute massages mentioned above far exceed the normal length of qualitative touch between ICU nurses and their patients. If nursing and touch are in themselves therapeutic, then benefits from many complementary therapies may be largely or solely due to nursing touch, rather than specific interventions. Thus, since Dunn *et al.*'s (1995) control group received only rest periods and were actually denied human touch, they might be expected to fare worse.

If the desired end effect of nursing is the comfort (in its widest sense) of patients and relatives, then utilitarian ethics can justify whatever means are used to gain that end. Placebos can therefore be justified ethically. However, deliberate misinformation (such as injecting water instead of analgesia) breaks duty-based codes, and is (at best) ethically dubious. Placebo use has been (largely anecdotally) condemned in the American nursing press; UK nursing has been disappointingly reticent about debating this issue. Professionalism makes all nurses accountable to their patients for their actions. Nurses should therefore know what they are giving, the likely effects and, ideally, follow informed consent from their patients. While placebos can produce significant beneficial effects, their use raises many ethical problems.

Nursing traditionally values 'doing'; complementary therapies provide sets of actions, which may provide nurses with a sense of achievement (placebo) regardless of actual patient benefit. Anecdotally, many complementary therapies appear beneficial, but they need to be rigorously and objectively tested against placebo effects.

Professional perspectives

The *Guidelines for Professional Practice* (UKCC 1996) stress individual accountability for all nursing actions, including the use of complementary therapies. If, as their proponents claim, complementary therapies are directly beneficial, then like any other drug or therapy, their use should be a team decision (UKCC 1996). Some complementary therapies rely on active chemicals (endogenous or exogenous), so that the effects of interactions with other therapeutic drugs should be discussed. Homeopathic and herbal medicines are subject to the Medicines Act of 1968 (UKCC 1992c), but most essential oils are outside the scope of legislation. Nevertheless, nurses should consider them as drugs, using them in accordance with the *Standards for the Administration of Medicines* (UKCC 1992c) and other professional requirements.

Most complementary therapies require the dedication of significant periods of time. If sufficient time cannot be allocated, it may be irresponsible to begin interventions that (knowingly) will not be completed. While complementary therapists can focus solely on their intervention, ICU nurses have multiple responsibilities to their patients. Nurses intending to practise complementary therapies should therefore ensure that they have sufficient time to complete their intervention.

Interest in complementary therapies has created some (as yet) unresolved questions for nursing, such as:

- What is treatment?
- Where does human touch end and therapeutic touch begin?
- How therapeutic is presence without direct skin touch?
- What is a massage? What is a wash?

Those interested in practising complementary modes are strongly advised to pursue their interests through specialist study; as is the case with most orthodox therapies, some of the effects of complementary therapies can be harmful. Those not wishing to practise therapies themselves should be aware of any options which colleagues or other professionals may be able to offer, and are advised to use any reasonable opportunity to experience for themselves available therapies.

Cautions/contraindications

Responsible practitioners of most complementary therapies have faced hostility from (among others) traditional medicine. Without definitive evidence, therefore, most reputable therapists apply therapies cautiously, creating extensive lists of contraindications and cautions for most therapies. While experienced practitioners may be prepared to treat patients in 'caution' groups, less experienced users are advised to avoid treating such patients (Rankin-Box 1988), both for the patients' safety and their own (for example, indemnity claims). Cautions would include most ICU patients (e.g. cautions for shiatsu should include AIDS, contagious diseases, operation sites, cardiac disease and high fever (Stevensen 1995)), so that while ICU nurses can benefit from insights into complementary therapies, 'dabbling' with interventions can be dangerous.

Dangers

The popularity of complementary therapies has encouraged the introduction of some unscrupulous products (these are usually very dilute, and so ineffective). Most of the cheaper products have little value, although high prices do not necessarily guarantee quality. The use of ineffective products can easily discredit the potentially worthwhile interventions.

The lack of regulation creates variable preparation for complementary therapy practice, ranging from 'how-to' books and single study days to degree and postgraduate courses. Selection can create dilemmas, the vested self-interests of writers and researchers sometimes decrying other, potentially valuable, approaches. As with any other aspect of their work, nurses should be constructively critical, remembering their individual professional accountability. Interest groups (e.g. RCN Complementary Therapies Specialist Interest Group) can offer valuable information; addresses for individual therapies can often be found in texts about that particular therapy.

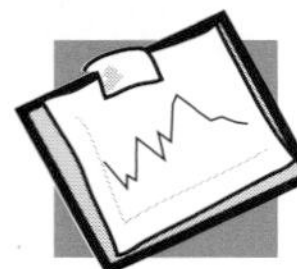

Implications for practice

- there is some (albeit limited) evidence of benefits from using some complementary therapies in ICU
- the proven knowledge-base for most complementary therapies is small
- complementary therapies may create undesired side-effects
- each nurse remains individually accountable for their own actions
- complementary therapies should therefore be practised by experienced therapists, or under their supervision
- aspects of some therapies (sedation grip; 'sea bands') have especial potential benefit in ICUs and merit further specialist study

Summary

The enthusiasm for complementary therapies in several areas of practice has helped many patients, but enthusiasm can exceed safe practice. This chapter offers insights into specialist application of some of the more widely used interventions, identifying some problems and professional issues surrounding the use of complementary therapies. Research into ICU application is most valuable when it is undertaken by, or in collaboration with, ICU nurses. Those wishing to practice complementary therapies, or use them themselves, should ensure a safe knowledge-base for practice, evaluating risks against benefits. The likely future regulation of complementary therapies may help to ensure their creditable practice and encourage a more reliable knowledge base.

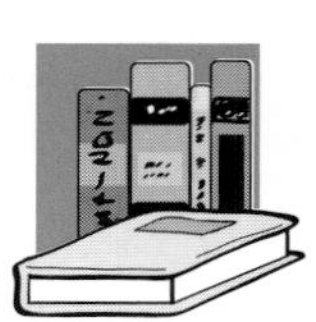

Further reading

There are many texts on the various complementary therapies, most written with much enthusiasm, although some with more bias than objectivity; Rossa *et al.* (1998) provides a useful balance. Rankin-Box has been instrumental in raising awareness of complementary therapies among UK nurses; her 1995 book summarises various interventions, giving useful addresses for each. The *Nursing Times* 1993 series of articles (since collected together in book form) also outlines many therapies.

Dunn *et al.* (1995) and any of Stevensen's articles (especially 1994) valuably describe ICU research studies, while Hill (1993) gives a useful review of ICU application. The journal *Complementary Therapies in Nursing and Midwifery* includes many useful articles.

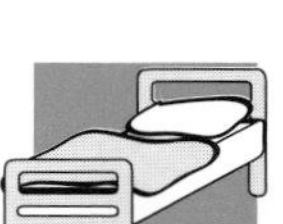

Clinical scenario

Duncan Munro, who is 46 years old, has been diagnosed with Guillain Barré Syndrome (GBS). He has been on ICU for two weeks and receives invasive ventilation via tracheostomy. He has become increasingly withdrawn and depressed, has difficulty sleeping and discomfort from paraesthesia in lower limbs.

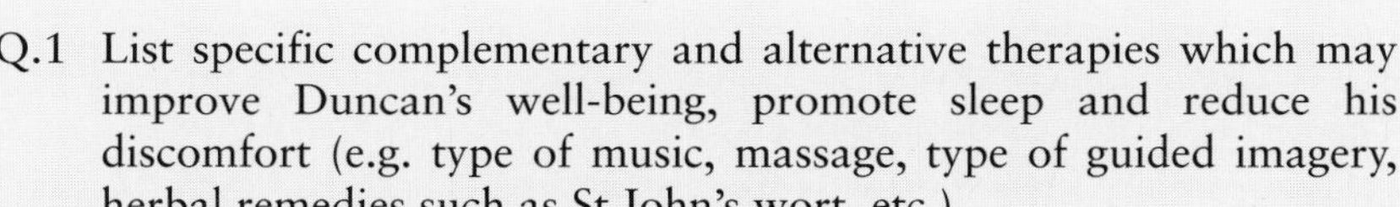

Q.1 List specific complementary and alternative therapies which may improve Duncan's well-being, promote sleep and reduce his discomfort (e.g. type of music, massage, type of guided imagery, herbal remedies such as St John's wort, etc.).

Q.2 Analyse the application of complementary therapies in ICU. From the list generated in Q.1, explain the therapeutic effects of each approach and how potential adverse effects and interactions are identified.

Q.3 Reflect on professional and/or role conflicts when using complementary therapies with ICU patients (consider accountability issues, effect on others, use of resources, skills and nursing time).

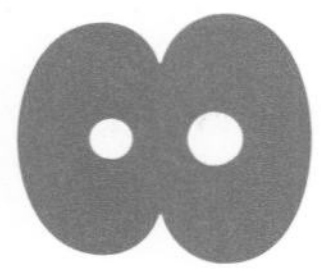
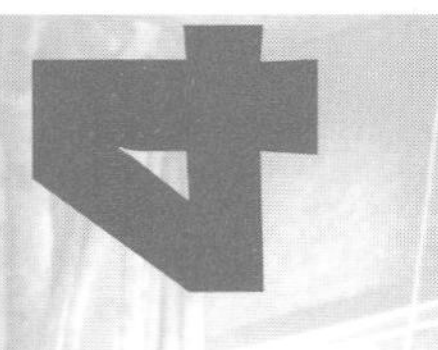
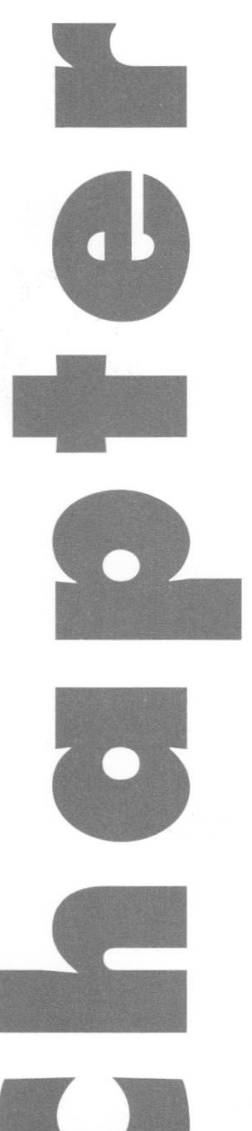

Chapter 48

Managing change

Contents

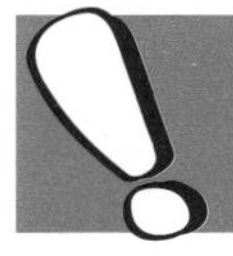

Fundamental knowledge

Individual Performance Review (IPR)
Management structure of the unit where you work

Introduction

Toffler (1970) suggested at that time that recent acceleration in the pace of change was likely to increase, so that change, rather than stability, would become the norm. In the thirty years since Toffler's work the pace of change has accelerated and the health service has seen frequent and major changes; since nursing and ICUs are part of wider political arenas, ICU nurses can be passively swept along by whatever changes occur (reactive), or actively try to control and manage change (proactive). Proactive management enables nurses to promote nursing values.

Nursing values may conflict with norms and values of other groups, and changes are not always successful, but planning helps achieve success. This chapter introduces change theory to help readers become change agents.

Asking basic questions helps to clarify issues and motives, and so this chapter adopts a what?-why?-how?-when? structure; such questions can help readers to develop their own plans of action. The initial time-out exercise can help readers to become proactive change agents.

Time out 1

Take a few minutes to jot down changes you have seen since you started working in ICU. Include changes on your own unit, within the hospital, and wider changes in healthcare.

Now identify a change you would like to see in your own workplace. As you read through this chapter, note down, section by section, how you would plan to bring this change about. After reading this chapter, you may have a workable plan which you can discuss with senior staff on your unit.

What?

Change for change's sake has few, if any, benefits. The requirements by managers and courses for introducing change have created some negative structures and outcomes; change should grow from convictions that it is needed. Ideas may be gained from courses, study days, reading, discussions with others, experience elsewhere, or (sometimes) out of the blue. Be clear about what you want to change (the exercise above should have crystallised your ideas).

Why?

Change may be prompted by internal or external stimuli. Internal stimuli are uncomfortable feelings that something can be improved. Internal stimuli depend on the motivation, ambition and values of the staff involved. Their success depends on the knowledge base they have or develop.

External stimuli may range from requirements by employers and demands by patients and purchasers to the requirements of professional bodies (UKCC) and government (Department of Health), and so performance indicators, IPR, quality control, patient satisfaction surveys, periodic re-registration, litigation and law may all cause change.

Rationales for change probably precede the identification of the precise nature of changes. Having clarified what you intend to do, reconsider your initial motivation, identifying the existing problems and benefits of suggested changes. Changes without clear benefits may not be worth the effort and trauma of introducing them.

Who?

Everyone is a potential change agent, capable of initiating, and possibly leading, change. Top-down change agents may be members of staff or outsiders; with bottom-up approaches, change agents are necessarily team members. Outsiders are usually authoritarian, although action research (Webb 1989), which has proved popular within nursing, helps people to reflect on and understand change better, and so aids the establishment of a change in practice (Pryjmachuk 1996). Outsiders need to establish either authority (power-coercive) or credibility (rational–empirical); insiders are usually already accepted group members.

Ketefian (1978) suggested that change agents should:

- diagnose need
- identify and clarify issues
- develop strategies and tactics
- establish and maintain working relationships with staff

This model recalls the nursing process, but usefully emphasises that interpersonal relationships are as important as the plan itself. Possible strategies include

- feedback
- education
- standards/guidelines/quality control

Ethical approval may be needed, especially if patients are involved in any research. Unit managers can advise on whether, and how, to obtain approval.

How?

Structured change management requires leadership from change agents. Wright (1998) suggests that most literature on leadership derives from sociology, industry or politics, but if nursing really is unique (as it is often claimed) it may need to develop its own unique management models. However, Surman and Wright (1998) follow most nursing literature in citing Bennis *et al.*'s three approaches:

- power coercive
- rational–empirical
- normative re-educative

Power-coercive approaches will be familiar to many: managers, from positions of power, make decisions, telling juniors to obey. Orders should be followed because managers are senior (coercive); no further reason is required, and discussion is usually discouraged.

Power-coercion is hierarchical, top-down, autocratic (Keyzer & Wright 1998), achieving strong, cost-effective leadership. Junior staff may not agree with the ideas, but know what those ideas are; change occurs quickly, and the power-base for decision-making is clear. National management of healthcare often adopts power-coercion, whether by government (Department of Health) or professional bodies.

Benner's (1984) novice may be more comfortable with clear power-coercive leadership; more advanced practitioners usually find power-coercion increasingly oppressive, with their own ideas and initiatives being cramped by others. Power coercion is grounded in behaviourism (see Chapter 2), with outward behaviours (action) being valued more than the inner feelings of individuals.

Rational–empirical management is also top-down (Keyzer & Wright 1998), but it invests power through knowledge rather than through appointed rank. Rational–empiricism assumes people are guided by reason, so that change agents only have to present rationales and others will follow (Keyzer & Wright 1998); motivation by self-interest was famously advocated by Hobbes (1962 [1651]).

Rational–empirical philosophy underlies:

health promotion (benefits from healthier lifestyles are described)
guidelines (where rationales are given)
audit

Unlike power coercion, rational–empirical philosophy respects individuals. However, people are not always logical (Sheehan 1990), and often continue with unhealthy lifestyles (e.g. smoking) despite knowledge. Thus, if people are irrational, those managing change should plan for irrationality.

Rogers (1951) suggests imposed structures are ineffective, relying on authority (and so presence) of whoever is in power. Once power-holders are away or leave, staff may ignore whatever they disagree with (while the cat's away, the mice play). Top-down change creates a 'shifting sand' effect: deep, quickly made impressions disappear with the next tide (Wright 1998).

Wright (1998) therefore argues that team ownership of change ('bottom-up' management) is essential for changes to survive. Unlike top-down approaches, *normative re-educative* change relies on normative cultures (majority rule) to reach decisions (Keyzer & Wright 1998). Ideally this would involve all staff (Keyzer & Wright 1998), although in practice shift work often prevents this; some staff may not wish to participate. Normative re-education relies on informed decisions of all staff, and so change agents should provide information and rationales, but be prepared to accept majority decisions (their 'good idea' may be rejected). Like rational–empirical approaches, normative re-education relies on others perceiving the need for change (Keyzer & Wright 1998).

Although normative re-educative change agents need not be senior members of staff, or someone appointed to make changes, they are more likely to succeed if they are supported by managers and/or existing structures. Staff wishing to make changes should discuss ideas at an early stage with senior staff. Clinical support structures (e.g. clinical supervision, IPR) can provide valuable opportunities for sharing ideas with all the team; quality circles, where staff of various grades (often multidisciplinary) discuss issues they consider important, facilitate bottom-up change.

Most people prefer to avoid change, so that motivating staff to become involved may prove difficult. Failing to involve the majority undermines the credibility of normative re-educative change, and so change agents should build co-operation and teamwork, not antagonise colleagues. The right of others to dissent should also be acknowledged: majority rule can oppress minorities (see Chapter 16).

Keyzer and Wright (1998) summarise the three styles above as

- 'telling' (power coercive)
- 'selling' (rational–empirical)
- 'participating' (rational–empirical, normative re-educative)
- 'delegating' (normative re-educative)

Such classifications, however, are oversimplistic, reflecting their bias towards normative re-education change; all four elements may be useful with each approach, just as elements of all three styles may be needed to achieve change in practice (Hancock 1996).

Adoption of change

Rogers and Shoemaker (1971) identify six groups that staff can fall into:

innovators
early adopters
early majority
later majority
laggards
rejectors

Innovators are change agents and allies (usually few in number) sharing enthusiasm for change; when planning change, identify your allies.

As momentum gathers, *early adopters* show interest and can help pilot change, serving as role models for others.

As change becomes accepted by most staff, the *early majority* establish it as the norm; further acceptance brings in the *later majority*.

This leaves two groups: the laggards and the resisters, both opposing the change. *Laggards* may be won over, albeit reluctantly, possibly attempting to undermine initiatives; superficial acceptance of change may be reversed at an early opportunity. Laggards may prove to be more problematic than the *rejecters*, who are usually open with their opposition and unlikely to be convinced.

Resistance may be active or passive. Active resistance is deliberate, but open; passive resistance is usually caused by apathy, with initiatives failing from lack of active support. Passive resistance can be difficult to overcome as it necessitates motivating others.

Resistance is usually caused by how change is introduced rather than by the change itself (Closs 1996). Change, and the unknown, are threatening; people fearing they will not cope seek refuge in, and defend, the status quo. Motivation for resistance should therefore be acknowledged and respected; belittling resisters increases the threat, damages morale, and may cause them to leave.

Involving resisters may make change less threatening and encourage acceptance. As their confidence develops, resisters may share ownership of change, gain a sense of achievement and join the (very) later majority. Planning change should therefore identify and involve potential resisters.

Change is not always beneficial; enthusiasm can blind change agents to any faults. Opposition can stimulate healthy debate, possibly even finding better ways forward. Change agents unwilling to consider that the change they have made might subsequently need changing become tyrants; resistance can usefully moderate misplaced enthusiasm (Wright 1998).

If change proves beneficial, and becomes the norm, continuing resistance may prove destructive. Once other avenues are exhausted, persistent resisters may leave; their resignation may be the best compromise for everyone.

Lewin's strategy

Lewin's (1952) classic work on change management includes:

- field theory
- stages of change

Lewin's *field theory* suggests that opposing forces both *drive* and *restrain* change. Identifying factors that help and hinder change (e.g. spidergraph, listing in columns, SWOT analysis) enables nurses to identify what they can use (driving forces), and what they need to resolve (restraining forces). Habit, often enshrined in rituals (Walsh & Ford 1989; Ford & Walsh 1994) is a major restraining force. A failure to identify restraining forces suggests superficial or naive planning.

More widely cited is Lewin's three *stages of change*:

- unfreezing (destabilising)
- moving (changing)
- refreezing (re-establishing)

Unfreezing, breaking habits and rituals, creates motivation for change. Wright (1998) suggests that unfreezing may occur when:

- expectations have not been met
- staff have uncomfortable feelings about something
- obstacles to change are removed ('psychological safety')

Moving occurs when change is planned and initiated.
Refreezing occurs once change is integrated and stability is restored.

Stability may have been possible when Lewin published his ideas in 1952, but if change and instability are now the norm (Toffler 1970), unfreezing may be unnecessary and refreezing impossible; change agents may only have to plan the moving stage.

Human needs

Change causes *stress* for everyone, including (often especially) change agents. Change agents should therefore consider their own limitations and abilities. Most ICU nurses already work an exhausting 37.5-hour week; the implementation of ambitious changes in addition to existing workloads may threaten personal and professional safety. Failed initiatives can leave change agents physically and emotionally exhausted, while 'shifting sand' quickly buries their ideas. Achieving small changes is better than failing with over-ambitious plans.

Familiarity breeds contempt (the 'wallpaper effect' (Wright 1998): we cease to notice familiar problems); change agents may become conservative, defending their own change against any subsequent developments.

Nursing and healthcare rightly places much emphasis on safety. However, safety needs should be balanced against the benefits of taking risks; this does not mean turning off ventilators each shift to see whether patients can breathe on their own, but it does include taking calculated risks when the likely benefits appear to outweigh the possible dangers.

Nursing has inherited a culture of negative criticism, which undermines the confidence of nurses who usually only receive feedback when they have done something wrong. Staff need to feel valued; management structures (e.g. IPR, clinical supervision) which emphasise *constructive feedback* can be used to support change by:

- giving credit and encouragement when staff achieve something;
- identifying specific achievements;
- ensuring that praise is genuine, but not routine – for nurses to automatically thank everyone at the end of shifts is in effect saying nothing in particular to anyone;
- avoiding clichés and sops

Many good ideas fail to be translated into practice because work or other pressures prevent potential change agents implementing them. Pressures should be recognised, and planned for; actions should be specific and timetabled, with achievable *targets* for everyone to work towards. It is necessary therefore to plan:

who will achieve something
by *what* date
how all staff will be made aware of changes
how they will be achieved, and
where specific events will occur

Plans which *remain flexible* and adaptable are more likely to succeed (Wilkinson 1994); targets may need modification later.

Evaluation

However good ideas may sound, their effects in practice, together with their strengths and weaknesses, should be evaluated and, if necessary, the ideas should be modified, developed further, or even abandoned. Evaluation should therefore be planned and timetabled (cf. nursing process). Evaluations may be achieved through questionnaires, interviews, or more informal approaches. Most texts on nursing research offer advice on designing evaluation feedback.

Time out 2

Look at the notes you have made of proposed changes. Check:

- Why (is the change needed)?
- Who (will make the change)?
- How (will it be made)?
- What problems can be anticipated?
- When will stages of change occur?

Beyond change

Having successfully seen through changes, staff should gain satisfaction (boosting morale) from positively contributing to practice. The benefits may also help nurses elsewhere. Experience may be disseminated within the hospital, and beyond – for instance, are there hospital-wide forums where you work? If not, consider the mounting of study sessions/days, or the publication of articles. Extending practice should be part of each nurse's professional development, and so relevant material, with written reflections on the process, can provide valuable additions to professional profiles.

Implications for practice

- change will occur, and the rate of change will increase
- nurses can either proactively manage change or reactively be managed by others
- any change forced on people against their will is usually overturned at the earliest opportunity
- change management should therefore seek to alter values
- bottom-up approaches are more likely to succeed, as they adopt the norms of majorities
- change is stressful for all concerned, and so should be carefully planned
- detailed planning, with specific target dates and achievable goals, helps to prevent procrastination
- change agents should facilitate informed decision making
- change agents should acknowledge their own and others' limitations
- all staff are likely to need support through the stressful time of change
- opposition to change can provide a forum for constructive debate
- change agents should pre-plan how and when their initiative will be evaluated, and be prepared to modify plans where necessary

Summary

The pace of change is accelerating; nurses and nursing can choose between managing change or being managed by others. Other chapters in this book may have triggered ideas that readers wish to translate into practice. Changes are more likely to succeed if carefully planned, and so this chapter has described models and strategies to help them succeed in introducing change.

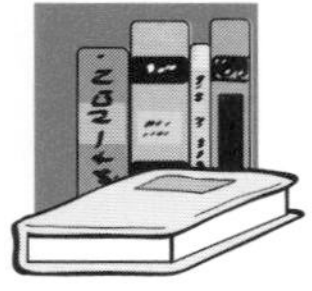

Further reading

Wright (1998) provides a practical description of change management; action research (Webb 1989) offers a way to develop change through practice.

Toffler (1970) remains challenging, developing wider perspectives (although providing little immediate help for nurses wishing to make changes). The problems of ritualised nursing are illustrated by Walsh and Ford (1989) and Ford and Walsh (1994).

ICU-specific material includes Wilkinson (1994) and Hancock (1996).

Journals specialising in nursing management frequently include articles on change management (e.g. McPhail (1997)).

Exercises

Q.1 Discuss the impact of the European Community on Working Time Regulations and the changes in UK employment law on nurses' duty shift patterns and workload in ICUs. How are nurses or other members of healthcare teams (doctors, pharmacists, cleaners, porters) affected by these changes?

Q.2 Analyse the process of how a new practice or policy was introduced into your area. Using your own example:

(a) Identify the style and approaches used (top-down, bottom-up, etc.)
(b) Examine key roles (change agent, innovators, laggards, resisters, etc.) taken on by colleagues and how these were expressed (verbally and with behaviours)
(c) How would you make this process more effective?

Q.3 Reflect on your understanding of clinical supervision. Evaluate how clinical supervision groups can help or hinder the change process.

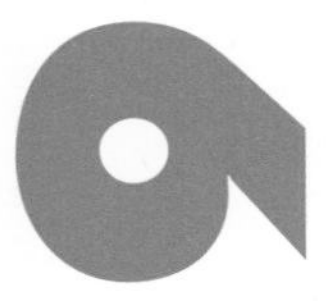
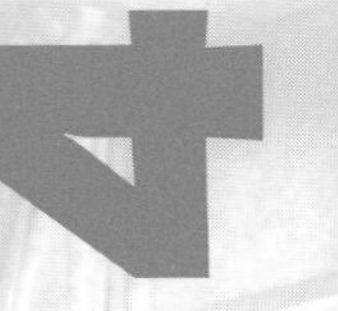

Chapter 49

Managing the ICU

Contents

Introduction

Staff who have gained the necessary bedside nursing experience, together with any required educational developments/qualifications, may plan managerial experience as part of their professional development; or they may find one day that they are the most senior person on duty (possibly due to sickness of senior staff) and so expected to manage the unit for that shift. This chapter provides a trouble-shooting introduction for staff not normally in charge of their units (hence the direct address to readers). The terms *manager* and *management* in this chapter normally refer to the nurse-in-charge of the shift, rather than to more senior management; where appropriate, senior management is specifically identified.

Many ICU staff have previous experience of working in, and often managing, other areas; the principles of management are similar, and so previous experience should be applied wherever possible.

Staff may look to a manager for direction. The manager therefore needs to have sufficient knowledge to provide information. Some information may be factual, but much of it will be a matter of sharing experience and ideas in order to help others make clinical decisions. There are often no right or wrong answers – just different ways of doing thing. Because of this, some readers may differ with the issues raised in this chapter. Hence, for the most part, options, rather than answers, are provided, and the issues will serve their purpose if they help readers to clarify their own values.

There is noticeably little literature in ICU nursing journals advising staff how to develop management skills; since many staff are unlikely to resource management journals unless undertaking management courses, this consigns the development of management skills to the 'sitting with Nellie' ethos which is so antithetical to evidence-based nursing.

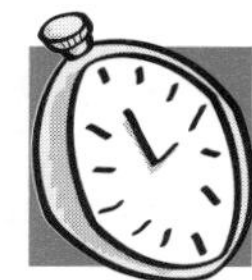

Time out 1

Compare your own previous experience of being in charge of wards or departments with how you have seen others manage the ICU where you work. Note down significant differences. Reflect on why these differences may be necessary.

Starting to manage

Much has been written about management, mostly from industrial perspectives, although there is a growing body of literature on health service management. Many of the principles of industrial management or managing other healthcare areas are applicable to ICUs.

Vaughan and Pilmoor (1989) suggest that management is getting the work done through people. Thus, the manager is an enabler, enabling other people to do their work. The nurse-in-charge should establish constructive working conditions at the start of the shift, enabling the development of the individual strengths and skills of staff, while recognising individual needs and limitations. Managers should individually assess and proactively plan and respond to needs for each shift, rather than seeking to impose their own agendas on staff.

You may remember most patients from your previous shift; if not, briefly assess patients before taking handover. You may need to walk through your unit to take handover, but if not a brief look at the unit can suggest both the number and dependency of patients (high-dependency patients usually have more equipment and people at a bedspace).

Since managers rely on their staff to achieve the work, staff are the manager's most important resource. Staff numbers are important – are there enough staff for patients already on the unit and the expected/potential admissions? In addition, the abilities and qualities of staff are also important. 'Skill mix' is more than simply counting numbers of staff at each grade. Some staff need more support than others; each has different experience, knowledge and skills to draw on. Most staff will probably be known to you and so scanning the off-duty roster helps your planning; with new or unfamiliar (e.g. agency) staff you may gain an insight into their qualities by asking about their experience and what they feel able and not able to do.

Allocation of staff may be guided by managerial structures such as named and team nursing; specific allocation should consider:

- the need to maintain patient safety
- the optimisation of patient treatment
- the development and support of staff.

Nurses unable to care *safely* for a patient should not be allocated to their care. All nurses are individually accountable for their actions and should acknowledge their limitations (UKCC 1992a, 1992b); however, staff are not always aware of their limitations, and so managers should actively assess the competence of each nurse. The most experienced member of staff may be able to give the *best care* to the sickest patient, but without gaining experience of nursing very sick patients, junior staff will be denied opportunities to develop their skills. If they are continually denied *developmental experience*, they may become demotivated and leave, or be unable to care safely for the sicker patients when more experienced staff are not available.

Safety during break cover should also be considered: two junior nurses may safely manage adjacent patients when both are present, but become unsafe if caring for two patients when covering each other's breaks. Nurse managers remain accountable for their actions, and unsafe allocation breaches the Code of Conduct (UKCC 1992a).

The Health and Safety at Work Act (1974) places specific requirements on managers (and employees) to ensure workplaces are safe; the nurse-in-charge also has wider moral responsibilities for the health and safety of their staff and patients. Fire exits should remain clear and accessible at all times, and safety and emergency equipment should be complete and in working order. Emergency equipment varies between units, but may include the resuscitation trolley, emergency intubation trolley and, on cardiothoracic units, thoracotomy pack. Any environmental hazards should be minimised and, where possible, removed.

The nurse-in-charge is responsible for all patients on their unit, even if some responsibilities are devolved to team/area sub-managers. Following handover, the nurse-in-charge should visit each patient to make their own assessment, identify the needs of each bedside nurse, and pass on any relevant additional information/expectations. Sufficient time should be allowed for bedside nurses to take individual handovers, complete their own safety checks and make their own patient assessment; seeking information before bedside nurses can fully assimilate it can create stress for the nurse without providing the manager with full information. Looking through each patient's notes gives bedside nurses time to complete their initial assessment and checks, while giving managers information that may have been missed in handover (relevant points should then be passed on to the bedside nurse).

The nurse-in-charge should ensure that imminent shifts are adequately covered by checking staff numbers and initiating the booking of any additional staff required. Many agencies provide their main service during office hours, and so planning should include all shifts until the agency's next 'working' period; on-call services may be able to provide emergency cover, but they often have few remaining staff to allocate. Other services (e.g. equipment suppliers/repairs) may also need to be contacted.

The nurse-in-charge may have to assume direct patient care. However, this can cause a conflict of roles between their responsibility to the unit as a whole (as manager) and individual responsibility to their patient; it also limits their availability to other members of staff. Instead, it may be reasonable to allocate two patients to one member of staff; the appropriateness or otherwise of assuming direct patient care necessarily remains an individual decision, based on resources available and remembering that the nurse-in-charge remains accountable for whatever decision is made.

Managers need to maintain clinical skills and credibility; with career progression and increasing management duties, staff may need to identify shifts when they assume direct patient care without unit management responsibilities.

Staff morale

Managers are responsible for enabling others to achieve their work goals, and so need to motivate and communicate (Drucker 1974). Nursing demands a high level of cognitive, affective and psychomotor skills, and the ability of staff to realise their potential is affected by their morale. Maintaining staff and unit morale is therefore an important management skill; loyal staff are more likely to support managers during crises.

It follows that managers need good interpersonal skills and respect for, as well as of, their staff. If aware of unsatisfactory practices, they should approach staff constructively, identifying why staff are acting that way (rationale, knowledge base), treating the incident as a developmental learning opportunity rather than a belittling and humiliating experience for the junior nurse (or possibly the manager); if patient safety is compromised, managers may need to act before any discussion.

Breaks from work provide a psychological coping mechanism. Delayed, compromised or missed breaks often cause dissatisfaction, so that ensuring the smooth (and safe) organisation of breaks for staff is an important duty of managers. Organising break relief varies between units and shifts; where units have a system that works and is familiar to staff, this should be followed. Managers may need to assume some direct patient responsibilities to cover breaks; this can also provide them with valuable opportunities to assess patients and the nurse's skills and needs. However, possible conflicts with managerial duties (see above) should be considered, especially if providing relief in inaccessible areas (e.g. side rooms).

When situations are particularly stressful, managers may be able to support staff by offering additional 'stress breaks', making themselves (and other experienced staff) available when necessary, and by acknowledging the stress of the situation.

ICU work is unpredictable; at times workload will exceed resources, and so managers and staff should identify priorities, accepting that some lesser priorities are not always achieved. Managers who are unable to offer ideal support to staff can still build team rapport and loyalty by acknowledging the stress of others. Opinions vary about staff consuming tea and coffee at bedsides; concerns usually include infection and professionalism. Ideally, staff should take breaks (at least every four hours) away from their workspace, but busy shifts (especially 12-hour shifts) may prevent this. If full breaks cannot be taken, providing refreshments at the bedside (this task could be delegated) may help staff to function safely, and also maintain morale. Anything brought into the bedspace may introduce infection, but, on the other hand, stressed nurses are more likely to work inefficiently, possibly skipping more important infection control measures (e.g. handwashing) under pressure of time. What is 'unprofessional' is a value judgement, but professional images may be less important than meeting the basic physiological needs of staff. Relatives, and patients who are able, may also be offered refreshments, and anecdotal experience suggests that they do not mind, or feel any less confidence in, nurses drinking at bedsides. Staff who are needing a break are likely to function inefficiently, give less empathy to others and be more difficult to motivate.

Staffing levels

UK ICUs usually aim to allocate one nurse to every patient, as recommended by the Intensive Care Society (Eddleston *et al.* 1996). This ideal is not always achieved, but if managers consider unit, patient or staff safety is compromised through inadequate staffing (or any other problem they are unable to resolve), they should inform senior managers, who have (higher) responsibility for the unit.

During the shift

The manager who has established mechanisms for staff to work effectively has achieved their most important role, but throughout the remainder of the shift managers should ensure that the unit continues to run smoothly, solving problems as they occur and providing a resource (knowledge, experience) for, and support to, more junior staff.

Staff need to have confidence in their manager; while managers usually have more experience and knowledge than their staff, each member of staff has potential to contribute knowledge, experience or values, and managers should be prepared to learn from, as well as guide and teach, their staff. Following the Code of Conduct (UKCC 1992a), managers should acknowledge the limits of their own knowledge and competence.

Staff also need to feel that they can approach their manager, so that managers should show positive attitudes and remain accessible (this includes spending most of their time in the main patient-care area).

The manager is a link between unit nurses and other hospital staff. If the medical review of patients does not involve bedside nurses, managers often become the links between medical and nursing staff. Similarly, information to and from other hospital departments, or telephone messages from family members, are often ciphered through the nurse-in-charge.

Managers may be pressurised to accept patients because there is an empty bed, there appears to be enough staff, or because the patient needs ICU treatment. Rationing is an unfortunate reality of healthcare, and when an 'ultimate' area such as an ICU is involved, the pressure cannot always be relieved through admission to other wards. While medical staff must decide whether patients require ICU admission, the nurse-in-charge must decide whether the patient can be safely nursed on the unit. This decision includes

imminent shifts
dependency of patients already on the unit
skills of staff available

The manager is professionally accountable for decisions about nursing management on the unit, but if faced with coercion or moral blackmail may need considerable skills in assertiveness.

Good managers may inspire loyalty in their staff, but being in charge can isolate managers from other support mechanisms. Managers also need their breaks: a stressed manager is less likely to be able to support their staff.

Time out 2

Using the cues below, jot down plans for your professional development over the next six months. Aims may be clinical, educational and professional. Be realistic, setting out sufficient aims to help you develop, but not too many to achieve (six aims is often a reasonable target, but the number and scope will vary between individuals). You may wish to share all or part of this with your manager/mentor/colleagues, or retain this as a private document in your professional profile. You may wish to divide aims between short term (a few weeks), medium term (up to six months) and long term (after six months), or cover all aims together. Long-terms aims will not be achieved fully by the time of your six-month review, but you may have partially progressed towards them. You will probably find that setting target dates for achieving aims is helpful.

Over the next six months I would like to achieve (include target times):
I would like to achieve these because:
To achieve these I will need (include people and resources):
I will know I have achieved these aims because (i.e. evaluation):
Possible problems I anticipate for myself/others are:
Ways to minimise these problems are:

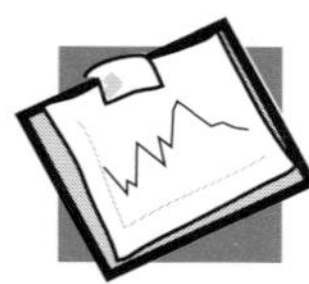

Implications for practice

- staff who have met the minimum criteria required to manage their unit should plan a structure to develop their skills before they find themselves unexpectedly in charge
- managers should enable their staff to work safely, efficiently and effectively
- managers rely on their staff, and so should encourage morale and meet the needs of their staff (professional development, support, breaks)
- managers should recognise potential role conflicts and priorities
- nurse managers, like all qualified nurses, are professionally accountable for their decisions and actions

Summary

This chapter has considered some of the practical issues for ICU nurses who are beginning to develop their management skills. Much has been written elsewhere on wider management issues and theory; nurses developing management careers may need to develop this knowledge further, but should first gain practical management skills through structured experiential programme. The nurse-in-charge is morally and professionally responsible and accountable for their managerial decisions.

Further reading

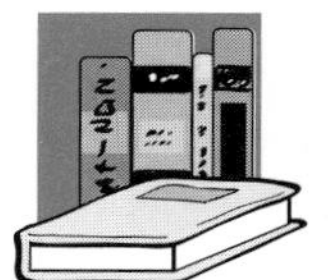

Most literature on management is written by non-nurses; Drucker (e.g. 1974, 1994) is an influential management theorist. Literature on nursing management is rarely ICU specific. Atkinson (1994) is one of the few texts by an experienced ICU nurse manager. The *Standards of Care for Critical Care Nursing* (RCN 1994) is an authoritative guide to prioritise and guide practice. Readers seeking self-help management texts should find Tschudin and Schober (1990) accessible and reliable.

Exercises

Q.1 Describe the role and list the responsibilities of the shift manager and overall unit manager within your own clinical practice area. (For example, specify responsibilities towards resource management, people management, monitoring standards and quality, etc.)

Q.2 Review the management style(s) on each shift within your own ICU. Are there differences in styles/behaviours used between different shift managers? Analyse any perceived differences in terms of leadership, relationship, personality and change theories.

Q.3 Formulate a training programme to prepare ICU nurses for shift and unit management. Propose and justify the selection criteria, basic nurse competencies required for managing the ICU, resources needed for training and the evaluation and feedback strategy.

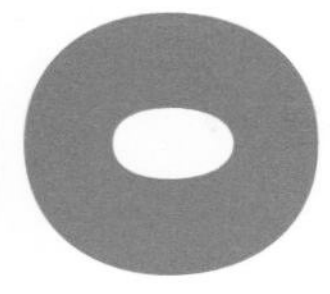
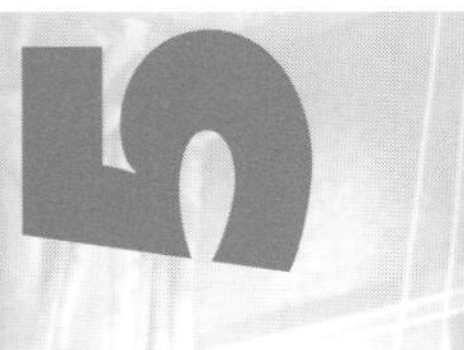

Chapter 50

Cost of intensive care

Contents

Introduction

ICU nursing has a high public profile, partly due to its high financial costs, but the humanitarian costs of ICU can also be high. Intensive care should be provided where beneficial consequences can be achieved at an acceptable cost (King's Fund 1989); defining and measuring 'beneficial consequences' and 'acceptable costs' is often problematic. Ironically, increasing financial pressures are paralleled by increasingly higher public expectations.

Subjectivity surrounds the human cost, and so there are seldom any absolute answers, but there are issues which all nurses (and other healthcare professionals) should consider. Having reached the end of this book, nurses developing their ICU careers should be grappling with the question: what price intensive care? Each nurse should use their own knowledge and values to decide whether the costs of intensive care are justified.

Spending on health

The UK spends less of its gross national product (GNP) on health than most developed countries, with a smaller proportion of what it does spend reaching ICUs (Bion 1995). Most developed countries spend 10.4 per cent of their GNP on health (Caldwell *et al.* 1998); the USA spends 14 per cent (Hudak *et al.* 1998); UK healthcare consumes a mere 6.9 per cent (5.9 per cent on the NHS) (Caldwell *et al.* 1998). Despite (or because) of this, UK ICUs have fewer beds than most developed countries: the average USA units have 24 beds (Endacott 1996), with critical care costing 22 per cent of hospital budgets (Halpern *et al.* 1994); UK units average 4.5 beds (Endacott 1996). The NHS is arguably the most cost-effective health service in the world, caring for sicker (Silvester 1994), thus more expensive, ICU patients on a fraction of the resources available elsewhere. These differences limit applicability of studies and literature from elsewhere to the UK, and may increase the humanitarian and financial costs of critical illness.

Budget

Intensive care inevitably incurs the greatest cost per patient day in almost all hospitals. Critical illness necessitates complex and multiple treatments (investigations and drugs) and high numbers of skilled staff. Intensive care is often at the forefront of technological and pharmaceutical developments, most of which are expensive. The economic microscope is therefore firmly focused on intensive care.

ICU costs have progressively increased against prolonged budget restrictions and increasing costs of healthcare litigation (see Chapter 45). Successful cures of simpler pathologies (e.g. single organ failure) have created more complex pathologies (e.g. MODS) which increase both cost per patient day, and length of stay. Financially, intensive care has become a victim of its own success.

Costing critical illness

Surprisingly, until the internal market forced cost quantification, ICU costs per patient day were largely anecdotal; Vandyk's (1997) telephone survey revealed ranges between £578 and £1,996, inevitably varying with treatments.

Treating non-survivors inevitably prolongs death, and so from humanitarian perspectives is undesirable; but the cost of treating non-survivors is also double the cost of treating survivors (Bion 1995), and so predicting survival could reduce both humanitarian and financial burdens of ICUs, but, at the same time, it raises ethical concerns about reliability and 'playing God'.

Scoring systems

There are various scoring systems, mostly developed for medical audit, and reviewed in many medical texts. Audit can help staff learn from experience, and inappropriate admission to ICU can cause excessive and unnecessary human suffering, but applying retrospective audit tools to prospective prediction may create dilemmas; Parkinson *et al.* (1996) suggest that most scoring systems have a 90 per cent accuracy in predicting survival in ICUs, but only 50–70 per cent accuracy in predicting mortality. The Ethics Committee of the Society of Critical Care Medicine (1997) recommend caution when applying such tools to individuals rather than populations, adding that while they measure survival, morbidity is not addressed. This echoes nursing debate around quality against quantity of life. Scoring systems have also been inappropriately used to predict nurse staffing requirements (Chellel *et al.* 1995).

The Acute Physiology and Chronic Health Evaluation (APACHE) is the most widely used scoring system in ICU nursing; its design is not too dissimilar to the Waterlow pressure scoring system. Most UK units use APACHE II (Knaus *et al.* 1985) – APACHE III (Knaus *et al.* 1991) requires the purchase of a computerised system from APACHE Medical Systems (Castella *et al.* 1995). APACHE III may (Cho & Wang 1997) or may not (Beck *et al.* 1997) be an improvement on APACHE II.

Although useful for retrospective audit, the accuracy of APACHE is affected by treatments and the application of American criteria to the UK (Rowan *et al.* 1993). Moving scores by two or three points can alter mortality prediction by up to one-quarter (Goldhill & Withington 1996; Rhodes *et al.* 1997), and so different users may score significantly different predicted outcomes on the same patient.

The *Riyadh Intensive Care Programme* (a computerised adaptation of APACHE II) captured media attention when used to determine admission. Public concerns centred on rationing by computer (especially the tasteless display featuring coffins for those not predicted to survive), although computers are arguably fairer than more subjective rationing by people. However, its poor predictive ability (often only 50 per cent accuracy) justifies the caution expressed by the Ethics Committee (above).

The Quality Adjusted Life Years system (QALYs) (Williams 1985) attempts numerical measurement of quality: one year of quality life scores one, death scores zero, and points are deducted for each disease/disability; scores below zero, implying quality of life worse than death, are possible. Whether life can be worse than death is debatable, but many ICU patients would achieve negative scores. QALYs have been used more for macro health economics than individual unit budgets, but Ridley *et al.* (1994) estimated that ICU patients incurred total hospital costs of £7,500 per QALY; the additional costs of non-survivors (necessarily scoring zero) highlight the costs of achieving quality outcomes with intensive care.

Measuring quality of life is problematic (North 1995). Seedhouse (1988) questions whether quality and value of life can (and should) be equated. However, even if measurement criteria are questionable, they focus debate of whether healthcare interventions achieve improvement on pre-morbid life.

Mortality

Mortality rates for general UK ICUs range between 11.2 and 31.3 per cent (MacDonnell *et al.* 1996), averaging 25–26 per cent (Rowan *et al.* 1993; Horton 1995). Mortality is usually measured to discharge from units; post-discharge measurements inevitably increase mortality. Goldhill and Sumner (1998) found UK ICU post-discharge mortality rates of 27.1 per cent (no time limit identified). Niskanen *et al.*'s (1996) Finnish study suggested that ICU patients' life expectancy was similar to that of the general population, but noted that approximately one-half post-discharge deaths had low predicted mortalities. The devolvement of budgets can create conflicts for senior doctors and nurses between balancing budgets and treating people. The premature transfer of patients to lower-cost areas can be false economies, increasing re-admission rates, long-term financial costs and mortality. Goldhill and Sumner (1998) conclude that patients are prematurely discharged from ICUs.

Death is often viewed as a medical failure (Sprung 1990), despite the recognition that not all patients will survive ICUs. Predicting those who will not survive is often difficult. Nevertheless the potency of ICU interventions is such that 72.6 per cent of deaths follow withdrawal of treatment (Mercer *et al.* 1998).

Morbidity

Although less quantifiable than mortality, morbidity indicates the human cost of intensive care. Follow-up clinics and studies reveal far higher morbidity costs than were previously suspected; White (1998) reports that four-fifths of patients had significant psychological problems three months after discharge, with most ex-patients not having resumed normal work. Among other changes, this study led to increased prescription of antipsychotic drugs on ICUs. While antipsychotic drugs may be useful, nurses should also consider all the non-pharmacological approaches available (e.g. reducing sensory imbalance – see Chapter 3) that can reduce or prevent post-discharge psychosis.

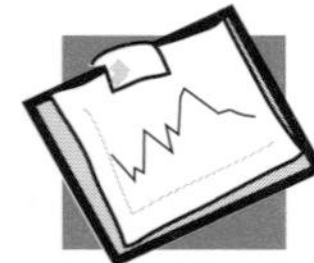

Implications for practice

- costs involve both financial and human aspects; human costs are subjective, including debatable issues such as quality of life, but are fundamentally central to nursing values
- medical outcome scoring systems are available, but predictive reliability for individuals is debated, and so rationing by scoring systems is ethically questionable
- post-discharge nursing visits/clinics can reduce the psychological cost of intensive care to ex-patients and identify areas of nursing practice that need development

Summary

This final chapter has revisited issues raised at the start of this book, namely:

- What fundamentally are we doing for our patients?
- What should we be doing?
- How should we be doing it?

There are many possible answers to these questions; discussion in other chapters should have developed readers' awareness of these issues in everyday practice. As professionals, ICU nurses need to evaluate both the financial and the humanitarian costs of intensive care to determine its ultimate value. Attempts to equate financial costs with humanitarian (morbidity) costs may help nurses to justify the value of their nursing, but may also create the danger that – to adapt Oscar Wilde – we know the price of everything, but the value of nothing.

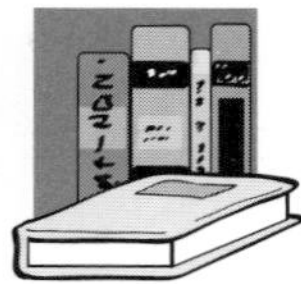

Further reading

As part of their continuing professional development, readers should understand the practice of their own clinical speciality within the provision of wider healthcare; sociological perspectives, such as Caldwell *et al.* (1998) can offer valuable insights to achieve this.

A number of recent medical articles evaluate ICU; Ridley *et al.* (1994, 1997) have taken particular interest in such fundamental re-evaluation. Much has been written about medical scoring systems; Knaus *et al.* (1985, 1991) and recent evaluations, such as Rhodes *et al.* (1997) or Beck *et al.* (1997), provide authoritative insights. Nursing has echoed the medical literature's interest in wider economic issues; Endacott (1996) provides a useful nursing perspective.

Exercises

Q.1 List the positive benefits of the critical care process and categorise these into:

(a) benefits to patients
(b) benefits to friends and family to health practitioners
(c) benefits to health practitioners
(d) benefits to society and the public

Q.2 Analyse the cost per day of a typical patient in your own clinical area. Break down this cost where possible into treatments, resources, staff, etc.

Q.3 Review the practical strategies that can be implemented by ICU nurses, and which can impact on the long-term survival of ICU patients once discharged home. Consider ICU nurses' role in community health, the feasibility of specialist community link nurses, advice booklets and follow-up/discharge clinics.

Answers

Answers

The following are the answers to questions to be found in the Clinical Scenarios at the ends of the chapters indicated.

Chapter 20, p. 218

The calculations for Q.2 are as follows:

CI = CO ÷ body surface area	Mrs Goodwin's CI = 3.0l ÷ 1.7 m^2 = 1.76 l/min/m^2
SV = CO ÷ HR	Mrs Goodwin's SV = 3,000 ml ÷ 125 = 24 ml
SVR = (MAP − CVP) × 79.9 ÷ CO	SVR = (68 − 11) × 79.9 ÷ 3.0 = 1,518 dyn/sec/cm^{-5}
PVR = (mPAP − PCWP) × 79.9 ÷ CO	PVR = (19 − 12) × 79.9 ÷ 3.0 = 186 dyn/sec/cm^{-5}

Chapter 24, p. 284

Q.1: ECG shows anteriolateral MI, coronaries which supply this area are: left coronary artery, anterior descending, and circumflex artery.

Chapter 26, p. 300

Q.1: TNFα, interleukins IL-1, IL-6, IL-8, transforming growth factor-*β*, platelet activating factor, thromboxane A, prostacyclin, bradykinin.

Symptoms associated with TNFα include fever, hyperglycaemia, hypotension, and capillary leak. (See Chapter 23.)

Glossary

The first occurrence of each of these terms in the main text is highlighted in **bold** type.

ABC of resuscitation Airway, Breathing, Circulation.

ACT Activated clotting times (normal 80–100 seconds).

anacrotic notch an abnormal notch occurring on the arterial blood pressure trace before the main pressure peak.

anthropometry measurement of body using relationships between height, weight and size.

anxiolysis Removing ('breakdown' of) anxiety.

arterial tonometry a noninvasive means of continuously measuring arterial pressure.

autologous from the same individual (e.g. autologous blood is the patient's own blood).

Babinski's sign normal flexor responses are replaced by extensor responses, big toe turns upwards; in adults this indicates upper motor neurone (pyramidal tract) pathology.

balloon tamponade inflation of balloon-tipped catheters (e.g. Sengstarken tube) places direct pressure on bleeding points; thus internal bleeding is stopped in the same way that nurses use digital pressure to stop bleeding after arterial lines are removed.

barotrauma damage to alveoli from excessively high (peak) airway pressure.

beta-lactam class of antibiotics (e.g. ceftazidime, penicillin).

Bohr effect acidosis – elevated blood hydrogen (pH) and carbon dioxide (pCO_2) – decreases oxyhaemoglobin saturation.

bradycardia heart rate below 60 beats per minute.

calorie (cal, c) amount of heat needed to raise one gram of water 1°C at atmospheric pressure (= small calorie).

Calorie (Cal, C) amount of heat needed to raise one kilogram of water 1°C at atmospheric pressure (= large calorie, kilocalorie).

capillary occlusion pressure the pressure at which capillary flow will be prevented, resulting in ischaemia, anaerobic metabolism and (eventually) infarction of tissue (e.g. pressure sore formation).

chemotaxis movement of cell/organism to/from chemical substance, so that chemotaxic chemicals enable phagocytic activity.

chronotherapy the science of giving drugs at certain times of the day to achieve optimum effect; this usually relates to interaction with endogenous hormones.

circadian rhythm the 'body clock', an endogenous rhythm around the day; a normal circadian rhythm takes about 24 hours, but abnormal rhythms can be longer or shorter. Circadian rhythm affects various endogenous hormone levels, so that a disturbed circadian rhythm results in various abnormal body responses (e.g. wakefulness at night).

coagulopathies disorders (pathologies) of clotting, such as DIC, sickle cell anaemia.

colloid osmotic pressure the osmotic pressure created by large molecules (e.g. proteins) that retain plasma in the intravascular space. Fluids with high colloid osmotic pressures therefore assist return of extravascular fluid (oedema) into the bloodstream.

commensal endogenous bacteria helping normal human functions.

cytokines secreted by cells of inflammatory and immune processes; interleukins, interferon, coagulation-stimulating factor, TNFα.

dalton (Da) unit of molecular weight.

d-dimer fibrinolysis product used to measure clotting.

depolarisation reduction of membrane potential to a less negative value.

dialysis movement of solutes through semipermeable membrane by concentration gradient.

dicrotic notch the notch normally seen on the downbeat of the arterial waveform; this represents closure of the aortic valve, which causes a transient slight increase in pressure.

diffusion solutes moving from greater to lesser concentration.

Ecstasy 3–4 methylenedioxymethamphetamine (MDMA).

eicosanoids fatty acid.

FiO_2 fraction of inspired oxygen (expressed as a decimal fraction, so that FiO_2 1.0 equals 100%, or pure oxygen).

Frank–Starling law the force exerted during each heartbeat is directly proportional to the length or degree of myocardial fibre stretch; thus increasing fibre length (e.g. with positive inotropes) increases stroke volume.

free radicals atoms with one or more unpaired electron in their outer orbit; this makes them inherently unstable, so they react readily with other molecules to pair the free electron.

General Adaptive Syndrome a reaction to stressors that causes generalised physiological responses throughout the body; first described by Hans Selye (see Chapter 46).

half-life the time taken for a chemical to lose half of its active effect.

heterotopic graft into a different site.

hydrostatic pressure exerted by fluids.

hypercalcaemia high serum concentrations of calcium (normal serum levels are 2.25–2.75 mmol/l).

hyperglycaemia high serum concentrations of glucose (normal serum levels are 4–8 mmol/l).

hyperkalaemia high serum concentrations of potassium (normal serum levels are 3.5–5.0).

hypernatraemia high serum concentrations of sodium (normal serum levels are 135–145 mmol/l).

hypertriglyceridaemia high serum concentrations of triglycerides; most animal and vegetable fats are triglycerides, and so this is the principle lipid found in serum (normal serum levels are 200–300 mg/dl).

hypo- low (thus **hypocalcaemia** is serum calcium below 2.25 mmol/l).

hysteresis literally, the difference between two phenomena; in a medical context, it usually refers to lung differences between inspiration and expiration (pressure/volume curve), where passive elastic recoil allows greater volume in relation to airway pressure during expiration than during inspiration; thus manipulating I:E ratio also manipulates mean airway pressure.

I:E ratio inspiratory to expiratory ratio (on ventilator).

inulin fructose derivative, not absorbed or metabolised, thus a useful biochemical marker.

interleukin a group of *cytokines*, many vasoactive, but often with opposing effects; they are known by numbers (e.g. interleukin 1 (IL-1) is a major mediator of SIRS/MODS; see Chapter 23).

joule (J) a unit to measure energy (=10^7 ergs or 1 watt second).

kilocalorie the amount of heat needed to raise one kilogram of water 1°C at atmospheric pressure (=Calorie, C)

kilodalton (kDa) molecular weight.

kilojoule 1000 joules.

Krebs' cycle (citric acid cycle) a chain of intracellular chemical reactions to metabolise fat for energy. Krebs' cycle is efficient at energy (adenosine triphosphate) production, but produces metabolic wastes (acids, ketones, carbon dioxide, water); see Chapter 9.

leukotrienes active compound contained in leucocytes; causes *chemotaxis* allergic and inflammatory response.

millivolt (mv) unit in which cell membrane action potential is measured.

mitochondria (single: mitochondrion) organelles within cytoplasm that provide the main source for the cells energy (often called the 'power-house' of the cell).

modified chest lead (MCL) this is used to assess ventricular aspects of ECG when only 3-lead ECG is available or is usually used with 5-lead continuous ECG monitoring in order to obtain waveform of one of the six chest leads (C1 to C6 on 12-lead ECG). MCL1 would need positive electrode to be positioned in C1 position on chest with MCL6 positioned in C6 position.

monoclonal antibodies antibodies (B leucocytes) that have been cloned (in a laboratory) from a single genetic strand; hence each monoclonal antibody is identical and specific to a particular antigen.

nosocomial infection an infection acquired in hospital (technically, at least 22 hours following admission).

oncotic osmotic pressure of colloids in solution.

orthotopic graft into normal anatomical position.

osmolality number of dissolved particles per kilogram of solvent.

osmolarity number of dissolved particles per litre of solution.

osmotic movement of solutes through a semipermeable membrane to form a concentration equilibrium on both sides.

ototoxic toxic to the ear (oto = ear); damage is caused to the eighth cranial nerve or the organs of hearing and balance. Many drugs (e.g. gentamicin) can be ototoxic.

parity number of pregnancies (including stillbirths/abortions/ miscarriages) reaching 20 weeks gestation.

permissive hypercapnia tolerating abnormally high arterial carbon dioxide tensions (pCO_2) to enable smaller tidal volumes, and so limit/avoid barotrauma and volotrauma.

***Pneumocystis carinii* pneumonia (PCP)** opportunist infection commonly causing respiratory failure with AIDS.

prostacyclin (PGI_2) an active arachidonic acid metabolite; inhibits angiotensin-mediated vasoconstriction, stimulates renin release, inhibits platelet aggregation (so used for anticoagulation).

prothrombin time a test to measure clotting; normal prothrombin time is 11–12.5 seconds; prolonged prothrombin time indicates deficiency in one or more clotting factors.

pulsus parodoxus (abnormal) decrease of over 10 mmHg in systolic BP on inspiration.

radicals an atom with an unpaired electron (see free radical).

repolarisation restoration of cell to its resting potential.

saturated fatty acid fats with univalent bonds joining all atoms; valency determines hydrogen binding capacity of molecules, and so saturated fatty acids contribute to hypercholestrolamia and cardiovascular (especially coronary) disease. Most animal fats are saturated.

serotonin tryptophan derivative found in platelets and cells of brain and intestine; vasoconstrictor and neurotransmitter.

shunt 'shunting' is a widely used medical term to describe a conduit between two body compartments. In respiratory medicine this is usually used to describe movement of blood from the venous to arterial circulation without effective ventilation, either from intrapulmonary problems, such as ARDS, but can also be caused by an atrial-septal defect allowing blood to pass between the atria without entering the pulmonary circulation. 'Shunt' can also be used to describe an abnormal conduit directly joining an artery to a vein, such as an arteriovenous shunt used for haemodialysis access, or a drain inserted to remove excess fluid (e.g. an intraventricular shunt to drain CSF from the ventricles of the brain, and so relieve intracranial hypertension).

sigh breath an occasional, especially large breath. At rest, people (and animals) take sigh breaths, which ventilate the lung bases, so helping to prevent atelectasis and infection; like most breaths, this usually occurs spontaneously and unconsciously. The benefits of physiological sigh breaths encouraged manufacturers to incorporate them into artificial ventilators, but sigh breaths during artificial ventilation do not appear to provide any benefits (see Chapter 4).

thromboxane A_2 (TXA_2) unstable derivative of PGG_2 (prostaglandin G_2), stimulates platelet aggregation.

transmembrane pressure the pressure across a membrane. Where artificial technologies replicate capillary function, such as the 'artificial kidneys' used for haemofiltration, excessive pressure may rupture the necessarily delicate membrane. Being artificial, damage is permanent and irreparable. As the surface area of the filter becomes progressively engorged with clots, filtrate is forced through a smaller area, increasing transmembrane pressure. Therefore measuring the transmembrane pressure should identify impending rupture of the artificial kidney. Stopping filters before maximum transmembrane pressure is reached enables blood in the circuit to be safely returned to the patient. (See manufacturers instructions for maximum transmembrane pressures of individual models.)

trimester pregnancy is divided into 3 trimesters: trimester 1 – up to week 12; trimester 2 – weeks 13–28; trimester 3 – week 29 to delivery.

ultrafiltration removal of fluid through a membrane under pressure.

volotrauma damage from alveolar distension (excessive volume; sometimes spelt volutrauma).

V/Q ratio (alveolar) ventilation to (pulmonary capillary) perfusion ratio; normal V/Q = 0.8.

xenograft transplant tissue from another species (e.g. pig heart valves).

References

Abbas, A.K., Lichtman, A.H. and Pober, J.S. (1994) *Cellular and Molecular Immunology*, 2nd edn, Philadelphia: W.B. Saunders.

Abbott, H. (1997) 'Complications of the puerperium', in B.R. Sweet (ed.) *Mayes' Midwifery: A Textbook for Midwives*, 12th edn, London: Baillière Tindall: 718–28.

Abman, S.H., Griebel, J.L., Parker, D.K. *et al.* (1994) 'Acute effects of inhaled nitric oxide in children with severe hypoxemic respiratory failure', *Journal of Paediatrics* 124(6): 881–8.

Abraham, E., Gallagher, T.J. and Fink, S. (1996) 'Clinical evaluation of multiparameter intra-arterial blood-gas sensor', *Intensive Care Medicine* 22(5): 507–13.

ACCP Consensus Conference (1993) 'Mechanical ventilation', *Chest* 104(6): 1833–59.

ACCP/SCCM (1992) 'Consensus conference: definitions for sepsis and organ failure and guidelines for the use of innovative therapies', *Critical Care Medicine* 20(6): 864–74.

Ackerman, M.H. (1993) 'The effects of saline lavage prior to suctioning', *American Journal of Critical Care* 2(4): 326–30.

Ackerman, M.H., Ecklund, M.M. and Abu-Jumah, M. (1996) 'A review of normal saline installation: implications for practice', *Dimensions of Critical Care Nursing* 15(1): 31–8.

Ackerman, N.B., Null, D.M. and deLemos, R.A. (1985) 'High frequency ventilation: history, theory and practice', in R.R. Kirby, R.A. Smith and D.A. Desautels (eds) *Mechanical Ventilation*, Edinburgh: Churchill Livingstone: 307–26.

Adam, S.K. (1994) 'Aspects of current research in enteral nutrition in the critically ill', *Care of Critically Ill* 10(6): 246–51.

Adam, S.K. and Osborne, C. (1997) *Critical Care Nursing: Science and Practice*, Oxford: Oxford Medical Publications.

Adams, D.H., Hughes, M. and Elliott, T.S.J. (1997) 'Microbial colonization of closed-system suction catheters used in liver transplant patients', *Intensive and Critical Care Nursing* 13(2): 72–6.

Addy, V.E., Waldemann, C.S. and Collin, C. (1996) 'Review of the use of intracranial pressure monitoring in a district general hospital intensive care unit', *Clinical Intensive Care* 7(2): 87–91.

Adelman, R., Berger, J. and Macina, L. (1994) 'Critical care of the geriatric patient', *Clinics in Geriatric Medicine*, 10(1): 19–30.

Adonat, R. and Killingworth, A. (1994) 'Care of the Critically Ill Patient: the impact of stress on the use of touch in intensive therapy units', *Journal of Advanced Nursing* 19(5): 912–22.

Ai, A.L., Peterson, C. and Bolling, S.F. (1997) 'Psychological recovery from coronary artery bypass graft surgery: the use of complementary therapies', *Journal of Alternative and Complementary Medicine* 3(4): 343–53.

Albarran, J.W. (1998) 'Managing the nursing priorities in the patient with an acute myocardial infarction', in J.W. Albarran and T.E. Price (eds) *Managing the Nursing Priorities in Intensive Care*, Dinton: Quay Books: 134–70.

Alcock, S.R. and Ledingham, I.McA. (1990) 'Prevention of infection in the medico-surgical intensive care unit', *Intensive Therapy and Clinical Monitoring* 11(2): 42–9.

Alexander-Williams, J.M. and Rowbottom, D.J. (1998) 'Novel routes of opiod administration', *British Journal of Anaesthesia* 81(1): 3–7

Ali, M.T. and Ferguson, C. (1997) 'Massive haemorrhage', in D.R. Goldhill and P.S.

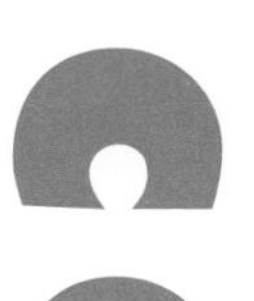

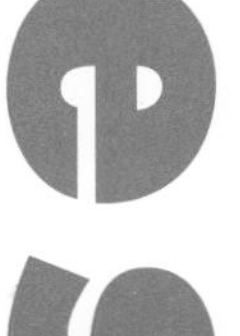

Withington (eds) *Textbook of Intensive Care*, London: Chapman & Hall: 21–6.

Allen, C.H. and Ward, J.D. (1998) 'An evidence-based approach to management of increased intracranial pressure', *Critical Care Clinics* 14(3): 485–95.

Allison, A. (1994) 'High frequency jet ventilation: where are we now? *Care of the Critically Ill* 10(3): 122–4.

Amoroso, P., Brunner, M. and Greenwood, R. (1992) 'Acute renal failure', *British Journal of Intensive Care* 2(2): 92–4.

Amyes, S.G.B. and Thomson, C.J. (1995) 'Antibiotic resistance in the ICU', *British Journal of Intensive Care* 5(8): 263–71.

Andrew, C.M. (1998) 'Optimizing the human experience: nursing the families of people who die in intensive care', *Intensive and Critical Care Nursing* 14(2): 59–65.

Appadu, B.L. (1996) 'Continuous, noninvasive, real-time monitoring of renal function: the ambulatory renal monitor', *Care of the Critically Ill* 12(5): 155–7.

Appel, P.L., Shoemaker, W.C. and Kram, H.B. (1991) 'Effects of prostaglandins E1 in postoperative surgical patients with circulatory deficiency', *Chest* 99(4): 945–50.

Armstrong, R.F. (1997) 'Burns and electrocution', in D.R. Goldhill and P.S. Withington (eds) *Textbook of Intensive Care*, London: Chapman & Hall: 671–8.

Armstrong, R.F., Bullen, C., Cohen, S.L. *et al.* (1992) 'Critical care algorithm: sedation, analgesia and paralysis', *Clinical Intensive Care* 3(6): 284–7.

Artigas, A., Bernard, G.R., Cartlet, B.J. *et al.* (1998) 'The American–European consensus conference on ARDS, Part 2', *American Journal of Respiratory Critical Care Medicine* 157(4,1): 1332–47.

Artinian, N.T., Duggan, C. and Millar, P. (1993) 'Age differences in patient recovery patterns following coronary artery bypass surgery', *American Journal of Critical Care* 2(6): 453–61.

Artnal, K.E. and Wilkinson, S.S. (1998) 'Fulminant hepatic failure in acute acetaminophen overdose', *Dimensions of Critical Care Nursing* 17(3): 135–44.

Arya, R. and Bellingham, A. (1997) 'Haemoglobin disorders', in D.R. Goldhill and P.S. Withington (eds) *Textbook of Intensive Care* London: Chapman & Hall: 577–83

Asensio, J.A., Demetriades, D., Berne, T.V. *et al.* (1996) 'Invasive and noninvasive monitoring for early recognition and treatment of shock in high-risk trauma and surgical patients', *Surgical Clinics of North America* 76(4): 985–97.

Ashurst, S. (1997) 'Nursing care of the mechanically ventilated patient in ITU', *British Journal of Nursing* 6(8): 447–54.

Ashworth, P. (1980) *Care to Communicate* London: RCN.

—— (1985) 'Intensive care nursing, a speciality developing – in which direction?' *Intensive Care Nursing* 1(1): 1–2.

Asmundsson, T., Johnson, R.F., Kilburn, K.H. *et al.* (1973) 'Efficacy of nebulizers for depositing saline in human lung', *American Review of Respiratory Disease* 108(3): 506–12.

Atkinson, B.L. (1994) 'Managing the critical care unit', in B. Millar and P. Burnard (eds) *Critical Care Nursing* London: Baillière Tindall: 128–44.

Atkinson, R.L., Atkinson, R.G., Smith, E.E. *et al.* (1996) *Hildegard's Introduction to Psychology* 12th edn, Fort Worth: Harcourt Brace College Publishers.

Aurrell, G. and Elmqvist, D. (1985) 'Sleep in the surgical intensive care unit: a continuous polygraphic recording of sleep in 9 patients receiving post-operative care', *British Medical Journal* 290, 6473: 1029–32.

Azar, G., Love, R., Choe, E. *et al.* (1996) 'Neither dopamine nor dobutamine reverses the depression in mesenteric blood flow caused by positive end-expiratory pressure', *Journal of Trauma* 40(5): 679–85.

Bailey, A. (1995) *United Kingdom Cardiac Surgical Register 1993/4* London: Society of Thoracic and Cardiovascular Surgeons of Great Britain and Ireland.

Baillie, L. (1993) 'A review of pain assessment tools', *Nursing Standard* 7(23): 25–9.

Bakker, J. (1996) 'Monitoring of blood lactate levels', *International Journal of Intensive Care* 3(1): 29–36.

Ball, C. (1990) 'Humanity in intensive care', *Intensive Care Nursing* 6(1): 12–16.

Banerjee, S., Straffen, A. and Rhoden, W.E. (1997) 'Value of qualitative Troponin T estimation in decision-making in patients with chest pain', *British Journal of Cardiology* 4(10): 414–18.

Banner, M.J., Jaeger, M.J. and Kirby, R.R. (1994) 'Components of the work of breathing and implications for monitoring ventilator dependent patients', *Critical Care Medicine* 22(3): 515–23.

Barden, C. and Hansen, M. (1995) 'Cold vs. warm cardioplegia: recognising haemodynamic variations', *Dimensions in Critical Care Nursing* 14(3): 114–23.

Barnett, M.I. and Cosslett, A.G. (1998) 'Endotoxin: a clinical challenge', *British Journal of Intensive Care* 8(3): 78–87.

Barrett, E. (1990) 'Pressure sores in intensive care', *Intensive Therapy and Clinical Monitoring* 11(5): 158–67.

Barrie-Shevlin, P. (1987) 'Maintaining sensory balance for the critically ill patient', *Nursing* 3(16): 597–601.

Barris, R.R., Israel, A.L., Amory, D.W. *et al.* (1995) 'Regional cerebral oxygenation during cardiopulmonary bypass', *Perfusion* 10(4): 245–8.

Bartlett, E.M. (1996) 'Temperature measurement: why and how in intensive care', *Intensive and Critical Care Nursing* 12(1): 50–4.

Bassion, S. (1996) 'Immunological reactions', in L.A. Kaplan and A.J. Pesce (eds) *Clinical Chemistry: Theory, Analysis, Correction* St Louis: Mosby: 213–49.

Bateson, S., Adam, S., Hall, G. *et al.* (1993) 'The development of a pressure area scoring system for critically ill patients', *Intensive and Critical Care Nursing* 9(3): 146–51.

Bauby, J-M. (1997) *The Diving-Bell and the Butterfly*, trans. J. Leggatt, London: Fourth Estate.

Baxby, D., van Saene, H.K., Stoutenbeek, C.P. *et al.* (1996) 'Selective decontamination of the digestive tract: 13 years on, what it is and what it is not', *Intensive Care Medicine* 22(7): 699–706.

Beal, A.L. and Cerra, F.B. (1994) 'Multiple organ failure syndrome in the 1990s: systemic inflammatory response and organ dysfunction', *JAMA* 271(3): 226–33.

Beale, R. (1994) 'Weaning from mechanical ventilation', *British Journal of Intensive Care* 4(5): 168–75.

Beale, R. and Bihari, D. (1992) 'The management of acute renal failure in the intensive care unit', *Current Anaesthesia and Critical Care* 3(3): 146–9.

Beauchamp, T.L. and Childress, J.F. (1994) *Principles of Biomedical Ethics* 4th edn, New York: Oxford University Press.

Beaumont, T. (1997) 'How To Guides: arterial blood gas sampling', *Care of the Critically Ill* 13(1): centre insert.

Beck, D.H., Taylor, B.L., Millar, B. *et al.* (1997) 'Prediction of outcome from intensive care: a prospective cohort study comparing Acute Physiology and Chronic Health Evaluation II and III prognostic systems in a United Kingdom intensive care unit', *Critical Care Medicine* 25(1): 9–15.

Benner, P. (1984) *From Novice to Expert* Menlo Park, CA: Addison-Wesley Publishing.

Bennett, P. (1995) 'Cutting the thread of life: legal guidelines for the withdrawal of treatment following the Anthony Bland case', *Care of the Critically Ill* 11(2): 62–4.

Bergman, J.S. and Yate, P. (1997) 'in D.R. Goldhill and P.S. Withington (eds) *Textbook of Intensive Care* London: Chapman & Hall: 84–94.

Bernard, G.R., Artigas, A., Brigham, K.L. *et al.* (1994a) 'Report of the American-European consensus conference on ARDS: definitions, mechanisms, relevant outcomes and clinical trial co-ordination', *Intensive Care Medicine* 20(3): 225–32.

Bernard, G.R., Artigas, A., Brigham, K.L. *et al.* (1994b) 'American-European consensus conference on ARDS: definitions, mechanisms, relevant outcome and clinical trial co-ordination', *American Journal of Respiratory Critical Care Medicine* 149(3,1): 818–21.

Bersten, A.D. and Oh, T.E (1997) 'Ventilators and resuscitators', in T.E. Oh (ed.) *Intensive Care Manual* 4th edn, Oxford: Butterworth-Heinemann: 256–65.

Betit, P., Thompson, J.E. and Benjamin, P.K. (1993) 'Mechanical ventilation', in P.B. Koff, D. Eitzman and J. Neu (eds) *Neonatal and Pediatric Respiratory Care* St Louis: Mosby: 324–44.

Bettany, G.E. and Powell-Tuck, J. (1997) 'Nutritional support in surgery', *Surgery* 15(10): 233–7.

Bewley, C. (1997) 'Hypertensive disorders of pregnancy', in B.R. Sweet (ed.) *Mayes' Midwifery: A Textbook for Midwives* 12th edn, London: Baillière Tindall. 533–47.

Bidani, A., Tzouanakis, A.E., Cardenas, V.J. *et al.* (1994) 'Permissive hypercapnia in acute respiratory failure', *JAMA* 272(12): 957–62.

Bion, J. (1995) 'Rationing intensive care', *British Medical Journal* 310(6981): 682–3.

Bion, J.F. and Ledingham, I.McA. (1987) 'Sedation in intensive care: a postal survey', *Intensive Care Medicine* 13(3): 215–16.

Bion, J.F. and Oh, T.E. (1997) 'Sedation in intensive care', in T.E. Oh (ed.) *Intensive Care Manual* 4th edn, Oxford: Butterworth-Heinemann: 672–8.

Bird, J. (1997) 'Intensive care problems in obstetric patients', *Care of the Critically Ill* 13(6): 241–4.

Birtwistle, J. (1994) 'Pressure sore formation and risk assessment in intensive care', *Care of the Critically Ill* 10(4): 154–9.

Biswas, C.K., Ramos, J.M., Agoyannis, B. *et al.* (1982) 'Blood gas analysis: effect of air bubbles in syringe and delay in estimation', *British Medical Journal* 284(6320): 923–7.

Black, D., Morris, J., Smith, C. *et al.* (1988) *Inequalities in Health* London: Penguin.

Blackwood, B. (1998) 'The practice and perception of intensive care staff using the closed suctioning system', *Journal of Advanced Nursing* 28(5): 1020–9.

Bloomfield, G.L., Holloway, S., Ridings, P.C. *et al.* (1997) 'Pre-treatment with inhaled nitric oxide inhibits neutrophil migration and oxidative activity resulting in attenuated sepsis-induced acute lung injury', *Critical Care Medicine* 25(4): 584–95.

Board, M. (1995) 'Comparison of disposable and glass mercury thermometers', *Nursing Times* 91(33): 36–7.

Bodenham, A., Knappett, P., Cohen, A. *et al.* (1994) 'Facilities and usage of general intensive care in Yorkshire: a six-months' audit', in Paediatric Intensive Care Society (UK) Conference Abstracts, *Care of the Critically Ill* 10(3): 129.

Boeing, M.H. and Mongera, C.O. (1989) 'Powerlessness in critical care patients', *Dimensions of Critical Care Nursing* 8(5): 274–9.

Bohm, S. and Lachmann, B. (1996) 'Pressure-control ventilation', *International Journal of Intensive Care* 3(1): 12–28.

Bohn, D. (1991) 'The current role of ECMO in paediatric practice', *Intensive Care World* 8(4): 162–6.

Boldt, J., Menges, T., Wollbruck, M. *et al.* (1994) 'Is continuous cardiac output measurement using thermodilution reliable in the critically ill patient? *Critical Care Medicine* 22(12): 1913–18.

Bolton, C.F. (1996) 'Sepsis and the systemic inflammatory response syndrome: neuromuscular manifestations', *Critical Care Medicine* 24(8): 1408–16.

Bone, R.C. (1994) 'Sepsis and its complications: the clinical problem', *Critical Care Medicine* 22(7): S8–11.

—— (1996) 'Toward a theory regarding the pathogenesis of the septic inflammatory response syndrome: what we do know and do not know about cytokine regulation', *Critical Care Medicine* 24(1): 163–72.

Bone, R.C., Balk, R.A., Cerra, F.B. *et al.* (1992) 'Definitions for sepsis and organ failure and guidelines for the use of innovative therapies is sepsis', *Chest* 101(6): 1644–55.

Bood, K. (1996) 'Coping with critical illness: the child in ICU', *Nursing in Critical Care* 1(5): 221–4.

Booth, B. (1993) 'Soft options', *Nursing Times* 89(34): 61–2.

Booth, R. (1997) 'Hepatitis C', *Professional Nurse* 12(4): 287–90.

Bourbonnais, F. (1981) Pain assessment: development of a tool for the nurse and the patient', *Journal of Advanced Nursing* 6(4): 277–82.

Boyer, T.D. and Henderson, J.M. (1996) 'Portal hypertension and bleeding esophageal varices', in D. Zakim and T.D. Boyer (eds) *Hepatology: A Textbook of Liver Disease*, 3rd edn, Philadelphia: W B Saunders: 720–63.

Brady, A.J.B. and Buller, N.P. (1996) 'Coronary angioplasty and myocardial ischaemia', *Care of the Critically Ill* 12(3): 83–6.

Braithwaite, M.A. (1996) 'Withholding or withdrawing intensive care', *British Journal of Intensive Care* 6(2): 51–4.

Brandstetter, R.D., Sharma, K.C., DellaBadia, M. *et al.* (1997) 'Adult respiratory distress syndrome: a disorder in need of improved outcome', *Heart and Lung* 26(1): 3–14.

Brazier, M. (1992) *Medicine, Patients and the Law*, 2nd edn, London: Penguin.

Brazzi, L., Pelosi, P. and Gattinoni, L. (1997) 'Oxygen delivery and consumption in intensive care unit practice: goal-directed therapy', *Current Anaesthesia and Critical Care* 8(6): 285–9.

Brett, S.J. and Evans, T.W. (1997) 'Acute lung injury', in D.R. Goldhill and P.S. Withington (eds) *Textbook of Intensive Care*, London: Chapman & Hall: 369–77.

Brewer, S.C., Wunderink, R.G., Jones, C.B. *et al.* (1996) 'Ventilator-associated pneumonia due to pseudomonas aeruginosa', *Chest* 109(4): 1019–29.

Bridel, J. (1993) 'The epidemiology of pressure sores', *Nursing Standard* 7(42): 25–30.

Bridges, M.J. and Middleton, R. (1997) 'Direct arterial vs oscillometric monitoring of blood pressure: stop comparing and pick one', *Critical Care Nurse* 17(3): 58–72.

Briggs, D. (1996a) 'Nasogastric feeding in intensive care units: a study', *Nursing Standard* 49(10): 42–5.

—— (1996b) 'What type of nasogastric tube should we use in the intensive care unit? *Intensive and Critical Care Nursing* 12(2): 102–5.

Briggs, M. (1995) 'Principles of acute pain assessment', *Nursing Standard* 9(19): 23–7.

Brimacombe, J., Berry, A., Brain, A.I.J. *et al.* (1997) 'The laryngeal mask airway – literature update', in L. Kaufman and R. Ginsburg (eds) *Anaesthesia Review 13*, New York: Churchill Livingstone: 121–38.

British National Formulary (BNF) (1998) *British National Formulary* No. 38 (September), London: BMA/Royal Pharmaceutical Society.

British Paediatric Association (1993) *The Care of Critically Ill Children: Report of a Multidisciplinary Working Party* London: British Paediatric Association.

Broughton, A.N. and Filcek, S.A.L. (1990) 'Dopexamine hydrochloride', *Intensive Therapy and Clinical Monitoring* 11(6): 202–8.

Brucia, J. and Rudy, E. (1996) 'The effect of suction catheter insertion and tracheal stimulation in adults with severe brain injury', *Heart and Lung* 25(4): 295–303.

Bruder, N., N'Zdghe, P., Graziani, N. *et al.* (1995) 'A comparison of extradural and intraparenchymatous intracranial pressures in head injured patients', *Intensive Care Medicine* 21(10): 850–2.

Brudney, K. and Dobkin, J. (1991) 'Resurgent tuberculosis in New York City: human immunodeficiency virus, homelessness and the decline of tuberculosis control programmes', *American Review of Respiratory Diseases* 144(4): 745–9.

Bruton, W.A.T. (1995) 'Infection and hospital laundry', *Lancet* 345(8964): 1574–5.

Buckley, P.M. and McFie, J. (1997) 'Enteral nutrition in critically ill patients: a review', *Care of the Critically Ill* 13(1): 7–10.

Budden, L. and Vink, R. (1996) 'Paracetamol overdose: pathophysiology and nursing management', *British Journal of Nursing* 5(3): 145–52.

Burglass, E.A. (1995) 'Oral hygiene', *British Journal of Nursing* 4(9): 516–19.

Burroughs, J. and Hoffbrand, B.I. (1990) 'A critical look at nursing observations', *Postgraduate Medical Journal* 66(775): 370–2.

Buswell, C. (1996) 'Beta thalassaemia', *Professional Nurse* 12(2): 145–7.

Byrne, C. (1995) 'Choosing a therapy', in D. Rankin-Box (ed.) *The Nurse's Handbook of Complementary Therapies*, Edinburgh: Churchill: 7–12.

Caldwell, K., Francome, C. and Lister, J. (1998) *The Envy of the World*, London: NHS Support Federation.

Califf, R.M. and Bengston, J.R. (1994) 'Cardiogenic shock', *New England Journal of Medicine* 330(24): 1724–30.

Calne, S. (1994) 'Dehumanisation in intensive care', *Nursing Times* 90(17): 31–3.

Calzia, E. and Radermacher, P. (1997) 'Airway pressure release ventilation and biphasic positive airway pressure', *Clinical Intensive Care* 8(6): 296–301.

Campbell, B. (1997) 'Arterial waveforms: monitoring changes in configuration', *Heart and Lung* 26(3): 204–14.

Campbell, I.T. (1997) 'Thermoregulation in critical illness', *British Journal of Anaesthesia* 78(2): 121–2.

Camsooksai, J. (1997) 'Inhaled nitric oxide: a possible therapy for ARDS', *Nursing in Critical Care* 2(5): 251–4.

Canavan, T. (1984) 'The psychology of sleep', *Nursing* 2(23): 682–3.

Caritas, S., Sibai, B., Hauth, J. *et al.* (1998) 'Low-dose aspirin to prevent preeclampsia in women at high risk', *New England Journal of Medicine* 338(11): 701–5.

Carlet, J. (1992) 'Selective decontamination of the digestive tract in ICU patients', *Intensive Care World* 9(3): 116–18.

Carleton, P.F. and Boldt, M. (1992) 'Coronary atherosclerotic disease', in S.A. Price and L.M. Wilson (eds) *Pathophysiology: Clinical Concepts of Disease Processes*, St Louis: Mosby: 421–46.

Carlson, K.K. (1995) 'Acute renal failure', in N.A. Urban, K.K. Greenlee, J.M. Krumberger *et al.* (eds) *Guidelines for Critical Care*, St Louis: Mosby: 501–09.

Carlson, P.C. (1997) 'Patient care and expectations for recovery after transmyocardial laser revascularization', *AACN Clinical Issues* 8(1): 33–40.

Carnevale, F.A. (1991) 'High technology and humanity in intensive care: finding a balance', *Intensive Care Nursing* 7(1): 23–7.

Caron, E.A. and Berlandi, J.L.H. (1997) 'Extracorporeal membrane oxygenation', *Nursing Clinics of North America* 32(1): 125–40.

Carroll, D. (1997) 'A non-pharmacological approach to chronic pain', *Professional Nurse Study Supplement* 13(1): S12–S14.

Case, R.B., Heller, S.S., Case, N.B. *et al.* (1985) 'Type A behaviour and survival after acute myocardial infarction', *New England Journal of Medicine* 312(12): 737–41.

Castella, X., Artigas, A., Bion, J. *et al.* (1995) 'A comparison of severity illness scoring systems for intensive care unit patients: results of a multicenter, multinational study', *Critical Care Medicine* 23(8): 1327–35.

Castillo-Lorente, E., Rivera-Fernandy, R. and Vasquez-Mata, G. (1997) 'Limitations of therapeutic activity in elderly critical patients', *Critical Care Medicine* 25(10): 1643–8.

Cathelyn, J.L. (1998) 'SvO_2 monitoring: tool for evaluating patient outcomes', *Dimensions of Critical Care Nursing* 17(2): 58–63.

Cavanagh, J.D. and Colvin, B.T. (1997) 'Bleeding and clotting disorder', in D.R. Goldhill and P.S. Withington (eds) *Textbook of Intensive Care*, London: Chapman & Hall: 545–54.

Cedidi, C., Myer, M., Kuse, E. *et al.* (1994) 'Urodilatin: a new approach for the treatment of therapy-resistant renal failure after liver transplantation', *European Journal of Clinical Investigations* 24(9): 632–9.

Chalfin, D.B. and Carlon, G.C. (1990) 'Age utilization of intensive care unit resources of critically ill cancer patients', *Critical Care Medicine* 18(7): 694–8.

Chalmers, A.G. (1991) 'Acute pancreatitis: radiological approaches', *Care of the Critically Ill* 7(4): 140–5.

Chatte, G., Sab, J-M., Dubois, J-M. *et al.* (1997) 'Prone position in mechanically ventilated patients with acute severe respiratory failure', *American Journal of Respiratory Critical Care Medicine* 155(2): 473–8.

Chellel, A., Dawson, D., Endacott, R. *et al.* (1995) 'Patient scoring systems in critical care', *British Journal of Intensive Care* 5(8): 250–4.

Chelluri, L., Pinsky, M.R. and Donahoe, M.P. (1993) 'Long term outcome of critically ill elderly patients requiring intensive care', *JAMA* 269(24): 3119–223.

Chitnavis, B.P. and Polkey, C.E. (1998) 'Intracranial pressure monitoring', *Care of the Critically Ill* 14(3): 80–4.

Cho, D.Y. and Wang, Y.C. (1997) 'Comparison of the APACHE III, APACHE II and Glasgow Coma Scale in acute head injury for prediction of mortality and functional outcome', *Intensive Care Medicine* 23(1): 77–84.

Chow, G., Roberts, I.G., Harris, D. *et al.* (1997) 'Stockert roller pump generated pulsatile flow: cerebral metabolic changes in adult cardiopulmonary bypass', *Perfusion* 12(2): 113–19.

Chudley, S. (1994) 'The effects of nursing activities on ICP', *British Journal of Nursing* 3(9): 454–9.

Clacy, J. (1998) 'The ultimate gift: organ donation the nurse's role', *Nursing Standard* 13(39): RCN Nursing Update Learning Unit 083.

Clancy, J. and McVicar, A.J. (1995) *Physiology and Anatomy: A Homeostatic Approach*, London: Edward Arnold.

Clapham, L., Harrison, J. and Raybould, T. (1995) 'A multidisciplinary audit of manual hyperinflation technique (sigh breath) in a neurosurgical intensive care unit', *Intensive and Critical Care Nursing* 11(5): 265–71.

Clarke, A.P., Winslow, E.H., Tyler, D.O. *et al.* (1990) 'Effects of endotracheal suctioning on mixed venous oxygen saturation and heart rate in critically ill adults', *Heart and Lung* 19(5, 2): 552–7.

Clarke, G. (1993) 'Mouthcare and the hospitalised patient', *British Journal of Nursing* 2(4): 225–7.

Clarke, G.M. (1997) 'Severe sepsis', in T.E. Oh (ed.) *Intensive Care Manual*, 4th edn, Oxford: Butterworth Heinemann: 525–39.

CLASP Collaborative Group. (1994) 'CLASP: a randomised trial of low-dose aspirin for the prevention and treatment of pre-eclampsia among 9364 pregnant women', *Lancet* 343(8898): 619–29.

Closs, M. 1996. 'Managing resistance: integrating nurse practitioner and nursing roles in a primary health care setting', *Nursing Practice* 21(2): 7.

Closs, S.J. (1992) 'Patients' night-time pain, analgesia provision and sleep after surgery', *International Journal of Nursing Studies* 29(4): 381–92.

Clutton-Brock, T.H. (1997) 'The assessment and monitoring of respiratory function', in D.R. Goldhill and P.S. Withington (eds) *Textbook of Intensive Care*, London: Chapman & Hall: 345–55.

Coad, S. (1996) 'Cardiovascular needs', in C. Viney (ed.) *Nursing the Critically Ill* London: Baillière Tindall. 77–119.

Coakley, J.H. (1997) 'Polyneuropathy', in D.R. Goldhill and P.S. Withington (eds) *Textbook of Intensive Care*, London: Chapman & Hall: 503–06.

Cobley, M., Atkins, M. and Jones, P.L. (1991) 'Environmental contamination during tracheal suctioning', *Anaesthesia* 46(11): 957–61.

Cochran, J. and Ganong, L.H. (1989) 'A comparison of nurses and patients perceptions of ICU stressors', *Journal of Advanced Nursing* 14(12): 1038–43.

Cochrane Injuries Group Albumin Reviewers (1998) 'Human albumin in critically ill patients: systemic review of randomised control trials', *British Medical Journal* 317(7153): 235–40.

Cockroft, S. (1997) 'Cardiac infection, inflammation and myopathy', in D.R. Goldhill and P.S. Withington (eds) *Textbook of Intensive Care*, London: Chapman & Hall: 287–97.

Coetzee, E.J., Dommisse, J. and Anthony, J. (1998) 'A randomised control trial of intravenous magnesium sulphate versus placebo in the management of women with severe pre-eclampsia', *British Journal of Obstetrics and Gynaecology* 105(3): 300–3.

Cohen, A.T. and Kelly, D.R. (1987) 'Assessment of alfentanil by intravenous infusion as a long-term sedation in intensive care', *Anaesthesia* 45(5): 545–8.

Cohn, E.G. and Gilroy-Doohan, M. (1996) *Flip and see ECG*, Philadelphia: W.B. Saunders.

Coleman, N.J. and Houston, L. (1998) 'Demystifying acid-base regulation', *Australian Journal of Nursing* 5(8): 23–6.

Comfort, A. (1977) *A Good Age*, London: Mitchell Beazey.

Conlin, C. (1995) 'Extracorporeal liver assistance device: hope for the future', *Critical Care Quarterly* 17(4): 73–8.

Conrad, S.A., Eggerstedt, J.M., Grier, L.R. *et al.* (1995) 'Intravenacaval membrane oxygenation and carbon dioxide removal in severe acute respiratory failure', *Chest* 107(6): 1689–97.

Cook, A. (1995) 'Ecstasy, MDMA: alerting users to the dangers', *Nursing Times* 91(16): 32–3.

Cook, D.J., Guyatt, G.H., Jaeschke, R. *et al.* (1995) 'Determinants in Canadian health care workers of the decision to withdraw life support from the critically ill', *JAMA* 273(9): 703–8.

Cook, S. and Palma, O. (1989) 'Diprivan as the sole sedative agent for prolonged infusion in intensive care', *Journal of Drug Development* 2(supplement 2): 65–7.

Cookson, B. (1997) 'Is it time to stop searching for MRSA? *British Medical Journal* 314(7081): 664–5.

Coombs, M. (1991) 'Motivational strategies for intensive care nurses', *Intensive Care Nursing* 7(2): 114–19.

—— (1993) 'Haemodynamic profiles and the critical care nurse', *Intensive and Critical Care Nursing* 9(1): 11–16.

Cornock, M.A. (1996) 'Making sense of arterial blood gases and their interpretation', *Nursing Times* 92(6): 30–1.

Cotterill, M.R.B. (1996) 'Helicobacter pylori', *Professional Nurse* 12(1): 46–8.

Cottle, S. (1997) 'Nurse's under-medication of analgesia in cardiac surgical patients: a personal exploration', *Nursing in Critical Care* 2(3): 146–9.

Coughlan, A. (1994) 'Music therapy in ICU', *Nursing Times* 90(12):35.

Coull, A. (1992) 'Making sense of pulse oximetry', *Nursing Times* 88(32): 42–3.

Cowan, M.J., Shelhamer, J.H. and Levine, S.J. (1997) 'Acute respiratory failure in the HIV-seropositive patient', *Critical Care Clinics* 13(3): 523–52.

Cowe, F. (1996) 'Living wills: making patients' wishes known', *Professional Nurse* 11(6): 362–3.

Cowley, H.C. and Webster, N.R. (1993) 'Management of liver disease on ICU', *Care of the Critically Ill* 9(3): 122–127.

Cox, C. and Hayes, J. (1998) 'Experiences of administering and receiving therapeutic touch in intensive care', *Complementary Therapies in Nursing and Midwifery* 4(5): 128–33.

Cox, P. (1992) 'Children in critical care: how parents cope', *British Journal of Nursing* 1(15): 764–8.

Creamer, J.E. and Rowlands, D.J. (1996) 'Electrocardiographic diagnosis of tachycardias', in D.J. Rowlands (ed.) *Recent Advances in Cardiology*, 12, Edinburgh: Churchill Livingstone: 115–43.

Crimlisk, J.T., Horn, M.H., Wilson, D.J. *et al.* (1996) 'Artificial airways: a survey of cuff management practices', *Heart and Lung* 25(3): 225–35.

Crippen, D. (1992) 'Stress, agitation and brain failure in critical care medicine', *Critical Care Quarterly* 15(2): 52–74.

Crosby, C. (1989) 'Method in mouth care', *Nursing Times* 85(35): 38–40.

Crouser, E.D. and Dorinsky, P.M. (1994) 'Gastrointestinal tract dysfunction in critical illness: pathophysiology and interaction with acute lung injury in adult respiratory distress syndrome/multiple organ dysfunction syndrome', *New Horizons* 2(4): 476–87.

Crowe, H.M. (1996) 'Nosocomial pneumonia: problems and progress', *Heart and Lung* 25(5): 418–21.

Cruz, J., Jaggi, J.L. and Hoffstad, O.J. (1995) 'Cerebral blood flow, vascular resistance, and oxygen metabolism in acute brain trauma. Redefining the role of cerebral perfusion pressure?', *Critical Care Medicine* 23(8): 1412–17.

Cubbin, B. and Jackson, C. (1991) 'Trial of a pressure area risk calculator for intensive care patients', *Intensive Care Nursing* 7(1): 40–4.

Cunningham, M. (1997) 'Ecstasy-induced rhabdomyolysis and its role in the development of acute renal failure', *Intensive and Critical Care Nursing* 13(4): 216–32.

Cureton-Lane, R.A. and Fontaine, D.K. (1997) 'Sleep in the pediatric ICU: an empirical investigation', *American Journal of Critical Care* 6(1): 56–63.

Curry, S. (1995) 'Identifying family needs and stresses in the intensive care unit', *British Journal of Nursing* 4(1): 15–21.

Curzen, N.P. and Evans, T.W. (1996) 'The endothelium and the vascular response to sepsis', in T.W. Evans and C.J. Hinds (eds) *Recent Advances in Critical Care Medicine*, 4, New York: Churchill Livingstone: 69–90.

Cuthbertson, B.H., Stott, S., Webster, N.P. (1997) 'Inhaled nitric oxide in British intensive therapy units', *British Journal of Anaesthesia* 78(6): 696–700.

Cutler, R. (1996) 'Acute respiratory distress syndrome: an overview', *Intensive and Critical Care Nursing* 12(6): 316–26.

Czarnik, R.E., Stone, K.S., Everhart, C.G.. *et al.* (1991) 'Differential effects of continuous versus intermittent suction on tracheal tissue', *Heart and Lung* 20(2): 144–57.

d'Amico, R., Pifferi, S., Leonetti, C. *et al.* (1998) *British Medical Journal* 316(7140): 1275–85.

Daffurn, K., Bishop, G.F., Hillman, K.M. *et al.* (1994) 'Problems following discharge after intensive care', *Intensive and Critical Care Nursing* 10(4): 244–51.

Dark, J.H. (1997) 'Lung: living related transplantation', *British Medical Bulletin* 53(4): 892–903.

Davidhizer, R.E., Poole, V.L. and Giger, J.N. (1995) 'What nurses need to know about sleep', *Journal of Nursing Science* 1(1/2): 61–7.

Davidson, J.A.H. and Boom, S.J. (1995) 'The significance of free radicals', *British Journal of Intensive Care* 5(5): 150–5; 5(6): 185–93.

Davidson, J.A.H. and Hosie, H.E. (1993) 'Limitations of pulse oximetry; respiratory insufficiency: a failure of detection', *British Medical Journal* 307(6900): 372–3.

Davis, I., Pack, G. and Logan, J. (1997) 'Promoting patient sleep: a critical but forgotten practice? *CACCN* 8(1): 12–17.

Davis, P. (1993) 'Opening up the gate control theory', *Nursing Standard* 7(45): 25–7.

Day, M. (1996) 'The bitterest pill', *Nursing Times* 92(7): 16–17.

Day, R. (1993) 'Mouth care in an intensive care unit: a review', *Intensive and Critical Care Nursing* 9(4): 246–52.

DBL (1991) 'Strong sterile dopamine hydrochloride solution' (data sheet), Warwick: Faulding.

de Beauvoir, S. (1970) *Old Age*, London: Penguin.

de Gregorio, J., Kobayashi, Y. and Albiero, R. (1998) 'Coronary artery stenting in the elderly: short-term outcome and long-term angiographic and clinical follow-up', *Journal of American College of Cardiologists* 32(3): 577–83.

de Jong, M.G. (1996) 'Medicinal devices single sterile use disposable', *International Journal of Intensive Care* 3(2): 73–5.

Deakin, C.D. (1997) 'Recent advances in cardiopulmonary resuscitation', in L. Kaufman and R. Ginsburg (eds) *Anaesthesia Review*, 13, New York: Churchill Livingstone: 139–62.

Dearden, N. (1991) 'Jugular bulb venous oxygen saturation in the management of severe head injury', *Current Opinion in Anaesthesiology* 2(4): 279–86.

deBono, D.P. (1990) 'Thrombolysis in the intensive therapy unit', *Intensive Therapy and Clinical Monitoring* 11(1): 25–8.

—— (1992) 'Coronary thrombolysis', in D.J. Rowlands (ed.) *Recent Advances in Cardiology*, 11, Edinburgh: Churchill Livingstone: 29–46.

Deby, C., Hartstein, G.D-D., Kamy, M. *et al.* (1995) 'Antioxidant therapy', in J. Bion, H. Burchardi, R. Dellinger *et al.* (eds) *Current Topics in Intensive Care* 2, London: Saunders (pp. 175–205).

Deitch, E.A. (1995) 'Tumour necrosis factor as the proximal mediator of sepsis – or this too will pass', *Critical Care Medicine* 23(9): 1457–8.

Dellinger, R.P., Zimmerman, J.L., Taylor, R.W. *et al.* (1998) 'Effects of inhaled nitric oxide in patients with acute respiratory distress syndrome: results of a randomised phase 2 trial', *Critical Care Medicine* 26(1): 15–23.

Depasse, B., Pauwels, D., Somers, Y. *et al.* (1998) 'A profile of European ICU nursing', *Intensive Care Medicine* 24(9): 939–45.

Desforges, J.F. (1992) 'The Guillain-Barré syndrome', *New England Journal of Medicine* 326(17): 1130–6.

Dickson, A. (1982) *A Woman In Your Own Right*, London: Quartet Books.

Diehl, C., Hass, J. and Schaefer, K.M. (1994) 'The brain-dead pregnant woman: finding meaning to help care', *Dimensions of Critical Care Nursing* 13(3): 133–41.

Dimond, B. (1995) *Legal Aspects of Nursing*, 2nd edn, London: Prentice Hall.

Dinsmore, J. and Hall, G.M. (1997) 'Metabolic emergencies: malignant hyperthermia and porphyria', in D.R. Goldhill and P.S. Withington (eds) *Textbook of Intensive Care*, London: Chapman & Hall: 603–10.

Dirkes, S. (1996) 'Liquid ventilation: new frontiers in the treatment of ARDS', *Critical Care Nurse* 16(3): 53–8.

DiRusso, S.M., Nelson, L.D., Safcsak, K. *et al.* (1995) 'Survival in patients with severe adult respiratory distress syndrome treated with high level positive end expiratory pressure', *Critical Care Medicine* 23(9): 1485–96.

Dobb, G.J. (1997) 'Gastrointestinal failure', in D.R. Goldhill and P.S. Withington (eds) *Textbook of Intensive Care*, London: Chapman & Hall: 467–76.

Dobson, F. (1993) 'Shedding light on pulse oximetry', *Nursing Standard* 7(46): 4–11.

Dobson, P.M.S., Edbrooke, D.L. and Reilly, C.S. (1993) 'The role of kinetic therapy in intensive care', *British Journal of Intensive Care* 3(10): 369–374.

Doebbling, B.N., Stanley, G.L. and Sheets, C.T. (1992) 'Comparative efficacy of alternative hand-washing agents in reducing nosocomial infections in intensive care units', *New England Journal of Medicine* 327(2): 88–93.

Doezema, D., Lunt, M. and Tandberg, D. (1995) 'Cerumen occlusion lowers infrared tympanic membrane temperature measurement', *Emergency Medicine* 2(1): 17–19.

Department of Health (DoH) (1959) *The Welfare of Children in Hospital: Report of the Committee on Child Health Services* London: HMSO.

—— (1977) *Health Circular* (HC 77, 22), London: DoH.

—— (1989) *A Strategy for Nursing*, London: DoH.

—— (1991) *The Patient's Charter*, London: HMSO.

—— (1992) *The Health of the Nation*, London: HMSO.

—— (1993) *Pressure Sores: A Key Quality Indicator*, London: DoH.

—— (1994a) *Nutritional Aspects of Cardiovascular Disease*, Committee on Medical Aspects of Food Policy: Report on Health and Social Subjects, 46, London: HMSO.

—— (1994b) *Report on Confidential Enquiries Into Maternal Deaths in the United Kingdom (1988–1990)*, London: HMSO.

—— (1995) *The Patient's Charter*, 2nd edn, London: HMSO.

—— (1996a) *Guidelines on Admission to and Discharge from Intensive Care and High Dependency Units*, London: DoH.

—— (1996b) *Report on Confidential Enquiries Into Maternal Deaths in the United Kingdom (1991–1993)*, London: HMSO.

—— (1997) *A Bridge to the Future: Nursing Standards, Education and Workforce Planning in Paediatric Intensive Care*, London: HMSO.

—— (1998a) *Our Healthier Nation*, London: HMSO.

—— (1998b) *Code of Practice for the Diagnosis of Brain Stem Death*, London: HMSO.

Doig, C.J., Sutherland, L.R., Sandham, J.D. *et al.* (1998) 'Increased intestinal permeability is associated with the development of multiple organ dysfunction syndrome in critically ill ICU patients', *American Journal of Respiratory and Critical Care Medicine* 158(2): 444–51.

Dolan, M. and Hughes, N. (1997) 'Hepatitis C: a bloody business', *Nursing Times* 93(45): 71–2.

Donnelly, T.J., Meade, P., Jagels, M. *et al.* (1994) 'Cytokine, complement and endotoxin profiles associated with the development of the adult respiratory distress syndrome after severe injury', *Critical Care Medicine* 22(5): 768–76.

Douglas, K.A. and Redman, C.W.G. (1994) 'Eclampsia in the United Kingdom', *British Medical Journal* 309(6966): 1395–1400.

Doverty, N. (1994) 'Make pain assessment your priority', *Professional Nurse* 9(4): 230–7.

Dowling, S., Martin, R., Skidmore, P. *et al.* (1996) 'Nurses taking on junior doctors work: a confusion of accountability', *British Medical Journal* 312(7040): 1211–14.

Downey, S. (1995) 'Acupuncture', in D. Rankin-Box (ed.) *The Nurse's Handbook of Complementary Therapies*, Edinburgh: Churchill Livingstone: 43–50.

Downie, R.S. and Calman, K.C. (1994) *Healthy Respect*, Oxford: Oxford University Press.

Doyle, B. (1990) 'Nutritional considerations in care of the elderly', in C. Eliopoulos (ed.) *Caring for the Elderly in Diverse Care Settings*, Philadelphia: Lippincott.

Draper, P. (1987) 'Not a job for juniors', *Nursing Times* 83(10): 58–62.

Drew, K., Brayton, M., Ambrose, A. *et al.* (1998) 'End-tidal carbon dioxide monitoring for weaning patients: a pilot study', *Dimensions of Critical Care Nursing* 17(3): 127–34.

Driessen, J.J., Dhaese, H., Fransen, G. *et al.* (1995) 'Pulsatile compared with nonpulsatile perfusion using a centrifugal pump for cardiopulmonary bypass during coronary artery bypass grafting: effects on systemic haemodynamics, oxygenation, and inflammatory response parameters', *Perfusion* 10(1): 3–12.

Drucker, P. (1974) *Management*, London: Butterworth-Heinemann.

—— (1977) *People and Performance: The Best of Peter Drucker on Management*, London: Heinemann.

Drummond, G.B. (1996) 'Mechanisms of breathing: effects of anaesthesia', in C. Prys-Roberts and B.R. Brown Jr. (eds) *International Practice of Anaesthesia*, Oxford: Butterworth Heinemann: 1/59/1–26.

Duckworth, G.J. (1990) 'Methicillin-resistant staphylococcus aureus', *Care of the Critically Ill* 6(6): 214–16.

Duke, G.J. and Bersten, D.A. (1992) 'Dopamine and renal salvage in the critically ill patient', *Anaesthetic Intensive Care* 23(3): 277–302.

Duke, G.J., Briedeff, J.H. and Weaver, R.A. (1994) 'Renal support in critically ill patients: low-dose dopamine or low-dose dobutamine? *Critical Care Medicine* 22(12): 1919–25.

Duke, J., Murphy, B. and Bell, A. (1998) 'Nurse's attitudes toward organ donation: an Australian perspective', *Dimensions of Critical Care Nursing* 17(5): 264–71.

Dunn, C., Sleep, J. and Collett, D. (1995) 'Sensing an improvement: an experimental study to evaluate the use of aromatherapy, massage and periods of rest in an intensive care unit', *Journal of Advanced Nursing* 21(1): 34–40.

Dunning, J. (1997) 'Artificial heart transplants', *British Medical Bulletin* 53(4): 706–18.

Dunstan, G.R. (1997) 'The ethics of organ donation', *British Medical Bulletin* 53(4): 921–39.

Dyer, I. (1995) 'Preventing the ITU syndrome, or how not to torture an ITU patient', *Intensive and Critical Care Nursing* 11(3): 130–9; 11(4): 223–32.

Earp, J.K. and Finlayson, D.C. (1992) 'Urinary bladder/pulmonary artery temperature ratio of less than 1 and shivering in cardiac surgical patients', *American Journal of Critical Care* 1(2): 43–52.

Earp, J.K. and Mallia, G. (1997) 'Myocardial protection for cardiac surgery: the nursing perspective', *AACN Clinical Issues* 8(1): 20–32.

Eastabrooks, C.A. and Morse, J.A. (1992) 'Towards a theory of touch: the touching process and acquiring a touching style', *Journal of Advanced Nursing* 17(4): 448–56.

Eburn, E. (1993) 'Monoclonal antibodies: the future of pharmacology', *Intensive and Critical Care Nursing* 9(1): 24–7.

Eclampsia Trial Collaborative Group (1995) 'Which anticonvulsant for women with eclampsia? Evidence from the Collaborative Eclampsia', *Lancet* 345(8963): 1455–63.

Eddleston, J., Cheetham, E. and Nightingale, P. (1996) 'Clinical audit in intensive care', *British Journal of Intensive Care* 6(1): 16–20.

Eddleston, J., Macdonald, I. and Littler, C. (1997) 'Withdrawal of sedation in critically ill patients', *British Journal of Intensive Care* 7(6): 216–22.

Edwards, D. (1997) 'Respiratory physiology', in D.R. Goldhill and P.S. Withington (eds) *Textbook of Intensive Care*, London: Chapman & Hall: 327–36.

Edwards, J.D. (1994) 'Technology responds to the challenge', *International Journal of Intensive Care* 1(3): 77.

Edwards, M. (1994) 'The rationale for the use of risk calculators in pressure sore prevention, and the evidence of the reliability and validity of published scales', *Journal of Advanced Nursing* 20(2): 288–96.

Edwards, S.L. (1998) 'Determining hypovolaemia using trans-oesophageal Doppler monitoring', *Nursing in Critical Care* 3(4): 176–81.

Elliott, M.W., Steven, M.H., Phillips, G.D. *et al.* (1990) 'Non-invasive mechanical ventilation for acute respiratory failure', *British Medical Journal* 300(6721): 358–60.

Ellis, A. and Cavanagh, S.J. (1992) 'Aspects of neurosurgical assessment using the Glasgow Coma Scale', *Intensive and Critical Care Nursing* 8(2): 94–9.

Ellis, M.F. (1995) 'Systemic inflammatory response syndrome, sepsis, and septic shock', in N.A. Urban, K.K. Greenlee, J.M. Krumberger *et al.* (eds) *Guidelines for Critical Care* St Louis: Mosby: 607–17.

—— (1998) 'Atrial fibrillation following cardiac surgery', *Dimensions of Critical Care Nursing* 17(5): 226–39.

Elpern, E.H., Larson, R., Douglas, P. *et al.* (1989) 'Long-term outcomes for elderly survivors of prolonged ventilator assistance', *Chest* 96(5): 1120–4.

Emmerson, A.M. (1997) 'Infection control in hospital and community settings', *Research and Clinical Forums* 19(6): 19–25.

Endacott, R. (1996) 'Staffing intensive care units: a consideration of contemporary issues', *Intensive and Critical Care Nursing* 12(4): 193–9.

Erickson, R.S. and Kirklin, S.K. (1993) 'Comparison of ear-based, bladder, oral, and axillary methods for core temperature measurements', *Critical Care Medicine* 21(10): 1528–34.

Erickson, R.S., Meyer, L.T. and Woo, T.M. (1995) 'Accuracy of chemical dot thermometers in critically ill adults and young children', *Image: Journal of Nursing Scholarship* 28(1): 23–8.

Ervine, I.M. and Milroy, S.J. (1997) 'Recent developments in renal physiology and pathophysiology: implications for therapy in acute renal failure', in L. Kaufman and R. Ginsburg (eds) *Anaesthesia Review*, 13, New York: Churchill Livingstone: 27–42.

Ethics Committee of the Society of Critical Care Medicine (1997) 'Consensus statement of the Society of Critical Care Medicine's Ethics Committee regarding futile and other possible inadvisable treatments', *Critical Care Medicine* 25(5): 887–91.

Evans, D. (1998) 'Inotropic therapy: current controversies and future directions', *Nursing in Critical Care* 3(1): 8–12.

Evans, J. (1997) 'HIV infection in children', *Care of the Critically Ill* 13(1): 21–3.

Evans, J.C. and French, D.G. (1995) 'Sleep and healing in intensive care settings', *Dimensions of Critical Care Nursing* 14(4): 189–99.

Fagan, E.A. (1995) 'Febrile granuloma', *British Journal of Intensive Care* 5(2): 59–66.

Farrell, M. and Wray, F. (1993) 'Eye care for ventilated patients', *Intensive and Critical Care Nursing* 9(2): 137–41.

Farrington, A. (1997) 'Strategies for reducing stress and burnout in nursing', *British Journal of Nursing* 6(1): 44–50.

Fawcett, J. (1997) 'Ventilator technology: safety and comfort for patients?', *Nursing in Critical Care* 2(1): 7–10.

Feest, T.G., Riad, H.N., Collins, C.H. *et al.* (1990) 'Protocol for increasing organ donation after cerebrovascular deaths in a district general hospital', *Lancet* 335(8698): 1133–5.

Feil, N. (1993) *The validation breakthrough*, Baltimore: Health Professionals Press.

Feldman, Z. and Robertson, C.S. (1997) 'Monitoring of cerebral haemodynamics with jugular bulb catheters', *Critical Care Clinics* 13(1): 51–77.

Feltham, E. (1991) 'Therapeutic touch and massage', *Nursing Standard* 5(45): 26–8.

Ferguson, J., Gilroy, D. and Puntillo, K. (1997) 'Dimensions of pain and analgesic administration associated with coronary artery bypass grafting in an Australian intensive care unit', *Journal of Advanced Nursing* 26(6): 1065–72.

Fiddian-Green, R.G. (1995) 'Gastric intramucosal pH, tissue oxygenation and acid-base balance', *British Journal of Anaesthesia* 74(5): 592–606.

Finocchiaro, D. and Herzfeld, S. (1990) 'Understanding autonomic dysreflexia', *American Journal of Nursing* 90(9): 56–9.

Fiorentini, A. (1992) 'Potential hazards of tracheobronchial suctioning', *Intensive and Critical Care Nursing* 8(4): 217–26.

Fitzgerald, J.D. (1992) 'Applied pharmacology of cardiovascular drugs', in J. Tinker and W. Zapol (eds) *Care of the Critically Ill Patient* New York: Springer-Verlag: 329–64.

Fitzpatrick, G. and Donnelly, M. (1997) 'Assessment of cardiac function', in D.R. Goldhill and P.S. Withington (eds) *Textbook of Intensive Care*, London: Chapman & Hall: 271–9.

Flapan, A.D. (1994) 'Management of patients after their first myocardial infarction', *British Medical Journal* 309(6962): 1129–34.

Fleck, A. and Smith, G. (1998) 'Albumin in intensive care', *British Journal of Intensive Care* 8(3): 89–95.

Forbes, A.M. (1997) 'Colloids and blood products', in T.E. Oh (ed.) *Intensive Care Manual*, 4th edn, Oxford: Butterworth-Heinemann: 754–9.

Ford, K. (1992) 'A seasonal depression: management of seasonal affective disorder', *Professional Nurse* 8(2): 94–8.

Ford, P. and Walsh, M. (1994) *New rituals for old*, Oxford: Butterworth Heinemann.

Fort, P., Farmer, C., Westerman, J. *et al.* (1997) 'High frequency oscillatory ventilation for adult respiratory distress syndrome – a pilot study', *Critical Care Medicine* 25(6): 937–47.

Foubert, L., Latimer, R.D. and Oduro, A. (1993) 'Vasodilators', *Current Opinion in Anaesthesiology* 6(1): 152–7.

Fox, J. (1989) 'Conjunctivitis, keratitis and iritis', *Nursing* 3(45): 20–3.

Foxall, M., Zimmerman, L., Standley, R. *et al.* (1990) 'A comparison of frequency and sources of nursing job stress perceived by intensive care, hospice and medical-surgical nurses', *Journal of Advanced Nursing* 15(5): 577–84.

Francome, C. and Marks, D. (1996) *Improving the Health of the Nation* London: Middlesex University Press.

Fraser, R.B. and Saunders, N.J. StJ. (1990) 'The obstetric management of severe pre-eclampsia/eclampsia', *Care of the Critically Ill* 6(1): 7–9.

Freeman, J.W. (1998) 'Solvent detergent treated plasma, viral safety and clinical experience', *British Journal of Intensive Care* 8(5): 172–5.

French, M.A.H. (1997) 'HIV infection and the acquired immunodeficiency syndrome', in T.E. Oh (ed.) *Intensive Care Manual*, 4th edn, Oxford: Butterworth Heinemann: 519–24.

French, S. (1989) 'Pain: some psychological and sociological aspects', *Physiotherapy* 75(5): 255–60.

Frid, I., Bergbom-Engberg, I. and Haljamae, H. (1998) 'Brain death in ICUs and associated nursing care challenges concerning patients and families', *Intensive and Critical Care Nursing* 14(1): 21–9.

Friedman, L.S., Martin, P. and Munoz, S.J. (1996) 'Liver function tests and the objective evaluation of the patient with liver disease', in D. Zakim and T.D. Boyer (eds) *Hepatology: A Textbook of Liver Disease*, 3rd edn, Philadelphia: Saunders: 791–833.

Fristoe, L.W., Merrill, J.H., Kangas, J.A. *et al.* (1993) 'Extracorporeal support with a cadaver liver as a bridge to transplantation', *Journal of Extra-corporeal Technology* 25(4): 133–9.

Frostell, C.G., Fratacci, M.D., Wain, J.C. *et al.* (1991) 'Inhaled nitrogen oxide: a selective vasodilator reversing hypoxic pulmonary vasoconstriction', *Circulation* 83(6): 2038–47.

Fuggle, P., Shand, P.A., Gill, L.J. *et al.* (1996) 'Pain, quality of life, and coping in sickle cell disease', *Archives of Diseases in Childhood* 75(3): 199–203.

Fulbrook, P. (1993) 'Core temperature measurement: a comparison of rectal, axillary and pulmonary artery temperature', *Intensive and Critical Care Nursing* 9(4): 217–25.

—— (1996a) 'The care of critically ill children in adult ICUs: the way forward', *Nursing in Critical Care* 1(6): 265–7.

—— (1996b) 'Advanced practice: do we know what it is?', *Nursing in Critical Care* 1(1): 9–12.

—— (1997) 'Core body temperature measurement: a comparison of axilla, tympanic membrane and pulmonary artery blood temperature', *Intensive and Critical Care Nursing* 13(5): 266–72.

Fulbrook, S.D. and Wilkinson, M.B. (1997) 'Xenotransplantation and the law', *British Journal of Theatre Nursing* 7(2): 21–24.

Fulgham, J.R. and Wijdicks, E.F.M. (1997) 'Guillain Barre syndrome', *Critical Care Clinics* 13(1): 1–16.

Gagne, R.M. (1975) *Essentials of Learning for Instruction*, New York: Holt, Reinhart & Winston.

—— (1985) *The Condition of Learning and Theory Instruction*, London: Holt, Reinhart & Winston.

Galvani, M., Ottani, F., Ferrini, D. *et al.* (1996) 'Coronary thrombolysis: what do the clinical trials tell us about the preferred approach? in D.J. Rowlands (ed.) *Recent Advances in Cardiology*, 12, Edinburgh: Churchill Livingstone: 3–26.

Ganong, W.F. (1995) *Review of Medical Physiology*, 17th edn, London: Prentice Hall.

Gardner, P.E. (1995) 'Hemodynamic monitoring', in N.A. Urban, K.K. Greenlee, J.M. Krumberger *et al.* (eds) *Guidelines for Critical Care*, St Louis: Mosby: 295–309.

Gaston-Johansson, F., Hofgren, C., Watson, P. *et al.* (1991) 'Myocardial infarction pain: systematic description and analysis', *Intensive Care Nursing* 7(1): 3–10.

Gattinoni, L., Bombino, M., Pelosi, P. *et al.* (1994) 'Lung structure and function in different stages of severe adult respiratory distress syndrome', *JAMA* 271(22): 1772–9.

Gattinoni, L., Presenti, A., Bombino, M. *et al.* (1993) 'Role of extracorporeal circulation in adult respiratory distress syndrome management', *New Horizons* 1(4): 603–12.

Gattinoni, L., Presenti, A., Mascheroni, D. *et al.* (1986) 'Low-frequency positive-pressure ventilation with extracorporeal CO_2 removal in severe acute respiratory failure', *JAMA* 256(7): 881–6.

Geary, M. (1997) 'The HELLP syndrome', *British Journal of Obstetrics and Gynaecology* 104(8): 887–91.

Gerlach, H. and Falke, K.J. (1995) 'The therapeutic role of nitric oxide in adult respiratory distress syndrome', *Current Anaesthesia and Critical Care* 6(1): 10–16.

Germon, T.J., Kane, N.M., Manara, A.R. *et al.* (1994) 'Near infrared spectroscopy in adults: effects of extracranial ischaemia and intracranial hypoxia on estimation of cerebral oxygenation', *British Journal of Anaesthesia* 73(4): 503–6.

Gerraci, E. and Gerraci, T. (1996) 'A look at recent hyperventilation studies: outcomes and recommendations for early use in the head-injured patient', *Journal of Neuroscience Nursing* 28(4): 222–4.

Gibbons, M. (1997) 'Transcutaneous oxygen monitoring in congenital diaphragmatic abnormalities', *Nursing in Critical Care* 2(3): 132–7.

Gibbs, W.W. (1996) 'Gaining on fat', *Scientific American* 274(8): 70–6.

Gibson, V. (1994) 'Does nurse turnover mean nurse wastage in Intensive Care Units? *Intensive and Critical Care Nursing* 10(1): 32–40.

—— (1996) 'The factors influencing organ donation: a review of the research', *Journal of Advanced Nursing* 23(2): 353–6.

Gimson, A.E.S., Ramage, J.K., Panos, M.Z. *et al.* (1993) 'Randomised control trial of variceal banding ligation versus injection sclerotherapy for bleeding oesophageal varices', *Lancet* 342(8868): 391–4.

Gin, T. and Ngan Kee, W.D. (1997) 'Obstetric emergencies', in T.E. Oh (ed.) *Intensive Care Manual*, 4th edn, Oxford: Butterworth Heinemann: 494–8.

Glass, G., Grap, M.J., Corley, M.C. *et al.* (1993) 'Nurses ability to achieve hyperinflation and hyperoxgenation with a manual resuscitation bag during endotracheal suctioning', *Heart and Lung* 22(2): 156–65.

Gluck, E., Heard, S., Patel, C. *et al.* (1993) 'Use of ultrahigh frequency ventilation in patients with ARDS', *Chest* 103(5): 1413–20.

Godard, C. and Gask, L. (1991) 'Problem drinking in the elderly', *Geriatric Medicine* 21(5): 18.

Goffman, E. (1963) *Stigma*, London: Penguin.

Goldhill, D.R. and Sumner, A. (1998) 'Outcome of intensive care patients in a group of British intensive care units', *Critical Care Medicine* 26(8): 1337–45.

Goldhill, D.R. and Withington, P.S. (1996) 'Mortality predicted by APACHE 2', *Anaesthesia* 51(8): 719–23.

Gomersall, C.D. and Oh, T.E. (1997) 'Haemodynamic monitoring', in T.E. Oh (ed.) *Intensive Care Manual*, 4th edn, Oxford: Butterworth-Heinemann: 831–8.

Gordon, P.A., Norton, J.M. and Merrell, R. (1995) 'Refining chest tube management: analysis of the state of practice', *Dimensions of Critical Care Nursing* 14(1): 6–12.

Gosheron, M., Leaver, G., Foster, A. *et al.* (1998) 'Prone lying: a nursing perspective', *Care of the Critically Ill* 14(3): 89–92.

Gosling, P. (1995) 'How to guides: blood gas analysis', *Care of the Critically Ill* 11(1): centre insert.

—— (1999) 'Fluid balance in the critically ill: the sodium and water audit', *Care of the Critically Ill* 15(1): 11–16.

Gosnell, D.J. (1973) 'An assessment tool to identify pressure sores', *Nursing Research* 22(1): 55–9.

Gotloib, L., Barzilay, E., Shustak, A. *et al.* (1984) 'Sequential haemofiltration in nonoliguric high capillary permeability pulmonary edema of severe sepsis: preliminary report', *Critical Care Medicine* 12(11): 997–1000.

Gould, D.J. (1994a) 'Nurses' hand decontamination practice: results of a local study', *Journal of Hospital Infection* 28(1): 15–30.

Gould, D.J. and Chamberlain, A. (1994) 'Infection control as a topic for ward-based nursing education', *Journal of Advanced Nursing* 20(2): 275–82.

Gould, I.M. (1994b) 'Strategies for antibacterial therapy in the ITU', in M. Rennie (ed.) *Intensive Care Britain (1993)*, London: Greycoat: 82–5.

Granberg, A., Enberg, I.B. and Lundberg, D. (1996) 'Intensive care syndrome: a literature review', *Intensive and Critical Care Nursing* 12(3): 173–82.

Grap, M.J., Glass, C., Corley, M. *et al.* (1994) 'Effects of level of lung injury on HR, PAP and SaO_2 changes during suctioning', *Intensive and Critical Care Nursing* 10(3): 171–8.

Graver, J. (1992) 'Inotropes: an overview', *Intensive and Critical Care Nursing* 8(3): 169–79.

Gray, J.E., MacIntyre, N.R. and Kronenberger, W.G. (1990) 'The effects of bolus normal-saline in conjunction with endotracheal suctioning', *Respiratory Care* 35(8): 785–90.

Gray, P.A., Bodenham, A.R. and Park, G.R. (1991) 'A comparison of low dose dopexamine and dopamine infusion to prevent renal impairment during liver transplantation', *Anaesthesia* 46(8): 638–41.

Graziano, C.C., Fox, S.J. and Ackerman, N.J. (1987) 'Evaluation of a closed suction system', *Critical Care Medicine* 15(5): 522–5.

Grech, E.D., Jackson, M.J. and Ramsdale, D.R. (1995) 'Reperfusion injury after acute myocardial infarction', *British Medical Journal* 310(6978): 477–8.

Green, A. (1996) 'An exploratory study of patients' memory recall of their stay in an adult intensive therapy unit', *Intensive and Critical Care Nursing* 12(3): 131–7.

Green, J.H. (1976) *An Introduction to Human Physiology*, 4th edn, Oxford: Oxford University Press.

Green, R.A. and Goodwin, G.M. (1996) 'Ecstasy and neurodegeneration', *British Medical Journal* 312(7045): 1493–4.

Greene, J.H. and Klinger, J.R. (1998) 'The efficacy of inhaled nitric oxide in the treatment of acute respiratory distress syndrome', *Critical Care Clinics* 14(3): 387–409.

Greenough, A. (1994) 'Extracorporeal membrane oxygenation', *Care of the Critically Ill* 10(1): 15–1.

—— (1995) 'Nitric oxide: clinical aspects', *Care of the Critically Ill* 11(4): 143–6.

—— (1996) 'Liquid ventilation', *Care of the Critically Ill* 12(4): 128–30.

Greenspan, J.S. (1993) 'Liquid ventilation: a developing technology', *Neonatal Network* 12(4): 23–34.

Griffiths, P. (1995) 'Reflexology', in D. Rankin-Box (ed.) *The Nurse's Handbook of Complementary Therapies*, Edinburgh: Churchill Livingstone: 133–40.

Grimble, G., Payne-James, J.J., Rees, R.G. *et al.* (1989) 'TPN: novel energy substrates', *Intensive Therapy and Clinical Monitoring* 10(4): 108–13.

Grimble, R. (1994) 'The modulation of immune function by dietary fat', *British Journal of Intensive Care* 4(5): 159–67.

Groeneveld, P.H.P., Kwappenberg, K.M.C., Kangermans, J.A.M. *et al.* (1996) 'Nitric oxide, NO) production correlates with renal insufficiency and multiorgan dysfunction syndrome in severe sepsis', *Intensive Care Medicine* 22(11): 1197–1202.

Groenveld, A.B.J. and Thijs, L.G. (1991) 'Is oxidative metabolism dependant on oxygen delivery in septic shock? *Care of the Critically Ill* 7(1): 14–18.

Grotte, G.J. and Rowlands, D.J. (1992) 'Long term management of patients with prosthetic heart valves', in D.J. Rowlands (ed.) *Recent Advances in Cardiology, II*, Edinburgh: Churchill Livingstone: 271–94.

Grover, E.R. (1993) 'The role of nitric oxide in the management of an acute lung injury', in M. Rennie (ed.) *Intensive Care Britain (1993)* London: Greycoat: 107–10.

Grubb, A., Walsh, P., Lambe, N. *et al.* (1996) 'Survey of British clinicians' views on management of patients in persistent vegetative state', *Lancet* 348(9019): 35–40.

Grubb, B.D. (1998) 'Peripheral and central mechanism of pain', *British Journal of Anaesthesia* 81(1): 8–11.

Grundstein-Amado, R. (1992) 'Differences in ethical decision-making processes among nurses and doctors', *Journal of Advanced Nursing* 17(2): 129–37.

Guenter, P.A., Perlmutter, S., Marino, D.L. *et al.* (1991) 'Tube feeding-related diarrhoea in acutely ill patients', *Journal of Parenteral and Enteral Nutrition* 15(3): 277–80.

Gunderson, L.P. and Stoeckle, M.L. (1995) 'Endotracheal suctioning of the newborn piglet', *Western Journal of Nursing Research* 17(1): 20–31.

Gunn, T. (1992) *The Man With Night Sweats*, London: Faber.

Gunning, K.E.J. (1997) 'Pancreatitis', in D.R. Goldhill and P.S. Withington (eds) *Textbook of Intensive Care*, London: Chapman & Hall: 477–82.

GUSTO Angiographic Investigators (1993) 'The effects of tissue plasminogen activator, streptokinase, or both on coronary-artery patency, ventricular function, and survival after acute myocardial infarction', *New England Journal of Medicine* 329(22): 1615–33.

Guyton, A.C. and Hall, J.E. (1997) *Human Physiology and Mechanisms of Disease*, 6th edn, Philadelphia: W B Saunders.

Hagler, D.A. and Travers, G.A. (1994) 'Endotracheal saline and suction catheters: sources of lower airway contamination', *American Journal of Critical Care* 3(6): 444–7.

Hall, C.A. (1997) 'Patient management in head injury care: a nursing perspective', *Intensive and Critical Care Nursing* 13(6): 329–37.

Hall-Lord, M.L., Larsson, G. and Bostrom, I. (1994) 'Elderly patients' experience of pain and distress in intensive care: a grounded theory study', *Intensive and Critical Care Nursing* 10(3): 133–41.

Hall-Smith, J., Ball, C. and Coakley, J. (1997) 'Follow-up services and the development of a clinical nurse specialist in intensive care', *Intensive and Critical Care Nursing* 13(5): 243–8.

Haller, M., Zollner, C., Briegel, J. *et al.* (1995) 'Evaluation of a new continuous thermodilution cardiac output monitor in critically ill patients: a prospective criterion standard study', *Critical Care Medicine* 23(5): 860–6.

Halliday, M.L., Kang, L-Y., Zhou, T-K. *et al.* (1991) 'An epidemic of hepatitis A attributable to the ingestion of raw clams in Shanghai, China', *Journal of Infectious Diseases* 164(5): 852–9.

Halpern, N.A., Bettes, L. and Greenstein, R. (1994) 'Federal and nationwide intensive care units and healthcare costs: 1986-(1992) *Critical Care Medicine* 22(12): 2001–7.

Hambley, H. (1995) 'Coagulation, II: clinical problems in coagulation disorder', *Care of the Critically Ill* 11(5): 203–5.

Hammond, F. (1995) 'Involving families in care within the intensive care environment: a descriptive study', *Intensive and Critical Care Nursing* 11(5): 256–64.

Hammond, J., Johnson, H.M., Varas, R. *et al.* (1991) 'A qualitative comparison of paper flowsheets vs a computer based clinical information system', *Chest* 99(1): 155–7.

Hampton, J.R. (1997a) *The ECG Made Easy*, 5th edn, Edinburgh: Churchill Livingstone.

—— (1997b) *The ECG in Practice*, 3rd edn, Edinburgh: Churchill Livingstone.

Hancock, H. (1996) 'Implementing change in the management of post-operative pain', *Intensive and Critical Care Nursing* 12(6): 359–62.

Hanley, D. (1997) 'Intracranial hypertension', in T.E. Oh (ed.) *Intensive Care Manual*, 4th edn, Oxford: Butterworth-Heinemann: 395–402.

Hanley, M.V., Rudd, T. and Butler, J. (1978) 'What happens to intratracheal saline installations', *American Review of Respiratory Diseases* 117: 124–6.

Hanson, G.C. (1990) 'Severe pre-eclampsia and eclampsia – hypotensive and anti-convulsant management', *Care of the Critically Ill* 6(1): 10–12.

Hanson, G. and Elston, R.A. (1990) 'Infection control over the next decade', *Intensive Therapy and Clinical Monitoring* 11(5): 153–7.

Hardy, G. (1991) 'Blood, fluids and electrolytes', *British Journal of Intensive Care* 1(5): 194–5.

Harper, N.C. and Collee, G.R. (1997) 'Poisoning, overdose and toxic exposure', in D.R. Goldhill and P.S. Withington (eds) *Textbook of Intensive Care*, London: Chapman & Hall: 687–96.

Harrahill, M. (1991) 'Pulse oximetry, pearls and pitfalls', *Journal of Emergency Nursing* 17(6): 437–9.

Harris, T.A. (1970) *I'm OK – You're OK*, London: Pan Books.

Hartstein, A.I., Denny, M.A., Morthland, V.H. *et al.* (1995) 'Control of methicillin-resistant Staphylococcus aureus in a hospital and an intensive care unit', *Infection control and hospital epidemiology* 16(7): 405–11.

Hatton-Smith, C.K. (1994) 'A last bastion of ritualised practice?', *Professional Nurse* 9(5): 304–8.

Hawker, F.H. (1997a) 'Hepatic failure', in T.E. Oh (ed.) *Intensive Care Manual*, 4th edn, Oxford: Butterworth-Heinemann: 343–53.

—— (1997b) 'Liver transplantation', in T.E. Oh (ed.) *Intensive Care Manual*, 4th edn, Oxford: Butterworth-Heinemann: 802–10.

Hayward, J. (1975) *Information: A Prescription Against Pain*, London: RCN.

Hazinski, M.F. (1992) *Nursing Care of the Critically Ill Child*, 2nd edn, London: Mosby.

Heals, D. (1993) 'A key to well-being', *Professional Nurse* 8(6): 391–8.

Health and Safety Executive (HSE) (1989) *Control of Substances Hazardous to Health Regulations*, London: HSE.

Heaton, N.D. (1997) 'Liver transplantation in children', *Care of the Critically Ill* 13(3): 90–5.

Heffner, J.E. (1993) 'Timing of tracheostomy in mechanically ventilated patients', *American Review of Respiratory Disease* 147(3): 768–71.

Heinz, J. and Yakovich, F. (1988) 'Washing with contaminated bar soap is unlikely to transfer bacteria', *Epidemiology of Infection* 101: 135–42.

Henderson, L. (1987) 'Haemofiltration', *The Kidney* 20(6): 25.

Henderson, V. (1980) 'Preserving the essence of nursing in a technological age', *Journal of Advanced Nursing* 5(3): 245–60.

Hendricks-Thomas, J. and Patterson, E. (1995) 'A sharing in critical thought by nursing faculty', *Journal of Advanced Nursing* 22(3): 594–9.

Herbert, R.A. (1991) 'The biology of human ageing', in S.J. Redfern (ed.) *Nursing Elderly People*, 2nd edn, Edinburgh: Churchill Livingstone: 39–63.

Herings, R.M.C., de Boer, A. and Stricker, B.H.C. (1995) 'Hypoglycaemia associated with use of inhibitors of angiotensin converting enzyme', *Lancet* 345(8959): 1195–8.

Herlitz, J., Karlson, B., Lindqvist, J. *et al.* (1997) 'Long-term prognosis in men and women coming to the emergency department with chest pain or other symptoms suggestive of acute myocardial infarction', *European Journal of Emergency Medicine* 4(4): 196–203.

Heuser, M.D., Case, L.D. and Ettinger, W.H. (1992) 'Mortality in intensive care patients with respiratory disease – is age important? *Archives of Internal Medicine* 152(8): 1683–8.

Hewlitt, P.E. and Machin, S.J. (1990) 'Massive blood transfusion', *British Medical Journal* 300(6717): 107–9).

Heyland, D.K. (1998) 'Nutritional support in the critically ill patient', *Critical Care Clinics* 14(3): 423–40.

Hickey, J.V. (1997a) 'Intracranial pressure: theory and management of intracranial pressure', in J.V. Hickey (ed.) *The Clinical Practice of Neurological and Neurosurgical Nursing*, 4th edn, Philadelphia: Lippincott: 295–328.

—— (1997b) 'Vertebral and spinal cord injuries', in J.V. Hickey (ed.) *The Clinical Practice of Neurological and Neurosurgical Nursing*, 4th edn, Philadelphia: Lipincott: 419–68.

Hickling, K.G. (1996) 'Acute lung injury: new concepts in ventilatory support', in T.W. Evans and C.J. Hinds (eds) *Recent Advances in Critical Care Medicine*, 4, New York: Churchill Livingstone: 20–43.

Hickling, K.G., Walsh, J., Henderson, S.J. *et al.* (1994) 'Low mortality rates in adult respiratory distress syndrome using low-volume, pressure-limited ventilation with permissive hypercapnia', *Critical Care Medicine* 22(10): 1568–78.

Hickman, K.M., Mayer, B.L. and Muswases, M. (1990) 'Intracranial pressure monitoring: review of risk factors associated with infection', *Heart and Lung* 19(1): 84–9.

Hill, C.F. (1993) 'Is massage beneficial to critically ill patients in intensive care units? A critical review', *Intensive and Critical Care Nursing* 9(2): 116–21.

Hillel, Z. and Thys, D.M. (1994) 'Electrocardiography', in R.D. Miller, R.F. Cucchiara, E.D. Miller *et al.* (eds) *Anaesthesia*, 4th edn, New York: Churchill Livingstone: 1229–52.

Hillman, D.R. (1997) 'Respiratory function tests', in T.E. Oh (ed.) *Intensive Care Manual*, 4th edn, Oxford: Butterworth-Heinemann: 839–47.

Hillman, K. and Bishop, G. (1996) *Clinical Intensive Care* Cambridge: Cambridge University Press.

Hilton, L., Uliss, A., Samuels, S. *et al.* (1983) 'Nosocomial bacterial eye infections in intensive care', *Lancet* 207(8337): 1318–20.

Hilton, P.J., Taylor, J., Forni, L.G. *et al.* (1998) 'Bicarbonate-based haemofiltration in the management of acute renal failure with lactic acidosis', *QJM* 91(4): 279–83.

Hinds, C.J. and Watson, D. (1996) *Intensive Care: A Concise Textbook*, 2nd edn, London: W B Saunders.

Hinwood, B. (1993) *A Textbook of Science for the Health Professions*, 2nd edn, London: Chapman & Hall.

Hipkiss, A. (1989) 'The production and removal of abnormal proteins: a key question in the biology of ageing', in A.M. Warnes (ed.) *Human Ageing and Later Life*, London: Edward Arnold: 15–28.

Hirschl, M.M., Binder, M., Gwechenberger, M. *et al.* (1997) 'Noninvasive assessment of cardiac output in critically ill patients by analysis of the finger blood pressure waveform', *Critical Care Medicine* 25(11): 1909–14.

Hlatky, M.A., Rogers, W.J., Johnstone, I. *et al.* (1997) 'Medical care costs and quality of life after randomalisation to coronary angioplasty or coronary bypass surgery', *New England Journal of Medicine* 336(2): 92–9.

Hobbes, T. (1962) [1651] *Leviathan*, Glasgow: Collins/Fontana.

Hockings, B.E.F. and Donovan, K.D. (1997) 'Acute myocardial infarction', in T.E. Oh (ed.) *Intensive Care Manual*, 4th edn, Oxford: Butterworth-Heinemann.

Hodgson, L.A. (1991) 'Why do we need sleep? Relating theory to practice', *Journal of Advanced Nursing* 16(12): 1503–10.

Hoffbrand, A.V. and Pettit, J.E. (1993) *Essential Haematology*, 3rd edn, Oxford: Blackwell Scientific.

Hohlfeld, J.M., Tiryaki, E., Hamm, H. *et al.* (1998) 'Pulmonary surfactant activity is impaired in lung transplant recipients', *American Journal of Respiratory and Critical Care Medicine* 158(3): 706–12.

Holloway, T. and Penson, J (1998) 'Nursing education as social control', *Nurse Education Today* 7(5): 235–41.

Holmes, S. and Mountain, E. (1993) 'Assessment of oral status: evaluation of three oral assessment guides', *Journal of Clinical Nursing* 2(1): 35–40.

Holowaty, L. (1995) 'Nitric oxide', *Neonatal Network: Journal of Neonatal Nursing* 16(6): 83–6.

Holtzclaw, B.J. (1992) 'The febrile response in critical care: state of the science', *Heart and Lung* 21(5): 482–501.

Hopkinson, R.B. and Freeman, J.W. (1988) 'Therapeutic progress in intensive care, sedation and analgesia', *Journal of Clinical Pharmacology and Therapeutics* 13(1): 33–40.

Hormann, C., Baum, M., Putensen, C. *et al.* (1994) 'Effect of kinetic therapy in patients with severe adult respiratory distress syndrome', *Critical Care Medicine* 22(1): A87.

Hornbein, T.F. (1994) 'Acid-base balance', in R.D. Miller, R.F. Cucchiara, E.D. Miller *et al.* (eds) *Anaesthesia*, 4th edn, New York: Churchill Livingstone: 1883–1400.

Horton, S. (1995) 'Support for bereaved relatives in ICU', *Professional Nurse* 10(9): 568–70.

Horvath, K.D., Gray, D., Benton, L. *et al.* (1998) 'Operative outcomes of minimally invasive saphenous vein harvest', *American Journal of Surgery* 175(5): 391–5.

Horwood, A. (1990) 'Malnourishment in intensive care units, as high as 50%: Are nurses doing enough to change this? *Intensive Care Nursing* 6(4): 205–8.

Hough, A. (1996) *Physiotherapy in Respiratory Care*, 2nd edn, London: Chapman and Hall.

House of Lords Judgement (1993) *Airedaile NHS Trust v. Bland HL*, 2WLR 317.

House of Lords Select Committee on Science and Technology (1998) *Resistance to Antibiotics and Other Antimicrobial Agents*, London: HMSO.

Howie, J.N. (1989) 'How and when should I respond to postop fever? *American Journal of Nursing* 87(7): 984–6.

Hudak, C.M., Gallo, B.M. and Morton, P.G. (eds) (1998) *Critical Care Nursing: A Holistic Approach*, 7th edn, Philadelphia: Lippincott.

Hudson, L.D. (1995) 'New therapies for ARDS', *Chest* 108(2): supplement 79S-91S.

Hug, C.C. Jr. and Shanewise, J.S. (1994) 'Anesthesia for adult cardiac surgery', in R.D. Miller, R.F. Cucchiara, E.D. Miller *et al.* (eds) *Anaesthesia*, 4th edn, New York: Churchill Livingstone: 1759–1809.

Humphreys, H. and Duckworth, G. (1997) 'Methicillin-resistant *Staphylococcus aureus*, MRSA: a re-appraisal of control measures in the light of changing circumstances', *Journal of Hospital Infection* 36(3): 167–70.

Hund, E.F., Borel, C.O., Cornblath, D.R. *et al.* (1993) 'Intensive management and treatment of severe Guillain-Barré Syndrome', *Critical Care Medicine* 21(3): 433–46.

Hund, E.F., Fogel, W., Krieger, D. *et al.* (1996) 'Critical illness polyneuropathy: clinical findings and outcomes of a frequent cause of neuromuscular weaning failure', *Critical Care Medicine* 24(8): 1328–33.

Hunt, G. and Wainwright, P. (1994) *Expanding the Role of the Nurse*, Oxford: Blackwell.

Hunt, J. (1993) 'Application of a pressure area risk calculator in an intensive care unit', *Intensive and Critical Care Nursing* 9(4): 226–31.

Hutchison, A.S., Ralston, S.H., Dryburgh, F.J. *et al.* (1983) 'Too much heparin: possible source of error in blood gas analysis', *British Medical Journal* 287, 6399: 1131–1132.

Idama, T.O. and Lindow, S.W. (1998) 'Magnesium sulphate: a review of clinical pharmacology applied to obstetrics', *British Journal of Obstetrics and Gynaecology* 105(3): 260–8.

Imai, H., Schaap, R.N. and Mortensen, J.D. (1994) 'Rate of thrombus accumulation on intravenacaval IVOX devices explanted from human clinical trial patients with acute respiratory failure', *Artificial Organs* 18(11): 818–21.

Intensive Care Society (1992) *Standards for Intensive Care Units*, London: Biomedica.

International Council of Nurses (1991), *Position Statement: Nursing Care of the Elderly*, Geneva: International Council of Nurses.

Isaac, J.L. and Manji, M. (1997) 'Hepatopulmonary syndrome', *Current Anaesthesia and Critical Care* 8(5): 237–40.

Isbister, J.P. (1997a) 'Blood transfusion', in T.E. Oh (ed.) *Intensive Care Manual*, 4th edn, Oxford: Butterworth-Heinemann: 741–53.

Isbister, J.P. (1997b) 'Haematological malignancies', in T.E. Oh (ed.) *Intensive Care Manual*, 4th edn, Oxford: Butterworth-Heinemann: 786–92.

ISIS-2 (1988) 'Randomised trial of intravenous streptokinase, oral aspirin, both or neither among 17,187 cases of suspected acute myocardial infarctions: ISIS 2', *Lancet* ii (8608): 349–60.

ISIS-3 (1992) 'A randomised trial of streptokinase vs tissue plasminogen activator versus alteplase and of aspirin plus heparin versus aspirin alone among 41,299 cases of suspected acute myocardial infarctions', *Lancet* 399: 753–70.

ISIS-4 (1995) 'A randomised factorial trial assessing early oral captopril, oral mononitrate, and intravenous magnesium sulphate in 58,050 patients with suspected acute myocardial infarction', *Lancet* 345(8951): 669–85.

Jackson, C. (1996) 'Humidification in the upper respiratory tract: a physiological overview', *Intensive and Critical Care Nursing* 12(1): 27–32.

Jackson, C. (1999) 'The revised Jackson/Cubbin pressure area risk calculator', *Intensive and Critical Care Nursing* 15(3): 169–75.

Jakobsen, C.J. (1995) 'Invasive cardiac output monitoring', *International Journal of Intensive Care* 2(2): 48–52.

James, I. (1991) 'Respiratory management in paediatrics', *Care of the Critically Ill* 7(2): 47–50.

Jamieson, E.M. and McCall, J.M. (1992) *Guidelines for Clinical Nursing Practice*, 2nd edn, Edinburgh: Churchill Livingstone.

Jansen, M.J., Hendriks, T., Knapen, M.F.C.M. *et al.* (1998) 'Chlorpromazine down-regulates tumor necrosis factor-alpha and attenuates experimental multiple organ dysfunction syndrome in mice', *Critical Care Medicine* 26(7): 1244–50.

Janssens, M. and Lamy, M. (1989) 'Laryngeal mask', *Intensive Care World* 10(2): 99–102.

Jeevaratnam, D.R. and Menon, D.K. (1996) 'Survey of intensive care management of severely head injured patients in the United Kingdom', *British Medical Journal* 312(7036): 944–7.

Jeffries, D.J. (1991) 'Zidovudine after occupational exposure to HIV', *British Medical Journal* 302(6789): 1349–51.

Jenkins, D.A. (1989) 'Oral care in the ICU: an important nursing role', *Nursing Standard* 4(7): 24–8.

Jenkins, M. (1997) 'Early extubation post-cardiac surgery – implications for nursing practice', *Nursing in Critical Care* 2(6): 276–8.

Jensen, L.A., Onyskiw, J.E. and Prasad, N.G.N. (1998) 'Meta-analysis of arterial oxygen saturation monitoring by pulse oximetry in adults', *Heart and Lung* 27(6): 387–408.

Johnson, C. (1992) 'The nurse's role in organ donation from a brainstem dead patient: management of the family', *Intensive and Critical Care Nursing* 8(3): 140–8.

Johnson, C.D. (1998) 'Severe acute pancreatitis: a continuing challenge for the intensive care team', *British Journal of Intensive Care* 8(4): 130–7.

Johnson, C.S. (1994) 'Knowledge of immunology is essential to plan effective nursing for immunocompromised patients', *Intensive and Critical Care Nursing* 10(2): 121–6.

Johnson, L.G. and McMahan, M.J. (1997) 'Postoperative factors contributing to prolonged length of stay in cardiac surgery patients', *Dimensions in Critical Care Nursing* 16(5): 243–50.

Johnson, M.I. (1998) 'Does transcutaneous electrical nerve stimulation (TENS) work? *Clinical Effectiveness in Nursing* 2(3): 111–20.

Jones, A. (1995) 'A brief overview of the analysis of lung sounds', *Physiotherapy* 81(1): 37–42.

Jones, C., Griffiths, R.D., Macmillan, R.R. *et al.* (1994) 'Psychological problems occurring after intensive care', *British Journal of Intensive Care* 4(2): 46–53.

Jones, C. and Griffiths, R.D. (1995) 'Social support and anxiety levels in relatives of critically ill patients', *British Journal of Intensive Care* 5(2): 44–7.

Jones, C. and Owens, D. (1996) 'The recreational drug user in the Intensive Care Unit: a review', *Intensive and Critical Care Nursing* 12(3): 126–30.

Jones, C., Macmillan, R.R., Harris, C. *et al.* (1997) 'Severe tracheal stenosis associated with reintubation', *Clinical Intensive Care* 8(3): 122–5.

Jones, C.V. (1998) 'The importance of oral hygiene in nutritional support', *British Journal of Nursing* 7(2): 74–83.

Jones, S.E. (1995) 'Getting the balance right: pulse oximetry and inspired oxygen concentration', *Professional Nurse* 10(6): 368–73.

Jørgensen, M., Gustafsen, K.B., Ernst, S. *et al.* (1992) 'Disseminated intravascular coagulation in critically ill patients – laboratory diagnosis', *Intensive Care World* 9(3): 108–14.

Joynes, J. (1996) 'An analysis of component parts of advanced practice in relation to acute renal failure in intensive care', *Intensive and Critical Care Nursing* 12(2): 113–19.

Juarez, V.J., Lyons, M. (1995) 'Inter-rater reliability of the Glasgow Coma Scale', *Journal of Neuroscience Nursing* 27(5): 283–6.

Juste, R.N., Panikkar, K., Soni, N. (1998) 'The effects of low-dose dopamine infusions on haemodynamic and renal parameters in patients with septic shock requiring treatment with noradrenaline', *Intensive Care Medicine* 24(6): 564–8.

Kalia, P., Webster, N.R. (1997) 'New modes of respiratory support', in D.R. Goldhill and P.S. Withington (eds) *Textbook of Intensive Care,* London: Chapman & Hall: 401–07.

Kallas, H.J. (1998) 'Non-conventional respiratory support modalities applicable in the older child', *Critical Care Clinics* 14(4): 655–83.

Kam, P.C.A., Kam, A.C. and Thompson, J.F. (1994) 'Noise pollution in the anaesthetic and intensive care environment', *Anaesthesia* 49(11): 982–6.

Kaplan, A.A. (1985a) 'Pre-dilution versus post-dilution for CAVH', *Transactions of the American Society of Artificial Organs* 31: 28–32.

—— (1985b) 'Acute fatty liver of pregnancy', *New England Journal of Medicine* 313(6): 367–70.

—— (1998) 'Continuous renal replacement therapy, CRRT) in the intensive care unit', *Journal of Intensive Care Medicine* 13(2): 85–105.

Kaplan, A.A. and Epstein, M. (1997) 'Extracorporeal blood purification in the management of patients with hepatic failure', *Seminars in Nephrology* 17(6): 576–82.

Karnik, A. and Freeman, J.W. (1998) 'Acute liver failure', *Care of the Critically Ill* 14(5): 148–54.

Kaufman, L. (1997) 'Medicine relevant to anaesthesia', in L. Kaufman and R. Ginsburg (eds) *Anaesthesia Review*, 13, New York: Churchill Livingstone: 5–26.

Kaye, C.G., Smith, D.R. (1988) 'Complications of central venous catheterisation', *British Medical Journal* 297(6648): 572–3.

Keely, B.R. (1998) 'Preventing complications: recognition and treatment of autonomic dysreflexia', *Dimensions in Critical Care Nursing* 17(4): 170–6.

Kelly, B.J. and Matthay, M.A. (1993) 'Prevalence and severity of neurologic dysfunction in critically ill patients', *Chest* 104(6): 1818–24.

Kelsey, S.M. and Colvin, B.T. (1997) 'Bleeding and clotting disorder', in D.R. Goldhill and P.S. Withington (eds) *Textbook of Intensive Care*, London: Chapman & Hall: 555–65.

Kennedy, J.F. (1997) 'Enteral feeding for the critically ill patient', *Nursing Standard* 11(33): 39–43.

Keogh, B.F. (1995) 'Modes of ventilation in adult respiratory distress syndrome', *Current Anaesthesia and Critical Care* 6(1): 17–24.

—— (1996) 'New modes of ventilatory support', *Current Anaesthesia and Critical Care* 7(5): 228–235.

Kerber, K. (1995) 'Hypovolaemic shock', in N.A. Urban, K.K. Greenlee, J.M. Krumberger *et al.* (eds) *Guidelines for Critical Care*, St Louis: Mosby: 601–06.

Kerr, M.E., Rudy, E.B., Weber, B.B. *et al.* (1997) 'Effect of short duration hyperinflation during endotracheal suctioning on intracranial pressure in severe head-injured adults', *Nursing Research* 46(4): 195–201.

Kesteven, P., Saunders, P. (1993) 'Disseminated intravascular coagulation', *Care of the Critically Ill* 9(1): 22–27.

Ketefian, S. (1978) 'Strategies of curriculum change', *International Nursing Review* 25(1): 14–24.

Keyzer, D., Wright, S. (1998) 'Change strategies: the classic models', in S. Wright (ed.) *Changing Nursing Practice*, 2nd edn, London: Arnold: 7–24.

Kiening, L., Unterberg, A., Bardt, T. *et al.* (1996) 'Monitoring of cerebral oxygenation in patients with severe head injuries: brain tissue pO_2 versus jugular vein oxygen saturation', *Journal of Neurosurgery* 85: 751–7.

Kilner, A.J., Janes, E.F. (1997) 'Intensive care in the elderly', *Current Anaesthesia and Critical Care* 8(3): 120–5.

Kilpatrick, S., Matthay, M. (1992) 'Obstetric patients requiring critical care', *Chest* 101(5): 1407–12.

Kimmings, A.N., Gouma, D.J., van Deventer, S.J.H. (1994) 'Endotoxin in the pathogenesis of gram negative sepsis', *Care of the Critically Ill* 10(4): 170–3.

King's Fund (1989) 'ICU in the United Kingdom: report from the King's Fund Panel', *Intensive Care Nursing* 5(2): 76–81.

—— (1992) *A Positive Approach to Nutrition as Treatment*, London: King's Fund.

Kingston, P., Hopwood, A. (1994) 'The elderly person in the Accident and Emergency Department', in L. Sbaih (ed.) *Issues in Accident and Emergency Nursing* London: Chapman and Hall: 165–82.

Kirby, S.A. and Davenport, A. (1996) 'Haemofiltration/dialysis treatment in patients with acute renal failure', *Care of the Critically Ill* 12(2): 54–8.

Kite, K. and Pearson, L. (1995) 'A rationale for mouth care: the integration of theory with practice', *Intensive and Critical Care Nursing* 11(2): 71–6.

Klein, D.G., Mitchell, C., Petrina, A. *et al.* (1993) 'A comparison of pulmonary artery, rectal and tympanic membrane temperature measurement in the ICU', *Heart and Lung* 22(5): 435–41.

Klintmalm, G.B. (1998) 'Liver transplantation for heptocellular carcinoma: a registry report of the impact of tumor characteristics on outcome', *Annals of Surgery* 228(4): 479–90.

Knaus, W.A. (1987) 'Too sick and old for intensive care', *British Journal of Hospital Medicine* 37(5): 381.

Knaus, W.A., Draper, E.A., Wagner, D.P. *et al.* (1985) 'APACHE II: a severity of disease classification system', *Critical Care Medicine* 13(10): 818–29.

Knaus, W.A., Wagner, D.P, Draper, E.A. *et al.* (1991) 'The APACHE III prognostic system: risk prediction of hospital mortality for critically ill hospitalised adults', *Chest* 100(6): 1619–36.

Knight, G.J. (1997) 'Sedation and analgesia in children', in T.E. Oh (ed.) *Intensive Care Manual*, 4th edn, Oxford: Butterworth-Heinemann: 907–11.

Knox, A.M. (1993) 'Performing endotracheal suction on children', *Intensive and Critical Care Nursing* 9(1): 48–54.

Konopad, E., Ker, J., Noseworthy, T. *et al.* (1994) 'A comparison of oral, axillary, rectal and tympanic-membrane temperatures of intensive care patients with and without an oral endotracheal tube', *Journal of Advanced Nursing* 20(1): 77–84.

Kootstra, G., Kievit, J.K., Heineman, E. (1997) 'The non heart-beating donor', *British Medical Bulletin* 53(4): 844–53.

Krachman, S.L., D'Alonzo, G.E. and Criner, G.J. (1995) 'Sleep in the intensive care unit', *Chest* 107(6): 1713–20.

Krafft, P., Metnitz, P., Fridrich, P. *et al.* (1997) 'Impact of inhaled nitric oxide on cardiopulmonary performances and outcome or ARDS patients: a literature review', *Clinical Intensive Care* 8(1): 27–32.

Kramer, M. (1991) 'Benefits of paracetamol antipyresis in young children with fever', *Lancet* 337(8739): 591–4.

Krieger, D. (1975) 'Therapeutic touch: the imprimatur of nursing', *American Journal of Nursing* 75: 784–7.

Krumberger, J.M. (1995) 'Acute pancreatitis', in N.A. Urban, K.K. Greenlee, J.M. Krumberger *et al.* (eds) *Guidelines for Critical Care*, St Louis: Mosby: 417–23.

Krumholz, W., Endrass, J., Hempelmann, G. (1995) 'Inhibition of phagocytosis and killing of bacteria by anaesthetic agents in vitro', *British Journal of Anaesthesia* 75(1): 66–70.

Kulkarni, V. and Webster, N. (1996) 'Management of sepsis', *Care of the Critically Ill* 12(4): 122–7.

Kuo, J. and Butchart, E.G. (1995) 'Sternal wound dehiscence', *Care of the Critically Ill* 11(6): 244–8.

Kuperberg, K.G. and Grubbs, L. (1997) 'Coronary artery bypass patients' perceptions of acute postoperative pain', *Clinical Nurse Specialist* 11(3): 116–22.

Kwan, J.T.C. (1997) 'Renal support in critically ill patients', in D.R. Goldhill and P.S. Withington (eds) *Textbook of Intensive Care*, London: Chapman & Hall: 441–6.

Kynman, G. (1997) 'Thrombolysis: the development of unit guidelines', *Intensive and Critical Care Nursing* 13(1): 30–41.

Laight, S.E. (1996) 'The efficacy of eye care for ventilated patients', *Intensive and Critical Care Nursing* 12(1): 16–26.

Laing, A.S.M. (1992) 'The applicability of a new sedation scale for intensive care', *Intensive and Critical Care Nursing* 8(3): 149–52.

Lakshmipathi, C., Pinsky, M.R. and Grenvik, A.N.A. (1992) 'Outcome of intensive care of the 'oldest-old' critically ill patients', *Critical Care Medicine* 20(6): 757–61.

Lally, I. and Pearce, J. (1996) 'Intensive care nurses' perception of stress', *Nursing in Critical Care* 1(1): 17–25.

Lamerton, M. and Albarran, J.W. (1997) 'Percutaneous balloon mitral valvuloplasty: advancing the nursing perspective', *Nursing in Critical Care* 2(2): 88–92.

Land, L., Mhaolrunaigh, S.N. and Castledine, G. (1996) 'Extent and effectiveness of the scope of professional practice', *Nursing Times* 92(35): 32–5.

Landis, C.A. and Whitney, J.D. (1997) 'Effects of 72 hours sleep deprivation on wound healing in the rat', *Research in Nursing and Health* 20(3): 259–67.

Lane, P.L. (1989) 'Nurse–client perceptions: the double standard touch', *Issues in Mental Health Nursing* 10(1): 1–13.

Lane, R.C. and Fontaine, D. (1992) 'Sleep in the pediatric intensive care unit', *Heart and Lung* 21(3): 287.

Langley, S.M. and Pain, J.A. (1994) 'Surgery and liver dysfunction', *Care of the Critically Ill* 10(3): 113–17.

LATE Study Group. (1993) 'LATE assessment of thrombolytic therapy efficacy: LATE study with alteplase 6–24 hours after onset of acute myocardial infarction', *Lancet* 342(8874): 759–66.

Lavery, J.F., Clapham, M.C.C. (1993) 'Acid-base balance using a blood gas analyzer', *Care of the Critically Ill* 9(2): 68–9.

Leathart, A.J. (1994) 'Communication and socialisation (1): an exploratory study and explanation for nurse–patient communication in an ITU', *Intensive and Critical Care Nursing* 10(2): 93–104.

Lee, B., Chang, R.W.S. and Jacobs, S. (1990) 'Intermittent nasogastric feeding: a simple and effective method to reduce pneumonia among ventilated ICU patients', *Clinical Intensive Care* 1(3): 100–2.

Lee, K. and Stotts, N. (1990) 'Support of the growth-hormone somatomedin system to healing', *Heart and Lung* 19(2): 157–64.

Leech, C.L., Fuhrman, B.P., Morin, F.C. III *et al.* (1993) 'Perfluorocarbon-associated gas exchange, partial liquid ventilation in respiratory distress syndrome: a prospective, randomised, controlled study', *Critical Care Medicine* 21(9): 1270–8.

Lehane, M. and Rees, C. (1996) 'When ecstasy means agony', *Nursing Standard* 10(37): 24–5.

Leighton, H. (1995) 'Paracetamol poisoning: a case study', *Intensive and Critical Care Nursing* 11(5): 280–2.

Leijten, F.S., De Weerd, A.W., Poortvliet, D.C. *et al.* (1996) 'Critical illness polyneuropathy in multiple organ dysfunction syndrome and weaning from the ventilator', *Intensive Care Medicine* 22(9): 856–61.

Lessig , M.L. and Lessig, P.M. (1998) 'The cardiovascular system', in J.G. Alspach (ed.) *Core Curriculum for Critical Care Nursing*, 5th edn, Philadelphia: W B Saunders: 137–337.

Lessing, M.P.A., Jordens, J.Z. and Bowler, I.C.J. (1996) 'When should healthcare workers be screened for methicillin-resistant *Staphylococcus aureus*? *Journal of Hospital Infection* 34(3): 205–10.

Levine, E. (1997) 'Jewish views and customs on death', in C.M. Parkes (ed.) *Death and Bereavement Across Cultures*, London: Routledge. 98–130.

Levy, B., Bollaert, P-E., Lucchelli, J-P. *et al.* (1997) 'Dobutamine improves the adequacy of gastric mucosal perfusion ephedrine-treated septic shock', *Critical Care Medicine* 25(10): 1649–54.

Levy, M., Miyasaki, A. and Langston, D. (1995) 'Work of breathing as a weaning parameter in mechanically ventilated patients', *Chest* 108(4): 1018–25.

Lewicki, L.J., Mion, L., Splane, K.G. *et al.* (1997) 'Patient risk factors for pressure ulcers during cardiac surgery', *AORN Journal* 65(5): 933–42.

Lewin, K. (1952) *Field Theory in Social Science*, London: Routledge & Kegan Paul.

Lewis, J.F. and Veldhuizen, R.A. (1996) 'Exogenous surfactant administration for ARDS', in T.W. Evans and C.J. Hinds (eds) *Recent Advances in Critical Care Medicine*, 4, New York: Churchill Livingstone: 45–68.

Lindsay, P. (1997) 'Complications of the third stage of labour', in B.R. Sweet (ed.) *Mayes' Midwifery: A Textbook for Midwives*, 12th edn, London: Baillière Tindall: 703–15.

Lip, G.Y.H. and Beevers, D.G. (1995) 'History, epidemiology and importance of atrial fibrillation', *British Medical Journal* 311(7016): 1361–3.

Lipman, J. (1997) 'Severe soft-tissue infections', in T.E. Oh (ed.) *Intensive Care Manual*, 4th edn, Oxford: Butterworth-Heinemann: 552–6.

Lisicka, J. (1997) 'The surgical management of portal hypertension', *British Journal of Theatre Nursing* 7(6): 4–15.

Liwu, A. (1990) 'Oral hygiene in intubated patients', *Australian Journal of Advanced Nursing* 7(2): 4–7.

Lloyd, F. (1990) 'Making sense of eye care for ventilated or unconscious patients', *Nursing Times* 86(1): 36–7.

Lloyd-Jones, N. (1994) 'Stress and burnout in critical care', in B. Millar and P. Burnard (eds) *Critical Care Nursing*, London: Baillière Tindall: 145–70.

Lockhart-Wood, K. (1996) 'Cerebral oedema in fulminant hepatic failure', *Nursing in Critical Care* 1(6): 283–5.

Loudon, I. (1994) 'Necrotising fasciitis, hospital gangrene, and phagedaena', *Lancet* 344(8934): 1416–19.

Loussert-Ajaka, I., Ly, T., Chaix, M. *et al.* (1994) 'HIV-1/HIV-2 seronegativity in HIV-1 subtype O infected patients', *Lancet* 343(8910): 1393–4.

Lowery, M.T. (1995) 'A pressure sore risk calculator for intensive care patients: the Sunderland experience', *Intensive and Critical Care Nursing* 11(6): 344–53.

Lowson, S.M., Rich, G.F., McArdle, P.A.. *et al.* (1996) 'The response to varying concentrations of inhaled nitric oxide in patients with ARDS', *Anesthesia and Analgesia* 82(3): 574–81.

Lowthian, P. (1997) 'Notes on the pathogenesis of serious pressure sores', *British Journal of Nursing* 6(16): 907–12.

Lynn-McHale, D.J., Corsetti, A., Brady-Avis, E. *et al.* (1997) 'Preoperative ICU tours: are they helpful? *American Journal of Critical Care* 6(2): 106–15.

Macallan, D.C. (1994) 'Intravenous nutrition in AIDS', *British Journal of Intensive Care* 4(9): 313–16.

McCaffery, M. and Beebe, A. (1994) *Pain: Clinical Manual for Nursing Practice*, UK edn, London: Mosby.

McCaffrey, P. (1991) 'Making sense of the Sengstaken tube', *Nursing Times* 87(36): 40–2.

McCann, U.D., Szabo, Z., Scheffel, U. *et al.* (1998) 'Positron emission tomographic evidence of toxic effect of MDMA, "Ecstasy" on brain serotonin neurons in human beings', *Lancet* 352(9138): 1433–7.

McClelland, P. (1993a) 'The use of haemofiltration in critical care', *British Journal of Intensive Care* 3(12): 449–55.

—— (1993b) 'Alternative therapies for sepsis', in M. Rennie (ed.) *Intensive Care Britain (1993)*, London: Greycoat: 89–93.

MacConachie, I. (1991) 'The ARDS and fluid therapy controversy: what we need and don't need', *Intensive and Critical Care Digest* 10(3): 59–61.

MacConnachie, A.M. (1996) 'Drug therapy review: Dopexamine', *Intensive and Critical Care Nursing* 12(4): 246–7.

—— (1997a) 'Eradication therapy in peptic ulcer disease', *Intensive and Critical Care Nursing* 13(2): 119–20.

—— (1997b) 'Ecstasy poisoning', *Intensive and Critical Care Nursing* 13(6): 365–6.

McDaniel, L.B. and Prough, D.S. (1996) 'Fluid therapy during and after anaesthesia', in C. Prys-Roberts and B.R.Brown Jr. (eds) *International Practice of Anaesthesia*, Oxford: Butterworth Heinemann: 1/47/1–17.

McDonald, A.H. (1997) 'Coronary heart disease', in D.R. Goldhill and P.S. Withington (eds) *Textbook of Intensive Care*, London: Chapman & Hall: 281–6.

MacDonnell, S.P.J., Sigston, P. and Coakley, J.H. (1996) 'A survey of post intensive care hospital deaths', *British Journal of Intensive Care* 6(7): 220–2.

McFie, J. (1996) 'Bacterial translocation and nutritional support', *British Journal of Intensive Care* 6(6): 195–201.

McGonigal, K.S. (1986) 'The importance of sleep and the sensory environment to critically ill patients', *Intensive Care Nursing* 2(2): 73–83.

McGuire, G., Crossley, D., Richards, J. *et al.* (1997) 'Effects of varying levels of positive end-expiratory pressure on intracranial pressure and cerebral perfusion pressures', *Critical Care Medicine* 25(6): 1059–62.

McGuire, P.K., Cope, H. and Fahy, T.A. (1994) 'Diversity of psychopathy associated with use of 3,4-methylenedioxymethamphetamine ('Ecstasy')', *British Journal of Psychiatry* 165(3): 391–5.

McHugh, M.I. (1997) 'Acute renal failure', *Care of the Critically Ill* 13(2): 55–7.

Macintyre, E., Bullen, C. and Machin, S.J. (1985) 'Fluid replacement in hypovolaemia', *Intensive Care Medicine* 11(5): 231–3.

MacKellaig, J.M. (1990) 'A review of the psychological effects of intensive care on the isolated patient and his family', *Care of the Critically Ill* 6(3): 100–2.

McKelvie, S. (1998) 'Endotracheal suctioning', *Nursing in Critical Care* 3(5): 244–8.

McLaughlin, A., McLaughlin, B., Elliott, J. *et al.* (1996) 'Noise levels in a cardiac surgical intensive care unit: a preliminary study conducted in secret', *Intensive and Critical Care Nursing* 12(4): 226–31.

MacLean, A. and Dunning, J. (1997) 'The retrieval of thoracic organs: donor assessment and management', *British Medical Bulletin* 53(4): 829–43.

Maclean, S.L. (1989) 'The decision-making process in critical care of the aged', *Critical Care Nursing Quarterly* 12(1): 74–81.

McMahon-Parkes, K. and Cornock, M.A. (1997) 'Guillain-Barre Syndrome: biological basis, treatment and care', *Intensive and Critical Care Nursing* 13(1): 42–8.

McNabb, M. (1997) 'Maternal and fetal physiological responses to pregnancy', in B.R. Sweet (ed.) *Mayes' Midwifery: A Textbook for Midwives*, 12th edn, London: Baillière Tindall. 123–147.

MacNaughton, K.L., Rodrigue, J.R., Cicale, M. *et al.* (1998) 'Health-related quality of life and symptom frequency before and after lung transplantation', *Clinical Transplantation* 12(4): 320–3.

MacNaughton, P.D. and Evans, T.W.. (1992) 'Management of adult respiratory distress syndrome', *Lancet* 339(8791): 469–72.

McPhail, G. (1997) 'Management of change: an essential skill for nursing in the 1990s', *Journal of Nursing Management* 5(4): 199–205.

Mahul, P., Perrot, D., Tempelhoff, G. *et al.* (1991) 'Short and long-term prognosis, functional outcome following ICU for the elderly', *Intensive Care Medicine* 17(1): 7–10.

Malago, M., Rogiers, X. and Broelsch, C.E. (1997) 'Liver splitting and living donor techniques', *British Medical Bulletin* 53(4): 860–7.

Mallett, J. and Bailey, C. (eds) (1996) *The Royal Marsden NHS Trust Manual of Clinical Nursing Procedures*, 4th edn, Oxford: Blackwell Science.

Malone, C. (1992) 'Intensive pressures', *Nursing Times* 88(36): 57–61.

Manley, K. (1994) 'Primary nursing and critical care', in B. Millar and P. Burnard (eds) *Critical Care Nursing* London: Baillière Tindall: 41–73.

Mann, R.E. (1992) 'Preserving humanity in an age of technology', *Intensive and Critical Care Nursing* 8(1): 54–9.

Manning, H. (1994) 'Peak airway pressure: why the fuss?' *Chest* 105(1): 242–7.

March, K. (1994) 'Retrograde jugular catheter: monitoring SjO_2', *Journal of Neuroscience Nursing* 26(1): 48–51.

March, K., Mitchell, P., Winn, R. *et al.* (1990) 'Effect of backrest position on intracranial and cerebral perfusion pressures', *Journal of Neuroscience Nursing* 22(6): 375–81.

Marian, R. (1997) 'Advance directive: refusal of treatment', *Care of the Critically Ill* 13(6): 212–13.

Marieb, E.N. (1995) *Human Anatomy and Physiology*, 3rd edn, Redwood City, CA: Benjamin/Cummings.

Marley, R. (1998) 'Postextubation laryngeal edema – a review with consideration for home discharge', *Journal of Perianesthesia Nursing* 13(1): 39–53.

Marsh, P. and Martin, M. (1992) *Oral Microbiology*, 3rd edn, London: Chapman & Hall.

Marshall, J.C., Cook, D.J., Christou, N.V. *et al.* (1995) 'Multiple organ dysfunction syndrome: a reliable descriptor of a complex clinical outcome', *Critical Care Medicine* 23(10): 1638–52.

Marshall, W.J. (1995) *Clinical Chemistry*, 3rd edn, London: Mosby.

Martin, C., Perrin, G., Gevaudan, M.J. *et al.* (1990) 'Heat and moisture exchangers and vaporizing humidifiers in the ICU', *Chest* 97(1): 144–9.

Martindale, W. (1996) *The Extra Pharmacopoeia*, 31st edn, J.E.F. Reynolds (ed.) London: Pharmaceutical Press.

Marty, C., Misset, B., Tamion, E. *et al.* (1994) 'Circulating interleukin-8 concentrations in patients with multiple organ failure of septic and nonseptic origin', *Critical Care Medicine* 22(4): 673–9.

Maslow, A. H. (1971) *The Farthest Reaches Of Human Nature*, London: Penguin.

—— (1987) [1954]*Motivation and Personality*, 3rd edn, New York: Harper & Row.

Mason, P. (1991) 'Campaigning fails to increase handwashing', *Nursing Times* 87(1): 8.

Matlhoko, d'A. (1994) 'Surface tension', *Nursing Times* 90(3): 60–7.

Matta, B.F. and Menon, D.K. (1997) 'Management of acute head injury', in L. Kaufman and R. Ginsburg (eds) *Anaesthesia Review 13*, New York: Churchill Livingstone: 163–200.

Maxam Moore, V.A. and Goedecke, R.S. (1996) 'The development of an early extubation algorithm for patients after cardiac surgery', *Heart and Lung* 25(1): 61–8.

Mayer, J.A., Dubbert, P.M., Miller, M. *et al.* (1986) Increasing handwashing in an intensive care unit', *Infection Control* 7(5): 259–62.

Maynard, N., Bihari, D., Beale, R. *et al.* (1993) 'Assessment of splanchnic oxygenation by gastric tonometry in patients with acute circulatory failure', *JAMA* 270(10): 1203–10.

Mead, G.E., Williams, I.M., McCollum, C.N. *et al.* (1995) 'Near infrared spectroscopy', *British Journal of Intensive Care* 5(6): 194–9.

Medical Devices Agency (1995) *The Reuse of Medical Devices Supplied for Single-Use Only*, London: Medical Devices Agency.

Meduri, G.U., Headley, A.S. and Golden, E. (1998) 'Effect of prolonged methylprednisolone therapy in unresolving acute respiratory distress syndrome: a randomized controlled trial', *JAMA* 280(2): 159–65.

Melzack, R. and Wall, P. (1988) *The Challenge of Pain*, 2nd edn, London: Penguin.

Menon, D.K. (1997) 'Monitoring the central nervous system', *Current Anaesthesia and Critical Care* 8(6): 254–63.

Mercat, A., Titiriga, M., Anguel, N. *et al.* (1997) 'Inverse ratio ventilation in acute respiratory distress syndrome', *American Journal of Respiratory and Critical Care Medicine* 155(5): 1637–42.

Mercer, M. (1996) 'Elimination needs', in C. Viney (ed.) *Nursing the Critically Ill*, London: Baillière Tindall: 215–44.

Mercer, M., Winter, R., Dennis, S. *et al.* (1998) 'An audit of treatment withdrawal in one hundred patients on a general ICU', *Nursing in Critical Care* 3(2): 63–6.

Merriman, H.M. (1981) 'The techniques used to sedate ventilated patients', *Intensive Care Medicine* 7: 217–24.

Methany, N. (1993) 'Minimising respiratory complications of nasogastric tube feedings: state of the science', *Heart and Lung* 22(3): 213–22.

Meyer, T.J., Eveloff, S.E., Bauer, M.S. *et al.* (1994) 'Adverse environmental conditions in the respiratory and medical ICU settings', *Chest* 105(4): 1211–16.

Michie, H.R. and Marley, R.T.C. (1992) 'Monoclonal antibodies in sepsis and septicaemia', in M. Rennie (ed.) *Intensive Care Britain*, London: Greycoat Publishing: 114–17.

Mihatsch, M.J., Kyo, M., Morozumi, K. *et al.* (1998) 'The side-effects of cyclosporin-A and tacrolimus', *Clinical Nephrology* 49(6): 356–63.

Mihissin, N.K. and Houghton, P.W. (1995) 'Occipital ulcer in a 45-year-old female', *British Journal of Intensive Care* 5(3): 90–1.

Millar, A. (1997) 'Gastrointestinal pharmacology', in D.R. Goldhill and P.S. Withington (eds) *Textbook of Intensive Care*, London: Chapman & Hall: 457–65.

Miller, O.J., Celermajer, D.S., Deanfield, J.F. *et al.* (1994) 'Guidelines for the safe administration of inhaled nitric oxide', *Archives of Diseases in Childhood* 70(3): F47–F49.

Miller, R., Kingswood, C., Bullen, C. *et al.* (1990) 'Renal replacement therapy in the ICU', *British Journal of Hospital Medicine* 43(5): 354–362.

Miller, R.F. and Roberts, C.M. (1991) 'Intensive care management of HIV positive patients and patients with AIDS', *Clinical Intensive Care* 2(1): 17–25.

Milliken, J., Tait, G.A., Ford-Jones, E.L. *et al.* (1988) 'Nosocomial infections in a paediatric ICU', *Critical Care Medicine* 16(3): 233–7.

Mimoz, O., Rauss, A., Rekik, N. *et al.* (1994) 'Pulmonary artery catheterization in critically ill patients: a prospective analysis of outcome changes associated with catheter-prompted changes in therapy', *Critical Care Medicine* 22(4): 573–9.

Miranda, A.D., Donovan, L.A., Schuster, L.L. *et al.* (1997) 'Malignant hyperthermia', *American Journal of Critical Care* 6(5): 368–74.

Mirski, M.A., Muffleman, B., Ulatowski, J.A. *et al.* (1995) 'Sedation for the critically ill neurologic patient', *Critical Care Medicine* 23(12): 2038–53.

Mitchell, C.J. and MacFie, J. (1991) 'Acute pancreatitis: a joint approach', *Care of the Critically Ill* 7(4): 134–136.

Mizock, B.A. and Falk, J.L. (1992) 'Lactic acidosis in critical illness', *Critical Care Medicine* 20(1): 80–93.

Molloy, A.R. Edmondson, S.J. and Hinds, C.J. (1992) 'High frequency jet ventilation in acute respiratory failure', *British Journal of Intensive Care* 2(3): 126–32.

Molnar, Z. and Shearer, E. (1998) 'Veno-venous haemofiltration in the treatment of sepsis and the multiple organ dysfunction syndrome', *British Journal of Intensive Care* 8(1): 12–20.

Molyneux, R. and Chadwick, C. (1997) 'Vancomycin-resistant enterococci: implications for infection control', *Professional Nurse* 12(9): 641–4.

Monger, E. (1995) 'Strategies for nursing conscious mechanically ventilated patients in Southampton and Amsterdam', *Intensive and Critical Care Nursing* 11(3): 140–7.

Moore, F., Feliciano, D., Andrassy, R. *et al.* (1992) 'Early enteral feeding, compared with parenteral, reduces postoperative septic complications', *Annals of Surgery* 216(2): 172–83.

Morgan, I. and Campanella, C. (1998) 'Transmyocardial laser revascularisation in Edinburgh', *British Journal of Theatre Nursing* 7(12): 4–9.

Morgan, S.P. (1990) 'A comparison of three methods of managing fever in the neurological patient', *Journal of Neuroscience Nursing* 22(1): 19–24.

Morgan, V. (1995) 'Brain stem death testing and consent for cadaveric organ donation', *Care of the Critically Ill* 11(1): 20–2.

Morris, A.H., Wallace, C.J., Menlove, R.L. *et al.* (1994) 'Randomised clinical trial of pressure-controlled inverse ratio ventilation and extracorporeal CO_2 removal for adult respiratory distress syndrome', *American Journal of Respiratory and Critical Care Medicine* 149(1): 295–305.

Morris, K. (1998) 'Synthetic blood substitutes safe in acute trauma', *Lancet* 352(9127): 551.

Morton, N.S. (1993) 'Extracorporeal life support in neonatology and paediatrics', in M. Rennie (ed.) *Intensive Care Britain (1993)*, London: Greycoat: 99–104.

Moss, J. and Craigo, P.A. (1994) 'The autonomic nervous system', in R.D. Miller, R.F. Cucchiara, E.D. Miller *et al.* (eds) *Anaesthesia*, 4th edn, New York: Churchill Livingstone: 523–75.

Moxham, J. and Goldstone, J. (eds) (1994) *Assisted Ventilation*, 2nd edn, London: BMJ Publishing.

Mudaliar, M.Y., Hunter, D.N., Morgan, C. *et al.* (1991) 'Extracorporeal gas exchange for respiratory failure', *Hospital Update* 17(5): 410–15.

Mulnier, C. and Evans, T. (1995) 'Acute respiratory distress in adults (ARDS)', *Care of the Critically Ill* 11(5): 182–6.

Mulvey, D.A., Mallett, S.V. and Browne, D.R.G. (1993) 'Endotracheal intubation', *Intensive Care World* 10(3): 122–8.

Murray, P.R., Kobayashi, G.S., Pfaller, M.A. *et al.* (1994) *Medical Microbiology*, 2nd edn, St Louis: Mosby.

Myburgh, J.A. and Oh, T.E. (1997) 'Disorders of consciousness', in T.E. Oh (ed.) *Intensive Care Manual*, 4th edn, Oxford: Butterworth-Heinemann: 357–80.

Myburgh, J.A. and Runciman, W.B. (1997) 'Inotropic drugs', in T.E. Oh (ed.) *Intensive Care Manual*, 4th edn, Oxford: Butterworth-Heinemann: 123–43.

Nadel, S., Levin, N. and Habibi, P. (1995) 'Treatment of meningococcal disease in children', in K. Cartwright (ed.) *Meningococcal Disease*, Chichester: Wiley: 207–43.

Naftchi, N.E. and Richardson, J.S. (1997) 'Autonomic dysreflexia: pharmacological management of hypertensive crises in spinal cord injured patients', *Journal of Spinal Cord Medicine* 20(3): 355–60.

Naik, S., Greenough, A., Giffin, F. *et al.* (1996) 'The effects of changes in PEEP on gas exchange', *British Journal of Intensive Care* 6(3): 82–8.

Neal, M. (1994) 'Necrotising fasciitis', *Nursing Times* 90(41): 53–4.

Neill, A.S. (1992) *The New Summerhill*, London: Penguin.

Nelsey, L. (1986) 'Mouthcare and the intubated patient – the aim of preventing infection', *Intensive Care Nursing* 1(4): 187–93.

Nelson-Piercy, C. and Hanson, G.C. (1997) 'Severe pre-eclampsia and eclampsia', in D.R. Goldhill and P.S. Withington (eds) *Textbook of Intensive Care*, London: Chapman & Hall Medical: 707–13.

Neoptolemos, J.P. (1992) 'Pancreatic disease', in R.E. Pounder (ed.) *Recent Advances in Gastroenterology*, 9, Edinburgh: Churchill Livingstone: 85–104.

Neuman, B. (1995) *The Neuman Systems Model*, 3rd edn, Norwalk: Appleton Century Croft.

Neville, K., Bromberg, A., Bromberg, R. *et al.* (1994) 'The third epidemic: multidrug resistant tuberculosis', *Chest* 105(1): 45–8.

Nightingale, F. (1980) [1859] *Notes on Nursing: What It Is, and What It Is Not*, Edinburgh: Churchill Livingstone.

Nightingale, P. and Campbell, I.T. (1998) 'Metabolic monitoring', *Care of the Critically Ill* 14(4): 134–7.

Nikas, D.L. (1998) 'The neurologic system', in J.G. Alspach (ed.) *Core Curriculum for Critical Care Nursing*, 5th edn, Philadelphia: W B Saunders: 339–463.

Nimmo, G.R. and Nimmo, S.M. (1993) 'Cardiogenic shock', *British Journal of Intensive Care* 3(8): 291–6.

Niskanen, M., Kari, A. and Halonen, P. (1996) 'Five-year survival after intensive care: comparison of 12,180 patients with the general population. Finnish ICU Study Group', *Critical Care Medicine* 24(12): 1962–7.

Norman, I.J. and Redfern, S.J. (eds) (1997) *Mental Health Care for Elderly People*, Edinburgh: Churchill Livingstone.

Norris, M.K.G., Fuhrman, B.P. and Leach, C.L. (1994) 'Liquid ventilation: it's not science fiction anymore', *AACN Clinical Issues in Critical Care Nursing* 5(3): 246–54.

North, B. and Reilly, P. (1994) 'Management and manipulation of ICP', *Current Anaesthesia and Critical Care* 5(1): 23–8.

North, N. (1995) 'Economics and health care', in G. Moon and R. Gillespie (eds) *Society and Health*, Routledge. London: 213–25.

Nowak, T.J. and Handford, A.G. (1994) *Essentials of Pathophysiology*, Iowa: Wm C. Brown.

Nunn, J.F. (1996) 'Oxygen consumption and delivery', in C. Prys-Roberts and B.R. Brown Jr. (eds) *International Practice of Anaesthesia*, Oxford: Butterworth Heinemann: 1/61/1–10.

Nursing Times (1993) *Complementary Therapy*, London: *Nursing Times*/Macmillan.

O'Conner, B. (1994) 'Hazards associated with the recreational drug "ecstasy"', *British Journal of Hospital Medicine* 52(10): 507–14.

O'Connor, L. (1995) 'Pain assessment by patients and nurses, and nurses' notes on it, in early acute myocardial infarction', *Intensive and Critical Care Nursing* 11(5): 283–92.

O'Grady, J.G., Wendon, J., Tan, I.K.S. *et al.* (1991) 'Liver transplantation after paracetamol overdose', *British Medical Journal* 303(6796): 221–3.

O'Hanlon-Nichols, T. (1998) 'The adult pulmonary system', *American Journal of Nursing* 98(2): 39–45.

O'Meara, S. and Glenny, A. (1997) 'What are the best ways of tackling obesity? *Nursing Times* 93(22): 50–1.

O'Shea, P. (1997) 'Altered consciousness and stroke', in D.R. Goldhill and P.S. Withington (eds) *Textbook of Intensive Care*, London: Chapman & Hall: 495–502.

O'Sullivan, G.F. and Park, G.R. (1990) 'The assessment of sedation in critically ill patients', *Clinical Intensive Care* 1(3): 116–22.

O'Sullivan, R.J. (1991) 'A musical road to recovery', *Intensive Care Nursing* 7(3): 160–3.

O'Toole, S. (1997) 'Alternatives to mercury thermometers', *Professional Nurse* 12(11): 783–6.

Odell, A., Allder, R., Bayne, R. *et al.* (1993) 'Endotracheal suction for adult, non-head-injured, patients', *Intensive and Critical Care Nursing* 9(4): 274–8.

Odell, M. (1996) 'Intracranial pressure monitoring, nursing in a district general hospital', *Nursing in Critical Care* 1(5): 245–7.

Oh, T.E. (1997) 'Oxygen therapy', in T.E. Oh (ed.) *Intensive Care Manual*, 4th edn, Oxford: Butterworth-Heinemann: 209–16.

Olleveant, N., Humphris, G. and Roe, B. (1998) 'A reliability study of the modified New Sheffield Sedation Scale', *Nursing in Critical Care* 3(2): 83–8.

Ommeslag, D., Colardyn, F. and Delaey, J. (1987) 'Eye infection caused by respiratory pathogens in mechanically ventilated patients', *Critical Care Medicine* 15(1): 80–1.

Ong, E.L.C. (1993) 'Infection with the Human Immunodeficiency Virus', *Care of the Critically Ill* 9(1): 7–10.

Osguthorpe, S.G. (1995) 'Acute myocardial infarction', in N.A. Urban, K.K. Greenlee, J.M. Krumberger *et al.* (eds) *Guidelines for Critical Care,* St Louis: Mosby: 146–62.

Palazzo, M. and Bullingham, A. (1994) 'Renal rescue in the critically ill: the Charing Cross Protocol', in M. Rennie (ed.) *Intensive Care Britain (1994),* London: Greycoat: 51–5.

Palmer, J., (1996) 'Exploring the psychological effects of intensive care on paediatric patients', *Nursing in Critical Care* 1(1): 26–30.

Palomar, M., Alvarez-Lerma, F., Jorda, R. *et al.* (1997) 'Prevention of nosocomial infection in mechanically ventilated patients: selective digestive decontamination versus sucralfate', *Clinical Intensive Care* 8(5): 228–35.

Papazian, L., Bregeon, F., Thirion, X. *et al.* (1996) 'Effect of ventilator-associated pneumonia on mortality and morbidity', *American Journal of Respiratory and Critical Care Medicine* 154(1): 91–7.

Parker, T.J. and Burden, P. (1998) 'Nosocomial pneumonia', *Care of the Critically Ill* 14: 163–6.

Park, G.R. and Evans, T.N. (1997) 'Albumin transfusions: transplanting the biochemical appendix?', *Clinical Intensive Care* 8(2): 81–2.

Park, G.R. and Navapurkar, V. (1994) 'Sedation in critically ill patients', *Care of the Critically Ill* 10(1): 5–9.

Park, G.R., Gunning, K.E. and Roe, P.G. (1996) 'Intensive care of patients after liver surgery', in C. Prys-Roberts and B.R. Brown Jr. (eds) *International Practice of Anaesthesia*, Oxford: Butterworth Heinemann: 1/75/1–11.

Parker, R.I. (1997) 'Etiology of acquired coagulopathies in the critically ill adult and child', *Critical Care Clinics* 13(3): 591–609.

Parkinson, E., Beale, R. and Bihari, D. (1996) 'Prediction of outcome in the ICU', *British Journal of Intensive Care* 6(2): 55–9.

Parobek, V. and Alaimo, I. (1996) 'Fluid and electrolyte management in the neurologically-impaired patient', *Journal of Neuroscience Nursing* 28(5): 322–8.

Parrott, A.C., Lees, A., Garnham, N.J. *et al.* (1998) 'Cognitive performance in recreational users of MDMA of 'ecstasy': evidence for memory deficits', *Journal of Psychopharmacology* 12(1): 79–83.

Payne-James, J.J. and Silk, D.B.A. (1992) 'Can artificial nutrition support for the critically ill be improved? in M. Rennie (ed.) *Intensive Care Britain (1992)*, London: Greycoat: 88–93.

Pearson, L.S. (1996) 'A comparison of the ability of foam swabs and toothbrushes to remove dental plaque: implications for nursing practice', *Journal of Advanced Nursing* 23(1): 62–9.

Peek, G.J., Moore, H.M., Moore, N. *et al.* (1997) 'Extracorporeal membrane oxygenation for adult respiratory failure', *Chest* 112(3): 759–64.

Pelletier, M.L. (1992) 'The organ donor family members perception of stressful situations during the organ donation experience', *Journal of Advanced Nursing* 17(1): 90–7.

Perrins, J., King, N. and Collings, J. (1998) 'Assessment of long-term psychological well-being following intensive care', *Intensive and Critical Care Nursing* 14(3): 108–16.

Phelan, D. (1995) 'Hopeless cases in intensive care', *Care of the Critically Ill* 11(5): 196–7.

Phillips, G.D. (1997) 'Pain relief in intensive care', in T.E. Oh (ed.) *Intensive Care Manual*, 4th edn, Oxford: Butterworth-Heinemann: 679–85.

Phillips, K. and Gill, L. (1993) 'A point of pressure', *Nursing Times* 89(45): 44–5.

Phillips, S. (1996) 'Labouring the emotions – expanding the remit of nursing work?', *Journal of Advanced Nursing* 24(1): 139–43.

Pierce, L.N.B. (1995) *Guide to Mechanical Ventilation and Intensive Respiratory Care,* Philadelphia: W B Saunders.

Pinger, R.R., Payne, W.A., Hahn, D.B. *et al.* (1995) *Issues for Today: Drugs*, 2nd edn, St Louis: Mosby.

Pinosky, M.L., Kennedy, D.J., Fishman, R.L. *et al.* (1997) 'Tranexamic acid reduces bleeding after cardiopulmonary bypass when compared to epsilon aminocaproic acid and placebo', *Journal of Cardiac Surgery* 12(5): 330–8.

Pitkin, A., Scott, R. and Salmon, J. (1997) 'Hyperbaric oxygen therapy in intensive care', *British Journal of Intensive Care* 7(3): 107–13.

Playle, J.F. (1995) 'Humanism and positivism in nursing: contradictions and conflicts', *Journal of Advanced Nursing* 22(5): 979–84.

Plowright, C. (1995) 'Needs of visitors in the intensive care unit', *British Journal of Nursing* 4(18): 1081–3.

Powell, H. and Paes, M.L. (1992) 'IVOX: a description of the device and early clinical impressions', *Care of the Critically Ill* 8(5): 189–90.

Powell, H. and Whitwam, J.G. (1990) 'New aspects of vasodilator therapy', *Care of the Critically Ill* 6(3): 109–15.

Powronznyk, A.V.V. and Latimer, R.D. (1997) 'Progress in monitoring and delivery of inspired nitric oxide therapy', *British Journal of Intensive Care* 7(4): 149–54.

Pratt, R. (1995) *HIV and AIDS: A Strategy for Nursing Care*, 4th edn, London: Edward Arnold.

—— (1998) 'HIV-related encephalopathy', *Nursing Standard* 13(7): 38–40.

Prencipe, L. and Brenna, S. (undated) *The Acid-Base Balance: Theoretical and Practical Aspects*, de V. Sabata (trans), Milan: Niguarda Hospital.

Preusser, B.A., Lash, J., Stone, K.S. *et al.* (1989) 'Quantifying the minimum discard sample required for accurate arterial blood gases', *Nursing Research* 38(5): 276–9.

Price, D.J. (1992) 'The intensive care of head injured patients', in J. Tinker and W.M. Zapol (eds) *Care of the Critically Ill Patient*, 2nd edn, New York: Springer-Verlag: 831–72.

Price, P. and Donahue, M. (1994) 'Warm heart surgery', *CACCN* 5(4): 16–20.

Price, T. (1996) 'An evaluation of neuro-assessment tools in the intensive care unit', *Nursing in Critical Care* 1(2): 72–7.

Price, T.E. (1998) 'Managing the nursing priorities in the patient with a cerebral insult', in J.W. Albarran and T.E. Price (eds) *Managing the Nursing Priorities in Intensive Care*, Dinton: Quay Books: 86–116.

Pritchard, A.J.N. (1994) 'Tracheostomy', *Care of the Critically Ill* 10(2): 66–9.

Pritchard, A.P. and Mallett, J. (eds) (1992) *The Royal Marsden Manual of Clinical Nursing Procedures*, 3rd edn, Oxford: Blackwell Science.

Pryjmachuk, S. (1996) 'Pragmatism and change: some implications for nurses, nurse managers and nursing', *Journal of Nursing Management* 4(4): 201–5.

Pugin, J., Auckenthaler, R., Lew, P.D. *et al.* (1991) 'Oropharyngeal decontamination decreases incidence of ventilator associated pneumonia', *JAMA* 265(20): 2704–10.

Puntillo, K.A. (1988) 'The phenomenon of pain and critical care nursing', *Heart and Lung* 17(3): 262–73.

—— (1990) 'Pain experiences of intensive care unit patients', *Heart and Lung* 19(5): 526–33.

Puntillo, K. and Weiss, S.J. (1994) 'Pain: its mediators and associated morbidity in critically ill cardiovascular surgical patients', *Nursing Research* 43(1): 31–6.

Purcell, S. (1997) 'Withdrawing treatment from a critically-ill child', *Intensive and Critical Care Nursing* 13(2): 103–7.

Purdy, F.R., Tweedale, M.G. and Merrick, P.M. (1997) 'Association of mortality with age of blood transfused in septic ICU patients', *Canadian Journal of Anaesthesia* 44(12): 1256–61.

Pyne, R.H. (1992) *Professional Discipline in Nursing, Midwifery and Health Visiting*, 2nd edn, Oxford: Blackwell Scientific.

Quinn, A. D'A. (1995) 'Acute upper gastrointestinal bleeding', in N.A. Urban, K.K. Greenlee, J.M. Krumberger *et al.* (eds) *Guidelines for Critical Care*, St Louis: Mosby: 470–79.

Quinn, A.C., Petros, A.J. and Vallance, P. (1995) 'Nitric oxide: an endogenous gas', *British Journal of Anaesthesia* 74(4): 443–51.

Quirke, S. (1998) 'A comparative study of the incidence of nosocomial colonisation in patients with closed suction catheter changes at 24 v. 48 hours', *Care of the Critically Ill* 14(4): 116–20.

Rachels, J. (1986) *The End of Life*, Oxford: Oxford University Press.

Raeside, F. revised Martin, J. (1996) 'Hepatitis A & B: the nurse's role. RCN nursing update', *Nursing Standard* 10(32): supplement.

Raftery, M.J. (1997) 'Renal physiology', in D.R. Goldhill and P.S. Withington (eds) *Textbook of Intensive Care* London: Chapman & Hall: 421–6.

Rahman, S., Kim, G. Matthew, A. *et al.* (1994) 'Effects of atrial natriuretic peptide in clinical acute renal failure', *Kidney International* 45(6): 1731–8.

Ralston, A.C., Webb, R.K. and Runciman, W.B. (1991) 'Potential errors in pulse oximetry', *Anaesthesia* 46(4): 291–5.

Ramos, M.C. (1992) 'The nurse–patient relationship: theme and variations', *Journal of Advanced Nursing* 17(4): 496–506.

Ramsay, M.A.E., Savege, T.M., Simpson, B.R.J. *et al.* (1974) 'Controlled sedation with alphaxalone-alphadolone', *British Medical Journal* ii: 656–9.

Randall, F. (1997) 'Why causing death is not necessarily morally equivalent to allowing to die: response to Ferguson', *Journal of Medical Ethics* 23(6): 373–6.

Randhawa, G. (1997) 'Enhancing the health professional's role in requesting transplant organs', *British Journal of Nursing* 6(8): 429–34.

Randolph, A.G. (1998) 'An evidence-based approach to central venous catheter management to prevent catheter-related infections in critically ill patients', *Critical Care Clinics* 14(3): 411–21.

Rankin-Box, D. (1988) *Complementary Health Therapies: A Guide for Nurses and the Caring Professions*, London: Croom Helm.

—— (ed.) (1995) *The Nurse's Handbook of Complementary Therapies*, Edinburgh: Churchill Livingstone.

Raper, S. and Maynard, N. (1992) 'Feeding the critically ill patient', *British Journal of Nursing* 1(6): 273–80.

Raphael, J.H. and Langton, J.A. (1995) 'Uses and abuses of the laryngeal mask airway', *Current Anaesthesia and Critical Care* 6(4): 250–4.

Rappaport, S.H., Shpiner, R., Yoshihara, G. *et al.* (1994) 'Randomized, prospective trial of pressure-limited versus volume-controlled ventilation in severe respiratory failure', *Critical Care Medicine* 22(1): 22–32.

Reading, J.S., Hargest, T.S. and Minsky, S.H. (1977) 'How noisy is intensive care?', *Critical Care Medicine* 5(6): 275.

Rebenson-Piano, M. (1989) 'The physiologic changes that occur with age', *Critical Care Nursing Quarterly* 12(1): 1–14.

Redfern, S.J. (1991) 'The elderly person: the challenge of an aged society', in S.J. Redfern (ed.) *Nursing Elderly People*, Edinburgh: Churchill Livingstone: 531–48.

Reece-Smith, H. (1997) 'Pancreatitis', *Care of the Critically Ill* 13(4): 135–8.

Reeve, W. and Wallace, P. (1991) 'A survey of sedation in intensive care', *Care of the Critically Ill* 7(6): 238–41.

Reich, D., Rothstein, K., Manzarbeitia, C. *et al.* (1998) 'Common medical diseases after liver transplantation', *Seminars in Gastrointestinal Disease* 9(3): 110–25.

Reid, J. and Morison, M.J. (1994a) 'Classification of pressure sore severity', *Nursing Times* 90(20): 46–50.

—— (1994b) 'Towards a consensus classification of pressure sores', *Journal of Wound Care* 3(3): 157–60.

Reilly, D.E. (1980) *Behavioral Objectives: Evaluation in Nursing*, New York: Appleton Century Crofts.

Rello, J., Torres, A., Ricart, M. *et al.* (1994) 'Ventilator-associated pneumonia by *Staphylococcus aureus*: comparison of methicillin-resistant and methicillin-sensitive episodes', *American Journal of Respiratory and Critical Care Medicine* 150(6): 1545–9.

Rennie, M. (1993a) 'Consensus workshop on enteral feeding in ICU patients', *British Journal of Intensive Care* 3(12): 438–47.

—— (1993b) 'EPIC: infection in intensive care in Europe', *British Journal of Intensive Care* 3(1): 27–36.

—— (1996) 'Increased prospects of rescue from acute renal failure', *British Journal of Intensive Care* 6(7): 217.

Rentoul, L., Thomas, V. and Rentoul, R. (1995) 'Understanding stress and its implications for health-care professionals', in J.E. Schober and S.M. Hinchliff (eds) *Towards Advanced Nursing Practice*, London: Edward Arnold: 154–81.

Resuscitation Council (UK) (1997) *The 1997 Resuscitation Guidelines for Use in the United Kingdom*, London: Resuscitation Council.

Rhodes, A., Lamb, F.J., Grounds, R.M. *et al.* (1997) 'The use of Apache III in Britain', *British Journal of Intensive Care* 7(6): 237–43.

Richardson, M.D. (1994) 'Systemic fungal infections', *Care of the Critically Ill* 10(6): 258–61.

Ridley, S., Biggam, M. and Stone, P.A. (1994) 'A cost utility analysis of intensive therapy II: quality of life in survivors', *Anaesthesia* 49(3): 192–6.

Ridley, S., Jackson, R., Findlay, J. *et al.* (1990) 'Long term survival after intensive care', *British Medical Journal* 301(6761): 1127–30.

Ridley, S.A., Chrispin, P.S., Scotton, H. *et al.* (1997) 'Changes in quality of life after intensive care: comparison with normal data', *Anaesthesia* 52(3): 195–202.

Riordan, S. and Williams, R. (1997) 'Bioartificial liver support: developments in hepatocyte culture and bioreactor', *British Medical Bulletin* 53(4): 730–44.

Rising, C.J. (1993) 'The relationship of selected nursing activities to ICP', *Journal of Neuroscience Nursing* 25(5): 302–8.

Rithalia, S.V.S., Farrow, P. and Doran B.R.H. (1992) 'Comparison of transcutaneous oxygen and carbon dioxide monitors in normal adults and critically ill patients', *Intensive and Critical Care Nursing* 8(1): 40–6.

Robb, J.A. (1995) 'Caring for children in an adult intensive care unit, Part 1', *Intensive and Critical Care Nursing* 11(2): 100–10.

—— (1997) 'Physiological changes occurring with positive pressure ventilation, Part 1', *Intensive and Critical Care Nursing* 13(3): 293–307.

Roberts, J.O., Fenton, O.M. and Peters, J.L. (1985) 'Necrotising fasciitis', *Hospital Update* 11(11): 829–41.

Robertson, G.S. (1995) 'Making an advanced directive', *British Medical Journal* 310(6974): 236–8.

Robinson, B.J., Buyck, H.C.E. and Galletly, D.C.V. (1994) 'Effect of propofol on heart rate, arterial pressure and digital plethysmograph variability', *British Journal of Anaesthesia* 73(2): 167–73.

Robson, W.P. (1998) 'To bag or not to bag? Manual hyperinflation in intensive care', *Intensive and Critical Care Nursing* 14(5): 239–43.

Rodrigus, I.E., Vermeyen, K.M., De Hert, S.G. *et al.* (1996) 'Efficacy and safety of aprotinin in aortocoronary bypass and valve replacement operations: a placebo-controlled randomized double-blind study', *Perfusion* 11(4): 313–18.

Roessle, M., Haag, K., Ochs, A. *et al.* (1994) 'The transjugular intrahepatic portosystemic stent-shunt procedure for variceal bleeding', *New England Journal of Medicine* 330(3): 165–71.

Rogers, C.R. (1951) *Client-Centred Therapy*, London: Constable.

—— (1967) *On Becoming a Person*, London: Constable.

—— (1980) *A Way of Being*, Boston: Houghton Mifflin.

—— (1983) *Freedom to Learn for the '80s*, New York: Merrill.

Rogers, E. and Shoemaker, F. (1971) *Communication of Innovations: A Cross-Cultural Report*, 2nd edn, New York: Free Press.

Rogers, M. (1992) 'Temperature recording in infants and children', *Paediatric Nursing* 4(3): 23–6.

Ronco, C., Tetta, C, Lupi, A. *et al.* (1995) 'Removal of platelet-activating factor in experimental continuous arteriovenous hemofiltration', *Critical Care Medicine* 23(1): 99–107.

Roper, N., Logan, W. and Tierney, A. (1996) *The Elements of Nursing*, 4th edn, Edinburgh: Churchill Livingstone.

Ross, A.P. (1993) 'Nursing interventions for persons receiving immunosuppressant therapies for demyelinating pathologies', *Nursing Clinics of North America* 28(4): 829–38.

Rossa, L., Rosa, E., Sarner, L. *et al.* (1998) 'A close look at therapeutic touch', *JAMA* 279(13): 1005–10.

Rossaint, R., Falke, K.J., Lopez, F. *et al.* (1993) 'Inhaled nitric oxide for the Adult Respiratory Distress Syndrome', *New England Journal of Medicine* 328(6): 399–405.

Roupie, E.E., Brochard, F. and Lemaire, F.J. (1996) 'Clinical evaluation of a continuous intra-arterial blood gas system in critically ill patients', *Intensive Care Medicine* 22(11): 1162–8.

Rowan, K.M., Kerr, J.H., Alperovich, A. *et al.* (1993) 'Intensive Care Society's APACHE II study in Britain and Ireland – II: outcome comparisons of intensive care units after adjustment for case mix by the American APACHE II method', *British Medical Journal* 307(6910): 977–81.

Rowlands, D.J. (1996a) 'Can coronary reperfusion be detected by clinical electrocardiograph?', in D.J. Rowlands (ed.) *Recent Advances in Cardiology*, 12, Edinburgh: Churchill Livingstone: 27–49.

—— (1996b) 'Percutaneous transluminal coronary angioplasty', in D.J. Rowlands (ed.) *Recent Advances in Cardiology*, 12, Edinburgh: Churchill Livingstone: 1–28.

Rowsey, P.J. (1997a) 'Pathophysiology of fever. Part 1: The role of cytokines', *Dimensions of Critical Care Nursing* 16(4): 202–7.

—— (1997b) 'Pathophysiology of fever. Part 2: Relooking at cooling interventions', *Dimensions of Critical Care Nursing* 16(5): 251–6.

Rowswell, M.K. (1997) 'Caring for the patient with a haematological disorder', in M. Walsh (ed.) *Watson's Clinical Nursing and Related Sciences*, 5th edn, London: Baillière Tindall: 340–98.

Royal College of Nursing (RCN) (1994) *Standards of Care for Critical Care Nursing*, London: RCN.

Ruggles, L. (1995) 'Auto-PEEP: measurement issues and nursing interventions', *Critical Care Nurse* 15(2): 30–8.

Rumbold, G. (1999) *Ethics in Nursing Practice*, 2nd edn, London: Baillière Tindall.

Runcimann, W.B. and Ludbrook, G.L. (1996) 'The measurement of systemic arterial blood pressure', in C. Prys-Roberts and B.R. Brown Jr. (eds) *International Practice of Anaesthesia* Oxford: Butterworth Heinemann: 2/154/1–11.

Rushton, C.H. (1992) 'Care-giver suffering in critical care nursing', *Heart and Lung* 21(3): 303–6.

Rutherford, I.A. (1996) 'Haemostasis and disseminated intravascular coagulation', *Intensive and Critical Care Nursing* 12(3): 161–7.

Ryan, C. (1995) 'Coronary artery bypass grafting', in N.A. Urban, K.K. Greenlee, J.M. Krumberger *et al.* (eds) *Guidelines for Critical Care*, St Louis: Mosby: 197–210.

Ryan, C.J. (1996) 'Betting your life: an argument against certain advance directives', *Journal of Medical Ethics* 22(2): 95–9.

Ryan, D.W. (1997a) 'Euricus-1', *Care of the Critically Ill* 13(1): 4.

—— (1997b) 'Octogenarians in an intensive care unit: a 15 year review', *Clinical Intensive Care* 8(1): 14–15.

—— (1998) 'How to Guides: BIPAP ventilation', *Care of the Critically Ill* 14(1): insert.

Ryan, D.W. and Pelosi, P. (1996) 'The prone position in acute respiratory distress syndrome', *British Medical Journal* 312(7035): 860–1.

Rykerson, S., Thompson, J. and Wessel, D.L. (1995) 'Inhalation of nitric oxide: an innovative therapy for treatment of increased pulmonary vascular resistance', *Nursing Clinics of North America* 30(2): 381–90.

Sachdeva, R.C, Guntupalli, K.K. (1997) 'Acute respiratory distress syndrome', *Critical Care Clinics* 13(3): 503–21.

Sagar, P., Sedman, P., Mitchell, C. *et al.* (1994) 'The clinical significance of gut translocation of bacteria', in M. Rennie (ed.) *Intensive Care Britain (1994)*, London: Greycoat: 95–9.

Saggs, P. (1998) 'Sedation scoring in a general ICU: comparative trial of two assessment tools in clinical practice', *Nursing in Critical Care* 3(6): 289–95.

Sair, M. and Evans, T.W. (1995) 'Acute respiratory distress syndrome', *Medicine* 23(9): 388–91.

Samples, J.F., Cott, M.L.V., Long, C. *et al.* (1985) 'Circadian rhythms: basis for screening fever', *Nursing Research* 34(6): 377–9.

Santamaria, J.D. (1997) 'Acute pancreatitis', in T.E. Oh (ed.) *Intensive Care Manual*, 4th edn, Oxford: Butterworth Heinemann.

Sasse, S.A., Chen, P.A. and Mahutte, C.K. (1994) 'Variability of arterial blood gas values over time in stable medical ICP patients', *Chest* 106(1): 187–93.

Sawatzky, J-A. V. (1996) 'Stress in critical care nurses: actual and perceived', *Heart and Lung* 25(5): 409–17.

Sawyer, N. (1997) 'Back from the twilight zone', *Nursing Times* 93(7): 28–9.

Say, J. (1997) 'Nutritional assessment in clinical practice: a review', *Nursing in Critical Care* 2(1): 29–33.

Sayre-Adams, J. (1994) 'Therapeutic touch: a nursing function', *Nursing Standard* 8(17): 25–8.

Scannapieco, F.A., Stewart, E.M. and Mylotte, J.M. (1992) 'Colonization of dental plaque by respiratory pathogens in medical intensive care patients', *Critical Care Medicine* 20(6): 740–5.

Schears, G.J. and Deutschman, C.S. (1997) 'Common nutritional issues in paediatric and adult critical care medicine', *Critical Care Clinics* 13(3): 669–90.

Schell, R.M., Cole, D.J., Schultz, R.L. *et al.* (1992) 'Temporary cerebral ischaemia. Effects of pentastarch or albumin on reperfusion injury', *Anaesthesiology* 77(1): 86–92.

Schewebel, C., Beuret, P., Pedrix, J.P. *et al.* (1997) 'Early nitric oxide inhalation in acute lung injury: results of a double blind randomised study', *Intensive Care Medicine* 23: supplement A2.

Schierhout, G. and Roberts, I. (1998) 'Fluid resuscitation with colloid or crystalloid solutions in critically ill patients: a systematic review of randomised trials', *British Medical Journal* 316(7136): 961–4.

Schinner, K.M., Chisholm, A.H. Grap, M.J. *et al.* (1995) 'Effects of auditory stimuli on intracranial pressure and cerebral perfusion pressure in traumatic brain injury', *Journal of Neuroscience Nursing* 27(6): 348–54.

Schmitz, T., Blair, N., Falk, M. *et al.* (1994) 'A comparison of five methods of temperature measurement in febrile intensive care patients', *American Journal of Critical Care* 4(4): 286–92.

Schobersberger, W., Hobisch-Hagen, P., Fuchs, D. *et al.* (1998) 'Pathogens of anaemia in the critically ill patient', *Clinical Intensive Care* 9(3): 111–17.

Schoenfield, P.S. and Butler, J.A. (1998) 'An evidence-based approach to the treatment of esophageal variceal bleeding', *Critical Care Clinics* 14(3): 441–55.

Schoenhofer, S. (1989) 'Affectional touch in critical care nursing: a descriptive study', *Heart and Lung* 18(2): 146–54.

Schofield, P. (1994) 'The role of sensation in the management of chronic pain', in R. Hutchinson and J. Kewin (eds) *Sensations and Disability*, Chesterfield: Rompa: 213–28.

Schwertz, D. and Buschmann, M. (1989) 'Pharmacogeriatrics', *Critical Care Nursing Quarterly* 12(1): 26–37.

Scothern, G.C., Jones, S. and MacFadyen, U. (1992) 'Young children in a general intensive therapy unit', *Care of the Critically Ill* 8(5): 208–9.

Scott, I. (1994) 'Effectiveness of documented assessment of postoperative pain', *British Journal of Nursing* 3(10): 494–501.

Sear, J.W. (1996) 'General pharmacology of intravenous anaesthetics', in C. Prys-Roberts and B.R. Brown Jr. (eds) *International Practice of Anaesthesia*, Oxford: Butterworth Heinemann: 1/15/1–21.

Seedhouse, D. (1988) *Ethics: The Heart of Health Care*, Chichester: Wiley (2nd edn, 1998).

Seers, K. (1987) 'Perceptions of pain', *Nursing Times* 83(48): 37–38.

Segatore, M. and Way, C. (1992) 'The Glasgow Coma Scale: time for change', *Heart and Lung* 21(6): 548–57.

Selby, I.R. and James, M.R. (1995) 'Severe metabolic and respiratory acidosis', *British Journal of Intensive Care* 5(7): 222–5.

Selective Decontamination of the Digestive Tract Trialists' Collaborative Group (1993) 'Meta-analysis of randomised controlled trials of selective decontamination of the digestive tract', *British Medical Journal* 307(6903): 525–32.

Seligman, M.E.P. (1975) *Helplessness: On Depression, Development and Death*, New York: Freeman.

Selye, H. (1976) *The Stress of Life*, 2nd edn, New York: McGraw Hill.

Semple, P. and Bellamy, M.C. (1995) 'Nitric oxide and acute lung injury in children: a report of two cases', *British Journal of Intensive Care* 5(3): 87–8.

Seymour, J. (1995a) 'Pain control: TENS machines', *Nursing Times* 91(6): 51–2.

—— (1995b) 'Counting the cost', *Nursing Times* 91(22): 24–7.

Shackell, S. (1996) 'Cooling hyperthermic and hyperpyrexic patients in intensive care', *Nursing in Critical Care* 1(6): 278–82.

Shah, S. (1999) 'Neurological assessment', *Nursing Standard* 13(22): 49–54.

Shapira, O.M., Alkon, J.D. and Aldea, G.S. (1997) 'Clinical outcomes in patients undergoing coronary artery bypass grafting with preferred use of the radial artery', *Journal of Cardiac Surgery* 12(6): 381–8.

Shaw, A.B. (1996) 'Non-therapeutic, elective) ventilation of potential organ donors: the ethical basis for changing the law', *Journal of Medical Ethics* 22(2): 72–7.

Sheehan, J. (1990) 'Investigating change in a nursing context', *Journal of Advanced Nursing* 15(7): 819–24.

Shelly, M.P. (1993) 'Sedation for the critically ill patient: current thoughts and future developments. in M. Rennie (ed.) *Intensive Care Britain*, London: Greycoat: 67–72.

—— (1994) 'Assessing sedation', *Care of the Critically Ill* 10(3): 118–21.

—— (1998) 'Sedation in the ITU', *Care of the Critically Ill* 14(3): 85–8.

Shelley, M.P. and Wang, D.Y. (1992) 'The assessment of sedation; a look at current methods and possible techniques for the future', *British Journal of Intensive Care* 2(4): 195–203.

Sheridan, R.L., Prelack, K. and Szyfelbein, S.K. (1997) 'Neuromuscular blockade does not decrease oxygen consumption or energy expenditure beyond sedation in mechanically ventilated children', *Journal of Intensive Care Medicine* 12(6): 321–3.

Sherry, K.M. (1997) 'The use of propofol for ICU sedation in patients following cardiac surgery', *British Journal of Intensive Care* 7(3): 91–6.

Sherry, K.M. and Barham, N.J. (1997) 'Cardiovascular pharmacology', in D.R. Goldhill and P.S. Withington (eds) *Textbook of Intensive Care*, London: Chapman & Hall: 245–53.

Sherwin, J.E. (1996) 'Acid-base control and acid-base disorder', in L.A. Kaplan and A.J. Pesce (eds) *Clinical Chemistry: Theory, Analysis, Correction*, St Louis: Mosby: 464–83.

Shields, P.L. and Neuberger, J.M. (1997) 'Hepatitis virology update', in L. Kaufman and R. Ginsburg (eds) *Anaesthesia Review 13*, New York: Churchill Livingstone: 43–64.

Shih, H-T., Miles, W.M., Klein, L.S. *et al.* (1996) 'Medical and surgical management of patients with Wolff-Parkinson-White syndrome', in D.J. Rowlands (ed.) *Recent Advances in Cardiology*, 12, Edinburgh: Churchill Livingstone: 171–97.

Shoemaker, W.C. and Beez, M.G. (1996) 'Relation of capillary leak to hypovolaemia, low flow, tissue hypoxia, oxygen debt, organ failure, and death. Part 2', *British Journal of Intensive Care* 3(4): 140–6.

Shoemaker, W.C., Appel, P.L. and Kram, H.B. (1988) 'Tissue oxygen debt as a determinant of lethal and nonlethal postoperative organ failure', *Critical Care Medicine* 16(11): 1117–20.

Shoemaker, W.C., Appel, P.L., Kram, H.B. *et al.* (1989) 'Comparison of hemodynamic and oxygen transport effects of dopamine and dobutamine in critically ill surgical patients', *Chest* 96(1): 120–6.

—— (1993) 'Sequence of physiologic patterns in surgical septic shock', *Critical Care Medicine* 21(12): 1876–89.

Shoemaker, W.C., Belzberg, H., Wo, C.J. *et al.* (1998) 'Multicenter study of noninvasive monitoring systems as alternatives to invasive monitoring of acutely ill emergency patients', *Chest* 114(6): 1643–52.

Sibai, B.M. (1994) 'Pre eclampsia – eclampsia', in J.T. Queenan (ed.) *Management of High Risk Pregnancy*, Boston: Blackwell Scientific: 377–85.

Sikes P.J. and Segal, J. (1994) 'Jugular venous bulb oxygen saturation monitoring for evaluating cerebral ischaemia', *Critical Care Nursing Quarterly* 17(1): 9–20.

Silvester, W. (1994) 'Outcome in terms of quality of life', *International Journal of Intensive Care* 1(3): 105–6.

Sim, K.M., Evans, T.W. and Keogh, B.F. (1996) 'Clinical strategies in intravascular gas exchange', *Artificial Organs* 20(7): 807–10.

Simmons, B.J. (1997) 'Management of intracranial hemodynamics in the adult: a research analysis of head positioning and recommendations for clinical practice and future research', *Journal of Neuroscience Nursing* 29(1): 44–9.

Simpson, T. (1991) 'Critical acre patients' perceptions of visits', *Heart and Lung* 20(6): 681–8.

Sinclair, M.E. and Suter, P.M. (1988) 'Detection of overdosage of sedation in a patient with renal failure by absence of lower oesophageal motility', *Intensive Care Medicine* 14(1): 69–71.

Skinner, B.F. (1971) *Beyond Freedom and Dignity*, London: Penguin.

Skowronski, G.A. (1997) 'Disorders of peripheral and motor neurons', in T.E. Oh (ed.) *Intensive Care Manual*, 4th edn, Oxford: Butterworth Heinemann: 428–33.

Slade, P. and Churchill, D. (1997) 'Recent advances in HIV therapy', *Care of the Critically Ill* 13(4): 156–60.

Sladen, R.N. (1994) 'Renal physiology', in R.D. Miller, R.F. Cucchiara, E.D. Miller *et al.* (eds) *Anaesthesia*, 4th edn, New York: Churchill Livingstone: 663–88.

Sloane, D., Shapiro, S., Kaufman, D.W. *et al.* (1981) 'Risk of myocardial infarction in relation to current and discontinued use of oral contraceptives', *New England Journal of Medicine* 305(8): 420–4.

Smith, D., Neal, J.J., Holmberg, S. and the Centres for Disease Control Idiopathic CD4+ T-lymphocytopenia Task Force (1993) 'Unexplained opportunistic infections and CD4+ T-lymphocytopenia without HIV infection', *New England Journal of Medicine* 328(6): 373–9.

Smith, J. (1980) 'The ideal of health', *Advances in Nursing Science* 3(3): 43–50.

—— (1998) 'Are electronic thermometry techniques suitable alternatives to traditional mercury in glass thermometry techniques in the paediatric setting?', *Journal of Advanced Nursing* 28(5): 1030–9.

Smith, M. (1994) 'Postoperative neurosurgical intensive care', *Current Anaesthesia and Critical Care* 5(1): 29–35.

Smith, P. (1991) 'The nursing process: raising the profile of emotional care in nurse training', *Journal of Advanced Nursing* 16(1): 74–81.

Smith, T.M., Steinhorn, D.M., Thusu, K. *et al.* (1995) 'A liquid perfluorochemical decreases the in vitro production of reactive O_2 species by alveolar macrophages', *Critical Care Medicine* 28(9): 1533–9.

Snell, C.C., Forthergill-Bourbonnais, F. and Durocher-Henriks, S. (1997) 'Patient controlled analgesia and intramuscular injections: a comparison of patient pain experiences and postoperative outcomes', *Journal of Advanced Nursing* 25(4): 681–90.

Snider, D.E. and Dooley, S.W. (1993) 'Nosocomial tuberculosis in the AIDS era with an emphasis on multidrug-resistant disease', *Heart and Lung* 22(4): 365–9.

Society of Critical Care Medicine's Ethics Committee (1994) 'Attitudes of critical care medicine professionals concerning distribution of intensive care resources', *Critical Care Medicine* 22(2): 358–62.

Sollars, A. (1998) 'Pressure area risk assessment in intensive care', *Nursing in Critical Care* 3(6): 267–73.

Sommers, M.S. (1998) 'Multisystem', in J.G. Alspach (ed.) *Core Curriculum for Critical Care Nursing*, 5th edn, Philadelphia: W B Saunders: 715–98.

Sontag, S. (1989) *AIDS and Its Metaphors*, London: Penguin.

Spencer, L. and Willats, S. (1997) 'Sedation', in D.R. Goldhill and P.S. Withington (eds) *Textbook of Intensive Care*, London: Chapman & Hall: 95–101.

Sprung, C.L. (1990) 'Changing attitudes and practices in foregoing life-sustaining treatments', *JAMA* 263(16): 2211–15.

Stanley, A.J., Lee, A. and Hayes, P.C. (1995) 'Management of acute liver failure', *British Journal of Intensive Care* 5(1): 8–15.

Stanski, D.R. (1994) 'Monitoring depth of anaesthesia', in R.D. Miller, R.F. Cucchiara, E.D. Miller *et al.* (eds) *Anaesthesia*, 4th edn, New York: Churchill Livingstone: 1127–59.

Stark, J.L. (1998) 'The renal system', in J.G. Alspach (ed.) *Core Curriculum for Critical Care Nursing*, 5th edn, Philadelphia: W B Saunders: 464–563.

Stechmiller, J.K. and Yarandi, H.N. (1993) 'Predictors of burnout in critical care nurses', *Heart and Lung* 22(6): 534–41.

Steel, A. and Hawkey, M. (1994) 'Moral dimensions', *Nursing Times* 90(37): 58–9.

Sternbach, R.A. (1968) *Pain: A Psychophysiological Analysis*, New York: Academic Press.

Stevensen, C. (1992) 'Holistic power', *Nursing Times* 88(38): 68–70.

—— (1994) 'The psychophysiological effects of aromatherapy massage following cardiac surgery', *Complementary Therapies in Medicine* 2(1): 27–35.

—— (1995) 'Shiatsu', in D. Rankin-Box (ed.) *The Nurse's Handbook of Complementary Therapies*, Edinburgh: Churchill Livingstone: 149–56.

—— (1997) 'Complementary therapies and their role in nursing care', *Nursing Standard* 11(24): 49–55.

Stewart, C.L. and Barnett, R. (1997) 'Acute renal failure in infants, children and adults', *Critical Care Clinics* 13(3): 575–90.

Stewart, F.S. and Beswick, T.S.L. (1977) *Bacteriology Virology and Immunology for Students of Medicine*, 10th edn, London: Baillière Tindall.

Stiegmann, G.V., Goff, J.S., Michaletz-Onody, P.A. *et al.* (1992) 'Endoscopic sclerotherapy as compared with endoscopic ligation for bleeding esophageal varices', *New England Journal of Medicine* 326(23): 1527–32.

Stockwell, M.A., Soni, N., Riley, B. *et al.* (1992) 'Colloid solutions in the critically ill: a randomised comparison of albumin and polygeline', *Anaesthesia* 47(1): 3–6.

Stoneham, M.D., Saville, G.M. and Wilson, I.H. (1994) 'Knowledge about pulse oximetry among medical and nursing staff', *Lancet* 344(8933): 1339–42.

Styrt, B. and Sugarman, B. (1990) 'Antipyretics and fever', *Archives of Internal Medicine* 150(8): 1589–97.

Suen, H.C., Johnson, R.G., Weintraub, R.M. *et al.* (1997) 'Minimally invasive direct coronary artery bypass: our experience with 32 patients', *International Journal of Cardiology* 62(Supplement 1): S95–S100.

Sung, J.J.Y. (1997) 'Acute gastrointestinal bleeding', in T.E. Oh (ed.) *Intensive Care Manual*, 4th edn, Oxford: Butterworth Heinemann: 329–36.

Sung, J.J.Y., Chung, S.C., Lai, C-W. *et al.* (1993) 'Octreotide infusion or emergency sclerotherapy for variceal haemorrhage', *Lancet* 342(8871): 637–41.

Surman, L. and Wright, S. (1998) 'Theory into practice: some examples of the application of change strategies', in S. Wright (ed.) *Changing Nursing Practice*, 2nd edn, London: Arnold: 25–38.

Sussman, N.L. (1996) 'Fulminant hepatic failure', in D. Zakim and T.D. Boyer (eds) *Hepatology: A Textbook of Liver Disease*, 3rd edn, Philadelphia: W B Saunders: 618–50.

Sutcliffe, J. (1997) 'Assessment of cerebral function', in D.R. Goldhill and P.S. Withington, (eds) *Textbook of Intensive Care*, London: Chapman & Hall: 631–7.

Suzuki, M.M., Cecka, J.M. and Terasaki, P.I. (1997) 'Unrelated living donor kidney transplants', *British Medical Bulletin* 53(4): 854–9.

Sweet, B.R. (ed.) (1997) *Mayes' Midwifery: A Textbook for Midwives*, 12th edn, London: Baillière Tindall.

Sweny, P. (1995) 'Management of acute renal failure in the intensive care unit', *Current Anaesthesia and Critical Care* 6(1): 25–8.

Sykes, M.K. (1986) 'Advantages in ventilatory support in acute lung disease', *Care of the Critically Ill* 2(2): 50–2.

Szaflarski, N.L. (1996) 'Preanalytic error associated with blood gas/pH measurement', *Critical Care Nurse* 16(3): 89–100.

Takala, J. (1997) 'Monitoring oxygenation', in T.E. Oh (ed.) *Intensive Care Manual*, 4th edn, Oxford: Butterworth Heineman: 848–53.

Talbot, D. (1998) 'Progress and regress in renal transplantation', *Care of the Critically Ill* 14(4): 124–6.

Tan, I.K.S. and Oh, T.E. (1997a) 'Mechanical ventilatory support', in T.E. Oh (ed.) *Intensive Care Manual*, 4th edn, Oxford: Butterworth-Heinemann: 246–55.

—— (1997b) 'Multiple organ dysfunction', in T.E. Oh (ed.) *Intensive Care Manual*, 4th edn, Oxford: Butterworth-Heinemann: 733–8.

Tatman, A. and Ralston, C. (1997) 'Assessment of pain in small children', *Current Anaesthesia and Critical Care* 8(1): 19–24.

Taube, D. (1996) 'Pathogenesis and diagnosis of acute renal failure in the intensive care unit', in T.W. Evans and C.J. Hinds (eds) *Recent Advances in Critical Care Medicine*, 4, New York: Churchill Livingstone: 213–30.

Taylor, L.F. (1978) 'An evaluation of handwashing technique', *Nursing Times* 174(2): 54–5.

Teare, E.L. and Barrett, S.P. (1997) 'Is it time to stop searching for MRSA? Stop the ritual of tracing colonised people', *British Medical Journal* 314(7081): 665–6.

Thangathurai, D., Charbonnet, C., Roessler, P. *et al.* (1997) 'Continuous intraoperative noninvasive cardiac output monitoring using a new thoracic bioimpedance device', *Journal of Cardiothoracic and Vascular Anaesthesia* 11(4): 440–4.

Thelan, L., Davie, J.K. and Urden, L.D. (1990) *Textbook of Critical Care Nursing*, St Louis: Mosby.

Thomas, C. (1997) 'Use of the prone position: the ventilator/perfusion relationship in ARDS', *Care of the Critically Ill* 13(3): 96–100.

Thomas, V. and Westerdale, N. (1997) 'Sickle cell disease', *Nursing Standard* 11(25): 40–5.

Thompson, D.R. and Webster, R.A. (1992) 'Nursing care of the patient with ischaemic heart disease', in P.M. Ashworth and C. Clarke (eds) *Cardiovascular Intensive Care Nursing*, Edinburgh: Churchill Livingstone: 91–110.

—— (1997) 'Caring for the patient with a cardiovascular disorder', in M. Walsh (ed.) *Watson's Clinical Nursing and Related Sciences*, 5th edn, London: Baillière Tindall: 261–339.

Thompson, P.L. (1990) 'Myocardial infarction', in T.E. Oh (ed.) *Intensive Care Manual*, 3rd edn, Sydney: Butterworths: 28–39.

Thomsen, G.E., Morris, A.H., Pope, D. *et al.* (1994) 'Mechanical ventilation of patients with adult respiratory distress syndrome using reduced tidal volumes', *Critical Care Medicine* 22(1): A205.

Tibballs, J. (1997) 'Equipment for paediatric intensive care', in T.E. Oh (ed.) *Intensive Care Manual*, 4th edn, Oxford: Butterworth Heinemann: 938–45.

Tibby, S.M., Brock, G., Marsh, M.J. *et al.* (1997) 'Haemodynamic monitoring in critically ill children', *Care of the Critically Ill* 13(3): 86–9.

Tighe, D., Bradley, C., Moss, R. *et al.* (1998) 'Alpha 1 adrenoceptor stimulation by dobutamine may amplify hepatic injury during sepsis', *British Journal of Intensive Care* 8(5): 150–6.

Tingle, J. (1997a) 'Pressure sores: counting the legal cost of nursing neglect', *British Journal of Nursing* 6(13): 757–8.

—— (1997b) 'Healthcare litigation: working towards a culture change', *British Journal of Nursing* 6(1): 56–7.

Tinker, J. and Jones, S.J. (1986) *A Pocket Book for Intensive Care*, London: Edward Arnold.

Tober, G. (1994) 'Drug taking in a northern UK city', *Accident and Emergency Nursing* 2(2): 70–8.

Todd, N. (1997) 'The physiological knowledge required by nurses caring for patients with unstable angina', *Nursing in Critical Care* 2(1): 17–24.

Toffler, A. (1970) *Future shock*, London: Pan.

Tombes, M. and Galluci, B. (1993) 'The effect of hydrogen peroxide rinses on the normal oral mucosa', *Nursing Research* 42(6): 332–7.

Tonnesen, A.S. (1994) 'Crystalloids and colloids', in R.D. Miller, R.F. Cucchiara, E.D. Miller *et al.* (eds) *Anaesthesia*, 4th edn, New York: Churchill Livingstone: 1595–1617.

Tooley, R., Hirschl, R.B., Parent, A. *et al.* (1996) 'Total liquid ventilation with perfluorocarbons increases pulmonary end-expiratory volume and compliance in the setting of lung atelectasis', *Critical Care Medicine* 24(2): 264–73.

Topf, M. and Davies, J.E. (1993) 'Critical care unit noise and rapid eye movement (REM) sleep', *Heart and Lung* 22(3): 252–58.

Topf, M *et al.* (1996) 'Effects of critical care unit noise on the subjective quality of sleep', *Journal of Advanced Nursing* 24(3): 545–51.

Torpy, D.J. and Chrousos, G.P. (1997) 'Stress and critical illness: the integrated immune/hypothalamic-pituitary-adrenal axis response', *Journal of Intensive Care Medicine* 12(5): 225–38.

Towers, S. (1997) 'Soap Box: "Sorted" ', *Accident and Emergency Nursing* 5(2): 113–16.

Tracey, K.J. and Cerami, A. (1993) 'Tumour necrosis factor: an updated review of its biology', *Critical Care Medicine* 21(10): S415–S422.

Treasure, T. (1995) 'Which prosthetic valve should we choose? *Current Opinion in Cardiology* 10(2): 144–9.

Trehan, N., Mishra, Y., Mehta, Y. (1998) 'Transmyocardial laser as an adjunct to minimally invasive CABG for complete myocardial revascularization', *Annals of Thoracic Surgery* 66(3): 1113–18.

Treloar, D.M. (1995) 'Use of a clinical assessment tool for orally intubated patients', *American Journal of Critical Care* 4(5): 355–60.

Treloar, D.M, Nalli, B.J., Guin, P. *et al.* (1991) 'The effects of familiar and unfamiliar voice treatments on intracranial pressure in head injured patients', *Journal of Neuroscience Nursing* 23(5): 295–9.

Trilla, A. (1994) 'Epidemiology of nosocomial infections in adult intensive care units', *Intensive Care Medicine* 20(supplement 3): S1–S4.

Tschudin, V. and Schober, J. (1990) *Managing Yourself*, Basingstoke: Macmillan.

Tsui, S.S.L. and Large, S.R. (1998) 'The current state of heart transplantation', *Care of the Critically Ill* 14(1): 20–4.

Tunstall-Pedroe, H., Kuulasma, K., Amouyel, P. *et al.* (1994) 'Myocardial infarction and coronary deaths in the World Health Organization MONICA project', *Circulation* 90(1): 583–612.

Turner, A. (1997) 'The holistic management of the patient with pre-eclampsia', *Nursing in Critical Care* 2(4): 169–73.

Turnock, C. (1990) 'Demystifying intensive care: Part 3', *Nursing Standard* 4(42): 32–3.

Twigley, A. and Hillman, K. (1985) 'The end of the crystalloid era?', *Anaesthesia* 40(9): 860–71.

Twycross, A. (1998) 'Perceptions about childrens' pain experiences', *Professional Nurse* 13(12): 822–6.

Tyler, P.A. and Ellison, R.N. (1994) 'Sources of stress and psychological well being in high dependency nursing', *Journal of Advanced Nursing* 19(3): 469–76.

Tzivoni, D., Banai, S., Schuger, C. *et al.* (1988) 'Treatment of torsades des point', *Circulation* 77(2): 392–7.

UK Central Council for Nursing, Midwifery and Health Visiting (UKCC) (1992a) *Code of Professional Conduct for the Nurse, Midwife and Health Visitor*, London: UKCC.

—— (1992b) *The Scope of Professional Practice*, London: UKCC.

—— (1992c) *Standards for Administration of Medicines*, London: UKCC.

—— (1996) *Guidelines for Professional Practice*, London: UKCC

—— (1997) *PREP and You*, London: UKCC.

UK Transplant Support Service Authority (UKTSSA) (1999) 'Transplant statistics', *Users' Bulletin*, Winter 1998/99 Issue No. 30, Bristol: UKTSSA.

Uldall, R. (1988) *Renal Nursing*, 3rd edn, Oxford: Blackwell Scientific.

Unsworth-White, M.J., Herriot, A., Valencia, O. *et al.* (1995) 'Resternotomy for bleeding after cardiac operation: a marker for increased morbidity and mortality', *Annals of Thoracic Surgery* 59(3): 664–7.

Valdix, S.W. and Puntillo, K.A. (1995) 'Pain, pain relief and accuracy of their recall after cardiac surgery', *Progress in Cardiovascular Nursing* 10(3): 3–11.

Valente, J.F., Anderson, G.L., Branson, R.D. *et al.* (1994) 'Disadvantages of prolonged propofol sedation in the critical care unit', *Critical Care Medicine* 22(4): 710–12.

Valtier, B., Cholley, B.P., Belot, J-P. *et al.* (1998) 'Noninvasive monitoring of cardiac output in critically ill patients using transoesophageal doppler', *American Journal of Respiratory and Critical Care Medicine* 158(1): 77–83.

van den Berghe, G. and de Zehger, F. (1996) 'Anterior pituitary function during critical illness and dopamine treatment', *Critical Care Medicine* 24(9): 1580–90.

van Saene, H.K.F., McClelland, P., Fox, M.A. *et al.* (1993) 'Where are we after one decade of selective decontamination of the digestive tract (SDD)?', in M. Rennie (ed.) *Intensive Care Britain (1993)*, London: Greycoat: 23–9.

Vandyk, R. (1997) 'Cash and carry', *Health Service Journal* 107(5551): 2–29.

Vanmaele, L., Noppen, M., Vincken, W.. *et al.* (1990) 'Transient left heart failure in amniotic fluid embolism', *Intensive Care Medicine* 16(4): 269–71.

Vaughan, B. and Pilmoor, M. (1989) *Managing Nursing Work*, London: Scutari.

Venables, C.W. (1991) 'The role of surgery in acute pancreatitis', *Care of the Critically Ill* 7(4): 137–9.

Verity, S. (1996a) 'Communicating with sedated ventilated patients in intensive care: focusing on the use of touch', *Intensive and Critical Care Nursing* 12(6): 354–8.

—— (1996b) 'Nutrition and its importance to intensive care patients', *Intensive and Critical Care Nursing* 12(2): 71–8.

Vilar, F.J. and Wilkins, E.G.L. (1998) 'Management of pneumocystis carinii pneumonia in intensive care', *British Journal of Intensive Care* 8(2): 53–62.

Vincent, J.L., Bihari, D.J., Suter, P.M. *et al.* (1995) 'The prevalence of nosocomial infection in intensive care units in Europe: results of the European prevalence of infection in intensive care', *JAMA* 274(8): 639–44.

Viney, C. (1996) 'Pain and sedation needs', in C. Viney (ed.) *Nursing the Critically Ill*, London: Baillière Tindall. 120–40.

Visser, L. and Purday, J. (1998) 'Management of cardiogenic shock in a district general hospital', *Care of the Critically Ill* 14(7): 240–4.

Vollman, K.M. (1997) 'Critical care nursing technique: prone position for the ARDS patient', *Dimensions in Critical Care Nursing* 16(4): 184–93.

Wahr, J.A. and Tremper, K.K. (1996) 'Oxygen measurement and monitoring techniques', in C. Prys-Roberts and B.R. Brown Jr. (eds) *International Practice of Anaesthesia*, Oxford: Butterworth Heinemann: 2/159/1–19.

Wainwright, P. (1994) 'Professionalism and the concept of role extension', in G. Hunt and P. Wainwright (eds) *Expanding the Role of the Nurse* Oxford: Blackwell Scientific.

Wake, D. (1995) 'Ecstasy overdose: a case study', *Intensive and Critical Care Nursing* 11(1): 6–9.

Waldmann, C. and Gaine, M. (1996) 'The intensive care follow-up clinic', *Care of the Critically Ill* 12(4): 118–21.

Waldmann, C.S. and Thyveetil, D. (1998) 'Management of head injury in a district general hospital', *Care of the Critically Ill* 14(2): 65–70.

Waldock, E. (1995) 'The pathology of Guillain-Barre Syndrome', *British Journal of Nursing* 4(14): 818–21.

Wall, P.D. and Melzack, R.W. (eds) (1994) *Textbook of Pain*, 3rd edn, Edinburgh: Churchill Livingstone.

Wallace, E. (1993) 'The effects of malnutrition in hospital', *British Journal of Nursing* 2(1): 67–71.

Walling, A., Tremblay, G.J.L., Jobin, J. *et al.* (1988) 'Evaluating the rehabilitation potential of a large population of post-myocardial infarction patients: adverse prognosis for women', *Journal of Cardiopulmonary Rehabilitation* 8: 99–106.

Walmrath, D., Schneider, T., Schermuly, R. *et al.* (1996) 'Direct comparison of inhaled nitric oxide and aerosolysed prostacyclin in acute respiratory distress syndrome', *American Journal of Respiratory and Critical Care Medicine* 153(3): 991–6.

Walsh, M. and Ford, P. (1989) *Nursing Rituals: Research and Rational Actions*, Oxford: Butterworth Heinemann.

Walters, S. and Brooks, H. (1996) 'Nutrition needs', in C. Viney (ed.) *Nursing the Critically Ill*, London: Baillière Tindall: 183–215.

Wardle, E.N. (1996) 'Prevention and treatment of septic shock, SIRS, ARDS and multi-organ failure', *Care of the Critically Ill* 12(5): 177–80.

—— (1997) 'New research findings in septic shock/endotoxaemia', *Care of the Critically Ill* 13(6): 222–4.

Waterlow, J. (1996) 'Operating table: the root of many pressure sores? *British Journal of Theatre Nursing* 6(7): 19–21.

Waterlow, J.A. (1985) 'A risk assessment card', *Nursing Times* 81(48): 49–55.

—— (1995) 'Pressure sores and their management', *Care of the Critically Ill* 11(3): 121–5.

—— (1996) 'Pressure sore assessment', *Nursing Times* 92(29): 53–6.

Watkinson, G.E. (1995) 'A study of the perception and experiences of critical care nurses in caring for potential and actual organ donors: implications for nurse education', *Journal of Advanced Nursing* 22(5): 929–40.

Watson, J.B. (1998) [1924] *Behaviorism*, New Brunswick: Transaction.

Watson, M., Hown, S. and Curl, J. (1992) 'Searching for signs of revival', *Professional Nurse* 7(10): 670–4.

Watt, B. (1996) *Patient*, London: Penguin.

Webb, A.R. (1991) 'Colloid osmotic pressure', *Care of the Critically Ill* 7(6): 213–17.

—— (1997) 'Fluid management in intensive care: avoiding hypovolaemia', *British Journal of Intensive Care* 7(2): 59–65.

Webb, C. (1989) 'Action research: philosophy, methods and personal experiences', *Journal of Advanced Nursing* 14(5): 403–10.

Webb, R.K., Ralston, A.C.and Runciman, W.B. (1991) 'Potential errors in pulse oximetry', *Anaesthesia* 46(3): 207–12.

Wedzicha, W. (1992) 'Nasal ventilation', *British Journal of Hospital Medicine* 47(4): 257–61.

Weekes, J.W.N. (1997) 'Poisoning and drug intoxication', in T.E. Oh (ed.) *Intensive Care Manual*, 4th edn, Oxford: Butterworth-Heinemann: 662–7.

Weinsten, R.A. (1991) 'Epidemiology and control of nosocomial infections in adult intensive care units', *American Journal of Medicine* 91(3b): 179s–84s.

Weller, I. and Williams, I. (1995) 'AIDS', in M.W. Adler (ed.) *ABC of Sexually Transmitted Diseases*, 3rd edn, London: BMA: 32–9.

West, S. (1996) 'How do nurses prevent sensory imbalance occurring in the intensive care unit?', *Nursing in Critical Care* 1(2): 79–85.

Westcott, C. (1995) 'The sedation of patients in intensive care units: a nursing review', *Intensive and Critical Care Nursing* 11(1): 26–31.

Weston, C.F.M. (1996) 'Current status of thrombolytic therapy', *Care of the Critically Ill* 12(3): 106–8.

Westrate, J.M.T. and Bruining, H.A. (1996) 'Pressure sores in an intensive care unit and related variables: a descriptive study', *Intensive and Critical Care Nursing* 12(5): 280–4.

Wheeler, A.P. and Bernard, G.R. (1999) 'Treating patients with severe sepsis', *New England Journal of Medicine* 340(3): 207–14.

White, B.S. and Roberts, S.L. (1991) 'Nursing management of high permeability pulmonary oedema', *Intensive Care Nursing* 7(1): 11–22.

White, P. (1998) 'Unit trust', *Nursing Times* 94(48): 36–7.

Why, H. (1994) 'Thrombolysis', *Nursing Standard* 8(49): 50–2.

Wilkinson, P. (1992) 'The influence of high technology care on patients, their relatives and nurses', *Intensive and Critical Care Nursing* 8(4): 194–8.

Wilkinson, P. (1994) 'Introducing a change of nursing model in a general intensive therapy unit', *Intensive and Critical Care Nursing* 10(1): 26–31.

Williams, A. (1985) 'Economics of coronary artery bypass grafting', *British Medical Journal* 291, 6491: 326–9.

Williams, P.F., Cartmel, L. and Hollis, J. (1997) 'The role of automated peritoneal dialysis (APD) in an integrated dialysis programme', *British Medical Bulletin* 53(4): 697–705.

Williamson, E.C.M. and Spencer, R.C. (1997) 'Infection in the intensive care unit', *British Journal of Intensive Care* 7(5): 187–97.

Williamson, L.M. (1994) 'Blood transfusion: a users' guide', *Care of the Critically Ill* 10(6): 267–70.

Willis, J. (1997) 'Shock absorbers', *Nursing Times* 93(24): 36–7.

Wilmoth, D.F. and Carpenter, R.M. (1996) 'Preventing complications of mechanical ventilation: permissive hypercapnia', *AACN Clinical Issues* 7(4): 473–81.

Wilson, A.P.R. (1985) 'Pseudomonas infection and the ventilated patient', *Intensive Care Nursing* 1(2): 107–10.

Wilson, J. (1997) 'Infection and diseases', in M. Walsh (ed.) *Watson's Clinical Nursing and Related Sciences*, 5th edn, London: Baillière Tindall. 102–26.

Wilson, V. (1983) *Cardiac Nursing*, Oxford: Blackwell Scientific.

Windsor, J. (1998) 'Haemodynamic monitoring', *Care of the Critically Ill* 14(2): 44–9.

Winer, J.B. (1994) 'Diagnosis and treatment of Guillain-Barre Syndrome', *Care of the Critically Ill* 10(1): 23–5.

Wingard, L.B., Brody, T.M., Larner, J. *et al.* (1991) *Human Pharmacology: Molecular to Clinical*, London: Wolfe.

Winkelman, C. (1995) 'Increased intracranial pressure', in N.A. Urban, K.K. Greenlee, J.M. Krumberger *et al.* (eds) *Guidelines for Critical Care*, St Louis: Mosby: 3–11.

Witrz, K.M., La Favor, K.M. and Ang, R. (1996) 'Managing chronic spinal cord injury: issues in critical care', *Critical Care Nurse* 16(4): 24–37.

Wolff, K., Hay, A.W.M., Sherlock, K. *et al.* (1995) 'Contents of 'Ecstasy'', *Lancet* 346(8982): 1100–1.

Wong, W.P. (1998) 'Acute respiratory distress syndrome: pathophysiology, current management and implications for physiotherapy', *Physiotherapy* 84(9): 439–50.

Wood, A.M. (1993) 'A review of literature relating to sleep in hospital with emphasis on the sleep of the ICU patient', *Intensive and Critical Care Nursing* 9(2): 129–36.

Wood, C.J. (1998) 'Endotracheal suctioning: a literature review', *Intensive and Critical Care Nursing* 14(3): 124–36.

Woodrow, P. (1998) 'An introduction to the reading of electrocardiograms', *British Journal of Nursing* 7(3): 135–42.

Woollons, S. (1996) 'Temperature measurement devices', *Professional Nurse* 11(8): 542–7.

Worthley, L.I.G. (1997) 'Acid-base balance and disorders', in T.E. Oh (ed.) *Intensive Care Manual*, 4th edn, Oxford: Butterworth-Heinemann: 689–99.

Wright, C. and Cohen, B. (1997) 'Organ shortages: maximising the donor potential', *British Medical Bulletin* 53(4): 817–28.

Wright, S. (ed.) (1998) *Changing Nursing Practice*, 2nd edn, London: Arnold.

Young, J.D. and Dyar, O.J. (1996) 'Delivery and monitoring of inhaled nitric oxide', *Intensive Care Medicine* 22(1): 77–86.

Young, J.D. and Sykes, M.K. (1994) 'Artificial ventilation: history, equipment and techniques', in J. Moxham and J. Goldstone (eds) *Assisted Ventilation*, 2nd edn, London: BMJ Publishing: 1–17.

Young, J.D., Brampton, W.J., Knighton, J.D. *et al.* (1994) 'Inhaled nitric oxide in acute respiratory failure in adults', *British Journal of Anaesthesia* 73(4): 499–502.

Young-McCaughan, S. and Jennings, B.M. (1998) 'Hematologic and immunologic systems', in J.G. Alspach (ed.) *Core Curriculum for Critical Care Nursing*, 5th edn, Philadelphia: W B Saunders: 601–46.

Zainal, G. (1994) 'Nutrition of critically ill people', *Intensive and Critical Care Nursing* 10(2): 163–70.

Zerbe, M. (1995) 'Obstetrical events in critical care', in N.A. Urban, K.K. Greenlee, J.M. Krumberger *et al.* (eds) *Guidelines for Critical Care*, St Louis: Mosby: 665–70.

Zimmerman, L., Nieveen, J., Barnason, S. *et al.* (1996) 'The effects of music interventions on postoperative pain and sleep in coronary artery bypass graft, (CABG) patients', *Scholarly Inquiry for Nursing Practice* 10(2): 153–74.

Index